THE INDIANA UNIVERSITY
SCHOOL OF MEDICINE

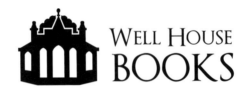

WILLIAM H. SCHNEIDER
with ELIZABETH J. VAN ALLEN, KEVIN GRAU, and ANGELA B. POTTER

The INDIANA UNIVERSITY

SCHOOL *of* MEDICINE

A HISTORY

INDIANA UNIVERSITY PRESS

This book is a publication of

Indiana University Press
Office of Scholarly Publishing
Herman B. Wells Library 350
1320 East 10th Street
Bloomington, Indiana 47405 USA

iupress.org

This book is printed on acid-free paper.

Manufactured in Canada

ISBN 978-0-253-05050-2 (cloth)
ISBN 978-0-253-05051-9 (ebook)

First printing 2020

In Memory of Pam Perry

CONTENTS

ACKNOWLEDGMENTS

A book, even as long as this, is somewhat like an iceberg with only a small portion visible. The complexities of a large institution plus the long time this project has run have required the work and support of a great number of people, all of whom simply cannot be acknowledged. Custom and full disclosure, in addition to gratitude, dictate recognition of financial support for the project. Earliest and foremost has been the Office of the Dean of the IU Medical School. Robert W. Holden, D. Craig Brater, and Jay Hess, as well as previous deans, have also provided encouragement while understanding the need for independent scholarship. In addition, the IU 200 Bicentennial Office, the Medical Humanities and Health Studies Program in the School of Liberal Arts at IUPUI, and several individual donors have contributed to support researchers. These donors include Richard B. Gunderman, C. Conrad Johnston Jr., Mary A. Maxwell, Richard T. Miyamoto, Robert M. Pascuzzi, Pamela Su Perry, Lawrence M. Roth, Richard L. Schreiner, James W. Smith, and John F. Williams Jr.

There have been numerous researchers, writers, and editorial collaborators who have made major contributions over the years. The most important of these include Elizabeth van Allen, who did major archival research and initial chapter drafts, plus Kevin Grau and Angie Potter, who did additional research and chapter revisions. Other research assistance has come from Kelly Gascoine, Melissa Dombrowski, Daniel Kinsey, and Monica Deck. Special thanks are also due to IU Press, including a series of directors and editors, who have persevered in supporting and bringing this project to its conclusion.

The archives of the medical school and university are extensive, and great thanks are due Steve Towne at IUPUI, plus Dina Kellams and Bradley Cook at IU Bloomington, as well as their assistants in special collections.

The IU Medical School Library and staff supported the project with their collections and work space, especially Gabe Rios, Sue London, and Coleen Method.

Numerous colleagues in the medical school and History Department too numerous to list offered advice and answered queries, but special thanks go to my History colleague Bob Barrows, who graciously read and provided suggestions for the final manuscript. I am also grateful to Tom Gannon, who helped navigate the administrative bureaucracy of the medical school and university.

Finally, the inspiration and long-serving shepherd of the project is undoubtedly Pam Perry, without whom the book quite simply would never have begun or been completed. Any errors or shortcomings are entirely my own, but kudos to all for their assistance.

William H. Schneider

THE INDIANA UNIVERSITY
SCHOOL OF MEDICINE

PART I
OUT OF MANY, ONE

*I*n the nineteenth century, at least twenty-four medical schools were started in Indiana, and twenty years after the Indiana University School of Medicine was started in 1903, there was only one. The numerous schools in the state reflected both the interest of those who wanted to become doctors and the willingness of practitioners to teach them. By 1900, the two largest schools in Indianapolis were also the most interested in meeting the emerging national standards of the medical profession. One of the key requirements was for medical schools to be part of a college or university with full-time faculty, and another was to teach scientific laboratory methods requiring expensive equipment. For these and other reasons, Indianapolis schools sought academic partners.

In fact, in 1871, only two years after the establishment of the forerunner of the Indianapolis schools (Indiana Medical College), it entered into an agreement with Indiana University in Bloomington, which in 1838 had been authorized to offer medical instruction. For a number of reasons, the partnership lasted less than ten years. Other colleges and universities attempted similar arrangements in subsequent decades, including Indiana Asbury (DePauw), Butler, and Purdue, but in the end, it was Indiana University and its new president, William Lowe Bryan, who successfully took over the two most important medical schools in Indianapolis. This occurred, however, after five complicated years of extensive negotiations, political lobbying, and what some described as academic warfare with its rival Purdue. The final outcome was sanctioned and funded by the state, and when the small medical school of Valparaiso closed in 1922, the Indiana University School of Medicine had a monopoly on medical education in the state for the next ninety years.

1

The Indiana Way of
Medical Education

*T*o paraphrase a John F. Kennedy quote, success has many fathers, and this oft cited judgment applies to the history of the Indiana University School of Medicine (IUSM). Now a $1 billion enterprise admitting over 340 medical students each year, the school had a late beginning and was the offspring of many parents, most significantly two proprietary medical schools in Indianapolis that joined Indiana University in 1908, a merger which the State of Indiana authorized and funded. This happened at the peak of medical education reform in the United States, which, as Kenneth Ludmerer has observed, responded to a number of developments in the nineteenth century.[1] Some were quite broad and cumulative, like the establishment of modern scientific medicine, professionalization of medical practice, and the creation of the American higher education system. Other changes were more specific, such as the need to teach new doctors about the flood of medical discoveries in diagnosis and treatment of illness, from anesthesia and antisepsis in surgery, to the germ theory and new field of bacteriology, as well as new technologies like X-rays.

The features of these reforms in medical education were adopted by such schools as Harvard, Pennsylvania, and Michigan by the beginning of the twentieth century—well before the American Medical Association (AMA) and the 1910 Flexner Report on medical schools in North America pushed hard for their adoption. They were most clearly embodied in the new Johns Hopkins University School of Medicine and included the establishment of entrance requirements and a four-year curriculum divided between medical sciences (e.g., anatomy and physiology) and clinical training. The latter were to take advantage of a teaching hospital, and all was to be done as part of a university, with full-time instructors.[2]

Existing and new medical schools such as the IU School of Medicine attempted to meet these standards with the local resources at their disposal. The specific circumstances in Indiana were not unique; rather, it was the combination of them that gave its medical school its distinctive character. These included the resources provided by the state and university, plus quite surprising and generous philanthropic support, focused in its early years on hospital construction and in later years also on support for medical research. This was crucial to the school's success, as was the case with other medical schools in the United States. Another distinctive feature of the IU School of Medicine, which shaped its subsequent history but set it apart from many of its peers, was the decision to keep its location at the site of the proprietary medical schools in Indianapolis, the capital and largest city of the state, which is fifty miles north of the campus of Indiana University in the small town of Bloomington (population of 6,400 in 1900). Although this was the case with some other medical schools where the home university was located in a small population center without sufficient hospitals for clinical instruction (for example, Colorado and Cornell), Indiana's response to this geographical situation was unique and played an important role in determining the history of the school.

Another feature of IUSM's history was its monopoly of medical education in the state until 2014. Among other consequences, this eliminated competition for state or philanthropic support, but at the same time, it placed constant demand on the school to produce more physicians and clinical care for citizens of the state. One result of this was the school's growth, which eventually gave it claim to the largest medical school enrollment in the country. This growth was fairly steady, but the school became a major provider of clinical care almost immediately after its creation with the construction of three new hospitals between 1914 and 1927. Research, on the other hand, developed much more slowly and initially depended on individual faculty interest. It was only after midcentury, as philanthropic and federal funding became available, that research played an important role in the school's operations.

These main features of state support, monopoly of medical education, location, and philanthropic support were crucial in determining how the new medical school in Indiana responded to the challenges of medical education reform faced by all US medical schools at the time. For example, the agreement to make the two proprietary schools part of Indiana University in 1908 obviously satisfied the requirement of medical schools to be part of universities that was stressed by the AMA and Flexner. Another key requirement was met surprisingly soon, when a local philanthropist donated funds in 1911 that were matched by the state legislature to build a university hospital. Reform of the curriculum took longer, however. As Flexner noted in his visit to Indiana in 1910, the school needed "to strengthen the laboratory equipment, [and] greatly to improve the organization and conduct of the clinical courses."[3] His first recommendation, however, was, "to employ full-time men," and that proved to be a goal that took much longer to achieve, given the resistance of faculty brought in from the proprietary schools, almost all of whom retained their private practice, and the need for significant additional funding. It took decades to replace part-time faculty, and it was only after the Second World War that deans were able to secure the funds to hire department chairs and faculty to meet this goal. The school's first accreditation report in 1954 listed one hundred full-time faculty.[4]

The IU School of Medicine was also shaped by its response to other major changes in medical practice and training during the course of the century, including the latest medical discoveries and the constant need for new equipment and other facilities for research and patient care. In the process, the medical school also faced unexpected but dramatic demands brought by the world wars and economic depression in the first half of the twentieth century, plus the need to adapt to broader social change that resulted in the entry of women and minorities into the field of medicine, especially after the 1960s and 1970s. One way to assess how the medical school mobilized resources to meet these challenges is in the balance of the school's efforts to fulfill its teaching, research, and service missions. Of these, the pressure to teach more medical students was perhaps the most constant and least surprising, although the way the school increased enrollments took a dramatic turn with the establishment of a multisite, statewide program in the 1970s.

Clinical service, as mentioned earlier, became a dominant responsibility surprisingly early thanks to the new hospitals the school had to manage. These included new children's and maternity hospitals, as well as the university hospital. Moreover, after the Second World War, the medical school made agreements to provide medical staff for the nearby City Hospital, as well as new VA and mental hospitals also constructed adjacent to the medical school. Then in 1995, the medical school agreed to combine its university and children's hospitals with the state's largest private hospital. The result was that although the purpose of the clinical mission was initially to provide opportunities to instruct students, the combination of philanthropic support and state demand created a substantial medical center with the school at its center. This inevitably shifted the appropriation of time and resources significantly toward this clinical care mission.

Research was initially much less important as a school mission, being left for all intents and purposes to the individual faculty member's interest and ability to obtain resources. In the last pages of Burton Myers's history of medical education in Indiana written in the 1940s, he admitted that "at no time was there the thought that Indiana University School of Medicine should develop chiefly as a research institute."[5] He continued, however, there was always hope "the day would come when the staff and physical facilities would be such as to provide time and encouragement for investigative work." Despite the delay during the war, which required emphasis on sped-up instruction, Myers concluded his book "with the happy conviction that the time long hoped for is at hand when research, which has been conducted under difficulties and inadequate support, is to be made a major objective of the Indiana University School of Medicine."[6] In fact, after the Second World War, philanthropy took the lead in inspiring and funding research, a development that was soon reinforced by government funding opportunities. In the 1954 accreditation report, the school indicated $686,000 in research grants, and the next review (1963) reported over $4.5 million.[7]

This is the first book-length history of the IU School of Medicine, although some shorter treatments have appeared over the years. Burton Myers's book was written from his perspective as the first medical faculty member hired by President Bryan in 1903 to teach anatomy. He began the book after his retirement in 1940, completing it just before his death in 1951, although it was published posthumously in 1956.[8] The first half of his book covers medical education in the state during the nineteenth century, Myers's initial interest. The later chapters on the establishment of the IU School of Medicine draw heavily from sections of the second volume of the *History of Indiana University, 1902–1937* that Myers wrote to follow the first volume on the university (1820–1902) by James Woodburn.[9] The coverage of the IU medical school in Myers's 1956 book on medical education in Indiana is sometimes uneven and episodic, especially the sections added for the decade after 1937.

At this same time, another effort to describe the history of the medical school in Indianapolis was published in a series of twenty-four monthly articles (four to five pages each) from January 1947 through December 1948, written by Thurman Rice in the *Monthly Bulletin [of the] Indiana State Board of Health*. Rice, a professor of bacteriology and public health who was also known as a strong proponent of eugenics and a national expert on sex education, selected as the running title for the series "History of the Medical Campus, Indianapolis, Indiana," indicating in a preface of the first article, "This is the story of the development of the *physical* plant. Any mention of persons or personnel is strictly secondary and is made only when necessary to understand the story." Despite the disclaimer, the series was quite thorough in covering the history of the medical school in Indianapolis to that date, providing discussion of the major people and programs and including numerous photographs.

Subsequent attempts to chronicle the medical school's history have been infrequent and largely commemorative. One in 1978 commemorated the seventy-fifth anniversary of the school. Another on the occasion of the school's ninetieth anniversary in 1993 was led by Dean Walter Daly, who authored and commissioned a number of unpublished booklets, department histories, and two overviews of the school's history.[10] Two more recent histories of Indiana University have treated the medical school differently. Thomas Clark's history of Indiana University (four volumes from 1970 to 1977) has three major chapters on the medical school. Ralph Gray's history of Indiana University—Purdue University Indianapolis (IUPUI) provides extended coverage only of the medical school's founding and its subsequent indirect influence on the nonhealth parts of the campus, with the understanding that a fuller study would come at the centennial of the medical school in 2003.[11]

The history that follows seeks to provide a fuller, in-depth account of the IUSM as an example of the development of medical education in a midwestern state that was typical of schools organized or reorganized at the beginning of the twentieth century. It shows the relation of local circumstances to broader developments in American medicine and society during the course of the twentieth century and the complicated organizational transition from proprietary to reformed medical school. Decisions about the location, as well as state and philanthropic support of the IUSM show the workings of local politics, plus the influence of social change and organizational entities that were peculiar to Indiana. This work, therefore, adds the record of an important and highly influential institution to understanding local and state history.

The book is organized using the terms of the deans of the school as benchmarks. This is not because these administrators were all-powerful. Indeed, despite the fact that deans of medical schools tend to have more influence than other deans within both their schools and the university, the long-range trend found in this study has been a decline in the influence of the deans as the school grew, and especially as individual faculty, departments, and research centers secured their own funding for clinical care and research.[12] Rather, IUSM had only seven deans during the century from 1911 to 2013, and all but two of their terms were long enough to be convenient for periodization, although there are some extra chapters and broader time coverage where necessary.

The first three chapters of "prehistory" introduce and outline medical education in Indiana in the nineteenth century as well as the complicated process by which the IUSM was established. This is especially important for understanding the nature of the two proprietary schools that joined Indiana University, and it helps explain the negotiations, rivalry, and sometimes bitter fight in the years during the school's creation from 1903 to 1908. The next chapters are organized by the terms of three deans who served from fifteen to twenty years each, during which time the foundations of the school were established. Two chapters are needed to examine these developments under Charles Emerson, the first dean recruited nationally and also the longest serving dean (1911–31). The next two chapters cover the medical school during the terms of the deans during the tumultuous times of the Great Depression, the Second World War, and the postwar period. The last four chapters are more topical, covering the establishment of the statewide medical education system in the 1960s, followed by the major changes in the last decades of the century, and more recent developments since a major hospital merger in 1995.

Virtually all of the over one hundred medical schools in the United States have accounts of their history, including dozens of books of varying style and scope. These range from commemorative, well-illustrated volumes (Maryland) to multivolume chronologies, especially for the older and more influential institutions (Harvard, Johns Hopkins). The main interest in all these histories is undoubtedly from a local audience with personal connections to their schools, although scholarly volumes have been very useful to professional educators eager to compare different experiences and results of medical reforms. Professional historians, as well as medical professionals, have also studied these highly influential components of higher education, which are so intimately connected to broader social change and the growing role that health has played since the end of the nineteenth century.

The audience for this book is both local and national, but the dilemma in writing any history of a medical school over a century old is the dramatic growth in size, complexity, and sources of that history. The approach of this volume is to provide a close analysis of developments in the formative decades of the school, examining the problems faced and decisions made as the two proprietary institutions were remolded into a university-based school with multiyear programs, including hospitals for clinical care and instruction. It is only possible to do a close analysis, however, for the first part of this history. The growth after the Second World War meant that the medical school added so many new people, centers, and institutes, plus relations to outside institutions, that it is necessary to select only the major and representative participants and developments. Fortunately, at this same time, the school was required to produce new reporting and summary materials for accrediting and administrative purposes that help describe the background and broader context during this period. Likewise, there are numerous oral histories that describe this period, as well as materials from medical students themselves, that reflect the human dimension and impact of these changes on all levels.[13]

Use of the word *success* can be justified in referring to the IU School of Medicine in many obvious ways. These include the number of physicians educated plus the residents and fellows trained. Its annual budget of over $1 billion makes the Indiana University School of Medicine one of the largest enterprises in the state, and its importance can be seen in the number of buildings that now make up the large medical center that has grown up around the school in Indianapolis, as well as newer centers in other parts of the state. This does not mean, however, that the school is without its critics, both today and throughout its history. The account that follows aims to present as complete a history as possible in the hopes it can provide lessons of missed opportunities and failures as well as success.

2

Learning and Practicing Medicine in the Nineteenth Century

*I*n May 1868, John S. Bobbs, best known as the first physician to perform surgery to remove gallstones (cholestcystotomy), addressed the Indiana State Medical Society as president and advocated the establishment of a new medical school in Indianapolis. In this inaugural address, Bobbs proclaimed ideals for medical education held by the state's early, leading doctors, which still hold true for medical educators today.

> What do we want with a medical school in Indiana, unless it be established on a scale and basis to compete in excellence, in eminence, in every appliance and means of instruction, with the very best schools of the age. It should assume, at once, a high rank. . . . It should be richly endowed, placing it quite beyond the influence of pecuniary considerations, and thus commanding teachers of the first order—vigilant guardians of professional character—providing against unworthy membership by enrolling only those of unquestionable fitness, and conferring degrees on merit only.[1]

Bobbs represented the best of the generation of frontier physicians who rose to become the first medical elite in Indiana. He was born in 1809 in Green Village, Pennsylvania, and trained with a local physician before attending Jefferson Medical College in Philadelphia. Bobbs came to Indiana in 1835, and his reputation grew such that in 1849, he served as the first dean and professor of anatomy and surgery at the short-lived Indiana Central Medical College. He served as a civilian doctor in Virginia and Indiana during the Civil War, and later in his life, he was faculty president and professor of surgery at the Indiana Medical College. Bobbs founded the Indianapolis and Indiana State Medical Societies and also served as a state senator. He was involved in a broad spectrum of reforms and was an organizer of the first two medical schools in Indianapolis. Bobbs was also an advocate for the establishment of City Hospital. He served as a member of the state commission that established Central State Hospital for the Insane, and he participated in the development of state schools for the blind and deaf.[2]

Although Bobbs proposed very high ideals for medical education to his colleagues, he was a realist. In fact, he made this speech at one of the lowest points in the history of medical education in the Hoosier state. In 1856, the last school remaining of those founded before the Civil War closed, and no medical school was opened in the state to replace it for almost fifteen years. At a time when these institutions were primarily commercial enterprises with bad reputations, Bobbs understood that the possibility of establishing a medical school such as the one he described remained remote. Neither was this the case only in Indiana. Up to that point in the nineteenth century, medical schools throughout the country

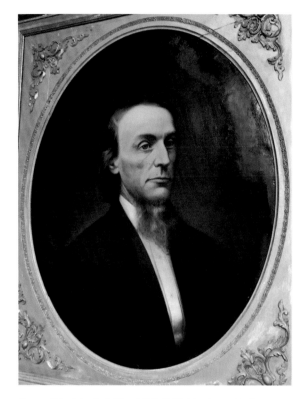

Figure 2.1. John S. Bobbs, 1809–1870. Courtesy of Indiana Medical History Museum.

had typically lowered admission and graduation requirements. Therefore, an institution that raised standards was unlikely to survive.[3] Nonetheless, in his speech before the State Medical Society, Bobbs declared that those gathered should establish a medical school even if it were not of the highest quality. During succeeding years, he argued, the school could take steps to make this institution competitive with the leading American medical schools. Bobbs's words inspired the organization of the Indiana Medical College created in Indianapolis in 1869, and its successor eventually became part of the Indiana University School of Medicine. This achievement took almost forty years, and to understand how that occurred, it is necessary to more closely examine the history of the nineteenth century medical schools in the state.

Practicing and Learning Medicine in the Nineteenth Century

Historians of medical education in the United States divide the nineteenth century at 1860 because of the medical education reforms that followed but also because of the Civil War and the socioeconomic and demographic growth of the country following that conflict.[4] The training of Bobbs exemplifies American medical education before 1860. According to historian William Rothstein, there were three ways a physician learned the trade: preceptorship (as apprenticeship was called) to a physician, attendance at a medical school, and self-instruction. The latter was always possible but diminished during the century as medical knowledge and practice improved and licensing was strengthened. Bobbs's combination of assisting a physician (for as long as three years for some applicants) before attending a medical school was more typical. These schools began on the East Coast (in 1820, ten of the thirteen schools in the United States were in New England, New York State, and Philadelphia), but their numbers grew rapidly to forty-seven by 1860. Any group of physicians could organize a private school and offer instruction, but there was also high turnover. Jefferson Medical College, the school Bobbs attended, was the second school established in Philadelphia in 1825, and it was able to survive and thrive.[5] The importance of preceptorship was underscored by the relatively short course of instruction in these schools, typically sixteen to eighteen weeks of lectures. Students could gain additional clinical experience afterward in the growing number of dispensaries and clinics, where patients came for immediate care. These had been created by philanthropists, physicians, and civic leaders following a British model developed in the seventeenth century as a less expensive way for poor patients to receive treatment rather than pay for home visits or stay overnight in hospitals, which were much more expensive to construct and operate.[6]

Because instruction was almost completely didactic, opening a medical school during much of the nineteenth century was not difficult or expensive. One needed a classroom for lectures, a back room in which to conduct dissection, and a minimum of four faculty members. Short term, half-year courses of study, didactic instruction, and no formal system of grading or evaluation characterized the way these proprietary medical schools served the needs of physicians who filled the open medical marketplace of nineteenth-century America. Schools granted credentials (degrees) to would-be physicians while providing additional income to established physicians who often served as both financiers and faculty for a medical school. Under these circumstances, the success or failure of these educational institutions largely depended on the entrepreneurial skills and persuasiveness of their organizers. Because of the competition, however, bankruptcy was a constant threat.[7]

The profession of medicine grew in the nineteenth century, but it started from a small client base, in large measure because effective treatments were limited. Physicians competed within a complicated medical marketplace containing allopathic physicians, sectarian physicians of various kinds, midwives, quacks, vendors of patent medicines, and, most important, family healers and folk traditions.[8] Moreover, for most people in the American Midwest, medical care usually happened at the bedside, and family members were the primary healers. Poor transportation, low population density, the high cost of professional care, and the inadequacies of nineteenth-century medical science contributed to a low demand for physician services despite the ever-present threat of diseases such as malaria, dysentery, whooping cough, scarlet fever, typhoid fever, smallpox, tuberculosis, and cholera. Where doctors were available, family members called them only as a last resort. Women customarily cared for members of the household and drew from a variety of sources, including regular and sectarian medicine, family recipes, and Native American traditions. In towns and new urban centers, the sick who could not afford a house call might find treatment at a dispensary.[9]

Adding to these difficulties, at this time regular medicine provided "heroic" remedies, so called because the goal was immediate results even at potential risk to the patient. These remedies included bleeding, heavy doses of mercury, and emetics, which ranged from being ineffective to lethal in the treatment of disease. Not until the turn of the twentieth century did American doctors' treatments become more likely to produce positive rather than negative results in the patients' outcomes.[10] Disagreements over therapeutic techniques due to the inadequacies of nineteenth-century medicine also gave rise to medical sects that caused deep divisions among America's physicians.

Practitioners chose training at a variety of alternative medical schools that arose during the 1800s largely in reaction to the widespread use of heroic therapeutics. Their graduates, plus those who had less education or who were denied access to hospitals and allopathic medical schools, could assert claims against the regular profession. Because of this competition in medical practice during the nineteenth century, doctors were motivated to differentiate themselves from others, make the services they provided distinctive, and above all appeal to a public that would pay. In Indiana, Bobbs noted with disdain in 1849 that some practitioners picked their medical factions based on the "remunerative probabilities." Although ultimately successful, nineteenth-century physicians faced rancorous antagonisms that for a long time prevented them from achieving the legitimacy and professional authority they desired.[11]

In this unregulated environment, those with little or no training could proclaim themselves doctors, such as some patent medicine manufacturers who adopted that title to give their products credibility and bolster their sales. These suppliers of "magic" tonics and remedies were usually charlatans; nevertheless, they managed to play a large role in the nineteenth-century medical marketplace. Bobbs commented on the "enormous amount of quack medicines" that were nothing more than "the refuse and sweepings of old warehouses" covered with cheap whiskey and dirty molasses.[12]

Practicing Medicine in Indiana

In Indiana, as in other parts of the country, relatively few of the numerous laws passed were effective in regulating individuals practicing medicine until the end of the nineteenth century. During its first session in 1816, the Indiana General Assembly passed a law that recognized each judicial district also as a medical district, and in each of these districts, a board of medical commissioners was to examine all those who wished to enter the practice of medicine. The act also provided for the formation of a state medical society, and in 1825 an amendment gave it the power to oversee medical education. Although the assembly enacted these laws "to regulate the practice of physic and surgery," they were ineffectual. They did not produce a permanent, strong, state medical society, and more important, they did not prevent the licensing of unqualified men or the operation of fraudulent medical colleges, such as the medical "diploma mill" in New Albany, reputedly one of the first in the United States.[13]

In 1843, the situation worsened when resistance to professional exclusivity, as well as the difficulty in enforcing laws regulating the professions, prompted the Indiana General Assembly to join state legislatures across the country in revoking laws that regulated the practice of medicine. Removing legal restrictions permitted any group to obtain a charter or business license, solicit funds, and engage a few reasonably learned people to teach a variety of individuals and groups. In this regard, medical schools were not unlike the numerous liberal arts colleges established at this time. New legislation regulating medical practice in Indiana did not take effect until 1885.[14]

Medical education in Indiana, like other areas of the Midwest, followed the national pattern, although as Bobbs's address indicates, it came with some delay. Until schools were established in the state, Bobbs and others

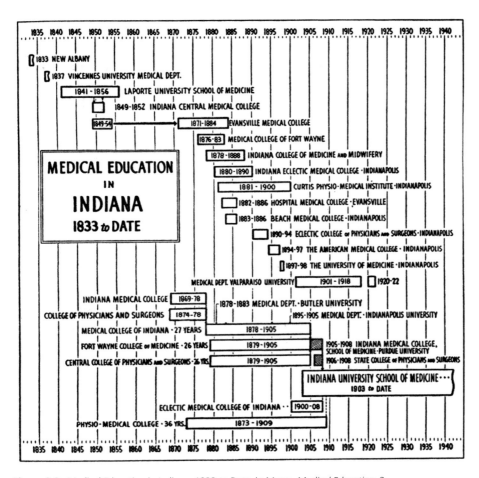

Figure 2.2. Medical Education in Indiana, 1833 to Date, in Myers, *Medical Education*, 3.

trained in the East, or at the first medical schools in neighboring states such as Kentucky (the Medical Department of Transylvania University, founded in 1799) and Ohio (the Medical College of Ohio in Cincinnati, founded in 1819). Through Bobbs's term, eleven of the first eighteen presidents of the Indiana State Medical Association graduated from Jefferson, Transylvania, or the Ohio medical colleges. They and their students then became the founders of at least twenty-four medical schools identified by Burton Myers that were chartered in Indiana prior to 1906.[15]

As figure 2.2 shows, most of the nineteenth-century medical schools in Indiana were short-lived and chartered after the Civil War. One exception of note was the LaPorte University School of Medicine, which began in 1841 and operated until 1856. Located in northern Indiana between

Gary and South Bend, the medical school was established the year after the legislature granted a charter to the university in 1840, thanks largely to the initiative of Robert Niles, a lawyer who settled in LaPorte in 1833, and Daniel Meeker, who instructed anatomy.[16] Within a few years the school was successful enough to attract over one hundred students from Indiana, Michigan, and Illinois, and it constructed its own medical building in 1847. Among its notable graduates was William Worral Mayo, who moved to Rochester, Minnesota, in 1863, where his two sons created the Mayo Clinic. Another was William H. Wishard, the father of William Niles Wishard, who became head of the Indianapolis City Hospital and was an early leader of the Indiana University School of Medicine (IUSM). Although initially Chicago had the only other medical school in the region (Rush Medical College, founded in 1837), the LaPorte school faced competition from the Indiana Central Medical College in Indianapolis (1849) and a new medical school at the University of Michigan (1850). Despite attempts to affiliate with Asbury College (later Depauw) and the Central Medical College, there are no records of instruction after 1851.[17]

Doctors who tried to establish medical schools usually lived in the rapidly growing towns and cities of Indiana following the Civil War. These included Evansville (population of 11,000 in 1860, which grew to 69,000 in 1900) and Ft. Wayne (18,000 in 1870, rising to 45,000 in 1900), but more often in the largest city and capital of Indianapolis (from 18,000 in 1860 to 170,000 people in 1900). One seeming exception that proves this rule was the failed attempt by Indiana University to establish a medical department in 1871 after the legislature chartered a new state-supported university in 1869 to teach agriculture and engineering in Lafayette using Morrill Land Grant funds and a donation from John Purdue. This is examined in more detail later, but of note here is the basic problem that hindered this plan of Indiana University and plagued its later attempts to establish and run a medical school in Bloomington, a small population center with few doctors and patients or hospitals. The effort in the 1870s sought to solve the problem by working with an established medical school in Indianapolis, in this case Bobbs's Indiana Medical College, but it was abandoned because of logistical problems and competing local interests. It proved to be the first of several unsuccessful attempts at an alliance, the solution to which became one of the defining features of the IUSM.

The many medical schools established in Indiana during the decades following the Civil War responded to the rising demand for physicians, but they needed to teach the growing knowledge that revolutionized the practice of medicine during the nineteenth century and fueled the call for reforms to ensure high standards. These included dramatic changes in such things as the practice of surgery, where the discoveries of anesthesia and antisepsis permitted more complicated operations with greatly reduced rates of infection. New discoveries in pathology (from anatamopathology to cellular pathology) produced a new concept of diagnosis that was accompanied by the introduction of new instruments—stethoscopes, thermometers, and ultimately X-rays—that required both more time for training and the purchase of expensive equipment. Most significant for medical schools was the need to lengthen the time of instruction and provide laboratories for training in microscopic and chemical analysis after the discovery of cells and germ theory.[18]

The need to teach these discoveries brought a call for higher admission standards and expansion of the curriculum. Some of the loudest voices came from new professional organizations, starting with the American Medical Association (AMA, established in 1847), the American Medical College Association (first founded in 1876 but reorganized in 1890 and later renamed the Association of American Medical Colleges, AAMC), and the AMA's Council on Medical Education (established in 1904).[19] As the nineteenth century came to an end, these reforms gained strength and were aimed at the rapid increase in medical schools. The largest number of new schools in Indiana were established in Indianapolis.

The Founding of Indiana Medical College

In April 1869, leading members of the Academy of Medicine of Indianapolis (created in 1865 following earlier attempts to promote "the study of medicine and its related sciences and in supporting the character of the profession"[20]) met with Bobbs in his office to discuss their plans. At this meeting, the physicians agreed to appoint a committee to carry out a strategy for the organization of a new school to be called the Indiana Medical College. Within a week, the committee wrote articles of association and bylaws for the new school and determined faculty positions. By late summer, they obtained and renovated a building, scheduled lectures, set the fees, and appointed the faculty. These first nine faculty members each invested $250 so that the school could operate privately. With this investment, each of them established a personal financial interest in its success.[21]

The organizers of Indiana Medical College realized that to compete for students and be successful, they had to offer clinical instruction "as the very best basis upon which the student can plant his educational interest."[22] Clinical instruction was a growing concern of all medical schools in the last half of the nineteenth century in response to the many changes in medical practice at a growing number of hospitals and dispensaries. As a result, unlike their predecessors, the Indiana Medical College faculty could take advantage of facilities available to them, including the new Indianapolis City Hospital, which opened in 1859 but soon was taken over by the army during the Civil War before returning to the city in 1865.[23]

In 1879, William Niles Wishard became superintendent of the struggling City Hospital and brought it into the modern era with improvements to operation and the buildings, linking it with charity care and education. Although he was superintendent only until 1888, the influence of Wishard's leadership and the hospital's commitment to modernization and medical education continued. Bobbs's death in 1870 also left a legacy of care and education; he bequeathed $5,000 to fund the development of a medical library and $2,000 to establish a free clinic as a gift to the poor, stipulating that these institutions remain under the control of the Indiana Medical College. With this bequest, the Bobbs Free Dispensary commenced operation during the latter part of the school's 1870–71 session. Indicative of the need for this institution, the dispensary treated fifteen hundred patients in the first year.[24]

With a large number of clinical subjects available, City Hospital and Bobbs Free Dispensary became the ideal places for clinical instruction. City Hospital treated approximately three thousand patients each year by the time the Indiana Medical College arranged for its students to be taught there during the school's first session. For the patient unable to afford medical care, the opportunity to receive treatment outweighed the invasion of privacy and discomfort in participating in these clinical exercises After completing their course of study, many graduates of the Indiana Medical College (and soon the Central College of Physicians and Surgeons) did additional training at Bobbs Free Dispensary and City Hospital, particularly in specialty areas of surgery. This was the origin of what came to be known as internship and residency, which was given the name "graduate medical education," as distinguished from the training in medical school resulting in an MD that came to be called "undergraduate medical education." Graduates also traveled to Europe to complete their education.[25]

Indiana University's First Medical Department

In 1871, there was a noteworthy, although brief, attempt by Indiana University to offer medical instruction in conjunction with the new Indiana

Medical College. This followed a pattern established by other American institutions of higher learning, such as the University of Pennsylvania, Harvard, Yale, Dartmouth, New York University, and the University of Michigan. Many of these affiliations were initially very loose, but after the Civil War, some university presidents, such as Charles Eliot of Harvard, sought closer relationships with their respective medical schools.[26] The motivation for Indiana University's interest in medical instruction grew out of the decision of the state of Indiana to participate in the federal Morrill Land Grant Act to support training in agriculture and the "mechanical arts." In 1869, the state selected Lafayette to be the home of the new Purdue University, to be chartered under the Land Grant Act, with classes beginning in 1874.

Following this decision, Indiana University President Cyrus Nutt sought a means for his institution to serve the state in a more practical way. In the 1838 legislation whereby Indiana College became Indiana University, the following was included: "There shall be and is hereby created and established a [university] for the education of youth in the American, learned and foreign languages, the useful arts, sciences [including law and medicine], and literature."[27] Nutt sought to take advantage of the addition of law and medicine to make medicine a professional course of study. The university's *Annual Report of 1870–1871* expressed Nutt's vision for the future based upon the direction in which American universities were developing as a whole. Departing from the rigid, narrowly defined traditional curriculum that emphasized classical languages, philosophy, theology, and mathematics, he saw the post–Civil War university as a dynamic institution for not only the transmission of ideas but also for their discovery and redefinition. By the second half of the nineteenth century, medicine fit into this new view of knowledge and its acquisition. Medicine was no longer a set body of information to be learned and handed down from master to apprentice, and during the last decades of the nineteenth century, it became one of the most important of the natural, experimental sciences and therefore was perfectly suited to the modern university curriculum.[28]

Following publication of Nutt's statement, the Indiana Medical College faculty realized that Indiana University might establish a rival medical school, and they did not want to compete for students with another school within the state, especially if it would benefit from the investment of public resources. Therefore, the faculty approached the IU trustees with the idea of concentrating the medical profession's efforts on one medical school in the state—an argument that recurred throughout the history of medical education in Indiana. In 1871, representatives from the medical college persuaded Indiana University's trustees to make Indiana Medical College the medical department of the university.[29] One persuasive argument to the trustees is indicated by enrollments in the annual report for the 1874–75 academic year. Of a total of 425 students, 107 were in the Medical Department in Indianapolis.[30]

Unlike other schools such as Harvard and the University of Michigan, Indiana University did not take immediate steps to integrate the medical college into the university or institute significant reforms; the connection between the Indiana Medical College and the university remained only nominal. That reforms were needed is indicated by the "Requirements for Graduation" from the Medical College listed in the 1874–75 university catalog. "Candidate for graduation must furnish proof of good moral character, that they have studied the science for three years, under the instruction of a competent preceptor, and that they have attended two full courses of lectures in a Medical College of good reputation, the last of which must have been in this department." The course of lectures that year for the Medical Department ran for five months from October 1874 through February 1875, and the catalog allowed "Four years of reputable practice [to be] considered equivalent to attendance upon one course of lectures."

Underlying the question of academic quality were fiscal problems. For example, according to the agreement between the two institutions, the physicians were to retain control of the medical college's assets until such time as the state legislature appropriated funds for the university to purchase them. Also, for its students to enjoy free tuition as did those in other departments at this time, Indiana University was supposed to provide funds to the medical college amounting to at least $8,000 per year. The IU trustees gained control of the medical school only after all of the requirements of this agreement had been met. Until that time, the physicians who taught in the college retained control of its management and operated it according to the same principles as before the affiliation.[31]

Given these conditions, within a few years the merger of the Indiana Medical College and Indiana University proved a failure. The university never could afford to pay the medical school the funds promised in the initial agreement, and despite such tactics as inviting state legislators to attend lectures at the school, the Medical Department never won the support of the Indiana General Assembly. In May 1874, the situation worsened when some members of the faculty (possibly because of discontent with the arrangement) decided to leave the Indiana Medical College to start a new school in Indianapolis, the College of Physicians and Surgeons (CPS). Finally, following the 1875–76 sessions, the Indiana Medical College faculty voted to terminate the relationship with Indiana University unless the university committed to "a definite and permanent paying basis of connection."[32]

The affiliation also did not meet the expectations of Indiana University officials. In the *Annual Report of 1876–1877*, Nutt's successor, Lemuel Moss, criticized the legislature and medical schools "for swelling the ranks of untrained and incompetent lawyers and physicians." As a member of the academic community, President Moss made it clear that he objected to the fact that the medical school operated like a trade school rather than a true professional school. Anticipating the future direction of medical education in the United States, Moss argued that medical schools should be graduate schools requiring college preparation. As he stated, "That men should be passed through these professional schools with little or no preliminary training, and little or no preliminary examination—ignorant of language, of literature, of history, of mathematics, of science, of philosophy, and almost wholly destitute of intellectual discipline—is to the disadvantage alike of good morals, good learning and good professional ability."[33]

Moss was not the only one to express disappointment with professional education. In 1877, echoing a broader public distrust, the Indiana General Assembly not only refused to sanction the medical school affiliation but also reduced support of IU's Law Department, declaring that it was "no duty of the people to help men into these easy professions."[34] As a result, the university ceased teaching in both schools. The Law Department reopened in 1889, and fourteen years later, with a new president, Indiana University made another attempt to add medical education.

In the meantime, the conditions that prompted the proprietary medical schools to seek a university partner continued. The Indiana Medical College had a small faculty and low admission standards. The five-month curriculum was not yet graded in a logical order or according to level of difficulty. In the early 1870s, graduation requirements increased to include some laboratory experience and dissection along with courses in anatomy and analytical chemistry. Otherwise, the Indiana Medical College merely required three years of study with a competent preceptor, proof of moral character, and attendance at two terms of lectures, which meant repeating the five-month curriculum. The students took tests at graduation only in subjects that the faculty considered fundamental to the practice of medicine.[35] In the next three decades, with advances in medicine and increasing call for reforms, proprietary schools were hard-pressed to keep up with these demands, which were of growing importance in order to keep up with their rivals.

Proprietary Medical School Rivalry in Indianapolis

The main reason the Indiana Medical College attempted to join Indiana University was to prevent the establishment of a competing medical school. In an unexpected sense, this worked because IU left the field after the failed merger. Again unexpectedly, the college's worst fears were nonetheless realized when disagreements, enmities, and jealousies among members of its own faculty soon resulted in the establishment of rival institutions. The strife within the field also raised questions about the status of the medical profession among the public and increased the call for state standards of training and licensure.

Before 1885, licensing of physicians was left to a "board of supervisors [doctors]" in each of three judicial districts in Indiana (changed in 1825 to the medical society there) who were to "examine and license to practice any applicant whom they might consider properly qualified."[36] The 1885 law was an attempt to provide better regulation, but its provisions reveal how vague and variable the term "properly qualified" remained. The law "required county boards to issue a license to practice medicine to anyone presenting a diploma from a 'reputable' medical school, or evidence of ten years of practice, or evidence of 3 years of practice if a full course of medical lectures was attended, even if diploma not obtained." The new law also helps explain why so many medical schools were established during this period, because they offered the quickest and easiest way to a license. Nor were they particularly rigorous; in 1874, Indiana Medical College's full course of lectures had only recently been extended to five months. Finally, in 1897, a state board was created because of differences between the county boards. Among other things, this law also tied Indiana to national reforms by relying on the Association of American Medical Colleges to set standards for admissions as well as the curriculum of medical schools.[37]

The situation was further exacerbated because sectarians, or irregular physicians, sought to increase their legitimacy by establishing their own schools. For example, in 1873, the physiomedicals organized the Physio-medical College of Indiana, located in Indianapolis. This was the result of a growing number of adherents to the medical sects, including eclectics and homeopaths, that had increased in the 1850s.[38] In turn, opposition to them grew among the regular physicians in Indiana. Ironically, part of the reason for stronger competition was that the eclectics and homeopaths believed in scientific training like regular doctors, and much of the curriculum taught at their schools differed little from that of the regular schools. Instead of attacking the irregulars for differences in medical doctrine, the

Indiana Medical College faculty, like other regular physicians, claimed that the homeopaths and eclectics violated professional ethics by "basing their practice on an 'exclusive' dogma, and actively proselytizing among both physicians and the lay public." The Indiana Medical College faculty joined other physicians across the country in prohibiting admission to individuals having any connection whatsoever with one of these medical sects, thereby limiting access to the profession.[39]

Meanwhile, the charges that physicians of the two regular medical schools in Indianapolis hurled at each other differed little from what they aimed at the sectarians. For example, from the time that physicians split off from the Indiana Medical College to establish the CPS in 1874, disagreements arose over each school's arrangements for holding clinics in City Hospital. In 1875, the two colleges agreed to share clinical privileges at the hospital equally, but during the following year, questions arose about the hospital's management. Rumors circulated that the hospital officials condoned the practice of homeopathy by CPS faculty.[40] In September 1877, the situation deteriorated to the point that the doctors associated with the Indiana Medical College took it upon themselves to gather "affidavits of various parties in reference to the irregular practices of members of the faculty of the College of Physicians and Surgeons" and resolved that they would have nothing further to do with City Hospital. Hence, the Indiana Medical College faculty were so hostile to any hint of sectarian medical practice by the faculty of the CPS that they were willing to give up access to one of its most important clinical facilities.[41]

In the meantime, matters were complicated further as liberal arts institutions like Indiana Asbury (later DePauw) and Butler sought relationships with medical schools to enhance their prestige. Likewise, association with a university was attractive to medical schools not only because of potential new resources but also because the prestige that came with a faculty position helped physicians to increase their private practices. Shortly following the notice that ties with IU were officially severed, the Indiana Medical College attempted to affiliate with Indiana Asbury University, but negotiations with this school ended in a legal deadlock in the winter of 1877. Only six months later, in March 1878, Butler University approached the Indiana Medical College and CPS faculties about the possibility of them becoming that university's medical department.[42] The Indiana Medical College faculty met with representatives of Butler and CPS, and after first rejecting the terms that Butler forwarded, they reconsidered. In July 1878, the Indiana Medical College and the CPS consolidated to become the Medical College of Indiana (MCI)/Medical Department of Butler University. The relative ease with which the faculties of the two rival medical schools entered into an agreement, especially considering the intensity of the animosity they had expressed so recently toward each other, suggests that the problems between them were caused more by petty jealousies than issues of any real substance. A similar, though much more complicated, scenario played itself out a quarter of a century later when the Indiana University School of Medicine was finally established.[43]

This consolidation with Butler, however, proved a fragile one and fell apart almost as quickly as it had been put together. There were not enough teaching positions in the new MCI to absorb the faculties of the two medical schools, and physicians such as Joseph Eastman believed that they had been excluded from prestigious positions within the new institution. For this reason, Eastman, who had been a member of the College of Physicians and Surgeons faculty, led a group of doctors who were dissatisfied with MCI to form the new Central College of Physicians and Surgeons (CCPS) in 1879. The continued rivalry between these factions of physicians dictated the history of much of medical education in Indiana throughout the rest of the nineteenth century.[44]

Attempts at Reform and Other Mergers

To set it apart from its rival, the opening announcement of the CCPS in 1879 stated that the school had "been organized with the view to an advanced standard of requirements." However, there were few differences in the way the two schools were conducted. "With such indifferent instruction and with such meager clinical material," recalled John Barnhill, who attended the CCPS in the late 1880s and later was a key participant in the establishment of the Indiana University School of Medicine, "one wonders what of value the student got that enabled him to go forth and practice successfully, as most Central students did."[45] The facilities Barnhill encountered were limited. By the time he enrolled, the Central College had moved from its location in the Ryan Building to its new site in the Hammond Block Building on Massachusetts Avenue, on the second floor above a meat market.

The school had a fairly good anatomy laboratory, but its other laboratories were ill equipped. Otherwise, the school's quarters contained little more than a few benches and a blackboard. MCI was no better equipped. In 1889, when the faculty began discussing the possibility of establishing a bacteriology lab, the school did not own a single microscope.[46]

The courses that Barnhill took were little different from those offered by the Indiana Medical College in the 1870s. Instruction was still almost entirely didactic; lectures began at 9:00 a.m. and continued until 5:00 p.m. Two afternoons each week, the MCI held clinics at City Hospital, also open to CCPS students. Although called clinics, these sessions consisted of lectures on the patients' illnesses, and students found the surgical lectures of little value because of the difficulty in observing an operation from a distance. In the late 1880s, germ theory was still a subject of debate among practitioners, although it was more widely accepted by academic doctors and researchers. In 1902, for example, MCI dean Thomas B. Harvey was not convinced about the significance of germ theory; nonetheless, the school presented demonstrations on bacteriology.[47]

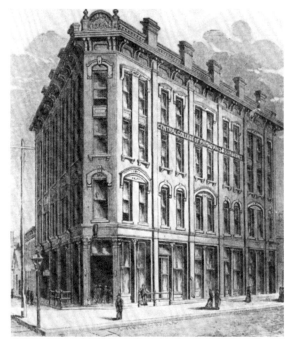

Figure 2.3. Central College of Physicians and Surgeons (engraving) was established under the leadership of Joseph Eastman in 1879 and moved to the Hammond Block Building in Indianapolis in the 1880s when John Barnhill attended. It remained there until constructing its own building in 1902. Thurman B. Rice, "The Hoosier Health Officer: A Biography of Dr. John N. Hurty: Chapter VIII," *Monthly Bulletin of the Indiana State Board of Health* 42 (August, 1939): 181.

Like many other physicians who attended medical school before the turn of the twentieth century, Barnhill contended that the experience he gained outside the formal classroom was the most important factor in preparing him to be a practitioner. A number of the faculty members were committed to education and often invited students to accompany them on their visits to private patients. During these home visits, where the majority of fee-for-service medical care still occurred, students had the opportunity to learn from interesting medical cases. In surgical operations, Barnhill assisted in the preparation of the patient, the administration of the anesthetic, and the operation itself.[48]

The introduction of a bacteriology laboratory at the MCI marked the beginning of a new era in medical education in Indianapolis. To keep up with the advances in laboratory medicine, MCI hired Theodore Potter (1861–1915), who represented a new generation of medical elite. Potter studied in Germany for a year after receiving his medical degree from the

Medical College of Ohio in 1887. An early exponent of the germ theory of disease, Potter was appointed as a demonstrator at MCI in 1889, "fresh from the labs and clinics of Germany [and] enthusiastic over the clinical significance and future of bacteriology." During summer and early fall 1889, he prepared the bacteriology laboratory by making cultures and staining solutions by hand, as well as pathological and histological specimens. In addition, he caged, fed, and inoculated the school's laboratory animals. When classes began in October 1889, Potter gave a four-week course in bacteriology followed by pathology and then histology. To teach these classes, however, he had to borrow microscopes from faculty members who owned them.[49]

In 1890, both MCI and the CCPS took another step toward reform by becoming charter members of the newly reorganized Association of American Medical Colleges (AAMC). Whereas before, medical schools could get by with having a lecture room, an anatomical laboratory, and some other makeshift laboratories, recognition by the AAMC required more space, equipment, and paid laboratory instructors. This meant that the MCI and CCPS now agreed to the AAMC requirement of a three-year graded course, although in the 1890s, many leading medical schools in the United States began to introduce compulsory four-year programs, and the Indianapolis schools soon followed.[50]

With these new requirements, the Indianapolis medical schools faced financial burdens they had never encountered before. In May 1890, the Ways and Means Committee of the MCI reported that the school had insufficient funds to defray the necessary expenses through the following term of lectures or "to procure such materials for equipping the various chairs and departments as [was] absolutely necessary to maintain the character of the college for good teaching." As a result, the school considered consolidation again with the newly renamed DePauw University (formerly Indiana Asbury). The faculty hoped that DePauw would be willing to meet the school's new financial needs.[51]

Instead, William Lomax, a physician from Marion, Indiana, and a strong advocate of medical education in the state, came to the MCI's rescue. In 1890, he bequeathed some property in and around Marion to the school. This proved to be a temporary solution because the property was not as valuable as either the donor or beneficiary first believed. Complicating matters, in early November 1894, a fire broke out at the medical college at its location at the Indianapolis Gas Company. Although the origins of the fire were never confirmed, there was widespread reporting that it started in the dissecting room of the medical college. Typically, the floors of anatomy laboratories were covered with sawdust, and a majority of the students smoked cigars as they worked to cover the smell of the dissecting room. In addition, medical students had a reputation for being rowdy, irreverent, and immature, so according to one theory, it was likely that a cigar stub carelessly disposed of by a medical student caused the fire, which not only burned down the medical college building but also damaged the gas company and many adjoining buildings.[52]

This fire completely destroyed the Bobbs Library, valuable specimens, and medical equipment. Although the Medical College of Indiana's fire loss was devastating, it proved to be only a temporary setback. Lomax's bequest was not large enough for an endowment, but it did provide enough funds to construct a new building for the college and to replace the books and equipment that were lost. Frank W. Hayes, who then served as the school's secretary, declared that this new building, which opened in 1895 opposite the statehouse at the corner of Senate Avenue and Market Street, made it possible for the faculty to operate a "more perfect" medical school than ever before. Hayes believed that it compared with the best facilities available in the United States at this time.[53]

While continuing to search for an endowment, in 1896, MCI joined an attempt to create the short-lived University of Indianapolis, an affiliation of four existing colleges in the city. This effort, which in some ways anticipated the successful creation of IUPUI in 1969, included MCI, Butler University, and two independent proprietary professional schools, the Indiana Law School and the Indiana Dental College.[54] Each institution maintained its own autonomy, the ownership of property, and internal management, but by honoring exchange courtesies, the schools hoped to gradually strengthen the bonds between them. In addition, the leaders of these schools thought that the idea of building a university in the state capital would gain enough confidence in the community to attract either state funding or a private endowment. These funds never materialized, however, in part because of opposition from other colleges and universities. For example, in 1900, the faculty of Central College of Physicians and Surgeons, along with friends of Indiana University, helped defeat legislation that would have diverted money away from the state university in Bloomington to finance the University of Indianapolis. Unable to procure state funding or a private endowment, the initial enthusiasm for the University of Indianapolis experiment faded, and the project never attained its objectives.[55]

As the role of the CCPS in the failure of the University of Indianapolis reveals, the bitter rivalry between the medical schools persisted. Although the MCI remained the larger of the two schools (it graduated 82 students in 1904 and 126 in 1906),[56] the CCPS grew in size and improved its teaching reputation in the last decade of the nineteenth century, thanks in part to a growing number of the professors who trained abroad. According to some ratings, the CCPS surpassed the MCI with an increasing percentage of matriculates holding college degrees.[57]

After having developed a good relationship with representatives of IU from their joint opposition to the University of Indianapolis bill in the legislature, the Central College faculty were encouraged to approach IU president Joseph Swain about making their school the university's medical department. Leaders of CCPS wrote to Swain in October 1900, stating that it had "been a long cherished hope" that the they might affiliate with IU, arguing that such an affiliation would be advantageous to both institutions. Those whom Swain consulted about the possibility of a merger with the CCPS disagreed, and their objections are worth examining in some detail because although in this case they prevailed, just a few years later, a new IU president ignored this advice.

Most of the letters Swain received expressed the opinion that although such an arrangement would benefit the Central College, it would not benefit the university. For example, the state librarian of Indiana, who was a former IU English professor, advised Swain not to merge with the CCPS unless the school's requirements were raised. Others objected that merger with the medical schools might renew demands that IU be moved from Bloomington to Indianapolis. Although some people believed that Central College at the very least equaled the MCI in quality, James W. Fesler, who was then a prominent Indianapolis attorney and IU alumnus, declared that it was the weaker of the two schools. The MCI, he pointed out, "had twice the students and graduates, a new building with laboratory equipment for the work, and above all the enthusiastic support . . . of the best specialists in the city."[58] In addition, Fesler criticized faculty member Joseph Eastman and his two sons, who owned a majority controlling interest of the Central College stock and whose "arbitrary and dictatorial management" had recently led several of the college's best lecturers to resign. Referring to the sharp and bitter rivalry between the Indianapolis medical schools, Fesler proclaimed that associating with the CCPS might do permanent injury to IU by antagonizing the faculty and graduates of the MCI. "We have never had the organized opposition of the doctors," Fesler told Swain. "Let's not invite it."[59]

Turned down for a merger with IU in 1901, the CCPS decided to proceed with plans to erect a new building. At the turn of the century, the commercial space the school rented was no longer appropriate to its needs, making it difficult for the Central College to compete with the MCI without a comparable modern structure dedicated to medical education. In early 1902, the college purchased a lot it designated for the building on Senate Avenue, just a few blocks north of the MCI. Unlike its rival, the CCPS found no generous donor to defray the costs of construction, so the faculty raised money for the building through subscription and had to take out a substantial mortgage, leaving the college in a vulnerable financial position.[60]

Then in late October 1902, just days before the new building of the Central College of Physicians and Surgeons was dedicated, the school's anatomy demonstrator, Joseph C. Alexander, and an intern at the school, J. C. Wilson, were indicted by a grand jury in a widely publicized grave-robbing scandal along with doctors who taught at two sectarian medical schools in Indianapolis, the Indiana Eclectic Medical College and the Physio-Medical College of Indiana. CCPS dean Allison Maxwell tried to make the best of the situation at the formal opening of the building: "We are very happy that the grand jury and the detectives have left as many of us outside as are here tonight."[61]

The problem was long in the making. Because laws did not permit an adequate supply of bodies for dissection, medical schools throughout the United States regularly engaged in practices that were not always legal to secure enough material to instruct students in practical anatomy.[62] As early as 1883, physicians connected to the medical schools in Indianapolis tried to get the anatomy laws of the state amended to eliminate the risk of involvement in any illegal dealings, but to no avail. Calling for the legislature to authorize provision of cadavers to medical schools met resistance because popular attitudes were opposed to the desecration of the human body and because access to cadavers would give physicians exclusive, private knowledge—an elite professional privilege that grated against democratic political sensibilities.[63]

Medical schools usually gave anatomy demonstrators complete control of dissecting rooms, including responsibility for obtaining bodies; hence, they were most vulnerable to lawsuits. Like Alexander at CCPS, the other medical school faculty arrested in the 1902 grave-robbing scandals worked as either anatomy demonstrators or as anatomy assistants. Although the charges were eventually dropped after a second trial of Alexander, the grave-robbing case was a grand, popular spectacle throughout 1902 and 1903. The visibility of the case drew much negative attention to the state and revealed the medical schools' need for a better way to legally obtain cadavers. In February 1903, while the grave-robbing trials were still pending, the Indiana General Assembly unanimously passed the Baird Bill, which created the state's first anatomical board, controlled by the medical schools. With the enactment of this law, an adequate supply of well-embalmed bodies reached the state's medical schools for the first time.[64]

Conclusion

The grave-robbing scandal was, at root, caused by the changes in medical understanding the preceding century and the rise in importance of anatomical instruction for medical students. However, this was just one of many growing fields such as bacteriology and physiology that required laboratories and other expenses, such that by the beginning of the twentieth century, the costs of operating a medical school were rising precipitously.[65] Like a majority of medical schools throughout the United States by the early 1900s, both of Indiana's largest orthodox colleges were committed to instituting reforms. They adopted a full, four-year, graded curriculum, and with increased requirements, the academic year lengthened from September to April. The MCI boasted that it had begun bedside medical clinics, following the methods of Johns Hopkins University School of Medicine and other medical colleges across the country, thus allowing their students to learn by doing rather than by listening, reading, and watching.[66]

To keep pace in the basic sciences, another educational reform that medical schools recognized was they could no longer depend on part-time local practitioners to teach these subjects. Yet at the turn of the century, professors at the Indianapolis medical schools continued to be doctors with private practices who devoted part of their time to teaching. The only full-time employees of MCI were its laboratory assistants; hiring professors to teach the basic sciences full-time would be much more costly. Even professors like Theodore Potter did not receive a full-time salary. The amount paid to laboratory assistants totaled $3,000 a year, and this was a significant proportion of the total $15,000–20,000 that the school earned in annual income from the fees of approximately three hundred students. With the increased demands, the student fees were not sufficient to pay salaries of qualified, full-time professors in the basic sciences or to supply the expensive equipment necessary for instruction.

One final feature of American medical education reform by the beginning of the twentieth century was for medical schools to be part of a university. As John Barnhill later recalled, the larger proprietary schools in Indiana "saw early that they must close their doors or join with a university."[67] At this time, the geographical, socioeconomic, and demographic features of the state resulted in the two largest private medical schools being in Indianapolis, the largest city with the most patients, hospitals, and clinics. The two largest institutions of higher education (Purdue and Indiana University), however, were located fifty miles from this city, and efforts to join the smaller, private colleges were unsuccessful, as was the approach to Indiana University by the CCPS in 1900, which again was declined. It took the appointment of a new IU president two years later to change the attitude of the university about medical education, but by then, Purdue University had also entered the picture. It took another five years and a change in the attitude of the public and the Indiana legislature before a lasting solution was found to meet the challenge proposed by John S. Bobbs, forty years before, to establish a medical school in Indiana that could "compete in excellence, in eminence, in every appliance and means of instruction, with the very best schools of the age."[68]

3

Making Medicine Modern, 1900–1912

What the people want is *open* paths from every corner of the state through the schools to the highest and best things which men can achieve.

William Lowe Bryan inaugural address,
Indiana University, January 22, 1903

One great department of education has been left for the most part to shift for itself and that precisely the one which concerns itself with the care of human life.

William Lowe Bryan to Henry Jameson, Dean,
Medical College of Indiana, May 25, 1904

*I*n 1900, there were six medical schools in the state of Indiana. Two decades later, there was one. The reason for this dramatic change was the establishment of the Indiana University School of Medicine and its merger with the Medical College of Indiana and the Central College of Physicians and Surgeons in 1908. What changed to make this possible so quickly? The appointment of William Lowe Bryan as president of Indiana University in 1902 is the most cited answer. The year following his appointment and just three years after his predecessor, Joseph Swain, had rejected an approach from the CCPS, Bryan persuaded the IU trustees to begin teaching the first two years of medical school, and he also entered merger negotiations with the Medical College of Indiana.

Bryan's appointment can legitimately be called the precipitating step, but despite his obvious importance, there are at least two reasons to view his influence as only part of the explanation for these changes. First, as the previous chapter has shown, changes in medical education in the state had been ongoing for decades as the proprietary schools adapted to the reforms that had arisen nationally. In fact, the two large schools in Indianapolis had begun to adopt many of the recommendations of the Association of American Medical Colleges (AAMC) and the American Medical Association (AMA) regarding admissions criteria, length of instruction, and inclusion of laboratory teaching. Both schools had also made efforts to meet another major reform, joining a university, although their previous efforts had failed. From this perspective, Bryan's new willingness to have his state university offer medical education was a significant new step in the long-building movement of medical education reform in Indiana.

The involvement of Purdue in consolidation of medical education in Indiana after 1900, however, shows that Bryan was not alone in pursuing this goal. The process, in fact, became quite complicated and dragged on for five years because in addition to the IU-Purdue rivalry, there were also two private medical schools involved in the negotiations, as well as the state legislature. The eventual consolidation after 1900 involved plans and beginnings of at least four viable schools in the first decade of the twentieth century: two four-year schools in Indianapolis, one planned in Bloomington, and a combined Purdue-Indianapolis school. The medical school that emerged at the end of the decade was partly the result of the resolve of the leaders in Indianapolis and Bloomington, but it was also the result of larger developments in the medical profession and state legislature.

Another indication that Bryan was following a well-trod path elsewhere was the consolidation of medical education around the country in the first decades of the twentieth century. The expansion of medical education in the United States peaked in 1906, when there were 162 schools of quite varying quality, but the number rapidly dropped off to 131 in 1910 and 95 in 1915. This resulted in the closing of many smaller schools but also the merger of proprietary medical schools with universities. Hence, some of the circumstances and developments in Indiana were similar to those in other places where private medical schools joined universities in cities, such as Cincinnati (1896), Chicago (University of Chicago in 1898 and University of Illinois in 1913), San Francisco (Stanford in 1908), and Louisville (1908).[1]

At stake for Indianapolis physicians such as John Barnhill and William Niles Wishard was control of their profession and their economic viability. At stake for Indiana University and President Bryan was the relevance and existence of the university and the values it embodied. For Bryan, medical education demonstrated the value of the research university while ensuring adequate enrollment for the undergraduate college. The tension between the needs of the university in Bloomington and the medical community in

Indianapolis produced a compromise that divided the resulting medical school to the complete satisfaction of no one and established a pattern of distributed education that helped define the Indiana University School of Medicine ever since.

The complicated history of the consolidation leading to the IUSM has been told numerous times from different perspectives. The first lengthy examination was in a 1929 master's thesis by J. H. Brayton, the son of A. W. Brayton, founder and longtime editor of the *Indiana Medical Journal* and faculty member of the Medical College of Indiana who joined the new IUSM. Figure 3.1 shows Brayton's effort to illustrate this history. Burton Myers, the first medical faculty member hired by Bryan, also included lengthy accounts of the consolidation in his volume on the *History of Indiana University* (1940) and his *History of Medical Education in Indiana* (1956). In the previous chapter, figure 2.2 summarizes Myers's even more extensive research. The second volume of Thomas Clark's updated history of Indiana University (1973) has a lengthy chapter on this story, and more recently former IUSM dean Walter Daly published an article focusing on the competition between Indiana and Purdue Universities that led to the establishment of the Indiana University School of Medicine.[2] This chapter examines the features of that history to show how they reflect the influences of the time and to provide background for the even more important subsequent events that instituted the changes promised.

Taking Medicine Public: The Medical Departments of IU and Purdue

When Bryan assumed the university presidency by unanimous vote of the trustees in June 1902, Indiana University's enrollment was well below one thousand students—and almost 90 percent of those were in the liberal arts.[3] Although earlier IU presidents, most notably David Starr Jordan, had done much to expand the curriculum and introduce a system of electives, Bryan wanted his institution to shed the last vestiges of the classical English academy tradition. To make IU a modern university, he first sought a medical school. Although earlier attempts at this by the university going back to the 1870s had failed, Bryan wanted to follow the example of such schools as Johns Hopkins and the University of Chicago in order to construct an institution that combined the ideals of research, teaching, and utility. A medical school most clearly exemplified these objectives. In late 1902, Bryan told the board of trustees he hoped that in the not too distant future, the university could establish a two-year medical department. Bryan realized that medical education was undergoing great changes and that medical schools were becoming an integral part of universities while increasing their standards and integrating emerging sciences in novel ways.[4]

When Bryan, an IU alumnus, was a young faculty member, Jordan encouraged him to study abroad in Berlin. Upon Bryan's return to Bloomington, he established one of only three psychological laboratories in the Midwest. In 1892, he earned a PhD in psychology at Clark University, where he met Franklin P. Mall, the influential anatomist, who was an adjunct professor at the school during the time that Bryan was studying there. In 1893, Mall became head of the Department of Anatomy at the new Johns Hopkins University School of Medicine. This relationship with one of the leaders in medical education reform at Johns Hopkins helped shape the direction of Bryan's plans and provided him with very important resources.[5]

By the time Bryan took over the presidency, the university had already developed many of the components necessary for medical instruction. Jordan had em-

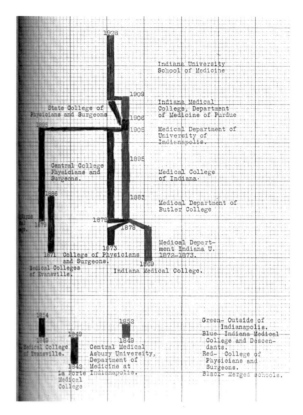

Figure 3.1. "Regular Medical Colleges of Indiana, 1842–1928," in Brayton, "Development of Medical Education in Indiana," 14.

phasized the importance of the sciences, particularly biology, and in 1891, when Jordan left Indiana to become president of Stanford University, IU established a medical preparatory course under the direction of Robert E. Lyons in chemistry and Carl H. Eigenmann in zoology. Many students who completed this course were able to enter medical schools with advanced standing.[6]

At the end of 1902, two major obstacles stood in the way of Bryan's goal to start a medical department. First was the overall inadequacy of the university budget. During Bryan's first year in office, total university appropriations amounted to less than $200,000, which precluded IU from providing "more than one year's work in medicine." Second, the state's deficient anatomical laws presented a barrier to securing cadavers for anatomical study, a hallmark of modern medical education. That was resolved the following year when sensational newspaper stories about the grave-robbing scandal mentioned in the previous chapter finally resulted in passage of the 1903 Indiana Anatomical Law that would allow IU to obtain the cadavers needed.[7] That same legislature increased university funding, thus enabling Bryan to plan for expansion of medical instruction.[8]

On March 27, 1903, at a meeting of the board of trustees, Bryan outlined his plan to establish the first two years of medical instruction in Bloomington. In addition to the existing medical preparatory courses, all that was necessary was to add anatomy and pathology to the curriculum and expand the number of classes taught in physiology. The university would have to hire only two additional faculty members, and he encouraged the board to authorize immediately the establishment of an anatomy department. By emphasizing elementary medical subjects in the science departments, Bryan contended, "It would be possible . . . to offer at once nearly, if not quite, two years of a four years' medical course." The IU trustees approved Bryan's plan to initiate the medical program and authorized him to start a search for an individual to organize a new anatomy department.[9]

In summer 1903, Bryan was presented with a chance at a shortcut toward his goal but with important complications. IU trustee James Fesler informed Bryan that Medical College of Indiana (MCI) dean Henry Jameson was "anxious to see him."[10] Jameson's motivation was that proprietary schools like MCI and the other medical school in Indianapolis, the Central College of Physicians and Surgeons (CCPS), increasingly needed to affiliate with universities to avoid losing students to schools with lower requirements and to gain access to resources for improving medical education. Such a consolidation would solve many of the independent medical schools' problems and enable Bryan to expand the university's medical course to a full four-year program by adding clinical instruction in Indianapolis to the two years of basic medical sciences to be offered in Bloomington.[11] Although this was eventually achieved, it was a complicated process that took years to work out.

Bryan strongly favored a merger, but he was also aware that the long history of rivalry between the Indianapolis medical schools posed a difficult obstacle to achieving his goals. The strength of Bryan's plan was that "scientific clinical work" could be better facilitated at the university because of its graduate education resources for science instruction, whereas the medical schools in Indianapolis had access to patients and physicians for clinical instruction. By July 1903, however, it became clear to Bryan that the personal and professional interests of the two medical school faculties prevented them from reaching an agreement, so he temporarily abandoned this plan.[12]

In the meantime, Bryan began his search for someone to start an anatomy department in Bloomington. For advice, he turned to Mall, who recommended a member of his own department at Johns Hopkins, Burton D. Myers. As a physician and scientist, Myers fulfilled perfectly Bryan's criteria for the job in Bloomington. Burton Dorr Myers was born in 1870 in Attica, Ohio. He received his bachelor of philosophy degree from Buchtel College (forerunner of the University of Akron) in 1893 and his master's degree from Cornell University in 1900. He earned his MD at the University of Leipzig in 1902, returned to Cornell as an assistant professor in physiology from 1898 to 1900, and moved to Johns Hopkins University in 1902–1903. In June 1903, Myers visited the IU campus and met with the trustees, who agreed to offer him the position of chair of the new Anatomy Department. Myers said that "he was impressed by the presence of outstanding men on the faculty and the excellent work of various departments," including chemistry, physiology, and embryology. Myers accepted the professorship at IU in early July 1903, stating, "The opportunity of taking an active part in the organization of medical education in Indiana on a basis equal to that of the eight leading medical schools of America, I find very attractive, and feel it a great and important work."[13]

Besides Myers, the other appointments in the Medical Department were faculty already at IU, so there was no delay in admitting students. The *Indiana Daily Student* newspaper declared that the Medical Department was "one of the most important additions . . . made to the institution in recent years."[14] Eighteen students enrolled in the new two-year program, including one woman, Sophia Augusta McKay, from New Albany, Indiana.

Despite this rapid start, the physical environment was a limitation to Bryan's plan. At this time, the entire campus in Bloomington comprised just ten buildings. Medical students attended chemistry classes in Wylie Hall and embryology classes in Owen Hall. The recently dedicated Science Hall housed anatomy and physiology. Plank and gravel walks led only to the campus's three main buildings. In inclement weather, the university administration made no provisions for clearing these walkways, making them unsafe and even at times impassable.[15] Although the *Daily Student* stated that the new medical school was "starting out under the most favorable auspices," Myers was unable to begin classes that involved human dissection in fall 1903 as he wished. He had to make do with students dissecting animals. These pioneer medical students studying anatomy in

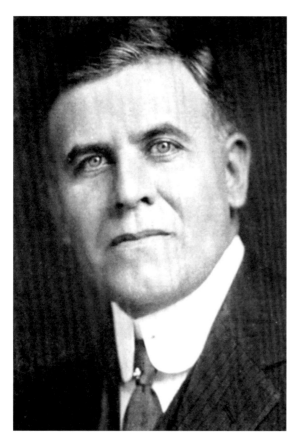

Figure 3.2. Burton Dorr Myers, professor of anatomy and first full-time medical faculty member at IU, *Arbutus* (1916): 281.

the attic rooms of Science Hall practiced dissecting cats until regular classes in human anatomy began in fall 1904.[16] Given these and subsequent developments, only three of the original eighteen students admitted were able to complete their MD in Indiana; the others likely completed their work at other four-year institutions.

Recognizing these limitations, Bryan resumed negotiations throughout 1904 with the medical schools in Indianapolis. At every turn, however, he encountered wariness about a new IU School of Medicine that might raise entry barriers for both faculty and students. In late November 1904, the trustees of the MCI and the CCPS scheduled conferences about merging with IU and then reported that they would not enter into a relationship with the university, again bringing all of the negotiations to a halt.[17]

At the beginning of 1905, the repeated failure of these negotiations and the limitations on the Bloomington campus made the medical school situation the most important and difficult question facing Indiana University. Official recognition of the two-year curriculum in Bloomington had been postponed by the AAMC at its April 1904 meeting. Approval was granted at the April 1905 meeting, but in the meantime, it placed the current students in peril for transfer to complete their clinical instruction elsewhere, and it jeopardized future enrollments. Bryan made it very clear to the board of trustees that the future of medical education at IU was at risk, and he even posed the possibility of dismantling the two-year medical program.[18]

Regardless of decisions in Bloomington, the dynamics of the Indianapolis medical marketplace quickly began to drive events. This became suddenly apparent on September 1, 1905, when, after three months of negotiations with MCI, Purdue officials announced an agreement in the executive offices of Indiana Governor J. Frank Hanly to make the medical school

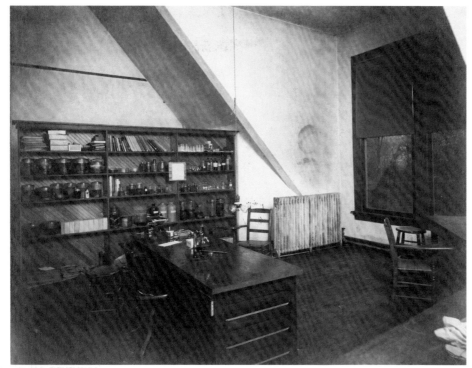

Figure 3.3a & b.
Medical Sciences
Bloomington 1910: (*top*)
Lindley Hall Anatomy
classroom for beginning
medical students, IUB
Archive photo collection
P0051848; (*bottom*)
Wylie Hall, IUB Archive
photo collection,
P0020555.

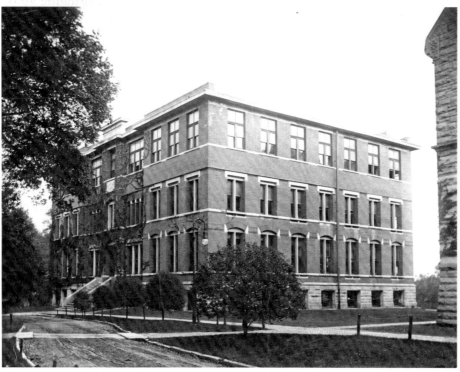

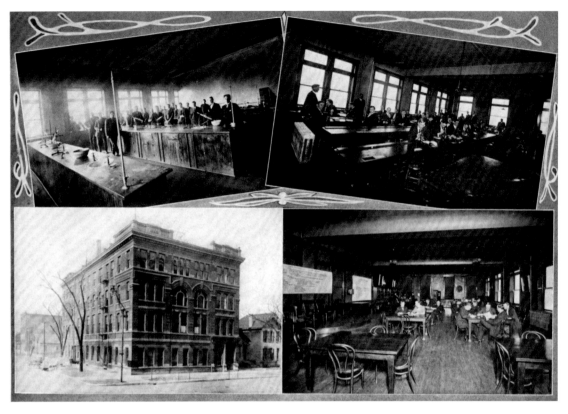

Figure 3.4. Indiana Medical College building and interior, constructed in 1895 at Senate and Market opposite the statehouse, *Arbutus* (1909): 210.

part of their institution. Hanly had lived in Lafayette and still had strong ties there. He was also an advocate of a number of progressive reforms and therefore supported bringing the medical school under state control through the auspices of Purdue. The president of Purdue, Winthrop Stone, felt that the time was ripe to unite all of the regular Indiana medical schools under Purdue's control, although the agreement reveals that the leaders of the MCI managed to achieve this consolidation on their own terms.[19]

Officials at the other Indianapolis medical school, CCPS, continued to play both sides by negotiating with IU and Purdue trustees. On the evening of September 24, 1905, the CCPS dean, George Kahlo, asserted to newspaper reporters that his faculty favored a consolidation with IU but admitted that if such an affiliation were accomplished, it might cause a contest between the two state universities in the upcoming session of the Indiana

General Assembly. The next day, Stone promptly called a meeting to urge the CCPS Board of Trustees to consolidate with the MCI as an interim step before joining Purdue and to act quickly so that the interests of the school's students could "be protected against the influence of uncertainty and unrest." By the end of the meeting, the Central College faculty and the board of trustees endorsed and approved Stone's plan. With this affiliation, the CCPS faculty united under the name of the Indiana Medical College.[20]

The CCPS announcement was almost as much a surprise as the Purdue/MCI merger. Bloomington authorities were "indignant over what they term[ed] sharp dealing and breach of faith on the part of Purdue University." Students enrolled at the CCPS were also displeased and threatened to refuse to transfer to the Indiana Medical College. In response, on September 28, President Stone gave a stirring address to the Central students professing the benefits of the union. According to newspaper accounts, as Stone concluded, the students in attendance loudly cheered and chanted the Purdue University yell, and over one hundred people marched to the Indiana Medical College building.[21]

Once this crisis had passed, another school joined the merger. The Fort Wayne College of Medicine, organized in 1879, was the third regular medical school operating in Indiana in the fall 1905. Leading state physicians like Alembert Brayton thought that such a merger would be very desirable for medical education in the state, and Fort Wayne dean Christian B. Stemen wanted to ensure that the Purdue merger did not leave out his school and told Stone that he was willing to immediately move his students to Indianapolis. On October 9, 1905, the faculty and students of the Fort Wayne College of Medicine closed their building and arrived in Indianapolis by train. Because few members of this school's faculty were willing to give up their private practices in Fort Wayne, they remained minor players in the combination.[22]

The merger with the Fort Wayne College of Medicine completed the amalgamation of proprietary schools that formed the new Indiana Medical College, which was to become the Medical Department of Purdue University. In four short months, Purdue accomplished what Indiana physicians had been striving to do since the late 1860s. Moreover, Stone had accomplished a task that eluded Bryan, in spite of the IU president's belief that establishment of a viable medical school was essential to the survival of his university. In the exuberance of their apparent victory, Stone, Purdue trustees, and members of the Indiana Medical College faculty underestimated their adversary.

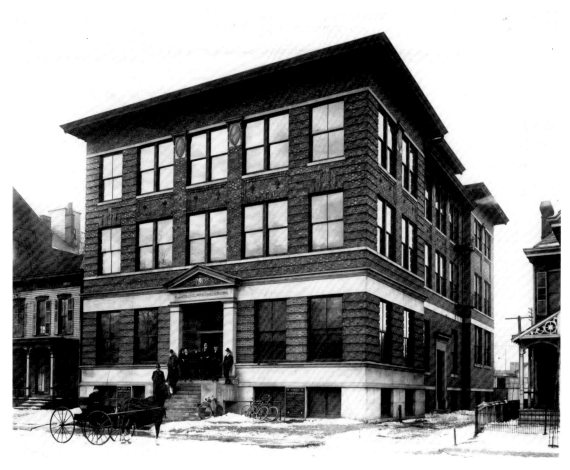

Figure 3.5. Central College of Physicians and Surgeons, building constructed in 1902 on Senate Avenue in Indianapolis, just north of the Medical College. IUPUI image UA024_000409.

The Hoosier "War" of Medical Education

On October 5, 1905, the same day Stone completed negotiations with the Fort Wayne College of Medicine, Bryan reacted to the Purdue medical college consolidation in a report to his board of trustees. He made it clear that the situation placed Indiana University in a state of crisis.

> The University stands immediately in the presence of the greatest danger in its history. . . . We are in danger of seeing nearly or quite everything which the state requires of a university done by the State elsewhere. The Department of Law is still ours, but if the Department of Medicine can be taken away in violation of our explicit rights, there is no reason why the Department of Law should not presently follow. . . . If these conditions

and tendencies hold, it requires no prophet to foresee the result. Within a few years Purdue will be in effect, if not in name, the University of Indiana, and Indiana University will be the name of an institution, which was once the University of the State as Corydon was once its capital.[23]

For Bryan, medical school consolidation with Purdue threatened to make Indiana University "superfluous." Far from marking the end of the period of "rivalry and antagonism" in medical education in Indiana as Stone predicted, the merger that created the Purdue School of Medicine kindled a battle between the two major state universities that was so hostile it has been described as a "war."[24] For Bryan especially, this fight meant the life or death of his institution.

IU was presented with a seemingly impossible roadblock in its path to creating a medical school as a result of the union of the three medical colleges that included dozens of respected and influential faculty, plus hundreds of alumni who, at first, fully supported the Purdue agreement. Moreover, enrollment at Indiana Medical College alone stood at over three hundred students, in striking contrast to the twenty-one students who attended class in the Medical Department in Bloomington. Yet Bryan saw one fortunate circumstance for his side: he had time. Official legislative sanctioning of the merger was necessary but not possible until the biennial General Assembly session of January 1907. This gave him time to carry out the lines of attack that he described in his board report of October 1905. Also in IU's favor was the fact that Purdue had neither a plan nor resources for the fundamental transformation of medical education that was needed. Nor had Stone established consensus among the physicians from Indiana Medical College and Central College about such a plan or governance and appointments within the new medical department. This gave ample opportunity and time for existing jealousies among the Indianapolis medical community to surface.[25]

The importance of the IU-Purdue conflict and the war metaphors for the people involved was that it took the decisions about medical education in Indiana solely out of the hands of the local Indianapolis professionals and made them statewide and public. Regardless of which university won the battle, the authority for medical education would shift from community practitioners to academic physicians. The result greatly diminished the importance of battles between the former faculties of the CCPS and the MCI because the agreement to consolidate medical education in Indiana would eventually make it part of a public university.

In late October 1905, Bryan took his first steps toward saving his plan by holding an initial meeting with Stone, where he presented his case.

According to Bryan, the Purdue president admitted that he should have consulted with Bryan and IU trustees before entering into negotiations with the Indianapolis medical schools. Bryan also noted that Stone acknowledged how important medical education was to Indiana University's future and how different his school's position was from that of IU. Bryan even thought that Stone might be willing to concede the field to IU if Purdue "could escape from this position honorably." Despite this surprisingly conciliatory attitude, there were many other points of dispute and rivalry, and in the end, the university presidents were unable to reach any kind of accord to end hostilities. Although Stone and Bryan agreed to meet again, the relationship between IU and Purdue deteriorated quickly in the months following this session.[26]

Given the heavy odds against the plans for medical education at IU, in the months that followed, the trustees considered a range of alternatives from adding the third and fourth years of medical school at Bloomington (even with few clinical facilities) to starting a school of engineering, perhaps by annexing Rose Polytechnic in Terre Haute.[27] Within weeks of the announcement of the Purdue merger, these were dismissed when other possibilities opened up thanks to signs that the Purdue consolidation was not as solid as it first appeared. Bryan reported a visit by faculty from the combined school who were disgruntled with the way Purdue and Indiana Medical College authorities handled the agreement between their old medical colleges and Purdue. A half dozen former faculty at the CCPS told him that "the union of schools was a union in name only" and that "the vastly too large number of professors created endless confusion." The faculty members present at this meeting "urged the establishment of a new medical college by Indiana University."[28]

Even more to the point, they revealed that following the terms of the agreement between their old medical college and Purdue, their building on North Senate Avenue was up for sale and could be purchased at a reasonable price. One of those present, Allison Maxwell, who had taught at CCPS since 1886, became dean in 1902, and notably was a grandson of the first president of the Indiana University Board of Trustees, urged Bryan to quickly arrange the purchase of the Central College building. Although he had not been in favor of the amalgamation of medical colleges with Purdue in September 1905, Maxwell had accepted a position, albeit an honorary one, in the new school. However, it was soon evident to Maxwell that the leaders of the Indiana Medical College, most notably Jameson, had no intention of honoring the promises that had been made to sixteen former CCPS faculty.[29]

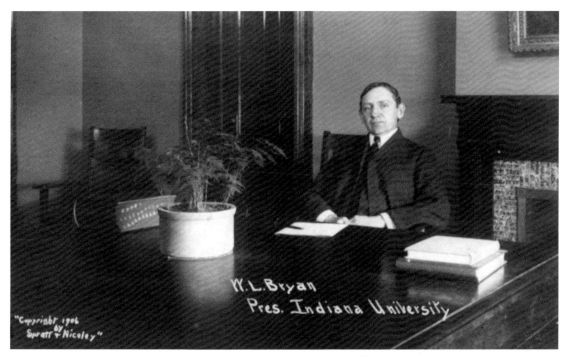

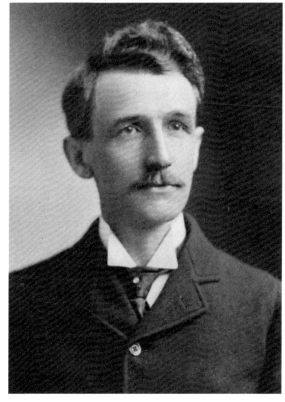

Figure 3.6a & b. The two new presidents: William Lowe Bryan (*above*), president of Indiana University (1902–37), photo from 1906, IUB Archive photo collection P0020474; Withrop Stone (*right*) in 1902, president of Purdue (1900–1921), Purdue e-archives PPH00941.

Buying the CCPS building offered a means to expand the IU Medical Department in Indianapolis, but it raised several questions. First was the relationship to teaching in Bloomington. The commitment to Indianapolis confirmed there would be no expansion to a four-year curriculum in Bloomington, something Bryan had decided earlier. There was also no desire to move the basic science instruction from Bloomington, so the logical plan was to convert the CCPS building for the third and fourth years of clinical instruction. Because they were challenging the Purdue merger, which provided four years of medical instruction at a well-established school (as was typically found in large cities), Bryan and Myers first had to justify the unusual arrangement they planned of teaching scientific laboratory courses at a different location from the third and fourth years of clinic.

To gather information and make their case, they sent a set of questions to over forty educators at medical schools around the country, the responses to which were compiled in a pamphlet that was distributed by the university in April 1906.[30] To the question "Do you believe there is time or reason for clinics during the first two years of the modern medical course?" they received forty negative answers. This was not surprising because it followed the medical reform of requiring scientific training before clinical instruction. The second question went more directly to their main point but in an obviously leading manner: "Do you believe the first two years of the medical course may be given effectively at a university located at some distance from the city in which the last two years of the course are given, as is done at Cornell, and the Universities of Nebraska, California, Kansas and elsewhere?" Statistics of all responses were not included, just excerpts from positive ones by a Cornell professor ("our Ithaca men . . . have proved themselves thoroughly prepared"), the president-elect of the AMA ("yes, provided they be given by [competent] men"), the dean of Ohio Medical University ("I do not see that it should make any difference"), and Frank Mall at Johns Hopkins ("the place that is best manned and best equipped will give the best course").[31]

Because Bloomington already was teaching the first two years, IU officials focused most of their attention on setting up clinical instruction in Indianapolis. Before finding the funds for this, however, there was first the problem that the university could not legally own property located outside Monroe County. To stay within the margins of the law, Bryan and Myers convinced a group of interested Bloomington citizens to buy the structure for the university. Then Bryan and members of the university's board of trustees faced the question of securing a faculty. In response, Maxwell submitted his resignation from the Indiana Medical College to Stone and began to confer with other leading Indianapolis physicians about forming a new medical school connected to Indiana University.[32] By the first weeks of 1906, it was very clear that the fight between Indiana University and Purdue over medical education was headed at least for the state legislature, if not also the courts.

Understandably, Purdue officials, especially members of the Indiana Medical College faculty, considered the purchase of the CCPS building by "Friends of Indiana University" a declaration of war.[33] To lay out its position to the medical community, legislators, and the press, Stone instructed Jameson to write a statement for wide distribution intended to restore consensus within the medical community. Addressing the advantages of the Purdue merger, the "three deans circular" (so called because it was also signed by former deans Kahlo of CCPS and Stemens of Ft. Wayne College of Medicine) allowed Stone to counter IU's actions with an official response not only to the Indianapolis medical community by publishing it in the *Indiana Medical Journal* but also by sending it to physicians, medical societies, legislators, newspapers, and even representatives of the American Medical Association (AMA). In his cover letter to the AMA, Jameson presented the document "as a fair statement of the conditions" leading to the merger of the three medical colleges with Purdue.[34]

Contrary to Stone's hopes, the reaction to the three deans' circular indicated that the Indianapolis medical community was not firmly united behind the new Purdue program. In addition, the purchase by IU "friends" of the CCPS building meant that Purdue could no longer claim a monopoly of medical education even in Indianapolis. As a result, throughout 1905 and 1906, the battle for control of medical education was fought in the press, county medical societies, the court, and the parlors of supporters and patrons of the schools, all of which eventually led to the legislature. In the contest, IU and Purdue battled mainly over three resources: students, patients, and legal authority.

Perhaps the most difficult challenge faced by Bryan and his allies was access to patients. This was because of a contract signed between the Purdue-affiliated Indiana Medical College and the Indianapolis Board of Health in March 1906, which gave the medical college exclusive rights to hold clinics at Indianapolis City Hospital (later Wishard and now Eskenazi Health) until January 1910. Because access to patients was so crucial for clinical education, Dean Jameson told Stone there is no other thing "that could have been done that will make it absolutely impossible for our adversaries to start a medical school at this point as this."[35] In effect, this contract made it very difficult, if not impossible, for the faculty of the IU-affiliated school to find enough patients for instruction in order to meet the requirements set by the Association of American Medical Colleges (AAMC).[36]

One response by Maxwell and fellow physicians like Simon P. Scherer was to question the legality of City Hospital to impede Indiana University's effort to establish a medical school in Indianapolis. In late February 1906, Scherer and Charles R. Sowder, who was affiliated with the former CCPS, filed suit in the Marion County Superior Court against Purdue University and the Indiana Medical College. As arguments in the case began in April, they claimed to represent a larger group of physicians determined to maintain their "property, rights, privileges and records, without the paternal care and protection of the Indiana Medical College." Joining Scherer and Sowder in their lawsuit were other CCPS alumni who complained that the Purdue medical school merger violated their legal rights. Bryan and other IU supporters knew this action risked miring the issue of the merger in the courts, but at the time, it represented the only way to challenge Purdue without taking the battle to the legislature. In fact, just the opposite occurred. The case was still in litigation when the medical school dispute was finally resolved by IU and Purdue in April 1908, and the legislature ratified it the following year.[37]

Meanwhile, after taking possession of the former CCPS building, a group of physicians still very small in number prepared for classes to begin in September 1906 despite the lack of patients for clinical instruction. Maxwell continued to recruit professors among former members of the CCPS faculty, beginning with John Barnhill, a clinical professor of otolaryngology, who was the first professor at the new Indiana Medical College to submit his resignation. Barnhill, more than most, was attracted by Bryan's vision to develop an integrated four-year program that would teach basic science and support research. He saw "no evidence of such authority or intention on the part of Purdue."[38] Eight more resignations from former faculty of the CCPS followed Barnhill's, driven as well by the sense that political influence had been more important to the Purdue merger than medical education. Within days after the Indiana Medical College finalized its City Hospital contract, the physicians of the proposed new IU/State College of Physicians and Surgeons announced their plans to open a free dispensary in the old Central College building on North Senate. By opening a clinic months before classes began, the physicians hoped that there would be enough patients for instruction by fall.[39] Finally, in April, the new school to be affiliated with Indiana University was officially incorporated as the State College of Physicians and Surgeons.[40]

The most immediate problem faced by the new school was the recruitment of students. The size of the challenge is reflected in the fact that in 1906, the Indiana Medical College had over one hundred students in its graduating class. To attract entering students, Indiana University followed a strategy of stressing the strength of its new, robust laboratory and science classes in Bloomington. For some new students, the chance to study in a modern medical program was immediately attractive. In addition, Bryan compiled a list of potential students through his connections in the state's secondary school system and directed Maxwell and Myers to get all the literature possible into their hands. This approach quickly showed results;

the program in Bloomington almost tripled its enrollment, from twenty-one students in 1905–1906 to fifty-seven students in 1906–1907.[41]

Although the search for entering students was successful, the problem of the clinical instruction in Indianapolis still had the potential to end the experiment. Indiana University officials and the State College faculty publicly claimed that either the free dispensary already established in the State College building or clinics at area private hospitals would provide enough experience with patients for students who entered in the fall, but in private they were in "despair" over their lack of clinical facilities. To make matters worse, university lawyers were concerned about their legal right to spend tax money to provide clinics, and in any case, there was little money available to keep the State College building open. As a result, the faculty periodically "passed the hat" to raise funds for immediate expenses.[42]

In June 1906, the organizers of the State College held a meeting at the Grand Hotel in Indianapolis to devise a way to secure clinics in area hospitals. They discussed various options but finally agreed to Scherer's plan to expand the dispensary in the State College building into a hospital. Because he was such a strong advocate of the Johns Hopkins University School of Medicine model, one of the few medical schools that controlled its own teaching hospital, Bryan enthusiastically agreed. Organizing such a hospital offered more than just a means of overcoming the obstacles that had prohibited the State College faculty from setting up clinics elsewhere. It also was a way for the school to make "staff appointments and organize its clinical teaching without the threat of outside interference."[43]

When the new hospital venture was announced, its proponents boasted that it would have a maximum capacity of one hundred beds and that it would be outfitted with the most up-to-date equipment, including X-ray and clinical laboratories, children's wards, adult medical and surgical wards, two operating rooms, and an amphitheater. Establishing these facilities in the State College building would create the ideal environment in which to hold medical school clinics, but $3,500 was needed immediately simply for renovating this space to make it ready for classes. Within a matter of days, enough money was raised "after strenuous effort" among friends in Indianapolis, and Myers spent most of summer 1906 in Indianapolis supervising the work.[44]

The State College of Physicians and Surgeons faculty now faced the challenges of establishing and running the hospital, including finding patients and hiring a nursing staff. The initial step toward solving the predicament of how to secure the first patients was made by the commanding medical officer of Fort Benjamin Harrison, a US Army installation that had been recently established on the outskirts of Indianapolis. One week before the fall term began, the officer contacted Scherer and asked him if the State College could take some of his typhoid fever cases, and on September 13, the hospital opened with thirteen patients. Within ten days, the hospital had forty patients, and by the first of October, it sometimes had to turn away patients.[45]

When the 1907 legislative session opened, the efforts by Indiana University and its allies had produced a formidable challenge to the Purdue merger. Stone naturally lauded his Indiana Medical College as the only school worthy of the state's approval, but the Purdue School of Medicine in many ways promised only to continue the late-nineteenth-century status quo in medical education rather than introducing real reforms. More concretely, the establishment of the State College of Physicians and Surgeons had thwarted Jameson's strategy to eliminate the fledgling Indiana University School of Medicine. The Purdue School of Medicine was no longer the only regular, four-year medical school in the state. Although neither the Bloomington nor Indianapolis part of the IU medical school had met the high standards that Indiana University officials had promised for medical education, their efforts accomplished far more than most people had thought possible. With a fight looming in the upcoming legislative session, Indiana University had greatly improved its prospects in medical education compared to only a few months before.[46]

The Legislative Failure and Final Success

As the time for fall 1906 legislative elections approached, both Indiana and Purdue Universities faced a prospect that no one (including the politicians) desired: a legislative decision about who would prevail in medical education. Nonetheless, both universities marshaled their forces for the impending showdown. The ranks of the Indiana Medical College, now the bulwark for Purdue's interests among physicians, included many of the state's most influential doctors, such as Health commissioner and Purdue alumnus John N. Hurty and William Niles Wishard. For his part, Stone met with not only representatives of the legislature but also Governor Hanly and Lieutenant Governor Hugh Th. Miller, the latter of whom assured Stone that he was Purdue's "friend" in the medical school matter.[47] At the same time, friends of Indiana University traveled throughout the state recruiting students for its medical school while also soliciting support in the legislature and the statehouse. IU trustee Nathaniel U. Hill was state treasurer, and his office became the headquarters of IU's delegation during the legislative session.[48]

Yet even as these preparations were underway, Stone made a final effort in late October 1906 to settle the medical school matter before it reached the General Assembly. He contacted Bryan, and the two men met at the Claypool Hotel in downtown Indianapolis as they had done one year before. Despite Stone's desire to reestablish harmonious relations with Indiana University, he stopped short of presenting any definite proposal to Bryan. Because neither one of them was ready to compromise, the university presidents could find no way to circumvent their dispute. After meeting with Bryan, Stone wrote to a colleague that Indiana University had not yet reached the "psychological moment" when the institution would "welcome any way by which she may be extricated [from the medical school conflict] in honor."[49]

The Indiana General Assembly's session began on January 10, 1907, with more fear than hope to resolve the medical school issue. Indeed, there were those who predicted that carrying the controversy into the legislature might "seriously injure both institutions in the very vital region of their respective appropriations." From the beginning, Bryan had been clear about the devastating consequences of losing the medical school fight, and some Purdue officials had doubts that the state would sanction the Indiana Medical College as constituted.[50]

On January 15, only a few days after the session began, Representative John H. Edwards, an 1891 graduate of Indiana University who practiced law in Mitchell, Indiana, introduced a bill that would allow his alma mater to teach medical courses in Indianapolis. The next day, Senator Will R. Wood from Tippecanoe County introduced a resolution that supported making the Indiana Medical College an official department of Purdue University and ratifying the 1905 merger agreement between Purdue and the three proprietary schools that formed the Indiana Medical College.[51]

A few days after the introduction of the competing bills, the judiciary committee in the House of Representatives reported the Indiana University medical bill favorably, by a vote of ten to one. In response, Jameson, who as dean of the Indiana Medical College directed much of Purdue's legislative campaign, urged Senator Wood to call a full investigation of both the Indiana and Purdue bills in a joint conference of the Senate Judiciary and Education committees. On the evening of January 22, "men and women packed the galleries and occupied every available foot of space on the floor" of the Senate chamber to witness the joint hearing.[52] The two university presidents differed on many issues, and one of the most telling was their testimony on the cost for the state to support medical education. Stone drew attention to the economic advantages of accepting the Indiana Medical College on behalf of the state. Responding to questions by Senate committee members about the need for future funding for the medical school, he claimed, "Indiana would at no future time be asked to make an appropriation on behalf of the proposed medical department." In his comments, Bryan critiqued Stone's view by arguing that a modern medical school could only be run in a responsible way with additional state appropriations, and he insisted that if Purdue "did not in time get appropriation from the State, it could not keep up to the standard or continue to exist."[53]

The day after the hearing, legislators predicted a very close vote, and when the House of Representatives took up the bill authorizing IU to establish a medical school in Indianapolis, it was rejected by a vote of fifty-one to forty-four. Observers interpreted this less as a rejection of IU's plan and more as an expression of dissatisfaction with the universities' inability to settle their differences. Either way, it was likely that Purdue's similar request of the legislature would meet the same fate, and this was borne out a few weeks later when the House of Representatives voted fifty to forty-two to postpone indefinitely the resolution to permit Purdue University to accept the gifts of the Indiana Medical College. For many of these legislators, the prolonged battle between Indiana and Purdue Universities threatened the state's involvement in higher education, and evidence of political damage was clear when the legislative budget committee denied increases in both universities' appropriations and cut their requests by a little over two-thirds.[54] Representative Thomas M. Honan spoke for many when he concluded, "This matter should be settled before we are all in an insane asylum."[55]

The legislature adjourned in March 1907, thus postponing indefinitely the question of state control of medical education. The result was to increase pressure on all parties to arrive at an agreement or face further erosion of their position in the next session. As evidence of the latter, some Indiana legislators began discussions about the need for a board of regents to supervise and control Purdue, Indiana, and the Indiana State Normal School in Terre Haute "so that they would act in harmony and advance all educational interests of the state."[56]

Following the close of the 1907 legislative session, prospects for conciliation between "the warring educational factions" seemed slim, but the attitudes of the two university presidents were quite different. Bryan remained implacable in his determination to build the IU Medical School, primarily because he had staked his entire career on the success of the project. Through the spring and summer of 1907, despite failing to persuade the legislature to support the medical school and suffering a reduction in total appropriations, Bryan continued to be optimistic and secured the unanimous support of the Indiana University Board of Trustees in August 1907 for an agreement that formally united the university with State College as its School of Medicine.[57] In contrast, the legislative defeat earlier in the spring discouraged Purdue president Stone, who feared that the conflict over the medical schools risked disaster. He was now willing to consider any proposal that both promoted the "the advancement of medical education" and protected the interests of the Indiana Medical College. In April, Stone sent a letter to the Purdue trustees in which he outlined three possible avenues. They could maintain the university's current association with the Indiana Medical College in anticipation of obtaining legislative approval; they could drop Purdue's affiliation with the Indiana Medical College; or, the option favored by Stone, they could seek a compromise agreement with Indiana University as long as any such agreement took the interests of the Indiana Medical College into account. The reaction of the trustees was inconclusive, so Stone was circumspect on the issue in his remarks to the medical school graduating class of May 1907.[58]

Over the course of the summer, both Purdue and Indiana Universities prepared for the new academic year, but both faced significant problems in addition to the unsettled political situation. Purdue's Indiana Medical College faced an unexpected enrollment decline to less than two hundred students in fall 1907 compared to a total of over three hundred students the previous year. Even more alarming to Purdue, the program in Bloomington was gaining in strength, thanks in part to the AAMC placing the State College of Physicians and Surgeons in the first rank of medical colleges in the United States.[59] The IU/State College in Indianapolis, however, had its own problems, specifically financial, because it remained illegal to utilize any university funds outside of Monroe County. Hence, support for the medical college was limited to student fees and contributions from faculty and friends of the institution. The State College struggled for survival, and leaders had to pool their own money to rescue the school from near economic disaster.[60] Nevertheless, State College officials boasted that the 1907–08 academic year began "with an increased enrollment of a high class of medical students," the majority of whom had completed their first two years of training in Bloomington. According to Myers, the number of students registered in all four years of the IU medical program in the 1907–08 academic year surpassed one hundred for the first time, at 111.[61]

The impasse between IU and Purdue began to break down when William Niles Wishard, who with Jameson had led the Purdue delegation during the 1907 General Assembly, asked Stone whether or not he could "be authorized in some tactful way to approach Indiana University on the question of a compromise." According to a later account, Wishard recalled he "had come to the generally accepted conclusion that legislative approval was not possible for either school and that in the interest of medical education," the separate concerns of the two universities should be laid aside. Serendipitously, in October, after Stone gave Wishard authority to negotiate on Purdue's behalf, John H. Edwards, the legislator who had sponsored the Indiana University medical school bill in the Indiana House of Representatives, consulted Wishard on a personal medical matter. Edwards stated he was disappointed that Indiana University had not obtained the medical school. In response, Wishard later recalled that he "expressed regret that the controversy had drawn out so long" and told Edwards that he thought Purdue might be willing to give up its participation in medical education if Indiana University agreed to maintain a complete four-year medical course in Indianapolis.[62]

Edwards approached Bryan, and negotiations began between the two schools on the question of a compromise.[63] The negotiations were complicated and centered around the division of instruction between Bloomington and Indianapolis. The faculty members of the Indiana Medical College were naturally concerned about their status, and a committee representing them declared that it could not recommend any compromise that did not include "permanent maintenance of a complete school of medicine in Indianapolis." In response, Indiana University promised that those individuals chosen to teach in the new united school would be selected "with due regard to the members of the present faculties." But the university's board of trustees initially opposed establishing a permanent four-year medical course in Indianapolis. On the other side, as late as March 1908, the Purdue board voted that a single medical school be established through the union of the two regular medical colleges in Indianapolis, and in addition that this school be governed by "a board consisting of representatives of Purdue University, Indiana University, and the State Medical Society." In order to eliminate the latter condition, Indiana's trustees offered a counterproposal, softening their stance on the question of maintaining a four-year course in Indianapolis. After a direct appeal by Stone to Indiana trustees Joseph Shea and Theodore Rosea, which was followed by additional hours of deliberation, the Indiana University trustees finally agreed "to the maintenance of a complete four years course in Indianapolis as well as the two-year course at Bloomington."[64] With these concessions, the Indiana Medical College faculty and Purdue's trustees accepted the terms, and during an evening session on April 4, 1908, the Indiana University Board of Trustees also accepted them.[65] On April 5, 1908, Bryan and Stone released a statement about the agreement, which was published in the Indianapolis newspapers the following day.[66] The medical school controversy that had caused the war between Purdue and Indiana universities for nearly three years was ended.

For Bryan and the friends of Indiana University, this agreement represented a major victory in the plan to make IU a major public state university. Bryan knew how close he had come to losing everything he had hoped to achieve for his institution. Years later, he looked at the series of events that enabled the Indiana University School of Medicine to survive "as a succession of miracles."[67] His successor, Herman Wells, said of Bryan in his memoirs, "Had he done nothing but secure the medical school for Indiana University, a step necessary to make the institution a true university, he would have achieved more than most university presidents do during their tenure." In the chapter of Thomas Clark's history of Indiana University entitled "The Long Step into Professionalization," which describes the medical school controversy, Clark stated, "At no time in its whole history did Indiana University come nearer the brink of political chaos, if not actual self-destruction of the university itself, than when it began the serious business of organizing a medical school."[68]

At the time, however, people across the state congratulated Stone as a peacemaker. "Everybody seemed pleased at the situation," Stone wrote to Harris the day after the agreement. "As for myself, I feel as if a great burden had been removed from my shoulders."[69] Unlike the medical school mergers attempted in Indiana going back well into the nineteenth century, this settlement united medical education in the state for the next century under the banner of the Indiana University School of Medicine. Although managing the new school in the following years continued to be a balancing act, medical education in the state started afresh, at least symbolically.

Indiana Enters Twentieth-Century Medical Education

After having bested its rival, Indiana University joined the growing list of colleges that attempted to work with the proprietary medical schools in their states. Bryan's success was due in part to his fundamental commitment to medical education reform, but now he had to follow through on his promises. In the weeks after the April 1908 agreement, Bryan set to work on reshaping the new medical school by appointing a Committee on Medical Organization to help guide the plan through this "most critical period of the school's life." Bryan and this committee traveled to the East Coast, where they spent a week visiting the top medical schools in the country—Johns Hopkins University, the University of Pennsylvania, Columbia University, Cornell University, and Harvard—with the intent of copying the best practices of each. This trip gave committee members, all of whom were leaders of the medical profession in Indiana, a broader perspective on the issues that immediately faced the newly reorganized medical school connected to IU.[70]

These issues can be summarized as follows. By far the most daunting task was reducing the number of part-time faculty from the large numbers at the two proprietary schools. Longer term, this was expensive because it required hiring more full-time faculty trained in the new scientific medicine. At the same time, retaining faculty with connections to local hospitals was important because a main reason for medical instruction in Indianapolis was the abundance of patients for clinical teaching. Eventually a teaching hospital would be needed to satisfy AAMC guidelines, but the city hospital and other facilities could be used in the meantime. Unlike Bloomington, basic science teaching in Indianapolis needed attention, but underlying all of these issues was securing state sanction and, if possible, additional resources.

Bryan recognized the importance of faculty appointments and asked former professors of both the Indiana Medical College and State College of Physicians and Surgeons to nominate physicians for teaching positions. Not unexpectedly, this yielded a faculty that was "preposterously large for working purposes," but Bryan made as few changes as possible, instead calling for every individual member "to use his influence for peace" and to work together for the "common good."[71] To assist in this effort, Bryan turned his attention to the selection of a dean who was "acceptable to most of the Faculty," loyal to Indiana University, and capable of steering the school "through the rocks" on the journey ahead. Many of the state's leading physicians supported Henry Jameson, former dean of the Medical College of Indiana, for this post, but on May 18, 1908, Jameson resigned from all positions he had occupied, citing his grievances with Bryan over the years, including dropping the name and traditions of the proprietary college.[72] Bryan's favorite candidate for the job was Samuel E. Smith, a psychiatrist who served as medical superintendent of the Easthaven State Hospital in Richmond. When Smith asked for an annual salary of $5,000, it revealed the financial challenges of the new medical school because it was a sum the university could not afford. The trustees instead hired Bryan's second choice for the position, Allison Maxwell, former dean of CCPS. He was a figure well-known to the Indianapolis medical community who promised stability following the previous political upheavals and in anticipation of the educational and institutional changes to come.[73]

During the summer of 1908, Bryan gave Myers the more immediate task of working with the faculty to plan the Indianapolis curriculum for the coming school year, thus drawing Myers away from his preference of teaching the first two years at Bloomington. Although the laboratory facilities in Indianapolis greatly needed attention, so too did the clinical course of study there. This was changed to require third-year students to spend part of each day at the hospital of the former State College building and in lectures on physical diagnosis and clinical microscopy. Fourth-year students also worked at the State College hospital and the City Hospital to gain experience in their specific areas of study. Clinical pediatric instruction was made possible by students seeing patients at the State College hospital and at the Eleanor Hospital for Children. The facilities available at Central State Hospital for the Insane, the city and state hospitals, and the Bobbs Dispensary made "it possible to outline a systematic and didactic course in Mental and Nervous Diseases." In gynecology, the operative clinics supplemented the didactic portion of instruction. Myers arranged classes in operative surgery and clinical medicine at the hospitals with groups of eight to ten students in each section. This system ensured more personal instruction than had been presented previously in amphitheaters.[74]

Besides organizing a new faculty and readying the curriculum, Bryan and the new medical school administration faced the even more immediate need of obtaining official sanction from the state legislature. Although legislators were relieved to see an end of the battle between the state's two largest universities, new objections arose from members of the unorthodox medical sects, including the physiomedicals, eclectics, and homeopaths. They threatened to disturb this process in the Indiana General Assembly because they had been excluded from the state's new medical school.[75] In response, Bryan appointed a special committee, including Maxwell, Wishard, and Wynn, which recommended that students electing to study sectarian medical principles should be permitted to take separate courses to prepare them to take the tests required in areas that deviated from orthodox therapeutics and practice. This was enough to secure sectarians' approval, and a bill passed the Indiana General Assembly on February 26, 1909, authorizing the Indiana University School of Medicine to conduct a medical school in Marion County.[76] Although an obvious milestone, by this time, after the earlier highly publicized disputes, legislative approval was anticlimactic.

In the end, the provisions for sectarian instruction were never used. Although the authorization bill provided for courses in alternative therapeutics at IU, they were optional, and as things turned out, no students were interested. Therefore in 1911, Myers told the physiomedical schools that he could not legally force students to take their courses if students did not elect to do so. This was, in fact, a reflection of larger trends. In 1908, the Eclectic Medical College of Indianapolis closed its doors, and in 1909, the Physiomedical College of Indiana met the same fate.[77]

With the passage of the 1909 Enabling Act, Bryan responded to the Indiana University Board of Trustees that he was continuing to implement the administrative and curricular reforms necessary to achieve the university's ambitious goals. For example, the school had already bolstered its admission requirements to require one year of college preparation for the 1909–1910 entering class, and the trustees voted the following year to require an additional year for the 1910–11 entering class.[78] This was expected to have short-term enrollment consequences, but a more serious, long-term budgetary problem was the commitment in the merger agreement to operate a full, four-year curriculum at Indianapolis as well as the first two years in Bloomington. Among other things, the school's budget for Indianapolis was insufficient to equip laboratories or pay basic science faculty adequate salaries. In addition, the State College Hospital, which had been created by IU as an alternative when its students were denied access to City Hospital, remained open and added significantly to the debt. As a result, in June 1909, the trustees suspended the hospital's operations.[79]

There was one important change in the 1908 agreement about the courses to be taught in both Bloomington and Indianapolis. The university bulletin tried to present this somewhat confusing feature in a positive light. "Students have the opportunity of taking the first two years of their medical course either at Bloomington or Indianapolis. In both places the work meets the requirements of the Association of American Medical Colleges. Tuition is the same at both places. Final examinations are also the same. The choice rests with the student."[80]

Change in this carefully negotiated arrangement came from a hitherto neglected party: the students. Initially, their choice of location was roughly equal for the first two academic years, with thirty to forty students each choosing their first and second years' coursework at each campus. In the fall of 1910, when the requirement began of two years collegiate work for entrance to medical school, there was a dramatic although anticipated decline from sixty-seven to twenty-six first-year entering students. This was highlighted by Myers in his *History of Medical Education,* as shown in table 3.1.

What was not expected was that all but six students chose Bloomington for the first year, and when the overall numbers rose to thirty-five the next year, all but four chose Bloomington. Wishard had warned against raising

Table 3.1. First and Second Year Enrollment at IUSM, 1908–1913

Year	Freshman		Sophomore	
	Bloomington	Indianapolis	Bloomington	Indianapolis
1908–09	34	35	35	42
1909–10	36	31	28	32
1910–11	20	6	23	35
1911–12	31	4	—	22
1912–13	42	—	—	34

Source: Myers, *Medical Education*, 159.

entrance requirements precisely because he feared the reduction in admissions. He was understandably sensitive to this possibility because of his experience as a faculty member of a proprietary school that could hardly afford such a step, unlike a university medical school. He also predicted the "disastrous effect upon the first two years' work at Indianapolis," a fear likely realized because students saw the value that the recently released and highly influential Flexner Report on medical education had placed on science-based course preparation before clinical experience. Indeed, Flexner's report specifically characterized the Bloomington medical courses as being of "such a character" that they were already "worthy of college-bred students." In addition, the ease of continuing from the baccalaureate college to the first year of medical school in Bloomington also helped produce the dramatic shift in enrollment to that campus.[81]

Equally surprising, all students chose Indianapolis for their second year of instruction in 1911–12. Faced with these unexpected developments, Bryan met with the faculty, who agreed to concentrate first-year instruction in Bloomington and suspend teaching the second year there the next fall. Accordingly, in the fall of 1912, all forty-two first-year students were taught in Bloomington, and all thirty-four second-year students in Indianapolis. Despite the decline in number of entering medical students, by raising the entrance requirements, the number of premedical students enrolled in Bloomington in 1915 rose to 329.[82] Thus, Bryan's goal of increasing non-liberal-arts students had been achieved. Nonetheless, the carefully negotiated agreement of 1908 about the division of instruction between the two sites was changed, with all students taking their first year of medical coursework in Bloomington and the rest in Indianapolis.[83] This remained the case for the next forty-five years, until changes in medical instruction, mounting criticism, and finally new facilities allowed the full four-year program to be offered in Indianapolis.

Flexner in the Heartland

Shortly after IU began to remake the medical schools it had taken charge of, the Carnegie Foundation announced that Abraham Flexner would be making a study of the condition of all the medical schools in the United States and Canada. This meant that in addition to consolidating the medical school's activities in two locations while raising standards, Bryan needed to prepare for a visit that would compare Indiana's efforts to over 130 other medical schools. Given such short notice, Bryan sent Myers to Indianapolis in November 1909 to prepare as best he could the old Indiana Medical College and State College buildings for Flexner's inspection. In the coming weeks, Myers worked often ten to twelve hours a day without a break to supervise all the renovations he thought necessary to make a decent impression on Flexner.[84]

Based on his visit to Indiana and the other medical schools, Flexner produced his famous report, *Medical Education in the United States and Canada*, published in 1910, which judged the quality of every medical school in North America against the most exemplary model: Johns Hopkins. Flexner, although not a doctor, was well-known as an educator and connected to medicine by his brother, who was director of the Rockefeller Institute for Medical Research. His report was commissioned by the Carnegie Foundation, whose head, Henry Pritchett, considered the teaching at medical schools to be a matter of education. By popularizing concerns about medical education, Flexner's report transformed the issue of improving the training of doctors into a broad national, progressive social movement.[85] Bryan had already accepted these high standards when he first proposed entering the field because of his contact with members of the academic medical elite, most notably Franklin P. Mall at Johns Hopkins. Thus, Bryan had an advantage over most others trying to reform their medical schools because IU had this goal from the beginning of its efforts in 1903.[86]

Despite Bryan's intention to make the new Indiana University School of Medicine into an innovative program of science-based, medical education, the school did not escape Flexner's criticism during his visit in 1909. He found that the program in Indianapolis in particular needed much improvement, although he recognized that the university had just secured complete control there. "It would appear necessary for some years to regard the needs of the Indianapolis department as a first lien on the increasing income of the university." Overall in his report, which generally treated medical schools throughout the country "with great severity," Flexner described the situation of the IU School of Medicine as "distinctly hopeful." Warning that "it will take time to work out faults," Flexner nonetheless concluded that to attract highly qualified students, the IU School of Medicine needed "(1) to employ full-time men in the work of the first two years, (2) to strengthen the laboratory equipment, [and] (3) greatly to improve the organization and conduct of the clinical courses."[87] Far from being upset at failing to meet Flexner's standards, Bryan saw the scathing criticism of other schools in the published report and was pleased that Flexner had noted, "If the university is to make good the ideals indicated by its entrance requirement . . . Indiana will be one of the few states that have successfully solved the problem of medical education."[88]

Bryan relied heavily on the preliminary findings of Flexner in a memorandum to the IU trustees calling for additional resources to solve the problems of faculty, administrative leadership, and facilities. They approved the memorandum on March 8, 1910, which Bryan promptly reported to Flexner in hopes of getting a more favorable review in the pending report. Flexner had already warned Bryan that he could not give the school credit for future plans. True to his word, Flexner made only one change in the comments about IU in the final draft, adding that he acknowledged that Indiana University had "formally committed" to the policies he advocated.[89]

Rather than being a distraction or roadblock, the Flexner Report was used by Bryan to advance his goals for the Indiana University School of Medicine by securing increased funding for the medical school, especially to reorganize the Indianapolis faculty and advance his plans for a teaching hospital. At the March 1910 trustees meeting, Bryan presented all of the criticisms and recommendations he had received from Flexner.[90] He first pointed out that the school had already raised its admission requirements to two years of college training, which was one of Flexner's standards. In addition, Bryan claimed that IU should make medical school appropriations a high priority in the state legislature in order to make provisions for a university teaching hospital and modernize all of the school's laboratories. With the Bobbs Dispensary and access to City Hospital, the school had good clinical facilities, but they had "been used to little advantage" because the school did not control them. A university hospital was the typical recommendation by reformers to solve this problem. To follow Flexner's recommendation about faculty, Bryan intended to replace local practitioners with highly qualified, full-time medical professors. Bryan summarized his goals as follows: "good laboratory facilities in Indianapolis, full-time scientific men there, a dispensary chief who has his whole time free for the dispensary work, and a fairly generous support of the whole establishment as so organized."[91]

The IU Board of Trustees acknowledged the "backward state of the medical department at Indianapolis" and the need to seek increased appropriations during the next legislative session. The overall goal, the trustees promised, was not to rest "until they established in the State a Medical School in which every department, whether at Indianapolis or Bloomington has been placed upon a thoroughly good university basis." To accomplish this goal, the trustees agreed to a plan guaranteeing that the dean supervised the school's daily operations in Indianapolis and that competent physicians be hired to direct the dispensary and hospital clinics full-time. They also resolved to provide "thoroughly modern equipment and instruction in all . . . laboratory courses." Finally, they pledged to select the "best available men for clinical positions as . . . the situation" permitted.[92]

Remedies for the inadequate condition of the school's facilities in Indianapolis reinforced the institutional distance between Bloomington and the state capital. Rivalry still existed even after the compromise on the school's two teaching locations resolved initial competition for new students. Although members of the Indianapolis faculty resented it, Bryan considered Myers's experience and training the ideal for making comparisons and judgments about the two locations. Myers was a product of the new, full-time academic medical elite, educated in the best schools and hospitals in the United States and abroad. In contrast, most of the Indianapolis professors were local practitioners who had been educated in proprietary schools.[93]

The cultural differences between the two campuses were even more obvious in the responses to Bryan's decision that a new dean was needed to replace Maxwell in Indianapolis. Early in 1909, Myers had informed Bryan that if one of the older faculty members remained dean, it was vital, at least, "that the educational management of the school should rest with the younger members of the faculty." He pointed out that important officers and committee members, including Maxwell, either contributed little to the school or were often unavailable. For Myers, it was clear that the political goal of consensus was compromising the drive for reform. As long as the situation in Indianapolis remained unchanged, Myers feared that there was "the greatest danger of the school becoming a parasite rather than an auxiliary" to Indiana University. Bryan finally brought the matter to the board of trustees after receiving another communication in early November 1909 from Myers about the need to search for a new dean, which concluded, "without it the School cannot succeed."[94] When he asked the trustees to take up the matter, however, they decided instead to increase the powers of the executive committee at Indianapolis. Thus, although the trustees had committed to transform the IU School of Medicine according to the ideals of Flexner, progress toward reaching this goal was slow.

The difficulty in making these changes was also evident in the even more pressing matter of faculty selection. Flexner's call to "improve the organization and conduct of the clinical courses" made the issue of a general reorganization and reduction of the faculty in Indianapolis urgent. Mindful of medical factionalism in Indianapolis, the Indiana University trustees and administrators resisted making cuts in the medical school faculty because of the possible political implications. For example, during 1909–1910, 175 physicians belonged to the IU School of Medicine teaching staff, ninety-one with the rank of professor. By the time the trustees met in March 1910, Myers and Wishard identified twenty-five individuals to be removed, including professors emeriti, lecturers, and those who had "never done any work in the school." Indeed, these were physicians who had never taught for the IU School of Medicine but nevertheless remained on lists in nearly every department. In a few cases, there was also clear evidence of either unethical behavior or professional incompetence. At its March 9, 1910, meeting, however, the trustees chose only to rule that doctors who engaged in fee-splitting deserved removal.[95]

The active professors for 1910–1911 were not only numerous but also inefficiently distributed. Some departments, such as the Department of Medicine, were understaffed, whereas other departments like Otolaryngology and Genito-Urinary Surgery had too many professors. The need to hire additional faculty in some departments, while at the same time dropping faculty members in others, further complicated the tense political situation among the faculty. In June 1910, the board of trustees again deferred authorizing a wholesale removal of names from the medical school faculty for a year and instead directed Myers to draw up a list that retained "those who . . . proved themselves most fit by training, ability, and fidelity in the service of the school."[96]

Work on this new active list was delayed by the absence of Myers and Barnhill, who both spent the summer doing research in Europe. It was therefore in mid-August 1910, only a few weeks before the start of the fall term, that the IU School of Medicine executive committee finally completed the list, which reduced the number of active professors by nearly one-fourth, from ninety-one to seventy, and decreased the total teaching staff, including lecturers, associates, and assistants, as well as professors, by almost one-third, from 175 to one 123.[97] Bryan announced the new list to the faculty and explained that from the very beginning, the faculty was too large and had to be reduced as soon as it was "practicable." Although some of the affected physicians understood the changing role of the medical school faculty and approved of the reorganization, Bryan's statements failed to appease many of the faculty targeted for elimination. Once removed from the active faculty ranks, they understood that they had little chance of returning. Dean Maxwell informed Bryan that at the first faculty meeting of the year, "the cutting off . . . of a number of . . . professors & assistants was discussed with some heat."[98]

Faculty, Students, and a New Dean of the IUSM, 1909–1912

The issue of faculty reorganization brought old jealousies as well as some new issues to the surface. For example, former faculty members of the CCPS thought that the Executive Committee was prejudiced against them. Of the 70 professors retained in active status, only 23, or about one-third, had been part of the Central College. One of these was Amelia R. Keller, a former Central College faculty member in the Department of Pediatrics who asked Bryan why those "who belonged to the faculty that fought the fight for the University [were] gradually dropped and our friends, the enemy, [became] so necessary, chosen for their 'fidelity' to the school!" Even more pointedly, Keller asked whether she had been dismissed from the Executive Committee because she was a woman: "Is it possible there is not a man on that committee big or broad enough to permit a woman to be the head of a department, however small that department might be? Alternatively, is it just 'friends' that were retained?"[99]

Ada Schweitzer was the only woman who remained on the faculty list for 1910–1911 as an associate professor of bacteriology. She was later appointed the director of the Division of Infant and Child Hygiene for the Indiana State Board of Health (ISBH) from 1919 to 1933.[100] The stories of these two women exemplify a broader trend not only at Indiana but also nationally. As the reform of medical education reduced the number and size of medical school faculties and produced a new set of standards, medical school faculty became more homogeneous. While the professional standards were perceived by the new leaders of medical education as technical, rational, and neutral, the transformation of the values associated with becoming a physician served to marginalize women and minorities in the profession leaving faculties "overwhelmingly white, male, and Christian."[101]

Historians have generally concluded that Flexner's report resulted in limited opportunities for minority and female applicants to medical schools in the United States, but the IU School of Medicine did not change the pattern set by the Indianapolis proprietary schools of admitting a few women and one or two African-Americans each year. Clarence Lucas, Sr., although admitted to a proprietary school, was the first African-American to receive an IU medical degree in 1908. As evidence of the kind of discrimination he suffered as a student, the administration refused to include his photograph with those of other members of his graduating class in the official portraits for that year.[102] The medical school also restricted the number of Jewish students it admitted. Nationally, Jews faced some of the most organized discrimination against their admission to medical schools. At Indiana, there was an unwritten quota for Jewish students, a pattern found at many medical schools across the country. Until the early 1940s, only about five percent of the students who earned medical degrees at IU were Jewish.[103]

Such unwritten quotas also existed for women. In 1909, Lillian B. Mueller, an Indianapolis native, was the first woman to graduate from the newly merged Indiana University School of Medicine. She was inspired to pursue a career in medicine by Amelia Keller, who was her physician as she grew up. When Mueller enrolled in Bloomington in 1905, she was the only woman in the freshman medical class. Indicative of the additional obstacles for women to become doctors even after graduating from medical school was the difficulty Mueller experienced finding an internship. "They didn't take women as interns in Indianapolis hospitals in those days—or in many others," Mueller told a newspaper reporter years later. As graduate medical education developed in the next fifty years, discrimination in internships and residency presented an even greater barrier than admission to medical school.[104]

Flexner's report had little impact on the minimal admission of women and minority medical students to the IUSM, but the year after its publication, two developments responded to his call for reforms that put the school in a better position than ever to recruit a dean with a national reputation. The first has already been mentioned: Bryan and the IU trustees finally began tackling the problem of faculty appointments, admittedly a long-term project. The second and more immediately helpful development was the announcement in January 1911 that Robert W. Long, a prominent Indianapolis physician and real estate investor who had taken Barnhill as a partner when the young doctor was just starting out in medical practice, proposed a gift to the state of property estimated at a value of $200,000, which he designated to build a teaching hospital for Indiana University. This development will be discussed in more detail in the next chapter, but one of the more immediate consequences was to prompt Bryan to finally persuade the trustees to hire a new dean. Even Maxwell was convinced the time was right; his response when Bryan informed him of the search was, "I am ready and have been ready to give up the position for a long while . . . [as] soon as someone capable and agreeable to all can be found."[105]

In June 1911, Bryan sent Myers east to find prospects, and after his visit, he recommended several men with connections to the Harvard University Medical School, the College of Physicians and Surgeons at Columbia, and

Johns Hopkins University School of Medicine. Following these initial interviews, two of the candidates came to Bloomington to meet with Bryan and the IU Board of Trustees. Although Joseph H. Pratt was recommended by the dean of the Harvard University Medical School, Bryan never really seriously considered him for the deanship because he did not have much administrative experience. In fact, Bryan brought him to Bloomington only out of deference to Flexner.[106]

Bryan's favorite was Charles P. Emerson, a Massachusetts native and 1899 MD graduate of Johns Hopkins. His credentials were impressive. Emerson had worked with eminent Hopkins professors, becoming an intern under Osler in 1903, and he also studied in Strasbourg, Basel, and Paris. He was in charge of the clinical laboratories during the time that he was a faculty member at Johns Hopkins. Drawing from his experience in this position, he wrote *Clinical Diagnosis*, the standard textbook in the field. As an internist, Emerson was persuaded that cultural, social, and environmental factors often played a major role in the causation of disease. He belonged to the emerging field of social medicine, a "vocal minority of socially oriented doctors" who advocated "increased intervention in the hospital patient's social milieu." Emerson's concern about the home environments of tuberculosis outpatients began while he was a student of Osler at Johns Hopkins, where Emerson and another medical student volunteered for the Baltimore Charity Organization Society so they could investigate the conditions in which these patients lived. As a result, Emerson organized medical social services at the university's teaching hospital. In 1908, Emerson left Johns Hopkins to become superintendent of the Clifton Springs Sanatorium in New York. While he was there, Emerson dedicated as much of his time as possible to research about the impact of social and environmental forces on health with particular attention to the causes of alcoholism.[107]

Before traveling east in 1911, Myers was already aware that Emerson had become dissatisfied with being a sanitarium superintendent. Emerson had found that he had little time for medical studies, and Myers reported to Bryan that Emerson might even be willing to take a cut in pay to assume a new position that "offered the hospital facilities necessary for investigation and opportunity for a consultation practice." When Bryan sent a letter to Emerson inquiring whether he would be interested in the deanship, Emerson wrote William Welch, former dean of the Johns Hopkins School of Medicine, asking for his advice. In response, Welch told Emerson that he should take the job if the university offered it to him.[108]

"This is the best compliment our School has ever received," Bryan wrote to Wishard when he learned that Welch had advised Emerson that he should accept the dean position at Indiana. With Welch's strong recommendation, Bryan had no doubt that Emerson was a "first-rate man" whom IU "should be fortunate in securing." Emerson met all of Bryan's requirements. There was "no doubt of his quality as a scientific physician." He was, "well trained in internal medicine" and "a superior executive" with "plenty of initiative." In addition, Emerson shared Bryan's ascetic and modest sensibility; both men followed a rigid moral code. Emerson believed that the school should not grant medical diplomas according to academic achievement alone; high standards of personal conduct were also required. In early July 1911, upon Bryan's recommendation, the IU trustees selected Emerson to become dean. The university president announced that Emerson's appointment was "the most important event in the history of the Medical School," which had made attracting such a highly qualified candidate for the position possible.[109]

The arrival of Emerson was both a real and symbolic milestone in the establishment of a modern medical school at Indianapolis. His appointment indicated that the cultural and institutional norms of twentieth-century academic medicine had taken root in Indiana. The successful faculty consolidation was a major step toward eliminating the vestiges of nineteenth-century factionalism in the Indianapolis medical community. The creation of a rigorous classroom and lab sequence in Bloomington provided the base for the new medical education. The resulting institution aspired to national professional goals in research and teaching while negotiating and accommodating the political and clinical realities of Indiana. After the tumult of its founding decade, the Indiana University School of Medicine emerged with a political and professional consensus supporting a modern medical school.

PART II
BUILDING A MEDICAL CENTER

As the previous section indicated, Indiana University School of Medicine's control of medical education was hardly inevitable, but the speed with which it developed and grew suggests that the setting was ripe for the reform and expansion of medical education and health care. Although enrollment at first declined because the school raised admission and teaching standards, a slow recovery followed, and by the 1920s, it was admitting as many students as the private schools before the merger, about one hundred per year. Equally as significant, ten years after the merger, the new school had built a teaching hospital and a new medical education building to relocate the school on a site adjacent to the City Hospital of Indianapolis, west of the city. In the next ten years, two more hospitals were added, one for children and another a maternity hospital. The school could legitimately claim to be the core of a medical center, providing training and care for not just the city but also the state of Indiana.

The medical center was well enough established to withstand the demands of the Great Depression and the Second World War and to take advantage of the opportunities during peacetime after 1945. Despite worsening economic conditions in the 1930s, the school kept up enrollment of medical students and care of patients. When federal funds were available for additional facilities, the university and state added to the medical center. The war required a significant increase in the number of students, even while faculty and nurses joined the war effort. In the postwar era, the school emerged from these trials and mobilized resources to make increased training of doctors permanent while for the first time securing significant research faculty and facilities, thanks to local philanthropy and greatly increased federal research programs.

4

Charles Emerson and the Creation of the Medical Center, 1912–1932

In medicine we realize that the future progress of our subject will be along two lines: first, the care of the individual patient; second community medicine in which society in general is the patient.[1]

Charles P. Emerson, May 8, 1923

By 1912, Indiana University had achieved in less than ten years some of the key goals called for by the American medical education reformers. Most important, it had made the private proprietary schools part of the public university and raised entrance requirements. Only the first steps were taken, however, in converting its faculty to being full-time and trained in science. These steps included two major new appointments, both trained at Johns Hopkins, which clearly showed the direction that President Bryan had in mind: Burton Myers, the chair of the Anatomy Department, and Charles Emerson, the dean. The university had also struck a compromise on dividing teaching between Bloomington and Indianapolis with surprisingly few objections, considering it had been a major bone of contention in the dispute with Purdue. Lingering resistance remained among the Indianapolis faculty, but there was no serious challenge for two decades. The clinical facilities of City Hospital and the Bobbs Dispensary were adequate but did not meet reform requirements of a university hospital. Ironically, this lower priority was the first to be met and exceeded in the years of Dean Emerson's tenure, thanks to new hospital construction.

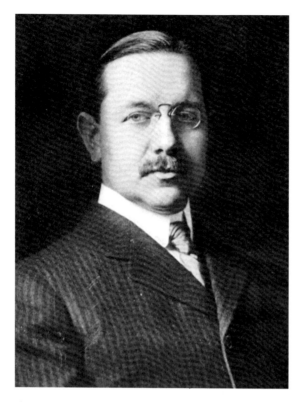

Figure 4.1. Charles P. Emerson, IUSM dean, 1911–32. *Arbutus* (1912): 284.

Nonexistent in 1903, rickety in 1905, and threatened in 1907, the school expanded during two decades of impressive growth under the leadership of Dean Charles P. Emerson to become one of the nation's twenty largest medical schools by 1930, built on a new medical campus built near City Hospital. To Emerson, however, the school in 1930 was a disappointment, despite its rapid growth. His expansive view of medical education and public health and his reformist zeal committed him to the goal of a deeper transformation of medical education based on a philosophy of healing both society and patients. Although he toiled to create a system that would produce doctors interested in changing the health service environment, he also oversaw the construction of a built environment including three hospitals. These embodied an ethos of medicine that eventually displaced his idea of community medicine based on a robust social service and environmental medicine program that he established shortly after his arrival in 1911. Meanwhile, a nationwide migration toward hospital-based teaching transformed not only medical education but also the hospital experience.[2] By 1930, Emerson's struggle to maintain the social service program, his battles with community physicians over access to patients and wards, and his confrontations with faculty who supported further specialization undermined his relationship with his patron, university president William Lowe Bryan.

This chapter focuses on the establishment of the new medical campus west of the city of Indianapolis and next to City Hospital. In addition to new hiring and programs started by Emerson, the school included three Indiana University hospitals, a dedicated building for the medical school, and other ancillary facilities that were built thanks largely to the initiative of private philanthropists in Indianapolis and around the state. The legislature and university were compelled to match these donations, without which it would have taken far longer to achieve such results. The next chapter will examine how these changes affected students, plus the later staffing and administrative changes that ultimately led to Dean Emerson stepping down.

The New Dean and Long Hospital

If the "war" between Indiana and Purdue universities determined the organizational home of the medical school in Indiana, the building of the new university hospitals established the physical location of what came to be known as the IU Medical Center. This alone makes the building of the first of these, Long Hospital, important. In addition, because it required the resources of philanthropy, the state government, and the university, the establishment of the new hospital provided a model for the subsequent development of the very large medical center that reflected and grew along with the enterprise of health in twentieth-century America. Because the role of Long Hospital in this process has been overshadowed by that of Riley Children's Hospital which followed, it is worth examining the Long Hospital story in some detail.

Once his work in selecting the new dean was completed, the chair of the Anatomy Department, Burton Myers, turned his attention back to laboratory instruction at the Bloomington campus. The division of teaching between Bloomington and Indianapolis meant that all first-year students who previously had been taught at both sites would have to be accommodated at expanded facilities in Bloomington. This required improvements to buildings such as Wiley, Owen, and Science Halls that had many undesirable features. Myers recommended that Owen Hall undergo a complete renovation, including the installation of a steel supported roof, raising the height of the third floor to fit its north wall with windows, and creating space in the basement suitable for "storage of cadavers." Myers told Bryan in 1910 that he strongly preferred to continue devoting all of his time to developing the resources of the Anatomy and Physiology Departments, but the gift of the Longs changed the school's priorities. As a result, Myers kept working in Indianapolis in order to help plan the new hospital.[3]

As a money-saving measure, the IUSM released its option on the old State College Hospital in February 1910, but IU president Bryan reported to Carnegie Foundation President Henry Pritchett that he and the school's officers had by no means given up on their goal "to provide as soon as possible . . . for a hospital entirely under the control of the University." Thanks to Dr. John Barnhill, first chairman of the Otolaryngology Department and a strident early advocate of university medical education, this objective became a reality.[4] In January 1911, Robert W. Long, a prominent Indianapolis

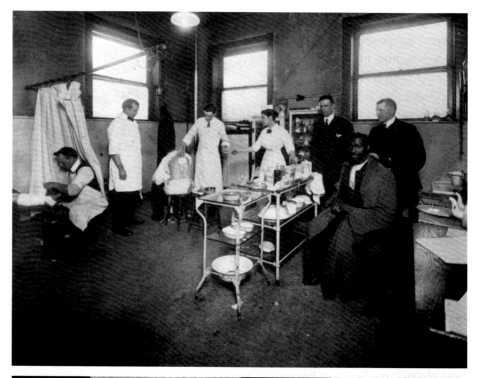

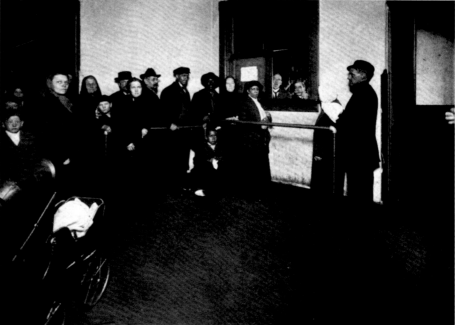

Figure 4.2a & b. Clinical facilities in Indianapolis hospitals before 1914 in photo essay on "A Senior Dilemma" by a graduating student of the IUSM class entering 1908: (*top*) picture titled "Surgery," *Arbutus* (1914): 135; (*bottom*) untitled picture of patients waiting for hospital admissions (presumably at City Hospital or Bobbs Dispensary, where medical students received clinical instruction), *Arbutus* (1914): 141.

physician and real estate investor who had taken the young Barnhill as a partner, proposed a gift of property to the state.[5] The land was valued at $200,000, and he wished to designate the proceeds of its sale to build a teaching hospital for Indiana University. Long had been contemplating making such a donation for some time. Through his extensive experience as a practicing physician, he realized that there were many indigents "who could be relieved from a life of suffering and prepared to support themselves instead of being dependent" on charity, "if they could afford to go to a good hospital." As a leader of the medical school faculty, Barnhill helped convince Long to donate his estate to the university in order to establish a teaching hospital that would accomplish Long's objectives.

In October 1910, Long met with Bryan to discuss the possibility of establishing a hospital in connection with the IU School of Medicine. The transformative power of a large capital gift appealed immediately to Bryan and his allies, who saw Long's donation as meeting the needs of the young school as well as the citizens of the state. First, although Indianapolis had its own city hospital, the lack of public hospitals in other cities in Indiana left a statewide need for an institution where "worthy persons of limited means from all parts of Indiana" could have access to health care from the best physicians. Second, having been trained at Rush and Jefferson Medical Colleges, Long personally appreciated the value of a good hospital for "the betterment of medical education." Making the hospital a clinical facility of the IU School of Medicine achieved both these goals. Long also hoped that his gift would inspire other donations for special wards or departments to enlarge the hospital. Within three months, IU officials and Indiana governor Thomas R. Marshall finalized the deal and announced the gift to the public in January 1911.[6]

Long's gift provided funds to build a hospital, but he made this gift contingent on the Indiana General Assembly's acceptance of terms that included state appropriations for the "permanent maintenance" of the hospital. Governor Marshall estimated that $25,000 in annual appropriations would be necessary to sustain the hospital and recommended that the legislature pass the enabling acts "at once," so that the Long endowment could be accepted.[7] The legislature had not increased the tax levy in the previous five years despite stagnant tax revenues and a profligate 1909 budget. This meant the 1911 General Assembly had to either reduce expenditures or raise taxes because it could not afford to turn down a gift of $200,000 that would benefit its neediest citizens. In fact, it would be the largest donation made to a public institution in Indiana by an individual. Within days, the Senate unanimously passed a bill accepting the contribution Long offered,

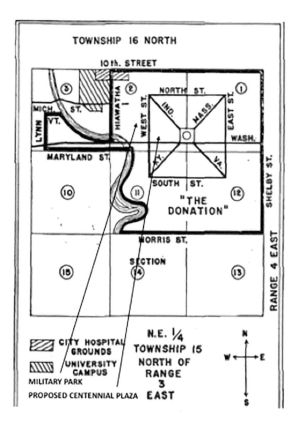

Figure 4.3. Robert W. Long's donation of property to the state to build a hospital. Based on map showing medical campus from Thurman Rice, "History of the Medical Campus, Chapter VI: Indiana University Chooses a Medical Campus," *Monthly Bulletin, Indiana State Board of Health* (February 1947): 37.

which included an annual appropriation of $25,000 for the proposed hospital's maintenance; approval by the House of Representatives quickly followed.[8]

When Dean Emerson arrived in the fall of 1911, he found that debates over the site of the hospital had delayed the groundbreaking. The argument centered on two locations, Military Park and a proposed Centennial Plaza, both of which ran into problems. Barnhill and other IU supporters feared that the glowing promises of a plaza to be built to the west of the statehouse to commemorate Indiana's centennial in 1916 would evaporate, or at best delay, the hospital's construction. With the gift in hand, they sought a location to break ground sooner rather than later at Military Park.[9] Behind the scenes, William Niles Wishard, as chairman of the IUSM Executive Committee, led the movement to locate the hospital at Military Park. University officers and many on the Centennial Committee favored this site because it would make it possible to "harmonize" the School of Medicine buildings with "a general plaza scheme" being developed for the area to the west of the Statehouse.

At the same time, there was opposition to the Military Park site because many children in this otherwise poor and industrial area used the park. Henry Jameson, the former dean of the Indiana Medical College and now president of the Indianapolis Park Board, opposed using Military Park for the School of Medicine hospital and asked the IU trustees to postpone their decision regarding the hospital site. Even Long was not convinced that Military Park was the correct place and thought that the strip of land that the legislature had designated was too narrow for the construction of a modern hospital. Moreover, university officials received no assurance that the state would permit other medical school buildings adjacent to the hospital at this site.[10] After consulting Long, the trustees agreed to Jameson's request to delay action on selection of a hospital site, especially if space could be obtained that would be better adapted "for both college & hospital."[11]

As the opposition to building in Military Park solidified, a third option was proposed when the Indianapolis city government approved construction of new facilities at City Hospital in excess of $1 million. Mayor Samuel L. Shank suggested that the Long Hospital be located on a tract of land near the expanded City Hospital because if the developments were carried out in conjunction, they "would be one of the most attractive and extensive groups of medical units in the United States." The IU trustees initially opposed the City Hospital area for the new hospital, which was near the confluence of Fall Creek and the White River. Although the area had seen much improvement, many residents still viewed the area west of City Hospital as unhealthy and swampy. The presence of a trash dump to the west of City Hospital only increased the trustees' concerns.[12]

In mid-December 1911, after investigating several available properties, a special committee appointed by Mayor Shank selected a nearby site for Long Hospital, located just southwest of City Hospital instead of in the river bottom lands directly to the west. It was a larger piece of ground and was more than sufficient to accommodate the School of Medicine for many years to come. Unlike the previous property, this tract fronted a paved road, West Michigan Street, and was only a mile from the city center and easily accessible by streetcar. The land had previously been part of a landfill, and it was also on higher ground than the site that the trustees had turned down a few weeks earlier. Governor Marshall urged the IU trustees to purchase the property and assured them that he would petition the legislature to reimburse them for the land when it came back in session. The trustees voted to proceed with the purchase of the site for $40,000. Although the land was far from desirable, the cheap price and proximity to the City Hospital ensured that the campus could continue to grow.[13]

Dean Emerson worked on the design of the hospital with the trustees and prominent local architect Robert P. Daggett to include the modern advances in design from a number of other hospitals. The facility was originally envisioned not only for adults but also for the children under the charge of the State Board of Charities. It was floored with linoleum to be easier on nurses' feet and was designed to save steps in treating and "making the patients as happy and comfortable as possible." To minimize distances, the beds were arranged in semicircles around two administrative centers. There were two large wards with sixteen beds each, four smaller rooms arranged in pairs with four beds to isolate noisy patients or those with similar diseases, and a center service room. The ward walls were made of two layers of hollow tiles with seaweed in between to deaden sound. They had ceiling lighting, with experimental floor lighting in one ward, and emergency buttons on the walls to shine green lights around the floor, as well as call buttons with a red signal.[14]

Throughout 1912, Bryan and Long's hospital began to rise from the swamp. After the groundbreaking, the construction was closely watched to ensure that no bodies from a nearby cemetery would be unearthed. Alice Fitzgerald, who became director of nursing in 1913, later recalled, "When I arrived in Indiana, the Hospital seemed so lonely and small." Daggett designed a four-story gray brick and steel construction with a normal capacity of 106 beds. The first floor was designed with rooms for eighteen private patients, medical offices of the executive staff, and a central reception room that protected paying patients' privacy.[15] He designed the second and third floors to operate independently with a laboratory and hydrotherapy bath on each floor. The fourth floor housed the surgical rooms. The basement housed kitchens, a dining room, storage, and engine rooms.[16]

The construction of the hospital faced delays and unexpected costs,[17] but on the afternoon of June 15, 1914, with Governor Samuel M. Ralston presiding, dedication ceremonies for Long Hospital began in the chambers of the Indiana House of Representatives. "This is a red letter day in the history of the medical profession in Indiana," the governor proclaimed in his opening remarks to the crowd. State and university officials, medical school faculty, and physicians from across Indiana gathered to witness this culmination of five years of work. Recognizing the school's aspirations, distinguished physicians attended from other university schools of medicine, including the University of Michigan, the University of Illinois, Western Reserve in Cleveland, and Washington University in St. Louis.[18]

Despite ill health, Long delivered remarks for the dedication. "It is a pleasure for me to live to see this hospital finished," he said as he officially turned the hospital over to the state. "I think it complete in every way." Expressing his gratitude to Bryan and others for their struggle to bring his dream to fruition, Long stated that he and his wife were "under lasting obligations to those who assisted . . . in [the hospital's] plans and arrangement." As the institution's chief guardian, Emerson promised to carry out Long's wishes. The medical school dean guaranteed that the poor of the state admitted to Long Hospital would receive "the best medical and surgical care Indiana University" could provide.[19]

The principal speaker for the event was Henry Pritchett, president of the Carnegie Foundation, who had commissioned the Flexner Report. In his speech, Pritchett described the state medical school as an institution "where practitioner and teacher, student and investigator mingled together

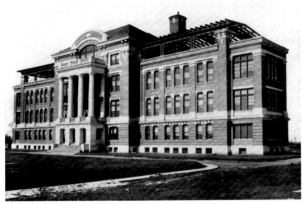

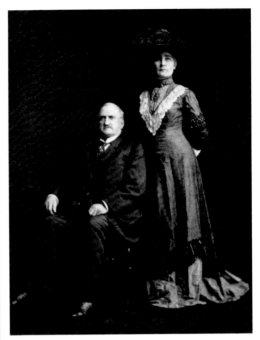

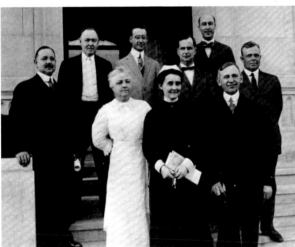

Figure 4.4a, b, & c. Long Hospital: (*clockwise from top left*) Long Hospital, 1914, IUB Archive photo collection P0031330; "The Longs," whose donation made Long Hospital possible, *Arbutus* (1911): 104; Ground breaking (back of photo: "Dedication Day, Robert Long Hospital June 16, 1914: Dr. Charles P. Emerson, IU School of Medicine, *extreme 1*; Robert Frost Daggett, architect, *extreme r*; Mrs. Sara J. Lowes, matron, Long Hospital, in white; Miss Alice Fitzgerald, director of nursing and School of Nursing (*in back*); Dr. William Lowe Bryan, president, IU, hat in hand (*in front*); *back row, 1to r*: Dr. Frank F. Hutchins, prof. of Neurology, IU School of Med; Robert E. Neff, Adm. Robert Long Hosp. Registrar School of Med Supt. Indpls City Dispensary; John W. Cravens, Registrar IU Blm. Secty Bd. of Trustees, UH; Smith, bursar"), IU, IUPUI Image, UA024_003976.

in an atmosphere charged not only with scientific skill but with the highest conception of patriotism." In Pritchett's view, and as reflected in the Flexner Report, American medical education was about to eclipse every other country in the world.[20]

Bryan had an ulterior motive for inviting Pritchett. Bryan had been appointed a trustee of the Carnegie Foundation late in 1910 and thought he was in a good position to persuade Pritchett and the rest of the organization's board that the IU School of Medicine was worthy of their beneficence. By bringing Pritchett to Indianapolis for the opening of Long Hospital, Bryan hoped to prove to the Carnegie Foundation president that there was no institution "in the country where an endowment of a million dollars for the advancement of medical education could be better placed." This was not merely wishful thinking. In June 1913, the foundation's president had suggested that IUSM was next in line after Vanderbilt University to receive funding for an endowment of "a half million or million dollars." Bryan was convinced that when Pritchett saw in person what the School of Medicine had accomplished, he would leave with an even more favorable view of the school.[21]

Despite these prospects, Bryan's hopes of Carnegie funding went unfulfilled. One reason was the general reluctance of both the Carnegie Foundation and the Rockefeller-controlled General Education Board to give money to state institutions. Even after policies regarding the funding of public institutions changed, the IUSM operated under too many handicaps to compete successfully for any major monies available from either foundation.[22] This included the lack of sufficient full-time faculty appointments and the medical school operations being divided between two locations. Above all, the greatest obstacle to receiving an endowment from these national foundations was a perceived lack of support from the state legislature. As public appropriations for higher education across the country grew significantly in the 1910s and 1920s, Indiana was not contributing as much to its universities as other states in the region. The Carnegie Foundation and the General Education Board usually required local matching funds as a condition of their benefaction. Therefore, as long as it appeared that the state was not doing enough to help complete the School of Medicine's transformation, the major foundations refused to support the institution. Beginning with Long, the IUSM began to receive significant donations from local philanthropists, thus enabling the construction of much needed medical facilities. However, the major foundations' officials were not convinced that the state would provide the funds necessary to sustain these efforts. In the end, Bryan's dreams of a major endowment proved illusory.[23]

Staffing Long Hospital and the Medical School

The new hospital soon showed its value as a clinical teaching resource, but it added significantly to the administrative responsibilities of Emerson, already burdened with the major task of transforming the medical school faculty. Long Hospital opened for patients on June 15, 1914, and because it was part of the School of Medicine, patient care fell under the Educational Committee, which selected patients for surgical or institutional care or active care, excluding mental or contagious disease cases. After selection and approval by the township trustee, patients had to be referred by the committee to doctors for admission by doctors before they left home.[24] The day-to-day operation of the hospital fell to three residents who were graduates of IUSM, as well as several graduate and student nurses. As was the case at other teaching hospitals, these residents, sometimes called house officers, were responsible for directing the routine care of patients and supervising the senior medical students who were assigned to wards in small groups. The medical students did patient histories and lab work, followed progress on cases, and made reports.

Long Hospital was under the supervision of Emerson, with two other administrators assisting him: Alice Fitzgerald, the nursing director, and Sarah Laws the business superintendent. Fitzgerald spent more than $40,000 equipping the hospital with all the best technologies, and she hired the nursing staff. Emerson looked for residents who were willing to accept three-year appointments to run the facility. The initial nursing staff was relatively small, consisting of one instructor, two head nurses, a night supervisor, an operating room supervisor, and seven staff nurses. The wards were designed so that one graduate nurse and her students could care for each floor, ideally forty to fifty patients.[25]

As was the case with many other large hospitals at the time, nursing staff was recruited by establishing a school. In fact, the IU Training School for Nurses opened just four days after Long Hospital. It was noteworthy as one of the first nurse training programs affiliated with a university, part of the professionalization of nursing that was underway. Fitzgerald (1874–1962) was a graduate of the Johns Hopkins Hospital School of Nursing in 1906, and she created and ran the new nursing program at Long Hospital from 1913 through 1915. Emerson recruited her because of her administrative experience at Bellevue Hospital in New York City and General Hospital in Wilkes-Barre, Pennsylvania.[26] She designed the school's curriculum, hired its first faculty, designed the uniforms, and oversaw the admittance of the first class of five nursing students. Admission required college credit and three years of coursework that conformed to the College of Liberal Arts at IU (College of Arts and Sciences after 1921). In addition to the course credits, the nurses needed a letter of reference, a certificate of clean health, and a personal interview.

The "Graduate Nurse Degree" was a three-year program provided to nurses in training with coursework following a sequence similar to the

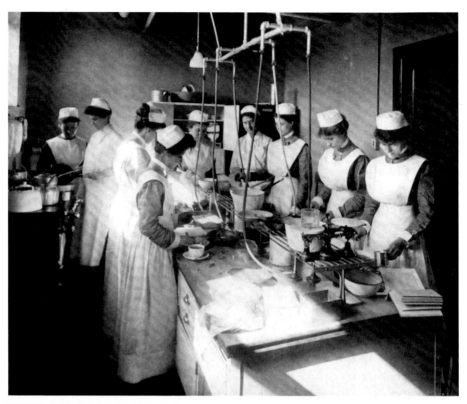

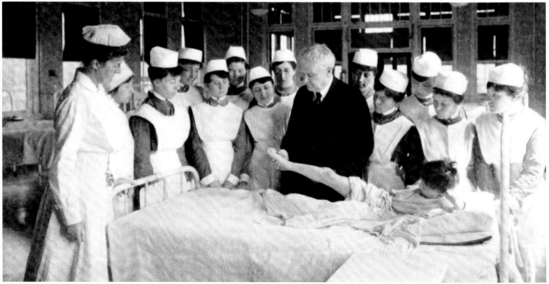

Figure 4.5a & b. Nurse Training School at the new Long Hospital: (*top*) Laboratory, *Arbutus* (1917): 217; (*bottom*) bedside training, *Arbutus* (1919): 161.

medical school program, as well as on-the-job training. Nursing students spent most of their time on the hospital wards, working under the supervision of the nursing supervisors. Initially housed in the hospital, they soon moved into the "nurses' cottages" east of the building until 1928 when a residence hall with a capacity for 165 nurses was built with funding from the Ball family of Muncie. The nursing program started small but grew steadily to the point where forty-seven nurses were admitted in 1928.[27] No fee was charged until 1928, and women received board, room, books, and uniform. In 1915, Ethel Clarke took over as director of the Training School for Nurses, a position she held until 1931.[28]

Even before the site selection controversy and staffing of Long Hospital played out very publicly in the press, Emerson faced other important internal problems, including the transformation of the faculty, who had been inherited from the proprietary schools. In November 1911, only a few months after he arrived, Emerson reported to the trustees that he needed "to get thoroughly acquainted with the situation himself before he recommend[ed] any radical measures." Therefore, during his first year, he planned "to hold rigidly to all promises or even partial understandings made before" his arrival.[29] By June 1912, the school's new dean was ready to give the trustees another report on the subject. According to Emerson, the state of the faculty was pretty grim. Although the faculty list was large, there were not enough physicians on the active list to fill all of the positions necessary for the school to succeed.[30] After he finished his investigation of the medical faculty, Emerson was more convinced than ever that it was essential to "collect a small nucleus of men" upon whom the school could depend. He contended that most of these men would have to be "called from other schools," and it was no accident that the dean's first two appointments, like Myers and Emerson himself, came from the Johns Hopkins University School of Medicine, although both had Indiana roots.

The first physician Emerson recruited to become a member of this dependable nucleus of professors was Willis D. Gatch. In the summer of 1911, Gatch contacted Emerson about applying for a position in the Department of Surgery at the IU School of Medicine. Gatch was interested in part because of dissatisfaction with a new position he had taken at Washington University School of Medicine in St. Louis but also because he was an Indiana native and an Indiana University graduate. Born near Aurora, Indiana, in 1877, he'd graduated from Indiana University in 1901. As a college student, Gatch had been in courses that Bryan had taught just before he'd become university president. Following graduation, Gatch taught science in an Indiana high school, but as the nephew of two Civil War surgeons, he decided to enroll at Johns Hopkins University School of Medicine, thus continuing the family tradition. He received his medical degree in 1907 and remained at Johns Hopkins through 1909 as an intern and resident, studying with the eminent surgeon William S. Halsted. During his time at Hopkins, Gatch invented the first adjustable hospital bed.[31]

Although Gatch demonstrated much surgical talent in addition to his impressive mechanical ingenuity, he was not admitted into the very selective Johns Hopkins residency program. Gatch remained long enough at Hopkins to be offered a surgical residency at Washington University. In addition, he had the respect of such men as William H. Welch, the first dean of the Hopkins Medical School, and Henry Mills Hurd, the first superintendent of Johns Hopkins Hospital. Welch described Gatch as "one of the ablest young men" to have graduated from Johns Hopkins and told Bryan that he represented "the . . . type of man best fitted for a clinical department—the teacher, investigator and good clinician." Hurd also identified Gatch as one of the "most promising surgeons" of his generation. In fact, Hurd admitted that he'd discouraged Gatch from moving to Indianapolis because the young surgeon had just been invited to join the newly reorganized medical faculty of Washington University, which Hurd believed was better than anything the IU School of Medicine could offer. Nevertheless, coming home to Indiana appealed strongly to Gatch, and he informed Emerson that he would accept a position at the IU School of Medicine.[32]

With Welch's recommendation, Bryan was eager to hire Gatch, and Emerson "persuaded him to cast his lot" with IU. In November 1911, the board of trustees appointed Gatch assistant professor of surgery "in charge of surgical laboratories." Gatch took the position with the understanding that there was a strong possibility that he would become chairman of the Department of Surgery as soon as the school had its own teaching hospital. Until that time, he agreed to work full-time for the university as "a laboratory man and teacher[,] attempting no private practice." Along with Emerson, Gatch helped to raise the prestige of the School of Medicine in national circles. "With two men like Emerson and Gatch," Welch told Bryan, "medicine and surgery would be splendidly represented . . . and the outlook would be most promising for a model medical school."[33]

Thanks to the new Long Hospital, immediately after hiring Gatch, Emerson was able to attract to the school another professor who had worked at Johns Hopkins: Indiana native George S. Bond, a pioneer in the use of electrocardiography. Emerson saw Bond as "one of the best . . . men in medical research" and part of a "nucleus of a good corps of workers in the future."

After receiving his medical degree from the University of Michigan, Bond went to Johns Hopkins, where he was one of the first individuals to operate an electrocardiograph machine in the United States, and he played an important role in the introduction of this technology into the institution's teaching hospital. Bond was willing to come back to Indiana to work for the university full-time as an assistant professor of internal medicine, with the understanding that he would be able to continue his work on cardiac disease. Emerson also relieved Bond from much routine teaching and hospital work in internal medicine to allow him to form his own Department of Cardiovascular and Renal Diseases.[34]

Long Hospital gave Emerson, Bond, and Gatch a space that supported the teaching style they had learned at Johns Hopkins, and they upheld the highest standards of medical practice. During this era, patients generally remained in the hospital for two to three weeks. At Long Hospital, senior medical students served as "externs," attending daily rounds and assisting the house staff. "Individual treatment" was the rule, and although medical students examined fewer cases at Long Hospital than they did at City Hospital, they had the opportunity to study each one of them in more depth. In addition to following cases, students served as surgical assistants and dressing clerks, helping to relieve the nursing staff. Externs at Long Hospital could see the course of disease, practice the principles of therapy, develop their communication skills with patients and their families, and see their contributions to patient care. They also continued to perform morning rounds at the Indianapolis Dispensary, which cared for more than forty thousand patients per year.[35]

While Long Hospital served its purpose to provide clinical instruction for students, the institution quickly posed administrative problems. In September 1914, Emerson informed Bryan that the hospital had been "very satisfactory" in fulfilling its statewide mission as a referral hospital. Counties throughout the state sent charity patients to Indianapolis, but the overall number of admissions remained rather limited. The third floor was vacant, even though no desirable patients had been turned away from the public wards. University officials sought more patients not only for educational reasons but also because they wanted to show members of the state legislature that hospital demand justified an increased appropriation, especially for charity patients.[36]

Because the state did not provide enough funds to support a hospital for charity care only, the building's design included space for patients who could pay as a way to provide a place for doctors' private patients and add to the budget income, as well as diversify patient clinical cases. This was made possible at the end of 1914, when adjacent cottages were completed to house nurses who had previously lived in the private patient rooms on the first and third floors of the hospital. Emerson hoped that the income generated from these private rooms would provide enough revenue so that the university could afford to open at least one-half of the hospital wards on the third floor for nonpaying patients. Members of the Educational Committee, which was responsible for directing professional medical work in the hospital, disagreed about whether or not to expand the admissions of paying patients.[37]

During discussions about the hospital's admission policy, Professors John H. Oliver and Frank Wynn argued that Long Hospital should be a charitable hospital. Oliver was the first chairman of the Department of Surgery, serving from 1908 to 1912. He was an Indiana native who completed his medical education at the State Medical College of Indiana, and then he studied in London, Paris, Vienna, and Berlin before leading IU's Department of Surgery.[38] Wishard sought a middle ground, arguing that patients who were able should be charged a "modest fee." But John Hurty, the secretary of the Indiana Board of Health, noted that in other state institutions (such as the tuberculosis sanitarium), patients who could pay already did so. Based in large part on Hurty's forceful argument, the Educational Committee voted to accept part- and full-pay patients at Long Hospital. Anticipating criticism from community practitioners, the school reminded doctors that the privilege of using private rooms in the university teaching hospital could "be extended to community physicians at the discretion of the Educational Committee." Nevertheless, some medical practitioners remained unalterably opposed to the policy because they believed it demonstrated a shift toward publicly subsidized medicine that would compete unfairly with them.[39]

The prospect of attracting paying patients was of particular interest to President Bryan, who was already quite concerned about the cost of operating Long Hospital. "I am deeply depressed by the financial estimate for the Medical School and Hospital," he wrote to Emerson in late November 1914. The one thing that troubled him most was the "proposed rate of maintenance." Bryan computed that the total actual cost per bed per day was almost four dollars rather than the two dollars twenty cents Emerson estimated. If Bryan's numbers were accurate, the teaching hospital would carry a deficit of about $13,000. Although he could cover that amount from his current surplus, Brian worried about recurring deficits.[40] Thus, the issue of hospital costs and income from patients, so evident in today's medical schools, was a concern from the very beginning of the first hospital of the IU School of Medicine.

The Social Service Department

Bryan was also concerned about another place responsible for rising costs: the Social Service Department.[41] This department, which proved to be an ongoing bone of contention between the dean and the president, was an early attempt by Emerson not only to teach medical students and do research about the broader causes and consequences of illness but also to provide services to hospital patients. This was the beginning of what has now become the fields of public health, hospital social work, and visiting nursing. Emerson had been involved in similar work at Hopkins and strongly supported it at IU.[42] In early 1909, Emerson was particularly interested in the social service department recently established at Massachusetts General Hospital by Professor Richard Cabot of Harvard University Medical School. According to Cabot, "beyond the special disease of a special child or adult," there was usually "a family problem, ultimately a community problem, poverty, bad housing, bad food, bad habits and associations, ignorance of the ways and means of making a clean and healthy life on scanty means." Serving as president of the National Commission of Mental Hygiene for eight years, Cabot said in 1921, "Hygiene and Preventive Medicine should be the crown of the medical course."[43]

Believing that this would be "the next move in Medicine," Emerson thought that IU should develop a medical curriculum that focused on environmental medicine, which would include hygiene, public health, and preventive medicine, in order to educate students who were public servants as well as physicians. In this way, Emerson believed IU could "take a leading part" in medical education in the United States.[44] The social service approach to medicine had an appeal to some faculty within the school as well as in the new hospitals, outpatient clinics, and dispensaries in Indianapolis, which were ideal places to hold educational lectures and other kinds of instruction to help correct social problems. Especially the encounter in the dispensary encouraged a style of medical practice that sought to understand the patient experience of disease not as an isolated encounter but more as a life event with social causes and social consequences. The social service model added follow-up visits by social workers and public health nurses with patients in their homes.

When Emerson arrived, he faced not only sympathy for his ideas but also the beginnings of a program to act on them. In fact, as early as 1909,

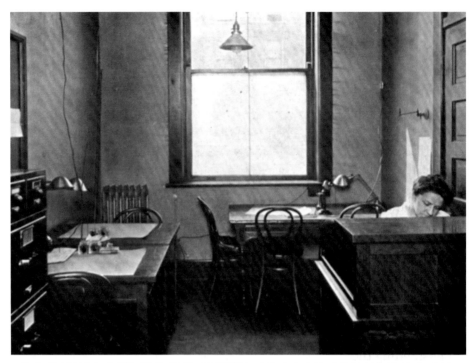

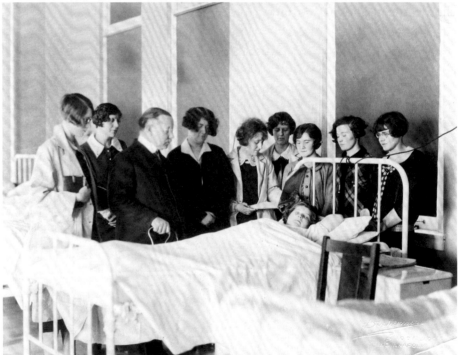

Figure 4.6a & b. Social Services Department: (*top*) Edna G. Henry, director of Social Service Department, *Arbutus* (1919): 165; (*bottom*) Charles Emerson making rounds with social service students at Long Hospital, 1920s, IUPUI Image UA024_002603.

Burton Myers in Bloomington had expressed interest in this approach and planned to apply "the principles of this social movement . . . in Indianapolis, working not merely in affiliation with the social organizations of Indianapolis but in cooperation with the affiliated societies of each county." Even more important than Myers was his colleague at Bloomington, Professor Ulysses G. Weatherly, head of the Department of Economics and Sociology, who was eager to collaborate. On June 17, 1911, the board of trustees authorized the IU School of Medicine Executive Committee to hire Edna Henry, the daughter of Charles L. Henry, a member of the IU Board of Trustees between 1894 and 1903 who had made his fortune in connection with Indiana's interurban system, to run the social service department. In fact, she started a program at the Medical School Dispensary with a modest budget of $800 just weeks before Emerson began his appointment.[45] Organizationally, Henry's position was put under Weatherly's department in Bloomington, but the medical school supplied the office space, supplies, and salary. After Emerson was hired, Weatherly asked him to supervise Henry in Indianapolis. The instruction of medical students (and soon nurses) was only part of her responsibility; most important was her work with patients, understanding their social and family background and explaining to them the treatment and prevention of their illness.[46]

This approach to medicine was a wellspring for some new and important approaches to health care, including the emerging fields of public health and social work. On the other hand, it also made common cause with the then influential eugenics movement. For example, Emerson was appointed a member of the Committee on Mental Defectives in Indiana, and IU Medical School faculty member Thurman B. Rice was author of *Racial Hygiene: A Practical Discussion of Eugenics and Race Culture.*[47] Emerson's more immediate task was supporting the Social Service Department's instruction of medical and nursing students. Although a separate bachelor's (and eventually graduate) degree was offered (with combined coursework in Bloomington and Indianapolis), the vast majority of the immediate work of the department was in conjunction with hospital patients.[48] This was not surprising given the volume of patients treated at the City Dispensary (more than thirty-five thousand in 1911), and even limiting intake only to referrals, Miss Henry had over 250 patients the first year. This increased to almost eight hundred patients the next year and double that the following year. Volunteers helped some, but by May 1913, the staff necessary for this work grew to include an assistant social worker, two stenographers, an office assistant, and a nurse supported by the Woman's Club of Indianapolis.[49] And all of this was before the opening of Long Hospital in June 1914.

The budget consequences of this growth led Bryan to conclude that a cap was necessary in service, and a reduction was needed in the budget. From its first year of less than $1,000, excluding the salary of Edna Henry, the Social Service Department budget rose to nearly $4,000 the following year as doctors at the Indianapolis City Dispensary gained confidence in the services and referred more patients. The department's budget for 1913–14 was a little over $7,000, and with the opening of Long Hospital, the department's services the next year extended to patients who came from all parts of Indiana. Therefore, the department requested another substantial budget increase to over $11,000 for the 1914–15 fiscal year.[50]

The expansion of the Social Service Department inevitably collided with the limited resources of the medical school because the department's budget came directly from state appropriations for the medical school and Long Hospital. In fact, by 1914–15, the Social Service Department used over 10 percent of the annual fund designated for the School of Medicine and its teaching hospital. The basic running of the new hospital was in competition with Emerson's drive to expand social service. An example of the clash of needs was when Emerson defended funding the social service program against the need to purchase much-needed X-ray equipment for Long Hospital. This prompted Bryan to warn Emerson about many faculty members' complaints concerning the Social Service Department.[51]

These budget increases led Bryan to conclude by the end of 1914 that the university "could not afford to establish a great bureau capable of dealing with all the patients in the city and state who present[ed] themselves." He therefore took two steps to solve the problem. The first was to make Social Services a separate department both to help identify expenses and so that Henry would no longer split her reporting between Weatherly and Emerson. In addition, Bryan declared that the department would have "to select and study a limited number of cases."[52] Although Bryan recommended an appropriation of $10,000 for the department for 1914–15, he informed Emerson that its budget would be cut in half in September 1915 to make provisions for a full-time faculty member in pharmacology.[53] Emerson agreed, telling Bryan that he recognized the need to bolster the school's teaching of the second year curriculum, and that Edna Henry would do her best to comply with his wishes to reduce the budget of the Social Service Department.[54]

Cutting the Social Services budget was only part of the bigger task that Bryan gave to Emerson in order to operate the hospital within the limits of the annual state maintenance fund of $50,000 (not counting income from paying patients). Bryan warned Emerson that without a "defensible budget," including more paying patients, the trustees would radically cut expenditures, "probably involving the discontinuance of the Nurses' School." Emerson replied, "I am not surprised that the financial estimate for the hospital was no[t] satisfactory for certainly it cannot be." But, he went on, "It is a mistake to run the hospital with so few patients[,] for the machinery of running it is very nearly the same as though one hundred patients were present. It is like trying to run a six-cylinder automobile on three cylinders." Emerson suggested that by moving the nurses from Long Hospital upon completion of adjacent housing, it would make beds available for additional patients. Then, once these rooms were "comfortably full," the university "would have sufficient income to pay the absolute increase in expense of maintenance and . . . should have even a little margin left for improvement of equipment." In response to Emerson's suggestions, the board of trustees ordered that the third floor of Long Hospital should be opened at once and that arrangements should be made to house the nurses outside the hospital as soon as possible so that the rooms they occupied could be used for paying patients. At the same time, to keep expenses down, the trustees indicated that they would not accept any increases in the hospital's salary roll, despite having a greater number of patients and workload.[55]

Finding places for all student nurses to live was easier said than done. It was already clear that the First Cottage would not be sufficient to accommodate them. Robert W. Long again came to the rescue. With his help, the university was able to purchase additional property adjacent to Long Hospital, east of the First Cottage right next to Hiawatha Street, so that it could be used as additional housing for nurses. Total purchase and renovation costs for what came to be known as the Second Cottage amounted to approximately $6,000. To demonstrate how much the cottages were needed, when they opened, they housed twenty-seven individuals.[56] By mid-December 1914, within a couple of weeks after opening the third floor of the hospital, it began to fill quickly with patients. At the end of the year, the hospital had nearly seventy-five patients, ten of whom were private. During the first quarter of 1915, the number of patients varied from about seventy-five to ninety a day. Therefore, Emerson could finally announce that Long Hospital was "comfortably full." Charity patients came from the state's various counties and now that there were more private rooms available, they were proving popular with physicians and their private patients.

Hiring More "Good Men," Wartime Conditions, and a New Medical Building

After making a few initial appointments of faculty, building and staffing Long Hospital, and starting a nursing school, Emerson returned to the task of recruiting more faculty members and eliminating those carried over from the medical school consolidations who were unsatisfactory. The dean was demonstrably responding to the hopes that the president and trustees of the university had placed in him, but he was about to face even more extraordinary challenges of fire, war, and epidemic in addition to an outright revolt of some faculty to his efforts. In the Department of Surgery, for example, Emerson attempted to reduce its dependence on community physicians who still formed the bulk of the faculty. The dean placed Gatch in position to lead this effort by promoting him to full professor in July 1912, less than a year after his initial appointment. Many members of the department resented the elevation of Gatch, who had so little seniority, even though physicians throughout the school realized that each new full-time, well-trained man like Gatch would "inevitably replace two or three of the old faculty" and that such men would be employed as rapidly as the university could afford to hire them. Gatch was equal to the task and played a key role in shaping the next generation of physicians.

More broadly, Emerson thought that a majority of the school's professors were "in a condition of constant dissatisfaction" because of the mismatch of their past training with the new expectations of this very different medical school. "I know no way of making them loyal," he reported to the trustees in 1916, because they did not share his vision of "a medical school with standards to which the faculty must conform, and from which they must expect to be dropped if they cannot meet these requirements or standards."[57] These professors especially begrudged the powerful Educational Committee's command of Long Hospital, which determined all physician privileges and the assignment of cases to the various members of the faculty. In particular, they severely criticized the Educational Committee for allowing Gatch to do so much of the surgery performed in the teaching hospital.[58]

Some physicians fought back by threatening the school's control of the City Dispensary and access to City Hospital. The school's relationship with city officials was sometimes tenuous, and a number of faculty who joined IUSM from the proprietary schools merger and also sat on the City Board of Health, including Thomas B. Eastman and G. B. Jackson, often worked to undermine the school's position. Emerson gave as one example their delaying action on City Board of Health matters that involved the medical school "until the very last minute," fruitlessly hoping that Emerson would "feel obliged to offer them something in the way of improved work, title, or some other advantage."[59]

In the fall of 1915, some of the dissatisfied faculty members, led by Eastman and Jackson, used their positions on the Indianapolis City Board of Health to create a crisis by disputing the university's right to make appointments to the City Dispensary. IU faculty member Frank Wynn warned Emerson that it would be "a detriment to the University's interests to take up a quarrel with the Eastmans." "I knew their father before them, and I know them," he told Emerson. "They are fighters who understand the game and have few equals." Emerson was not inclined to back down. He complained in no uncertain terms to Bryan that doctors like Eastman and Jackson "have been pirates from the very first." As a result, he concluded, "they know that they cannot hold their position through reason but must do it through that which corresponds to force."[60]

In November 1915, the dispute reached a crisis when the board of health took the City Dispensary out of the hands of the IUSM and suspended the school's privilege of holding clinics at City Hospital.[61] The latter was even more ominous because City Hospital was the primary provider of charity care and had a strong internship program dating back to an agreement in the late nineteenth century with the two IUSM predecessor schools, the Medical College of Indiana and the College of Physicians and Surgeons. In 1905, the still nascent IUSM and City Hospital entered into a teaching affiliation agreement authorizing school faculty to serve as hospital staff physicians, and as many as one-third of its students rotated through City Hospital for clinical experience.

IUSM could not, therefore, survive long without access to the hospital because the school would immediately be in serious danger of losing its Class A rating by the American Medical Association. Long Hospital was too small to offer all of the clinical advantages required to remain in this top category. Although the university tried to downplay the problems these circumstances might cause by defining them as an "inconvenience," long-term consequences would have been dire. Fortunately for the medical school, the City Hospital was not in the strongest position to assert its independence. It had recently begun to improve its facilities thanks to a donation in 1913 from Alfred Burdsal, who willed his estate worth $700,000 to the city in part for the expansion and improvement of the hospital. The adult and pediatric wards opened in 1914 and were designed according to the latest theory in hospitals including natural light, tile floors, and public art in patient wards. This increase in funding for infrastructure only compounded the need for the staffing resources of the growing IUSM. Without such support, City Hospital could not keep up with medical advances, and the new Burdsal wards would deteriorate.[62]

Within a month, IUSM and the Board of Health resolved their differences and signed a new contract that allowed the School of Medicine "to furnish all consulting and visiting medical and surgical" staff for the City Hospital and Dispensary. The new contract placed City Dispensary under the joint control of the City Board of Health and IUSM, until it became part of City Hospital in 1929. In a concession, however, the school's administrators agreed to submit their nominations for these positions to the City Board of Health for approval.[63]

Although this settled the controversy with the City Board of Health, the situation demonstrated to Emerson how vulnerable the school was to the influence of practitioners who were antagonistic to its aims. He was not convinced that the trustees fully appreciated either the dangers of retaining poorly trained physicians as instructors or "the inevitable hostility" which the dean faced daily. He maintained that the school could progress only as fast as the university could afford to hire more "good men." Up to this point, IUSM attracted a handful of first-rate professors; the possibility of continuing to do so was increasingly remote, according to Emerson, because word had spread throughout the national medical community that the university's administration in Bloomington was not behind the medical school. As a result, in June 1916, Emerson urged the trustees to dispel this perception by pledging to provide a new medical school building adjacent to Long Hospital on Michigan Street and much closer to City Hospital. He feared "for the future of the school" without an upgrade in the teaching facilities. The Educational Committee reiterated many of Emerson's arguments and warned that in addition to its location the downtown medical school building, which had housed the old proprietary schools, was "a dangerous fire trap."[64]

As it happened, the Educational Committee's fears were confirmed within months. On December 7, 1916, a fire that started in the incubators in the pathology laboratory destroyed nearly all of the third and fourth floors of the old Indiana Medical College building. Water damage rendered many rooms on the lower floors unusable. The insurance company determined that the "building was unsuited, inadequate, and could not be made tenantable," and approved $17,000 for replacement. The school estimated damages at $350,000, so the insurance adjustment was not nearly enough to cover repairs.[65]

Replacing the structure was now an emergency. Before the fire, facilities at the medical school building already had been inadequate, but now the situation was desperate. In the interim, only the first floor of the old medical school building remained functional, so the school held classes for nearly one hundred students in Shortridge High School, Indiana Dental College, and the basement of City Hospital. They relocated the third- and fourth-floor offices and laboratories to City Hospital and a corridor in Long Hospital. The situation was exacerbated because the premedical program in Bloomington had grown slowly to over two hundred students, which led Dean Emerson to ask, "Where will these young men study medicine?" As feared by Emerson, the state legislature's reluctance to replace the building sent a message that the state was "not behind its Medical School."[66]

IU developed plans based on its estimate for a new $350,000 medical and classroom building, assuming that the university turn over to the state the old medical school building, which, although badly damaged, was still valued at over $250,000. During the 1917 General Assembly session, the governor's intention to limit education spending bogged down the funding of the building, and the session ended without passing a bill.[67] The governor informed IU trustee Fesler that "certain persons in the House and Senate were absolutely opposed to it, and he was unable to do anything" to save it. The medical school faculty was "thoroughly disheartened or worse," Bryan told the board of trustees. "They hold that if we find no way of assuring in the near future a new medical building or a unit of such a building and if we ask them to go on under conditions which all know to be intolerable, the school will go to wreck." Members of the faculty were convinced that without the prospect of a new classroom and laboratory building, students would not stay and few new ones could enroll.[68]

What fire and overcrowding could not do, however, war helped achieve later in the spring of 1917. With the entry of the United States into World War I, Governor Goodrich and other members of state government could not ignore the medical school's needs for very long. When war broke out in Europe in 1914, some medical schools and hospitals, notably on the East Coast, organized hospital units to support the Allied war effort. Although the United States was neutral, the American Red Cross anticipated the entry of the country into the war and urged local chapters to make plans for medical assistance. In February 1917, the Indianapolis chapter of the Red Cross, thanks in large part to a $25,000 donation by Josiah K. Lilly Sr., began making plans for what came to be known as Base Hospital 32. The five-hundred-bed hospital was opened in January 1918 in several hotels of the resort town of Contrexeville behind French lines and was directed by Edmund D. Clark of the Medical School Surgery Department.[69] According to Benjamin Hitz's 1922 history, the hospital cared for almost ten thousand patients until it was closed in January 1919.

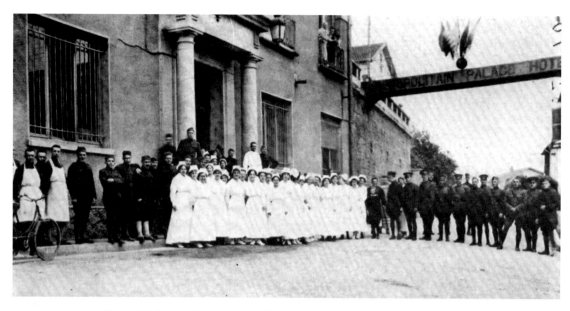

Figure 4.7. Personnel of Hospital A of Lilly Base Hospital 32, Contrexeville, France, during World War I, from *A History of Base Hospital 32* (including Unit R) by Benjamin D. Hitz, compiled in 1922, 100.

Back home, the medical school's contribution to the war effort greatly strengthened its case for a new medical building. Bryan pointed out to the governor that at this time, the university could render the government the "most immediate and . . . greatest service" through its medical school. The exigencies of war bore this statement out by soon demonstrating a dearth of competent physicians and surgeons and revealing a desperate need for better health care. The US Armed Forces found that 29 percent of draftees examined were rejected on medical grounds.[70] Within weeks of the declaration of war, the Council on National Defense called Emerson and other deans to Washington, DC, to confer about what the government expected medical schools to do to meet the increased demand for medical personnel. Eventually, twenty-eight School of Medicine faculty members entered the military service, and all the medical students who passed their physical examination enlisted and were placed on the medical reserve list. University officials agreed that the institution should adopt an accelerated program to graduate two medical school classes each year.[71]

On May 8, 1917, less than a month after the United States entered the war, the IU trustees met with Governor Goodrich to discuss the immediate need for a medical school building. Following this conference, the governor announced support for construction of the new facility. "A building which will be adequate to the needs of the school will be erected," IUSM's Barnhill stated to a reporter. "All doubt . . . was wiped out at today's conference with the Governor." The new building was to be two to three times larger than the old Indiana Medical College. The newspaper predicted that ground would be broken at the site near Long Hospital during summer 1917, even without securing the financing.[72]

As had happened with the construction of Long Hospital, this pronouncement was premature because the means of financing the project had not yet been determined. It was only in March 1918, a full year after the original bill, that the State Finance Committee voted appropriations for construction of a new medical school building from the state's emergency fund, but the amount was only $130,000. In return, the old Indiana Medical College building would be turned over to the government so that it could be used for state offices.[73] In the end, the state provided only $125,000, hardly adequate when the lowest bid for the building totaled over $386,000. Because construction costs during the war were so high, the trustees decided that the university should not attempt to build the entire structure. Therefore, the school sought bids for erection of only a portion of the building, lowering the cost to $238,000. To fill the gap, the governor brought together a group of prominent Indianapolis citizens who joined him in advancing $175,000 in credit to fund construction. These men did so with the understanding that during the next meeting of the General Assembly in 1919, Goodrich would support a bill that would provide an appropriation for the medical school building and release them as guarantors.[74]

The lack of suitable quarters made expanding the IUSM's wartime enrollment program difficult. Nevertheless, the school pressed ahead to institute an accelerated course beginning in July 1918 so that students could graduate in a little less than three years. The war emergency meant that adequate facilities for the medical school had eclipsed the arena of local and state interests and had become a matter that was also vital to national defense. "The need for medical science," Goodrich declared in his speech at the medical school building groundbreaking on June 18, 1918, "is clearly illustrated by the number of men called for military service who have been rejected on account of physical defects." He continued, "Not only from a humanitarian standing, but from a point of self-interest all citizens should stand behind the medical school." Goodrich had already shown his personal support by making a financial pledge to the medical school building project.[75]

Against the dramatic backdrop of these world-changing events, Governor Goodrich delivered his message to the 1919 Indiana legislature, recommending that the state purchase the old Indiana Medical College building from Indiana University so the private investors could be reimbursed. Notwithstanding a number of fights over appropriate sources for higher education funding, at the end of the legislative session, the appropriations bill was passed and enabled Indiana University "to repay the advanced credit underwritten" by the group of "public-spirited citizens who had responded to the war emergency need for a new and more adequate medical [school] building."[76]

Because the university had started construction the year before with this unusual funding, the building was complete enough by the start of the new school year in late September 1919, only a few months after the legislation was passed, for Emerson to hold an informal dedication.[77] An article in the *Indianapolis Star* announced that "this handsome structure, alongside . . . Long hospital," was destined to become part of a "great medical center in Indianapolis." The early use of the term "medical center" is noteworthy for a number of reasons, not the least of which is that most histories give Columbia Presbyterian Hospital credit for coining the term in 1928, and it was not until 1936 that the IU trustees voted that "the official name of the Indianapolis campus be Indiana University Medical Center."[78] Emerson used the term despite the building having only one wing. But the new structure was located adjacent to Long Hospital and close to City Hospital, and because other hospitals were soon added, they vindicated Emerson's characterization.

More immediately, the Medical Building was a vast improvement over the old Indiana Medical College facility, with the most up-to-date equipment, reported the *Indianapolis Star,* to make "it one of the most modern medical school buildings in the country."[79] The building was four stories high and contained three laboratories, research rooms, and three lecture rooms that were large enough for a hundred students. In 1928, the rear T-wing was added to include a library with 7,500 volumes, administrative offices, and an auditorium that accommodated 160 students and featured a moving picture projector with stereopticon. Classrooms and laboratories were available to teach students microscopy, general pathology, bacteriology, biochemistry, and pharmacology. The basement contained a department of illustrations, a bookstore, and a cafeteria.[80] In 1961, the Medical Building underwent long-needed renovations and was renamed Emerson Hall in honor of the dean who oversaw its construction.[81]

The complexities of managing the growing facilities and programs of the medical school prompted the board of trustees in 1923 to have Bryan appoint Samuel E. Smith to a newly created position of provost of the

Indianapolis campus. Smith was a leader in psychology and the asylum movement in Indiana. He was selected as provost due to his success working with the state legislature on the expansion of mental asylum construction throughout the state.[82] During the five years of Smith's tenure, he and Emerson attempted to improve salaries and compensation to attract new faculty to the School of Medicine. The low salaries were a constant problem and caused the loss of professors, particularly in the basic sciences. Over the years, Myers repeatedly complained about the salaries he and his colleagues in Bloomington received. Unfortunately, attracting strong, full-time faculty members in the clinical departments required large increases in the budgets of the various IU School of Medicine departments, but throughout the 1920s, the university's economic circumstances made this impossible. Because of this situation, the problem of replacing the retiring medical school faculty continued to be "disquieting" to Emerson.[83] In the meantime, the forces pushing for new hospitals continued to grow.

A Tribute by the "Friends of Riley"

Shortly after the dedication of the Medical Building in 1919, the medical school found its priorities rearranged when it was approached by an influential philanthropic group interested in funding a children's hospital. Pediatrics was a concern of Emerson's, but it had not been one of his top priorities following the war. The establishment of the Riley Memorial Association to support the construction of a new pediatric hospital offered him both the resources and opportunity for the school to be part of this growing field of medicine. This initiative had begun following the death of Indiana poet James Whitcomb Riley in 1916, when a group of his friends met to consider establishing a memorial that would celebrate his contributions to the state. During his lifetime, Riley had achieved nationwide recognition as a poet and performer and, through his widespread fame, had become the state's "ambassador to the rest of the United States and, for that matter, to the rest of the English-speaking world." His works depicted a sense of Indiana's cultural identity, but he also captured the mood of many in the country at the end of the nineteenth century by writing poetry about nature and childhood. In a world that was undergoing rapid industrialization and urbanization, these idealized messages about an imagined world of simple values and virtues, now lost, spoke to a segment of the public who yearned to escape modern anxieties.[84]

The "friends of Riley" met in the summer of 1917, and among the suggestions they considered was one by Lafayette Page, an IUSM otolaryngology faculty member, who urged the group to establish a children's hospital in Riley's name. The self-named Riley Memorial Committee unanimously agreed "that the endowment of a children's hospital would be the most fitting tribute that could be paid to the man whose genius created 'Little Orphan Annie,' and 'The Raggedy Man.'" Near the end of August 1917, the *Indianapolis News* reported that "definite steps toward . . . raising of money for an endowment of approximately $2,000,000" had already been taken.[85]

These men as well as the medical community were responding to a new consciousness about the state of child health across the country in the late nineteenth century. The perils of poverty, environment, and contagion were increasingly construed as a collective crisis to be resolved through a variety of responses from education and medicine to public health and eugenics. There was much reason for concern. In 1900, child mortality in the United States remained very high. More than 12 percent of all infants died before reaching their first birthday, and more than 18 percent died before age five. The Indiana State Board of Health reported that the infant mortality rate for white males was 10 percent, whereas 29 percent of African-American males died during their first year. Further evidence was found in physicals given to draftees during World War I, where more than one-fourth of the men were found unfit for military service, and physicians on draft boards traced many of the defects "to childhood malnutrition or to problems that should have been corrected in their youth."[86] Emerson was a member of the Indiana Committee on Mental Defectives, established in 1916 as part of the state's eugenics efforts, and it reported that "approximately 3 per cent of the school population is definitely feebleminded in varying degrees and another 3 per cent is borderline in intelligence (sub-normal)." Other reports found up to 20 percent were "slow" or "backward."[87]

Although there had been an earlier effort to care for children in 1895 when the Indianapolis Flower Mission opened the Eleanor Hospital for Sick Children, named for the deceased daughter of Colonel Eli Lilly, the thirteen-bed facility closed in 1909 when City Hospital opened a children's unit.[88] The Riley Memorial Committee recognized that a children's hospital with more resources was needed, and Indiana was not alone. Throughout the United States, health-care facilities dedicated to children were few. A 1914 Russell Sage Foundation study identified only ten pediatric hospitals and fourteen pediatric convalescence homes operating nationwide.[89] The Riley committee intended to provide an institution that would fit this description in "closest co-operation" with the IU School of Medicine, and this recognition of a public need intersected with a professional need in shaping the building project. For some time, pediatrics had been a weak area in the school's curriculum. Emerson repeatedly told Bryan and the trustees that Long Hospital was not caring for as many children as it should. "The demand from all over the State for space for children is more urgent," he said in 1917, "than in the case of all other groups of patients." Although City Hospital had a pediatric ward, Long Hospital had space for only ten cots to care for children who lived outside the state capital. As a result, pediatric patients were often scattered among the adult wards. Due to the lack of adequate facilities, Emerson reported that he could not recruit a head for the school's Department of Pediatrics. A separate children's hospital working closely with the school would enable the dean to attract a strong candidate to head the pediatrics department and to develop the area as a specialty for which the school could become well-known.[90]

Despite a promising start, construction of the children's hospital was soon deferred until the close of World War I; nor was the project immediately revived after the war. Many of the prominent citizens who had supported the project in 1917 had grown wary of the idea of erecting another hospital in connection with IUSM due to the less-than-generous attitude of the state legislature toward Long Hospital and the new medical school building. Nevertheless, the men who initiated the project wished to proceed "with a campaign of education to enlist the support of citizens living in every part of the state." Pledges of substantial support reportedly had already been received so that construction could proceed quickly as soon as the conflict ceased. In fact, some, including author and humorist George Ade and Indianapolis businessmen Louis C. Huesmann and Hugh McK. Landon, were the same men who had advanced credit to the school for the medical school building in 1918.[91]

In December 1920, the Riley Committee again began to hold formal meetings to investigate how to establish a pediatric hospital in the poet's honor. Within weeks, the group that soon incorporated to become the James Whitcomb Riley Memorial Association voted to work in partnership with the ISUM and the Indiana Child Welfare Association.[92] In late January 1921, representatives from the Riley Committee and the university conferred with Indiana Governor Warren T. McCray, who supported the hospital, although he requested that the committee work out "some plan for unified action" with the other organizations. The pediatric hospital's operation was to be supervised by the IU trustees, "with the Riley Memorial Association serving in an advisory capacity."[93]

The committee submitted a draft of the proposed bill to McCray, which was modeled after a law that established a children's hospital at the University of Iowa in 1917. The Riley Hospital legislation called for "an appropriation of $250,000 to construct the hospital, $150,000 a year for two years for maintenance and equipment, and $50,000 a year thereafter for maintenance." Because lawmakers believed that "nothing could have greater effect in insuring a better citizenship than . . . an institution such as the one provided for in the [Riley Hospital] bill," the measure passed both houses of the legislature with only five dissenting votes. Although in the process the lawmakers cut the appropriation in half, the responsive chord it struck is exemplified by Representative Chester A. Davis, of Jay County, who only two years earlier had been vehemently opposed to providing a maintenance fund for Long Hospital but now sponsored the bill. "This hospital is not being established at the behest of physicians," Chester declared when he explained the measure. "It is purely a memorial to the revered Hoosier who devoted so much of his time and his efforts toward pleasing the little ones. The children need the hospital. Considering the benefits to be derived from its establishment, the state is being put to little expense."[94]

Indiana University officials were disappointed in the reduction of the requested state appropriations, but they thought it would be better to make a start on the project. To solve this problem, the Riley Committee members declared that they would raise $250,000 to begin construction.[95] They also resolved that the hospital should be "constructed and managed by a committee having equal representation from IU and the Riley Association." University officials had no objection to such a joint executive committee due to the wording of the state statute that placed the "ultimate authority in the board of trustees." The Riley Memorial Association was officially created on April 9, 1921. Bryan and Fesler, who had become president of the trustees in 1919, "welcomed the fullest cooperation of the Riley Memorial Association in the entire undertaking of raising funds and making plans for the hospital." Bryan told Samuel E. Smith, "It is surely a red-letter day for us to be able to begin at once the erection of the Hospital for $375,000."[96]

The Joint Executive Committee met weekly throughout 1921. They quickly hired as project architect Robert Frost Daggett, son of the designer of Long Hospital, and then they traveled to visit other children's hospitals.[97] Next, after inspecting sites adjacent to Long Hospital, the committee decided to build Riley Hospital on land located just northwest of the existing medical school buildings. Following some difficult negotiations, the association also convinced the City of Indianapolis to purchase land east of the Riley Hospital site for a convalescent park.[98]

The university was encouraged by the Riley Memorial Association's agreement to make up the funding shortfall created by the legislature, in fact so much so that once they received these assurances, the IU trustees on the Joint Executive Committee asked them to consider underwriting part of a larger project for the development of the campus. This plan had been proposed in 1920 by the Committee on University Interests, chaired by Myers, which studied Indiana University's future physical needs in Indianapolis as well as Bloomington. Its members concluded that ideally, within the next decade, ten new buildings should be added in Indianapolis to meet the increasing demands of the medical school, including a large general hospital, a medical laboratory, a nurses' dormitory, and a psychiatric hospital, in addition to the children's hospital. The estimated cost of this expansion in Indianapolis alone totaled over $3 million. Among the projects in the Joint Executive Committee's report that the Riley Memorial Association was asked to support was a pediatric orthopedic clinic, designed to care for children with clubfoot, cleft palate, and curvature of the spine. At that time, children with these conditions required several months convalescence. The committee anticipated that Riley Hospital would care for a large number of orthopedic patients, but adequate provisions had not been made for their convalescence period. The Riley Memorial Association agreed to incorporate a special building for convalescents and a nurses' home in the overall plan for the Riley Hospital complex to make IUSM competitive with other states.[99] Thus, almost from the start, the philanthropic support for the children's hospital was changed from a one-time construction fund-raising effort to what proved to be an organization that provided ongoing support for the hospital and pediatrics as the field and the medical school grew.

The school broke ground on July 11, 1922, with architect Daggett estimating that the entire Riley project's cost could reach nearly $2 million and take several years. The first building alone would cost approximately $500,000 to construct and equip.[100] To raise the overall sum needed, the Riley Memorial Association planned a statewide campaign that followed the model used for fundraising during World War I. The committee set fund-raising quotas for each county to help all Hoosiers see the hospital as a state resource. The committee assigned the largest quota of $700,000 to Marion County and Indianapolis, with fifty Indianapolis businessmen pledged to make significant contributions. Wealthy individuals like George A. Ball of the Ball Corporation in Muncie and Frederick M. Ayres of the L. S. Ayres department store in Indianapolis made substantial contributions to the hospital fund. Indiana service clubs and fraternal organizations such as the Junior League, Rotary, Kiwanis, Kappa Kappa Kappa, and Psi Iota Psi also named the hospital as their major charity. School children also participated, raising over $17,000 "on behalf of their less fortunate peers."[101] By the time the building campaign ended and the hospital opened in 1924,

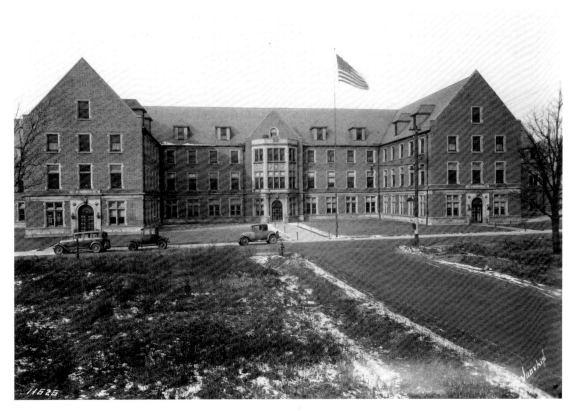

Figure 4.8. Riley Hospital, 1925. IUPUI image UA024_004150.

more than forty-four thousand Hoosiers had contributed. The *New York Times* estimated that this amounted to "one person in every hundred" Indiana residents.[102]

However, not everyone was enthusiastic about Riley Hospital. Some people complained about the additional expenditures that taxpayers would have pay to support the new institution. The Riley Committee also heard objections from Indianapolis doctors who were concerned with another "free hospital" cutting into their practices. More specifically, physicians feared that Riley Hospital would attract patients away and force them to provide medical care at bargain prices, thus tending "to pauperize communities." They identified the hospital as "another link in the chain of evidence which show[ed] the drift toward socializing medicine." Other objections came from physicians outside of Indianapolis, who feared that Riley Hospital would help only the capital and "feather the nests of a very few medical men, at the expense of the rank and file of the medical profession of the state."[103] This concentration of resources at the emerging medical center in the state's largest city was another example of the long-term consequences of the creation of the medical school in Indianapolis.

In response to these criticisms from the medical profession, the Joint Committee directed Judge Ira Batman to explain the terms of the 1921 law that created the hospital for the public. Batman made it clear that the law dictated that only those children who suffered from a disease, defect, or deformity that could be benefited by treatment in Riley Hospital "and whose parent or legal guardian [was] not financially able to defray the necessary costs of such treatment" were entitled to admission. The Joint Committee also directed that all publicity refer to Riley as a "hospital for poor children," and Emerson wrote a letter to members of the Indiana medical profession emphasizing that Riley Hospital would not be in conflict with local community hospitals because the new institution would care for patients that private physicians "could not handle to advantage."[104]

Riley Hospital was dedicated on the anniversary of its namesake's birth, October 7, 1924, and the hospital officially opened and admitted its first patient a little more than one month later on November 19, 1924.[105] During its first year of operation, twelve hundred children from eighty of Indiana's ninety-two counties were treated in Riley Hospital. The average age of these patients was nine years, and most were admitted due to orthopedic problems or accidental injuries. Many of them suffered from polio, tuberculosis, chronic tonsillitis, and malnutrition. By September 1925, a waiting list for admission existed, demonstrating the need for additions to the facility.[106] John H. Oliver, Lafayette Page, and John F. Barnhill were appointed to direct the medical and surgical services of the facility, and eight recent graduates of the IU School of Medicine were appointed as residents in the new pediatric hospital, two of whom were women.[107] In another case of some priorities of the medical school (in this case, hiring of full-time faculty) lagging behind others (in this case, construction of facilities), the School of Medicine was unable to attract a full-time pediatrician to direct this first-class children's hospital for another seven years, when Lyman T. Meiks was hired in the fall of 1931.[108]

Coleman Hospital for Women

The third hospital built in the years following the establishment of IU's Medical School in Indianapolis served the need for obstetric services. Emerson ranked this lower than other needs such as an expanded children's clinic, orthopedic surgery, and psychiatry, but once again the preference of donors changed the school's priorities. As was the case with Long and Riley hospitals, the construction of Coleman Hospital for Women was made possible by a philanthropic gift combined with the reluctant but eventual support from the Indiana state legislature. Part of the reason for the lower priority was that the provision of obstetric care was bound up with broader social attitudes regarding sex, birth, and marriage, plus the medical profession's ongoing efforts to extend medical authority over the birth process. By the late 1920s, obstetrics was contested ground—both over notions of morality and the medicalization of childbirth and motherhood.

The typical practice at the time was for medical school physicians and students to attend home births, also called the "outdoor obstetrical service." Long Hospital had a small obstetrical department, but it had become so overcrowded by 1923 that it was one of the main reasons the New York Board of Regents refused reciprocal registration to the graduates of the IU Training School for Nurses. In response to this criticism, the Educational Committee recommended that Cottage Number One, the nurses' dormitory located just to the west of Long Hospital, should be adapted and expanded for "the care of obstetrical cases and the teaching of medical students and student nurses." Although Emerson feared that Cottage Number One would "not be a very satisfactory department for obstetrics," he thought that it would be "good enough" and would "certainly serve as an invitation to somebody to give . . . a new building."[109]

Another reason for the relative neglect of obstetrics was that it was seen as an easier subject to teach—that is, it typically did not require hospital admission. "Outdoor obstetrics" was, in fact, how Emerson himself had learned the practice in Baltimore, and it became a rite of passage for several generations of IUSM students. During the first half of the 1920s, juniors and seniors spent three weeks in obstetrics training, during which time they were required to attend a minimum of nine obstetric cases in the home. Most of these deliveries were carried out in residences close to campus on the west side of Indianapolis; and many of the mothers and babies were African Americans. The underlying reason for this practice was that pregnant women and their families viewed the home as the right place for childbirth. This meant that only unsupported or desperate expectant mothers would make use of a lying-in hospital, and the association of this clientele with such a hospital meant, according to Emerson, "the legislature would naturally look with considerable criticism on a building erected for the care of young unmarried girls, and, of course, the majority of patients in a hospital obstetrics ward belong to this group."[110]

The establishment of a lying-in hospital for the university was made possible by a gift from the third major donor for a hospital in ten years.

In December 1924, Indianapolis businessman William H. Coleman, along with his wife, proposed a donation of $250,000 for construction of a hospital in memory of his stepdaughter, Suemma Coleman Atkins, who had died of complications connected to her pregnancy. William Coleman was born in Pennsylvania and moved to Indianapolis in 1880, where he started a large lumber business. Because of the fate of their daughter, the Colemans were eager to help prevent such maternal deaths. They favored a hospital connected to Indiana University because as a teaching hospital, it would help train physicians and nurses "who would carry [its] beneficent influence . . . throughout the state and nation." Similar to the contingencies attached to previous major donations, the trustees voted to accept this gift on the condition that the legislature provide sufficient maintenance funds.[111]

In a conference with Bryan and other university officials, Indiana Governor Emmett F. Branch and Governor-elect Edward L. Jackson approved Coleman's generous proposal. University officials also met with the chairman of the Legislative Visiting Committee, Senator Robert L. Moorehead, who assured them that the legislature would provide "the necessary maintenance fund." Despite these assurances, as had happened with previous promises of funding for the medical school, the 1925 Indiana General Assembly was not very quick to support the operation of another hospital. State Representative Russell V. Duncan, of Marion County, introduced a bill to accept the gift, which included $75,000 in annual maintenance to the new hospital, but this bill never reached the floor of the House. Many legislators were reluctant to fund an institution that they perceived, as Emerson rightly predicted, would be used to care for pregnant, unmarried girls. Evidence that the university and medical school had reached the limit of what the legislators would support is the fact that they also refused to consider a bill that would have provided for a psychiatric hospital on the IU School of Medicine campus. Even more threatening, they froze appropriations for the maintenance of Long and Riley Hospitals and made no provisions to cover expenses for any increases in enrollment either in Bloomington or Indianapolis. Due to this retrenched fiscal policy, Bryan and the trustees expected the next two years to be difficult ones.[112]

Despite being disappointed by the legislature, university officials were determined to find a way to build the women's hospital. Provost Smith met with Governor Edward L. Jackson and members of the Budget Advisory Committee to secure an agreement that the 1927 legislature would recommend annual appropriations of at least $50,000 for Coleman Hospital. Smith explained that "with such an assurance," Coleman would make a gift to Indiana University that would allow it to start building the hospital at once. In accord with the Budget Advisory Committee, Jackson promised

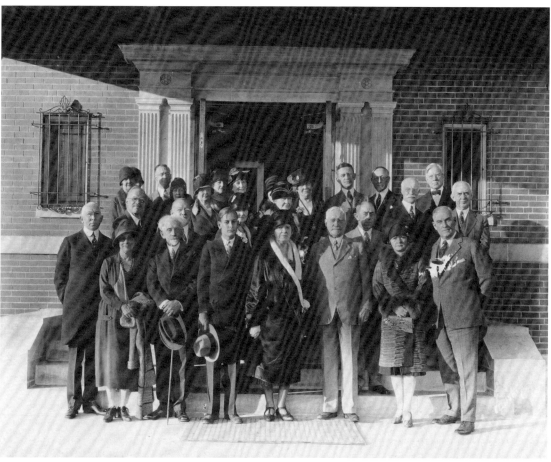

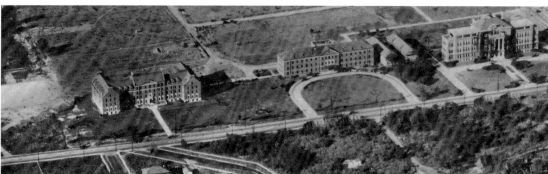

Figure 4.9a & b. Coleman Hospital dedication, 1927. (*Top*) Attached to photo: "Mrs. Miles Chapman, Dr. Burkhardt, Dr. Emerson, Rev. Dr. Taylor (First Baptist Church), Daughter Ferguson, Jr. Ferguson, Coleman Atkins, Mrs. W. H. Coleman, William H. Coleman, Mrs. Atkins, Will Atkins, Will Fesler, S. Earp, Dr. [?] Milner," IUPUI Image UA024_001095; Aerial view of Coleman Hospital ca. 1931, (*bottom*) between Ball Residence and Long Hospital (second building from left), IUPUI Image UA024_002460.

that the recommendation for Coleman Hospital would "be properly presented to the next session of the General Assembly." The word of the governor was, indeed, enough for Coleman, who at the beginning of 1926 gave the university a piece of property to be sold, which he estimated to be worth $175,000. He also gave $75,000 in cash and securities so that preparations for constructing William H. Coleman Hospital could begin.[113]

In June 1926, the architect Daggett presented tentative plans for this hospital to the board of trustees. The building was designed to include sixty-four beds, exclusive of the nursery, with twenty-two in private rooms. Following the pattern in the other hospitals, the legislature eventually voted to support the operation of the new facility. By the time the hospital was dedicated on October 20, 1927, Coleman had donated over $300,000 to build it. It was described as "one of the best modern examples of a well arranged and equipped hospital for lying-in patients." Each year from 1927 to 1934, the department interns worked at Colman as well as outdoor obstetrical service and dispensaries included in the internship rotations.[114]

In subsequent years, the hospital came to replace the home as the site of childbirth in America. The building of the IU hospitals (particularly the construction of Coleman Hospital in 1927) was therefore well timed to accommodate this shift and usher in a new era for the Obstetrics Department. The size and number of procedures began to increase in 1937 and expanded greatly after World War II. The department also took the lead on social justice issues, including care for the poor, reducing the cost of health care, access to family planning services, and overall women's health. The Coleman Hospital remained the university's women's hospital until 1973. During its forty-seven-year history, seventy thousand babies were born there. Over twenty-five hundred student nurses received their maternity training in the hospital, and all IU School of Medicine students between 1928 and 1973 "learned to do their first normal deliveries at Coleman." In 1979, obstetrics and gynecology services moved to the new University Hospital, and the Coleman building was adapted almost entirely for the use of the Division of Allied Health.[115]

Conclusion

In 1908, after half a dozen years of bitter rivalry about which university in Indiana would have charge of medical education, no one would have predicted what the Indiana University School of Medicine would look like twenty years later. Most expected a failure, like every other effort before it to affiliate private medical schools with colleges and universities. But by

1928, the medical school not only still existed but had also established a nationally recognized medical center just west of downtown Indianapolis and adjacent to City Hospital, with a new classroom building, a nurse training school, and three new hospitals. In addition to the perseverance of IU President Bryan, this success can also be attributed to his selection of a dean familiar with the leading reforms of medical education in the country, as well as some judicious compromises that avoided controversies about location of instruction and speed of replacement of faculty from the proprietary schools. Perhaps most important and surprising was the extent of support from private philanthropy, which helped obtain grudging but crucial additional funding from the state of Indiana in support of the medical school and especially its hospitals.

Yet within a few years, Emerson was out. The next chapter, after examining the operations of the school from the viewpoint of the students and faculty, will show how the new hospitals and postponed decisions about faculty became a source of disagreement between the president and dean. The end result of this led to the dean relinquishing his position in 1932.

5

New Medical Education, 1912–1932

In its first twenty years, the IU School of Medicine replaced half a dozen proprietary schools in the state, built a new medical building for instruction, and constructed three new hospitals to enhance clinical care and instruction. In the process, it created a new medical center on the west side of Indianapolis. The new university-based medical school in Bloomington and Indianapolis enforced tough entrance requirements, although its evolution into an institution that employed full-time faculty committed to research and teaching took much longer to complete.

The pedagogical rationale for the establishment of three university hospitals by the IUSM was to provide a suitable variety of patients for clinical instructions of students. One of the earliest calls for such an arrangement was by French Enlightenment physician Philippe Pinel, who is better known for his reforms in the humane care of patients in mental asylums.[1] It was new German medical schools that adopted this practice during the nineteenth century and in turn provided the model for American medical education reform. These hospitals could be constructed in Indiana only thanks to funding from the state and private donors, which in turn obligated the university to provide more and better hospital care for the citizens of the state. The result, as part of the previous chapter showed, was to divert attention away from, if not overshadow, the medical school's concern with teaching. This chapter looks more closely at students and faculty during this period of establishing the medical center while Charles Emerson was dean. Then it returns to how the growing responsibilities of hospital care and administration led to increased disputes between the dean and his faculty that were contentious enough to strain relations between President Bryan and the dean, such that Emerson was involuntarily replaced.

Students and Faculty

Having access to university teaching hospitals was crucial to accommodating growth in enrollment in Indianapolis. By the fall of 1914, after the change in requirements temporarily reduced admissions, the number of students registered in the last three years of medical school stood at just over one hundred students, an increase of 15 percent from the previous year.[2] Walter Daly has written an unpublished paper analyzing the nature of medical education from records for the years 1914–15.[3] The curriculum for these students, which was developed by the faculty who remained from the

Table 5.1. Summary of Time in Class by Year in Medical School, 1914–1915

	Lecture	Laboratory	Clinics	Total
Freshman Year				
Anatomy	63	597		660
Physiology	90	170		260
Chemistry	60	120		180
Total	**213**	**887**		**1,100**
Sophmore Year				
Pathology and Bacteriology	146	480		626
Pharmacology, Materia Medica, and Toxicology	73	172		245
Applied Anatomy	33			33
Clinical Pathology	33	77		110
Physical Diagnosis	11	55		66
Topographical Anatomy	55			55
Total	**351**	**784**		**1,135**
Junior Year				
Pathology	22			22
Therapeutics	66			66
Medicine	242	132	276	650
Surgery	142	107	210	437
Obstetrics and Gynecology	77	18	84	77
Dermatology and Syphilology	22			22
Total	**571**	**239**	**486**	**1,296**
Senior Year				
Medicine	176	24	365	565
Surgery	176	20	163	437
Obstetrics and Gynecology	66	18	84	168
Eye, Ear, Nose and Throat	55		90	145
Dermatology	11		49	60
Therapeutics			33	33
Total	**484**	**62**	**784**	**1,330**

Source: Daly, "Essay on Medical Education: Historical Perspective."

proprietary schools plus new leadership, was typical of US medical schools adopting reforms at the beginning of the twentieth century.

Coursework was heavy on lectures and anatomy. Table 5.1 also shows that typical of the reformed curriculum, laboratory and science instruction was in the first two years, and direct patient care was in the third and fourth years, largely in the outpatient clinics and "outdoor obstetrics." Class time included conventional professorial lectures and smaller, professor-led discussion groups. According to Daly, the students' time was fully occupied with scheduled activities—something that made their heavy moonlighting obligations, necessary for income to live on, all the more remarkable.

The guiding principle of the reform curriculum was to expand laboratory and clinical experiences to replace didactic teaching, but from the students' perspective, the change was not appreciated as much as the medical school faculty and administration hoped. Reflecting back, William Day, who matriculated in 1923, described the first year as "purely didactic." He remembered that it was not until his junior year that students got any practical experience, and then it was a "smattering of clinical work, but nothing like they do today." Durand Paris, a student in the 1930s, began clinics only in his senior year. Edith Schuman, who matriculated in the late 1920s, recalled that she did have clinical work in both her junior and senior years, but she felt that she only got realistic experience once she began her internship.[4] Despite these complaints, students experienced very personal contact with a number of professors quite attuned to contemporary educational methods and dedicated to teaching.

Although there were a few "full-time" appointments as called for by Flexner-inspired reforms—and they taught as much as thirty hours per week—faculty from the old proprietary schools continued to be important in regular teaching despite their private consulting practices at downtown Indianapolis offices. The classes in medicine, which took up almost half of the third and fourth years, were under the charge of Dean Emerson, George Bond, and Frank Wynn. Surgical teaching, about one-third of the last two years of instruction, was supervised by John Oliver and Willis Gatch, who also directed an animal laboratory that furnished specimens for surgical instruction. Because of his interest in the clinical laboratory, Emerson taught the course in Methods and Interpretation while Bond taught Physical Diagnosis, both of which took advantage of the new Medical Building.[5]

Gross anatomy and cadaver dissection were hallmarks of the beginning year. As one medical student put it, "Well, it's a little hard to adjust to the dead bodies and the smell [of] the formaldehyde. I think all of the students, [at least] some of them, made them a little sick. And of course you don't

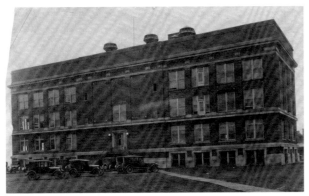
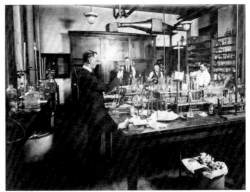
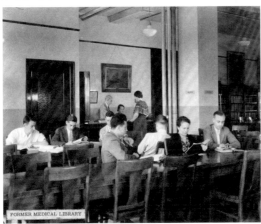
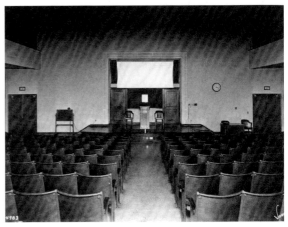

Figure 5.1a, b, c, & d. Medical Building (now Emerson Hall), featured in *Arbutus* (1919): 148: (*clockwise from top left*) first construction phase in 1924, before addition of auditorium, IUPUI image UA024_003751; laboratory scene, third floor (*far left*) Bernard B. Turner-Pathology, (*far right*) Rolla Harger, IUPUI image UA024_000416; medical library, IUPUI image UA024_001120; auditorium included in second phase, IUPUI image UA024_003753.

ever let on that you feel a little squeamish. Eventually you get used to it." Margaret M. Newhouse, who graduated in 1932, remembered some boys playing tricks on her by bringing a white mouse from the laboratory and turning it loose on the cadaver table. As the professor walked across the room, she grabbed the mouse, put it into her white coat pocket, and held it while he questioned them on what they were doing, which prevented her from acknowledging the prank. In the 1920s, third- and fourth-year medical students divided their time between medical and surgical clinics in Long Hospital, City Hospital, and the City Dispensary, devoting most of their time to surgery, internal medicine, gynecology, pediatrics, obstetrics, and psychiatry. A smaller amount of time was dedicated to such clinical specialties as urology, neurology, ophthalmology, anesthesiology, and orthopedics.[6]

Often lost in the narratives celebrating the arrival of modern scientific medical education were some new barriers that came with the effort to improve it. Part of that change was the reduction of the total number of positions available in American medical schools in the early twentieth century following the Flexner report. As the number of positions declined, the number of students entering American medical education from underrepresented groups such as women and blacks was also reduced. The higher standards and restrictions on admission resulted in far fewer, less socially and economically diverse physicians being graduated from medical school, even if they were "better trained."[7] In Indiana, this problem had first occurred when the proprietary schools merged with Indiana University. In its last years, Indiana Medical College graduated 82 students in 1904 and 126 in 1906, whereas only 35 students graduated from IUSM in 1915. After 1920, however, there was a steady growth in the number of graduates from a few over 50 in 1923 to over 100 in 1931.[8]

After the shift of all first-year medical students to Bloomington, Burton Myers was responsible for selecting students for admission to the school for the next thirty years. Students' transcript records contain admission requirement checklists of high school graduation proof of and at least two years of college with premedical coursework credits in general chemistry, physics, biology, embryology, English, foreign language, and mathematics. Only course credits were evaluated, not grades. Myers's requirements paralleled the Indiana State Board of Medical Registration and the Association of American Medical Colleges as they then existed. He vigorously tried to recruit promising undergraduates and persuade the uncommitted to enter medical school to fill the classes, as opposed to selecting from many applications.[9]

The number of students in the medical school varied quite a bit in the first ten years as both students and faculty from the proprietary schools were integrated into the new medical school. There were always a few women and black men admitted to IUSM, but a handful at most at any given time in the first half of the 1900s. Daly found no women or blacks in the entering classes of 1914 and 1915, but four women were admitted in 1916. One African-American student had already been admitted and graduated in 1919. From 1914 to 1923, there were a total of eleven female and six African-American graduates from IUSM.[10]

From the records of the over ninety IU medical school students in the 1914 and 1915 admissions, table 5.2 provides a profile of some of their

Table 5.2. Cohort Profile, IUSM Admissions, 1914 and 1915 Combined

Admitted	94
Indiana residents	90
Taught public school before medical school	17
Transferred to other medical schools	12
Dropped from medical school	11
Graduated on time	54

Source: Daly, "Essay on Medical Education: Historical Perspective."

background and medical education experience.

Students who matriculated at IUSM in those years were in classes of forty-eight and forty-six students, respectively. Barely a majority of those ninety-four students graduated in four years. Twelve transferred to another medical school, and records show, in Daly's terms, they were "among the best of their class."[11] Eleven dropped out completely, nine graduated late, and eight had to repeat a year. These were perhaps not quite the stellar statistics that the IUSM hoped for five years after taking over the two proprietary medical schools and raising standards for admission, but fifty-four students did graduate and become doctors.[12]

Doctors who attended IUSM the following decade later recalled the hard work they put into medical school. Durward W. Paris remembered that he spent all his time studying. Edith Schuman also recalled, "There was no relaxation. There was no play. Every minute went into memorizing what you had to know. And of course, in those days we had to learn *Gray's Anatomy*, that great big book, almost by heart." Professors questioned students in class, although Indiana physician George W. Macy found the faculty to be friendly and approachable. However, Medical school archives contain several petitions signed by students asking for changes in class work, most often requesting more direct patient contact. On at least one occasion, in 1918, the discontent exploded when a group of medical students "smashed furniture and broke windows." The cause was not reported, but it coincided with complaints about Indiana Health commissioner and faculty member John Hurty, who gave only Cs and Ds in his hygiene (public health) class that year. In contrast to Hurty's reputation, Myers was described as a "fair and good teacher and a good doctor," although others recalled that Myers frequently reminded them of his medical training in Germany. Despite the long hours spent studying for medical school and extra hours of employment, medical students always found some room for fun. George W. Macy, entering the class of 1928, said that, "It was an annual practice for the whole class to quit medical school and go down to the Burleyque" (a burlesque theater) once each year.[13]

As mentioned previously, medical students often worked at outside jobs. Tuition in 1914 and 1915 amounted to $100 each for the freshman and sophomore years, rising to $130 each for the junior and senior years. By

1927, tuition had increased to $150 per year. The *School Bulletin* outlined living expenses as five dollars each week in Bloomington and nine dollars in Indianapolis. Ten one-year scholarships of $100 were available each year. Students also often worked to save money before starting medical school. As table 5.2 shows, of the ninety-four students admitted in the 1914 and 1915 years, seventeen had taught in public schools before entering medical school—one as long as nine years. Daly cites a 1917–18 medical school survey that reported 84 percent of students engaged in outside work. One example was Thurman Rice, an IUSM graduate who went on to become chair of the Pathology Department and an officer of the Indiana State Board of Health. Rice taught in public schools for six years prior to entering medical school in 1917, and thereafter he worked as a laboratory assistant to help pay his expenses.[14]

The medical school received other complaints related to the cost of tuition from students during the 1924–25 school year, many of whom challenged the out-of-state tuition and fees they were charged, arguing that they should be considered in-state students. They claimed that they lived in Indiana prior to matriculation and had not been alerted to the extra fees prior to the start of school. As an example of how strictly the school interpreted the matter of residency, one student pointed out, "I enlisted in the United States Army from Madison, Indiana, as my honorable discharge shows. The state of Indiana considers me as one of her soldiers; I hope that Indiana University can consider me as one of her residents." It took a formal vote by the Finance Committee for him to be reclassified as an in-state resident.[15]

The Great Depression brought hardship for all the medical students. Edith Schuman recalled that often one student would purchase a course textbook, and several students would share it. Sometimes the students would simply take very good class notes and skip buying the textbook altogether. Students worked even more in outside jobs during the Great Depression in order to attend medical school. In fact, Schuman reported, "My whole class in medical school worked during the Depression, so much so that Dean Gatch made a ruling soon after our class [graduated] that [students] couldn't work as much as we did."[16]

In addition to teaching in the public schools, the outside work of medical students (ranging from ten to seventy hours per week but averaging twenty-five) was at a variety of venues, including restaurant wait staff and work in doctors' offices, laboratories, and drug stores. Many reported employment in the undertaking field. Some had paper routes, and others reported doing clerical work, playing music, working for the telephone company and the police station, and officiating at football matches. One

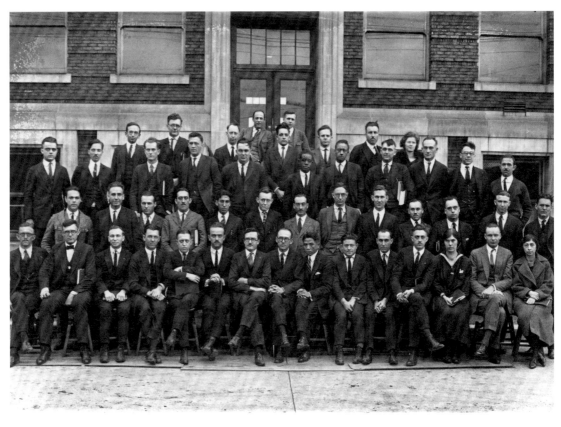

Figure 5.2. School of Medicine graduating class of 1924. IUPUI image UA024_000269.
In front of Emerson Hall before 1928 addition. Note three female and likely at least two black male students.

enterprising student bragged (or complained) that he did canvassing, managed Indianapolis' Riverside amusement park, was a deputy assessor, and worked at the post office while attending medical school.[17]

The views of the male students about the few women were mixed. One male student in the 1920s recalled that medical students thought that their fellow female medical students were "old hens," and the men "didn't see how they'd ever become doctors." On the other hand, Frank P. Albertson, who matriculated in 1930, stated of his fellow female medical students, "Oh, we treated them well. I more or less felt like they were my sisters." Edith Schuman's recollections were similar: "We weren't, I wasn't aware, honest to goodness, I wasn't aware of being treated in any special way except in the way Dr. Myers picked on me." The reason Dr. Myers "picked on" Edith Schuman, as she recalled, was to explain the definitions of the medical vocabulary because her Latin was so much better than her fellow students.[18]

Other women who enrolled described varying levels of discrimination and harassment from male colleagues and faculty. Mary Keller Ade, who graduated in 1932, recalled, "The girls were harassed some. Mostly being made fun of or they [male students] tried to make us feel that we could [not] take it . . . particularly in anatomy class. They got a bit rough sometimes." She continued, "Well, they were just teasing us that we might faint or that we might [drop out]." Whatever the level of teasing or harassment, women had to be resilient because there was little recourse if they complained. They feared the faculty might think that they could not handle the pressure of medical school or the rigors of being a physician. However, women did find acceptance from some students and faculty. Newhouse reported a story of a blue book exam, where she finished first. Her professor's response was, "That's the reason we have let women in medical school." She earned an A on the test.[19]

Naomi Dalton also attended medical school in the early 1930s and recalled that her father was very supportive of her decision and career. She never felt any harassment from fellow students or professors. However, she did remember a situation when she was a senior, and a male junior was paired with her during outdoor obstetrics. "I had a junior man who was very upset because he was junior to a woman. And at first he just didn't like it." Ade worked closely with the male students, such as those working in her pharmacology laboratory group, who "were very kind and helpful and considerate and never condescending in any way." Ade also fondly recalled the support offered by women doctors at the time she was a student. Ade stated, "And I remember the few women doctors who were practicing in Indianapolis did sort of take us under their wing and they had [deletion] a girls' medical sorority which we all belonged to."[20]

In addition to the four years of medical school, graduate medical education in the United States also changed greatly during this period thanks to hospital expansion, the rise of medical specialization, and changes in the medical licensure procedures. Although they share some similarities, the graduate and undergraduate experiences differed in a number of ways. For example, unlike undergraduate medical education, which was on its way to becoming controlled by universities when the Flexner report accelerated the process, graduate medical education was not widespread enough to be included in Flexner's study. Moreover, it involved complicated and conflicting relationships between hospitals, specialty and licensing boards, national regulators, and universities. At first, during the initial decades of the twentieth century, hospitals and universities generally referred to those doing professional training after medical school as house officers. Over time, the first clinical year after graduation was increasingly called an internship, which was followed by a two- to three-year residency to obtain specialist certification. Various fellowships and subspecialty residencies could extend this training period to more than a decade.[21]

Interns and residents occupied a precarious position as both doctors who had graduated from medical school and students continuing their specialized education.[22] Most of the graduates from the 1918–19 IUSM classes served internships, the largest number at the Indianapolis City Hospital, and six at the new Robert Long Hospital.[23] The program grew in the 1920s with expansion of the academic medical center and bears the imprint of many influences—universities, professional associations, state and federal governments, and the residents themselves.

These early internships were intended to prepare doctors for general practice. With the growth of new facilities and full-time faculty, however, opportunities expanded for residents to staff these services. For example, the obstetrics residency program began in 1927 with one or two residents per year, covering Coleman, Long, and the City Dispensaries services. By 1927, the graduating class of 110 competed for twenty-seven local internships increasingly viewed as necessary for training, although not yet required at this point. Histories of residency describe many challenges, but the subsequent careers of residents demonstrate that close faculty relationships led to successful and productive practice. Several IUSM residents became leaders in their fields. Among these was a president of the Central Society for Clinical Records, a president of the American Heart Association, a master of the American College of Physicians, and a member of the Association of American Physicians.[24]

The growth of undergraduate and graduate medical education, plus the addition of new hospitals and faculty, meant that the administration of departments in the medical school became increasingly important, with department chairs exercising greater control over many operations of the school. After the merger of the medical schools to form IUSM, the original departments of Anatomy, Physiology, Medicine, and Pathology expanded to include the clinical departments of Obstetrics/Gynecology, Ophthalmology, Surgery, Urology, and Otolaryngology. The university added the departments of Microbiology and Pharmacology & Toxicology in 1915 based on the increasing importance of testing and pharmaceuticals in patient care. Table 5.3 shows the change in number of faculty members by department from 1915 to 1932.

Table 5.3. Faculty, Instructors, and Assistants, 1915 and 1932

	Faculty, Instructors, and Assistants 1915	Faculty, Instructors, and Assistants 1931–32
Anatomy	3	8
Physiology	2	7
Cardiovasuclar—Renal Disease		5
Chemistry	2	7
General Inderdepartmental Laboratory		8
Pathology and Bacteriology	4 (New department)	
Pharmacology, Materia Medica, Theraputics	4 (New Department)	5 (Biochemistry & Phamacology)
Medicine	32	40 (Dispensery, Radiology, Anaesthiology)
Surgery	27	28
Obstetrics	5	10
Pediatrics	5*	15 (separate department)
Mental and Mervous Disease	7*	12 (separate department)
Gynecology	8	Division of Surgery
Genitourinary Surgery	8	10
Rhinology, Otology, Largology (1909)	8*	23
Opthamology	5	12
Dematology	4*	8 (Dermatology and Syphilis)
Total	**124**	**205**

* Subdepartment or division
Source: School of Medicine, Indiana University, Bulletin, 1915–16 and 1931–32.

Adding to the complexity from this growth, by the 1920s, the interests of increasing professional organizations and specialization led to debates within the departments over their control of certain fields. Table 5.3 reflects numerous examples of these changes, but one of the most controversial of these was the unit that Dean Emerson viewed as the School of Medicine's greatest asset, the Social Services Department. As mentioned in the previous chapter, its work grew rapidly, and so did its budget, but for a number of reasons, Bryan kept it organizationally under the Economics and Sociology Department in Bloomington. This was despite all the work being done at the hospitals and medical school in Indianapolis, with office space plus salaries initially paid from Emerson's budget. By 1921–22, its budget had grown to $14,000, and in 1929–30 it was over $17,000.[25] The following year, Emerson requested an additional $6,000 for a Bureau of Social Research. This was part of the dean's plan to pursue the research on the causes of alcoholism that he had begun at his prior post as superintendent of Clifton Springs Sanatorium. He viewed this research as an essential part of medicine that, if pursued rigorously, could offer benefits on a par with laboratory research.[26] In reporting and requesting funds, however, Emerson's efforts were seen to be in direct competition with the goals of faculty who followed the much more traditional approach to medicine that focused on the patient and on the cause and cure for specific diseases. Moreover, as a newly established medical school, Emerson's institution was in great need of funding basic infrastructure—something that places like Harvard and Johns Hopkins already possessed.[27] As described below, these conflicting goals were at the root of the controversy that eventually led to Emerson's departure.

Emerson's unusual interest in research is noteworthy because it reflects the relative lack of such activity at the medical school. This is not surprising because, like most other US medical schools at the time, teaching and clinical care were the institution's primary responsibilities. As a result, funds for research were very limited. To the extent they existed, as had been the case with the new hospitals, private philanthropy stepped in to provide support but on a much smaller scale. In 1925, Eli Lilly contributed the first outside research funds to the school, designating $1,200 annually for this purpose for a five-year period. During 1925–26, these funds were used to employ Harold M. Trusler, a top graduate of the class of 1924, as a research fellow to aid Gatch in his surgical investigations.[28] In October 1926, after the death of Indianapolis businessman Louis C. Huesmann, the Riley Memorial Association established a fund in his memory to support research. By 1932, with these funds in place, the IU School of Medicine still had only $18,000 available annually for research purposes, mostly in the area of pediatrics.[29]

Disagreements and the Retirement of Emerson

Emerson had been Bryan's man since the president had brought him to Indiana in 1911, and together they accomplished a great deal. This included the construction of hospitals and a new medical instruction building that became the core of a modern medical center quite different from the proprietary schools that the university took over. The two men had their differences, including one that was very personal when, in 1920, Bryan's wife, Charlotte, became sick with a "nervous condition." In fact, she became so ill that Bryan decided to take her to Clifton Springs Sanitorium in New York, where Emerson had been superintendent between 1908 and 1911. Bryan and Charlotte stopped overnight at the Fletcher Sanitarium in Indianapolis, where they saw Emerson, who told Bryan that because of her condition, Clifton Springs would not admit Charlotte. Instead, she should remain at the Fletcher Sanitarium. Bryan left her there for two months in the care of an inexperienced guardian, and Charlotte rapidly grew worse. Finally, according to Bryan and much to his horror, Emerson "gave her case a frightening name, said that she was incurable, and that she must spend the rest of her life" in a mental institution.[30] In defiance, Bryan brought Charlotte home, "where Dr. E[merson] said she could not remain three days." Instead, she "grew better with astonishing rapidity." About one month later, Bryan and his wife met Emerson at the Claypool Hotel in downtown Indianapolis. Emerson was "dumbfounded." He later recalled that "He then contritely confessed that [his] diagnosis & treatment had been 'tragically wrong.'" Due in great part to Bryan's attentive care, Charlotte remained at home until she died in August 1948. "Whatever I have done or failed to do in this world," Bryan later confessed, "I saved my wife from tragic death in spite of the doctor."[31]

Despite this unfortunate experience, throughout most of the rest of the decade, Bryan and Emerson continued to work together to expand and strengthen the medical school. By 1928, they had overseen the construction of what could legitimately be called a medical center on the west side of Indianapolis while fostering the growth of the medical school in both the state capital and Bloomington. Yet in the process, an increasingly strained relationship developed that led the university president to question the professional judgment of his dean. Emerson himself had also come to question the outcome of the building and growth process that now defined the life of the medical school. Originally, he saw the teaching hospitals as one aspect of a broader vision of medical education. Like so much of modern infrastructure, the availability of the hospital beds in an academic medical center served to create more demand for services and facilitated more calls to increase hospital capacity. Now the care and feeding of these facilities drove much of the school's decision making and priorities toward the more widespread and practical needs of obstetrics and pediatrics and away from other important fields of medical teaching and research.

Increasingly in the late 1920s, disputes arose over the operations of the hospitals and the needs of the growing departments in the medical school, all of which eventually caused Bryan to lose confidence in Emerson, whom he ultimately forced to retire as dean in 1931. The immediate roots of the break originated in a change in leadership in the Department of Surgery, one of the busiest and most prestigious departments. John H. Oliver had run the Department of Surgery since the establishment of the university medical school and oversaw the expansion of services into all

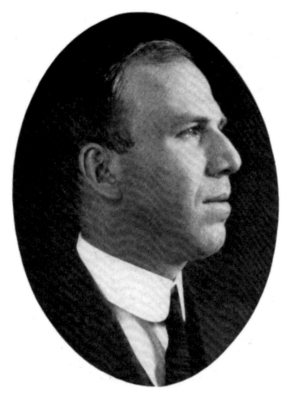

three of the new hospitals. Oliver's logical successor following the older surgeon's death in 1927 was Gatch, whom Emerson had personally recruited as an example of one of the first of the "new" faculty that the dean hoped to lead the new school. Gatch was an Indiana native who trained at Johns Hopkins University, where he completed a surgical residency with William S. Halsted. He later returned to IU in 1912 as a professor of surgery, also developing a large practice in the city. He was a pioneer in the use of nitrous oxide in anesthesia, had interest and did research in hypotensive shock, and worked to develop the adjustable bed that bears his name, the Gatch Bed.[32]

The dispute over Gatch becoming the new chair arose in part because of

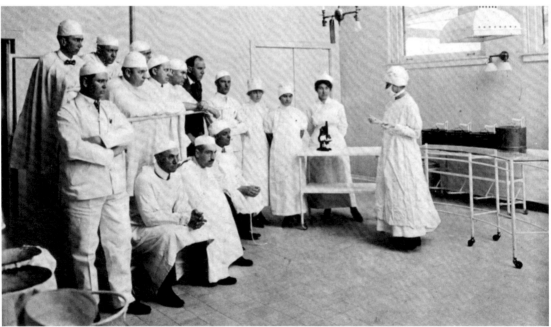

Figure 5.3a & b. (*top*) Professor of surgery Willis Gatch in 1916, shortly after Emerson recruited him to the medical school, *Arbutus* (1916): 292; (*bottom*) Gatch with students in surgical section of Long Hospital, *Arbutus* (1918): 210.

misunderstandings about the reorganization of the Department of Surgery. Oliver had been chairman of all of the surgical groups in the department, including at the time such areas as orthopedics, obstetrics, and gynecology. Following Oliver's death, Emerson wanted to create separate departments for each division, keeping only some areas such as gynecology, which he believed belonged in the realm of general surgery. According to Emerson's plan, Gatch would become head of the Department of General Surgery.[33]

Emerson's plan was taken by some university officials as reluctance to name Gatch as Oliver's successor in any capacity. University Provost Smith criticized Emerson for having "any doubts on the matter." Smith's attitude toward Emerson had always been colored by his sense that the board of trustees lacked full confidence in the medical school dean. Indeed, the trustees installed Smith as provost, in part because they perceived that Emerson could not handle the administration of the medical center as it became increasingly complex. Whatever the reason, Bryan told Emerson in a note he sent to the dean in December 1927 that he and the trustees saw objections to Gatch heading surgery as unwarranted.

> We are all of one mind that Dr. Gatch and no one else should be considered for this position. It was yourself who taught us in the first place to recognize in him one of the rising surgeons of the United States, and now as we all know he has risen. We do not know what objections you have to him and shall be glad to hear. We feel however that no matter who should be selected there would be objections from some quarters. We have no doubt of his [Gatch's] cooperative spirit and that he can and will add essential strength to your own work in the School of Medicine.[34]

Emerson agreed to recommend Gatch as Oliver's successor, but with the understanding that surgical obstetrics should maintain its independence.[35] Despite the fact that Smith immediately indicated his disagreement,[36] Emerson expressed surprise in February 1928 to learn that Gatch had been appointed head of the Department of Surgery and that this included obstetrics as well as gynecology and orthopedic surgery. "In effect," it made these areas "united into one single department." When Emerson presented his objections to Bryan, however, he chose not to focus on the organization and responsibilities but rather on the qualifications of Gatch, whom Emerson claimed had not "yet proven himself able to head even one small group. . . . Therefore, to enlarge this with the disorganized remnants of two other departments place[d] them in jeopardy." According to Emerson, some of the decisions Gatch had already made proved that he was not ready to handle his new responsibilities. Emerson also disapproved of some things Gatch did in his private practice, which the dean claimed only served to antagonize members of the local medical community. "Nobody can have a higher opinion of Dr. Gatch's personal qualities than can I," Emerson concluded, "but he has been unsuccessful in working with professional rivals in his own field."[37]

Emerson went one step further and exacerbated the situation when he asked Gatch to voluntarily give up some of the power and responsibilities the trustees had just given him. Emerson now naturally focused on the department reorganization rather than Gatch's qualifications, arguing that general surgery, orthopedic surgery, and gynecology should not have been "hooked up" as "practically one department" and that Gatch should be in charge of only general surgery. Gatch, who had been waiting to assume Oliver's position almost since the time he came back to Indiana in 1912, was personally insulted. The relationship between the dean and the surgeon was irreparably broken, which isolated Emerson further as the trustees and the president increasingly questioned his judgment.[38]

With confidence in Emerson on the wane, the dean of medicine found his decisions more frequently questioned about budget matters as the complexity and costs of the medical school hospitals increased by the end of the 1920s and the accompanying struggles over maintenance funds became more fraught.[39] Moreover, the financial emergency of the Great Depression beginning in late 1929 caused university officials to scrutinize Emerson's decisions even more closely, in particular the dean's continued insistence on maintaining the large budget of the Social Service Department. As mentioned earlier, the faculty, especially in the basic sciences, viewed the maintenance of Social Service as coming at the expense of the first two years of the school curriculum. This was despite the fact that the department was administered by the Economics and Sociology Department in Bloomington, and the budget came separately from the University General Fund.[40] Nonetheless, the fiscal reports were filed with the medical school and hospitals, and between 1921–22 and 1929–30, disbursements for the activities associated with this department grew from a little under $14,000 to almost $17,000 with an additional $8,000 to support a training course for social workers. In 1928–1929, the staff alone for Social Service in the hospitals included two faculty, six social workers, a secretary, and three stenographers.[41]

Despite being a separate budget coming directly from Bloomington, the increase in funding of Social Services was seen by medical faculty to be in stark contrast to the inadequate support for clinical medical education and hospitals in Indianapolis. This was especially the case for teaching of the first two years of basic sciences in the medical school program in both Indianapolis and Bloomington. Even before the budget constraints of the Great Depression, in June 1928, Emerson admitted that the second year was "in the greatest need of strengthening."[42] However, he never shifted enough money to the departments involved to make real improvements. As a result, the Departments of Pathology, Pharmacology, and Bacteriology remained understaffed. By 1930, the inadequacy of Owen Hall at IU Bloomington led to a serious problem accommodating the increases in class size (see table 5.4), resulting in severe overcrowding in teaching the first-year medical students.

Table 5.4. Admission of First-Year Students, IUSM, Selected Years, 1910–1933

Academic Year	Number of Students
1910–11	26
1915–16	45
1925–26	116
1930–31	134
1931–32	121
1932–33	125
1933–34	140

Source: Myers to Bryan, January 4, 1933; March 4, 1935, C286, InU-Ar.

"For some years," Myers warned Bryan, the school had received "more applications for matriculation . . . than the University of Illinois or the University of Chicago." He went on, "I worry about the unfavorable comment which I fear must arise from the further crowding of inadequate Owen Hall."[43]

These budget problems prompted Bryan to take concrete actions. First, having been made aware "that the first two years of medicine [were] in serious danger of injurious criticism from national authorities because . . . [of] inadequate support," Bryan once again turned to "cutting down less important services in [Emerson's] Social Service Department" so that more could be done for the parts of the curriculum that were "more essential." In 1931, after an outside reviewer stated that it would take a minimum of $50,000 a year to run the Social Service Department properly, the School of Medicine's Finance Committee decided it was unwilling to continue its operations in the same mode, suggesting a reorganization.[44]

The financial constraints of the 1930s and the decision to eliminate the Social Service Department thus brought to an end the tension that had existed since 1914 between supporting the social medicine model and funding the hospitals. It also ended Emerson's dream of a medical education where social medicine played a central role, although this was not exclusively an Indiana phenomenon. Social medicine and social service were increasingly viewed as only ancillary support for the main goals of modern American medical schools: to teach and do research on diagnosis and treatment of disease. No other medical school in America had a dean who had served so long and was so closely associated with social medicine. As a result, young faculty and trustees increasingly saw Emerson's views as outdated and outside the mainstream of academic medicine.[45]

Bryan took the final steps leading toward Emerson's departure in reaction to reports about his management of the hospitals. In June 1930, Fesler directed Bryan to investigate "the manner in which the hospitals [were] being administered with special reference to the attention given to patients and the general morale of the hospital." He was convinced that the university would "suffer incalculably unless radical changes" were made in the staff of Long Hospital "with as little delay as possible." This gave Gatch an opportunity to offer his view of Emerson's performance when he informed Fesler that the university hospitals were not managed well. He charged, for example, that forty-two nurses were on the payroll, "whereas half the number could do the work." In addition, the hospital administrator's office also had too many employees. Supposedly, fifteen women were doing work better done by four clerks. In addition to these financial issues, "a good deal of dissatisfaction [had] arisen among doctors because of rules the Dean [had] promulgated in . . . Coleman [Hospital]." Further eroding confidence in Emerson's ability to administer the School of Medicine, Gatch also told the university trustees that he thought "the Dean would go to any length to complicate the situation." Fesler concluded, "Many things have been done by the Dean . . . wholly beyond explanation or any rational basis." In his opinion, Emerson needed to be "superseded."[46]

This criticism of Emerson was reinforced as cases of patient injury and death at the hospitals accumulated and appeared to be linked to management practices. A dramatic example came in February 1931, when Fesler's sister died at Coleman Hospital, and it appeared to her family to have happened "without sufficient attention on the day of her death." Dean Emerson, in writing about the case to President Bryan, admitted a series of mistakes in carrying out medical orders that were associated with overcrowding and short staffing. The letter reveals a hospital operating on very thin margins of competence and authority, but by 1931, this was no longer viewed as a problem of resources but rather a problem of leadership.[47]

An opportunity to facilitate Emerson's departure arose at the end of February 1931. The dean was "being pressed" to travel to China as part of the American mission to certify doctors in that country. Taking this post would require Emerson to spend the 1931–32 academic year investigating medical education and hospitals in the Far East, necessitating a leave of absence.[48] Perhaps Emerson saw this as a way of escaping the accumulation of events and criticisms, but in any case, when the board of trustees granted

Emerson's request for leave, they began discussing who should take over his duties. In June 1931, the trustees informed Emerson that the board had "reached the conclusion that the best interests of the University would be served by a change in the office of the Dean."[49] Bryan permitted Emerson to retain the title of dean during his mission to Asia, and upon his return, the university announced that Emerson had "retired from active administrative duties to become research professor of medicine." Gatch officially became dean of the IU School of Medicine in June 1932.[50]

Conclusion

Emerson's tenure as dean of the IUSM encountered biblical trials of flood, plague (the global influenza pandemic), and (world) war. Yet in the face of these challenges, he led the school to a solid place in the rankings of medical schools with some of the largest entering classes in the country, only to be dismissed primarily as a result of the mundane tasks of hospital administration.[51] In assessing the work of Emerson and the first twenty years of the IU School of Medicine, it is obvious that the dean never abandoned his goal, which was also the main reason Bryan selected him: to raise the standards of the IU School of Medicine to be an institution on the forefront of medical education. In the process, the school converted medical education in the state from what was an effort based on the proprietary model to one that followed the standards advocated by the Flexner Report in line with other leading medical schools of the country. This involved increasing the number of full-time clinical faculty organized in growing departments reflecting new specialties, and whose teaching, clinical work, and research were done within a university at a campus in Indianapolis with new hospitals and other facilities that served growing numbers of students and patients.

This was impressive but by no means unique because other medical schools across the country achieved similar results, albeit by different paths. In Indiana, there were two features of notable difference in the establishment of its new medical school, one a problem that was postponed and the other an opportunity that was missed. The problem postponed was the existence of the medical campus in Indianapolis, fifty miles away from the university in Bloomington. The situation was not unique; Illinois, Colorado, and Iowa faced similar geographical problems whereby the state universities were not located in large population centers with the hospitals and patients that were essential to the new medical schools. Bryan and the trustees of Indiana University postponed the problem by keeping the initial year of medical instruction in Bloomington while putting most new resources into growing the Indianapolis campus, including faculty and the buildings needed for clinical instruction and care. They later also took advantage of the opportunities presented by the availability of the resources of the state government and private philanthropy in the state capital and largest population center of the state.[52]

The missed opportunity was in the field that Emerson thought was the best way available for IU to become a top US medical school: concentrating its efforts in the Social Service Department. At the time, its greatest impact was to play a role in Emerson's undoing because the results obtained were expensive and not clear or obvious enough to justify the growing cost. This was at the same time that other compelling needs were growing in the new medical school, and by the late 1920s, financial support was cut because of the economic crisis. In addition, by the 1930s, Emerson's goals in social medicine increasingly came into conflict with those of the faculty who were "captivated by the promise of science and the hunt for diseases and their causes" and who dismissed his interest in the further development of environmental medicine and the Social Service Department as peripheral and nonmedical. In their opinion, Emerson was insisting on maintaining an "expensive social service department," which not only rendered "no service commensurate" with its costs but also caused other parts of the school to be "neglected and starved."

Emerson's failure to convince his faculty and administration to support the Social Service Department resulted in a backlash that prompted the trustees to eliminate the department. It was reestablished in 1944 as the Division of Social Service, administered under the Indiana University Graduate School but with a very different focus, as indicated in 1973, when it became a separate school and then took the name School of Social Work.[53] The longer term, and perhaps more significant, result of Emerson's failed experiment with the Social Service Department was the negative reaction (or at least limiting of support) it produced among medical faculty and administrators for what was emerging as the field of public health. At other medical schools, efforts such as Emerson's to improve the overall health and welfare of the population resulted in departments and eventually schools of public health. The missed opportunity in Indiana may also be related to Emerson's, along with John Hurty's and their protégé Thurman Rice's interest in eugenics.[54] The reason for Emerson's inability to establish support for a unit in the school to deliver public health instruction requires further research, but the opportunity was there, as will be seen in a later chapter, given the strong ties that Hurty and his protégé Rice had with the Indiana Board of Health.[55] In fact, the opportunity continued in subsequent decades, but the reaction against Emerson's Social Service Department efforts lingered and contributed to the long delay before a Department of Public Health was established in the IU Medical School in the 1990s, and finally a separate School of Public Health in Indianapolis in 2012.[56]

Despite this disappointment, during Emerson's tenure, the enrollment of the School of Medicine more than doubled to become one of the twenty largest medical schools in the United States. In spite of the resource limits that constantly restricted the ability of the school to hire and retain faculty, the School of Medicine entered the 1930s with instructional facilities and hospitals that were unimaginable to the medical leadership of Indiana twenty-five years before. More than anyone else, Emerson had brought the School of Medicine to maturity, although it was not the institution he'd imagined in its infancy. Like other medical schools across the United States during this same period, the school grew in "size, complexity, and wealth." After Emerson, the School of Medicine faced the tumult of the 1930s and 1940s on foundations secured by his labor.

6

Leadership Change and the Great Depression, 1932–1941

I have no doubt that the next twenty years will bring about almost as great a change in the work of our medical center, as the last twenty years have done in the transformation of the public dump, upon which it stands. But the first and greatest problem now is to survive and save what we have achieved. Of course, we shall all dig out of this period but not before day after tomorrow.[1]

James W. Fesler to Burton D. Myers, 1934

When James Fesler wrote to Burton Myers in 1934 about the future of the medical center, it reflected the mood in the depths of the Great Depression. He also must have realized that others, besides himself and Myers, would take the lead in saving what the medical center had achieved. Fesler had served for almost twenty years as the president of the Indiana University Board of Trustees, having first been elected as an alumnus trustee at the start of the Bryan era in 1902. By 1934, Burton Myers had served even longer—thirty years—in the medical program and medical school, and both of them ended their service within a few years. They were not alone. Just two years earlier, Charles P. Emerson had stepped down after two decades as dean of the medical school, and in 1937, William Lowe Bryan ended almost four decades' service as president. At all levels of leadership—board, university, and medical school—the 1930s were a time of generational transition under trying conditions.[2]

As the new dean of the IUSM, Willis Gatch played a crucial role in facing these times of worldwide turmoil, beginning with the Great Depression and ending with the Second World War. These changes would be a great challenge to any institution, but the medical school had been remarkably

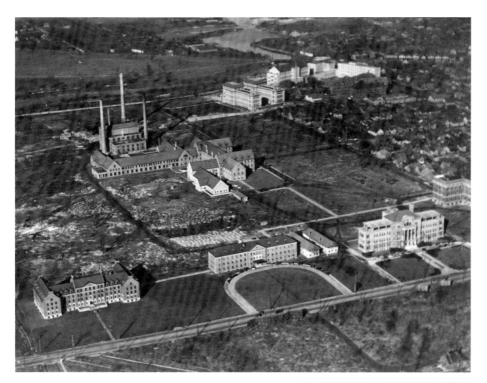

Figure 6.1a & b. (*top*) Aerial view of medical center when Gatch became dean, just prior to new building for Dental School that joined IU in 1925, IU Archives Bloomington P0029849; "Indianapolis," *Arbutus* (1933): 319; (*bottom*) heading of sixty-three-page section on IU programs (mainly health) in Indianapolis, including: Medical School, Dietary Department, Outpatient Department of City Hospital, Nurses Training, and Dental School.

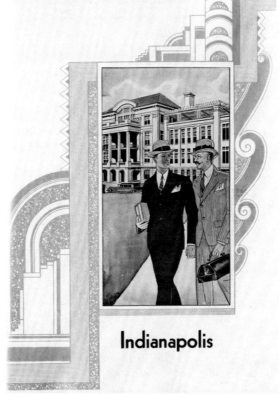

successful in establishing itself as a center for training and medical care during the first twenty-five years since the merger of 1908. The school graduated one hundred physicians and over fifty nurses a year. To be sure, new construction was much more limited than it had been in the 1920s, but even in the midst of the Depression during the 1930s, new buildings were constructed at the medical center. In addition to a facility for the proprietary dental school in Indianapolis that had earlier joined the university, a significant clinical facility was added to Long Hospital as well as a building for the State Board of Health, thanks to funding from the federal New Deal. The direct influence of the US government was a new development in the history of the medical school during this period, but it foreshadowed even greater influence during the war for obvious reasons, and to the surprise of many, this continued after 1945.

This chapter examines the operations of the medical school as well as its response to these wider changes leading up to the entry into war. In the two decades since the opening of Long Hospital, that facility and the other Indiana University hospitals had become an integral and essential part of medical care in the Hoosier state. One obvious indication of this was the growing waiting lists that confronted patients referred to Long, Riley, and Coleman Hospitals throughout the 1930s. Simultaneously, the pathway to becoming a doctor was changing; expectations for incoming students were rising, and increasing specialization fostered the growth of graduate medical education, internship, and residency.[3]

The new IU president, Herman Wells, was not as closely attached to the medical school as Bryan. Organizationally, except for the first year of instruction, the school and medical center functioned largely independent from the Bloomington campus. (The curtailment of the Social Service Department in 1931 ended the only other significant collaboration.) Much of Wells's work was to secure governmental funding for the school.[4] By 1936, not counting the program in Bloomington, the medical school in Indianapolis now covered forty acres, and the facilities were increasingly referred to as the Indiana University Medical Center to reflect not only the numerous buildings but also the multifaceted training offered. In addition to nursing education, which was established when Long Hospital was created, new programs started in allied health fields such as dietetics and occupational therapy. Moreover, in 1925 Indiana University acquired an existing proprietary dental school that had begun in Indianapolis in 1879. Similar to the merger in 1908, the Indiana Dental College (which had ties to both Eli Lilly and John Hurty) had difficulties keeping up with rapid changes in the field, and the medical center saw an opportunity to expand its health services. In 1933, a new building was constructed for the school across Michigan Street from Long Hospital.[5]

The New Dean and the New Deal

Upon Emerson's return from Asia in the summer of 1932, the title of dean of the medical school was formally transferred to Gatch, who had filled the role the previous year. The appointment of Gatch reflected the deep concern of Bryan and the trustees that stability was essential to the future of the medical school. This was because of the management issues identified at the end of Emerson's tenure that resulted from the challenges of operating increasingly complex clinical facilities with a limited budget and expanding demand for services. Gatch had been a persistent member of the loyal opposition to Dean Emerson within the medical school almost since his arrival in 1912. While a fierce advocate for public, university-based medical education, he was more sympathetic than Bryan or Emerson to the views of physicians in Indianapolis. For example, throughout his career at IU, Gatch opposed the division of the medical school that required the first year of instruction at Bloomington.[6]

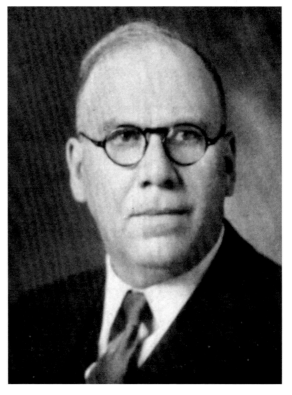

Figure 6.2. Willis D. Gatch, IUSM dean, 1932–46, *Arbutus* (1932): 384.

Gatch's desire to unify the school in Indianapolis was a signal that the problem of the Bloomington-Indianapolis rift had not disappeared. Any of Bryan's concerns about Gatch's opinion on this, however, were outweighed by Gatch's long experience in the Department of Surgery. This included his work overseeing all the surgical services since the departure of John H. Oliver in 1927, which gave Gatch intimate experience with the university's growing medical school and hospital operations. In addition to the new dean's record of service to the university, he enjoyed a reputation as an effective and frugal manager with an excellent understanding of operational details, and he had strong relationships with the Indianapolis medical community. His appointment as dean also set a precedent of promotion from within that was followed for the next six medical school deans.

Gatch was well aware that he faced serious financial problems. As Bryan put it, university officials were "obliged to recognize the fact" that there was "no more money to spend in the hospitals" and that there was "no assurance of relief before 1933, if then." His solution was, "We must tighten our belts . . . and secure improvement by better administration." Gatch's experience and temperament fit these new demands well, and he followed a course of action that had most recently been spelled out in a 1931 survey done at the request of the trustees, who were concerned with the rising costs of the operation of Long, Riley, and Coleman Hospitals. When Gatch became acting dean of the School of Medicine in July of that same year, he immediately set out to solve these problems and improve the efficiency of the IU Medical Center. One of his first actions was to eliminate the controversial Social Service Department and reduce its remaining staff to one social worker, a clerk, and stenographers, who helped some of the patients with transportation, medications, and treatments. Any medical school funds used to support the department were reassigned to the hospital administrative funds.[7]

Like Maxwell and Emerson before him, Gatch's position as dean was initially only part-time. In addition to maintaining a private practice, he retained the chairmanship of the Department of Surgery and remained involved in teaching. Many students and faculty felt that Gatch, as the new dean, took a direct, no-nonsense approach to administering the School of Medicine, as he had during his time as head of the Department of Surgery. "He was not tall, but was quite stocky with a round face," recalled one of his students, but he "always had a very determined look [that] commanded attention and respect."[8]

In spite of growth over the previous twenty years, the number of faculty and students on campus was still small enough to permit personal, intimate, collegial relationships. Each class still had less than one hundred students who met Gatch in surgery classes during their junior year, and they saw him again during surgery clinics in their fourth year. He regularly challenged his students and was just as demanding of his faculty. A student who graduated in 1933 recalled one encounter with Gatch that illustrates this. "He kept me up there [i.e., standing] for about 20 minutes answering questions. And when I got through, he said, 'Well Dr. Van Buskirk it's obvious you didn't read the book. But you answered all the questions correctly.'"[9] There were still few full-time faculty in the School of Medicine, most of whom met daily for lunch in a small dining room at Riley Hospital. Gatch conveyed the impression of being aware of all of their activities. As Donald E. Bowman, who joined the Department of Pharmacology and Biochemistry during Gatch's administration, remembered, "Missing a Clinico-pathological Conference on a cold and snowy Friday night might well bring the Dean to your laboratory to administer a direct quiz (to say the least) on a topic of his choice. . . . It took time to learn that the Dean had to be on your back to be properly appreciated."[10]

Although he always let his staff know who was ultimately in charge, Gatch became known at the Medical Center for his ability to delegate tasks and authority. At the beginning of his tenure, he believed that the administrative committees of the School of Medicine had become too unwieldy. Moreover, so many vacancies occurred among members of the school's committees that they were no longer representative bodies. Therefore, Gatch decided to create a new Medical Council in place of the Educational Committee. The dean appreciated that if the Indiana University School of Medicine were to progress, it was necessary to appoint men to this council who belonged to a new generation of leaders at the Medical Center as well as some who had a great deal of seniority. The council was another manifestation of the generational change that Gatch brought with his appointment as dean.[11]

Throughout the 1920s, Emerson had raised concerns about the increasing need for improving graduate education for physicians following medical school. Dean Gatch formalized the school's efforts by creating a committee that appointed interns and arranged for their instruction. He believed the internship programs at Indiana University's hospitals had been "sadly neglected" and was concerned that the medical school's reputation was becoming just as dependent on the quality of its internships and residencies as it was on the quality of its undergraduate work. The growth of graduate medical education at hospitals not affiliated with undergraduate medical schools created additional problems of organization, standards, and certification. Without direct faculty supervision, these unaffiliated residencies were little more than underpaid hospital staff who would not be prepared to work in increasingly demanding specialties.[12]

Financial constraints, hospital operations, and undergraduate and graduate education defined the broad scope of Gatch's work. Although he advocated during the next fifteen years for increased funding for research, it nonetheless remained beyond the interest of the state legislature, which was much more concerned with the number of doctors trained to serve Hoosiers and the care they received at the university's hospitals. State funding for teaching and care therefore comprised the bulk of the medical school's budget, especially in a time of fiscal crisis. Gatch continued to respond to the changing demands on the school in the face of deteriorating economic conditions while political change altered policies and resources available to the medical school.

The political changes of the Depression and New Deal hit Indiana hard, particularly because of the politics in the preceding decade. In 1932, the depths of economic crisis in Indiana and across the nation created ferment for political change in the state, and federal elections produced changes in the next budget cycle that exceeded Bryan's fears. The political failure and scandal-driven collapse of the Ku Klux Klan in the 1920s left Indiana uniquely ill prepared culturally, philosophically, and politically for the economic crisis that began in 1929. After winning the gubernatorial election of 1916, the Republican Party in Indiana controlled the governor's office for the next sixteen years.[13] The 1932 fall election campaign was an extended debate over the proper response to the growing national crisis of the Great Depression.

While Franklin Roosevelt campaigned for the presidency offering fundamental change to a beleaguered nation, the Hoosier state sat on the precipice of its own homegrown radical change. Paul V. McNutt, the charismatic Hoosier veteran and dean of the Indiana University Law School, brought an attractive, righteous fury to the campaign from the moment he took the podium at the state Democratic convention at Cadle Tabernacle in Indianapolis. When the votes were tallied on election day, McNutt's victory mirrored the national Democratic landslide and put him in the governor's office with huge Democratic majorities in the General Assembly.[14] For his new administration, McNutt declared, "the purpose must be restoration rather than destruction, healing rather than harm." If there were doubts that the governor intended anything less than sweeping change that would consolidate power in the executive branch, the next few weeks eliminated them.[15] And the impact was felt directly by the medical school.

Promoted as a means of making government more efficient and economical, McNutt's Executive Reorganization Act of 1933 gave more responsibility to the medical school for state services. For example, the reorganization of the State Board of Health included combining its laboratories with those of the university hospitals. Clyde Culbertson became director of the two laboratories. Thurman B. Rice, who had been a member of the Department of Pathology and Bacteriology since 1920, was appointed assistant secretary of the Board of Health and given the additional title professor of bacteriology and public health. Although the overt goals were efficiency and economy, these changes also reduced perceived threats to the power of physicians. For example, McNutt closed the Division of Infant and Child Hygiene and involved the medical school directly in the State Board of Health's operations. As a result, the Executive Reorganization Act took away power from what had been perceived to be more radical, left-leaning elements within both agencies. It also removed predominantly female public health authorities and restored the predominantly male physician leadership.[16]

At the federal level, the Roosevelt administration and its alphabet soup of new agencies offered unprecedented financial resources for public projects. Although the new governor of Indiana was an alumnus and former faculty member of Indiana University who understood the needs of the university, the federal programs required an understanding of the operation and priorities of a novel and distant bureaucracy that neither McNutt nor President Bryan immediately appreciated. University administrators were experienced in lobbying state legislators, but now they had to confront a growing federal bureaucracy that itself was feeling its way through this new world. Early Civil Works Administration (CWA) and Federal Emergency Relief Administration (FERA) projects were started and stopped repeatedly throughout 1933 and early 1934.

With the end of the CWA and FERA, the university finally turned to the Public Works Administration (PWA) for assistance, beginning with a personal letter from Bryan to Harold Ickes, Secretary of the Interior. Even then, Bryan did not fully recognize the potential of the newly organized PWA to assist the construction of new university buildings. When he made his first appeal in April 1934, Bryan asked for only $400,000 to erect a new building in Bloomington, which set a pattern of seeking federal aid for the Bloomington campus. Thanks to the work of numerous trustee and political allies, especially Judge Ora Wildermuth, Bryan and Wells secured federal funding for numerous buildings constructed on the campus. By 1940, these included the Medical Building, Bryan Hall, Woodburn Hall, the auditorium, and the School of Music.[17]

There was a similar timid response later that same year when Gatch asked Bryan to approach Governor McNutt to support a new building at the medical school to relieve overcrowding in Long Hospital, one of Gatch's top priorities. The space was needed for the expansion of radiology and research, as well as more space for patient care. Gatch wrote, "I believe that we have the support of the governor and of [a] great many influential people." Moreover, if PWA funds were utilized, he concluded, "A small state appropriation could be supplemented by a large [one] from the federal government" for the structure. Although Bryan said he recognized how great the need was for a new medical building, he warned Gatch that it was unlikely McNutt would support increased funding for new facilities, because more cuts in the state budget would have to be made.[18] This modesty of aspiration fit Bryan's character but did not match the new political world inaugurated in 1933.

In contrast, Bryan's successor, Herman B Wells, lacked neither modesty of vision nor appreciation of the opportunities at hand. Since his appointment to the faculty of Indiana University in 1930, Wells had served the state and Indiana University as both an educator and administrator. Following the Executive Reorganization Act, Wells served as secretary for the Indiana Commission for Financial Institutions, supervisor of the Division of Research and Statistics at the Indiana Department of Financial Institutions, and bank supervisor for the same state agency. In 1935, Bryan appointed Wells dean of the School of Business Administration. Two years later, Wells was named acting president, and upon Bryan's resignation, he became president in 1938.[19]

Of all the changes to the university administration that impacted the school of medicine, none equaled that of the departure of Bryan and arrival of Wells in 1937. The acting president had already begun examining the operations of the university in the new era. One of his first steps was to commission a self-study that was the foundation of many of his subsequent reforms of the university and medical school.[20] During his twenty-five years in office, between 1937 and 1962, he helped to integrate the medical school into the university as it never had been before. In this process, and during the tenure of just two deans, the IU School of Medicine was transformed from a respectable professional school dominated by part-time faculty who focused primarily on teaching and patient care into a burgeoning research institution dominated by full-time academic medical professionals with a broad scientific perspective.

The Weiskotten Report and Divided Medical Education

At the same time that Gatch became dean of the medical school, he was faced with national scrutiny of the program. Following a report on medical education in 1932 by the American Association for Medical Education (AAMC), the AMA's Council on Medical Education decided "that the time was ripe for a comprehensive resurvey of . . . medical schools . . . in order that the public, the profession, the licensing boards and prospective medical students might know which schools were advancing in accord with the prevailing standards of teaching and which were lagging."[21] After an immediate decline following the Flexner Report in 1910, medical school enrollments rose steadily across the United States from 1921 to 1931. Likewise, as seen in the previous chapter, enrollment at the Indiana University School of Medicine during this same period rose from 80 to 126 students, an increase of nearly 70 percent. The growing number of students at the School of Medicine severely overburdened its faculty and facilities. Yet despite this growth, the number of doctors per thousand residents in Indiana continued to decline. This was due in part to the increase in the overall state population during the period but more significantly to the number of students leaving the state after graduation.[22]

It was in this setting that in 1934, Herman G. Weiskotten, dean of the Syracuse University College of Medicine, directed an evaluation of medical schools in Canada and the United States on behalf of the Council on Medical Education of the American Medical Association. This was the first comprehensive survey of medical schools since the Flexner Report of 1910, and all medical deans were understandably anxious about the findings. This was despite the fact that the AMA planned to keep individual school assessments confidential while making a more general report to the public.[23] The individual reports went to the schools, including university presidents and trustees with whom Weiskotten and his team met during their visits. Gatch feared that facilities constraints at IU would weigh heavily against the evaluation of his medical school, and as predicted, Weiskotten and his team noted the strain of the increased enrollments when they visited Indiana in late March 1935. They told Burton Myers that Indiana was "a fine school" but that it was "overcrowded and undermanned."[24]

There was another criticism in the report, however, that fed Gatch's concern about first-year instruction in Bloomington. Even though the full report was not published until 1940 and individual assessments of each school were kept confidential, Edmund D. Clark, a faculty member who was then president of the Indiana State Medical Association, learned much earlier that William D. Cutter, secretary of the Council on Medical Education, had indicated an even greater problem than overcrowding. As Clark stated in a letter to Bryan in 1937, "The separation of the first year from the real center of the medical school at Indianapolis" was the "most serious handicap" under which the IU School of Medicine operated.[25]

His view was reinforced by the 1940 Council on Medical Education (CME) report of general findings. which stated that this kind of separation made it "difficult to maintain a completely satisfactory interchange of influence between the members of the clinical and preclinical departments." In addition, the council reported that this division also threatened to imperil "the unity and sequence in the curriculum, continuity of teaching effort, availability of patients for illustrative teaching in the preclinical departments, availability of fresh material for study in histology, pathology, and biochemistry, and cooperative research."[26]

This was not a problem unique to Indiana. The CME report reminded readers that many of the country's medical schools had begun independently in cities where clinical facilities existed and only later joined universities, a number of which had been established in small centers of population. The result was that a total of nineteen medical schools (of the sixty-six four-year schools evaluated) were "located more or less remote from the other schools of the university." Moreover, six of these, including Indiana, "conducted part of their instruction in one city and part in another."[27] As proof of the "educational disadvantages" of medical schools being separate from the rest of the university, let alone dividing medical instruction, the report stated that of the fifteen schools (unnamed) receiving the highest rankings, eight were centralized, and only one was completely decentralized. In contrast, among the fifteen ranked lowest, six were completely decentralized, and only one was "located on a university campus."

Clark, as president of the state medical association, took action on his conviction that the entire medical course should be given in Indianapolis.[28] Interpreting Gatch's reluctance to share specific information in the council's report with the State Medical Association as affirmation that conditions at the School of Medicine were deficient, Clark asked that the State Medical Association appoint a committee to make a detailed investigation of the situation. As to its purpose, Clark said, "This committee . . . should ascertain whether it is true the Council on Medical Education and hospitals of the American Medical Association feel it is a detriment to have a medical school divided."[29] It was no surprise that when the special committee to investigate Clark's allegations made its report in 1938, it recommended a plan to consolidate the IU School of Medicine in Indianapolis that "would have obvious teaching advantages . . . and would be in line with current medical education." Moreover, "consummation of the plan would require only one new building in Indianapolis," which the school would soon need anyway for research and teaching.[30]

To be sure, this recommendation reopened an argument going back to negotiations about the merger of the Indianapolis proprietary medical schools with Indiana University, which had been laid to rest by the compromise of 1911. Now, the case for consolidation was rekindled and bolstered by the rising national standards for medical education, which Bryan had used as a rationale for starting anatomy and physiology instruction at the Bloomington campus in 1904. However, the tables were turned as the argument was made that the latest advances in medical practice could best be taught where all resources were concentrated, at the medical school in Indianapolis. Despite the new impetus from the Weiskotten report and the State Medical Association recommendation, there was little chance for immediate action. Although Bryan had been replaced by Wells, who had less of a stake in the compromise, one of the first buildings constructed with PWA funds on the Bloomington campus in 1937 was to house expanded facilities to teach the first-year medical students.[31] In addition, the outbreak of war immediately concentrated attention elsewhere as far as medical instruction was concerned. As will be seen later, however, with the war's end, proponents of consolidation were quick to bring up the proposal again.

Although consolidation of the medical school was not immediately feasible, a symbolic and real indication of the importance and weight of Indianapolis came when Burton Myers retired in 1940. To replace him as chairman of the Department of Anatomy in Bloomington, Gatch chose Edwin N. Kime, a private practitioner in Indianapolis who had "been doing nearly all of the teaching in Anatomy in Indianapolis" but who was listed as a member of the Department of Surgery. The reaction from Myers was swift, telling Wells that he "felt that a person of this type should not be chosen." Despite the reaction of Myers and the rest of the Bloomington preclinical faculty, Kime became chairman of the Department of Anatomy in July 1940, thus reflecting the authority of Gatch and the Indianapolis campus, as well as how anatomy, which had once reigned supreme in the medical school, had declined in importance.[32]

Gatch was understandably anxious about the Weiskotten Report, but he attempted to make the best of the situation in a report to the board of trustees about rumors of a negative review. "In size of budget, in cost of buildings and in salaries to faculty we cannot compete with Harvard, Yale, Chicago, or with most other schools," Gatch admitted. "We are in great need of more room and more money." But he added, "we can compete in quality of work, in the training of students and in research. Fortunately for us success in these does not depend entirely on money." Gatch assured the trustees that Weiskotten's team had confided in him that because of the economic hardships of the Depression, if they declared that schools like the IUSM were below acceptable standards, then they "would not have twenty schools left in the United States."[33]

Teaching and Learning, 1932–1941

While dramatic changes affecting the Indiana University School of Medicine were taking place in state and national politics as well as the university administration, the quotidian tasks of teaching medical students and caring for patients continued within the fiscal realities of the economic crisis. For example, despite the lack of facilities, admissions grew at IUSM in contrast to many medical schools around the country, which continued to raise admissions requirements that limited enrollment. These included standardized tests such as the Medical Aptitude Test (MAT) and admission quotas to make admission decisions. In addition to academic records, other criteria used in admissions decisions by schools included alumni and family connections, geographic proximity, and ability to pay tuition. Whereas IUSM admitted most applicants, the national admissions rate was approximately 75 percent, with some minority groups having admission rates fewer than 10 percent.[34] In addition, as had been the case from the start, IU admissions rested almost entirely in the hands of Myers and remained so until his retirement in 1940.[35]

Gatch had some concerns, however. "I am thoroughly convinced that unless we reduce the number of students to about seventy-five in a class," Gatch wrote to Bryan in 1935, "we shall have trouble with the American Medical Association." In addition, he argued, by taking immediate steps to elevate admission standards, the anticipated limit on enrollment would better fit the institution's physical capacity.[36] In response, in June 1935, the IU Medical Council passed a resolution that mandated three years of college preparation for all entering freshmen medical students starting in 1937–38. This resolution also called for lowering the number of admissions for 1936–37 to 110 students, including limiting the number of women enrolled. This did not immediately reduce the number of medical school graduates, which continued at approximately one hundred students per year, and then the outbreak of World War II ended any chance of reduction.[37]

When Burton Myers retired in 1940, the School of Medicine had the opportunity to change admissions procedures for the first time since the beginning of the school. Myers had interviewed each student who applied for admission to the school and spent hours examining their records. The new system initiated by the school's executive committee in July 1940 was more objective and, for the first time, gave members of the Indianapolis faculty the chance to be included. Twelve faculty members representing both campuses were appointed by the dean to the new Admissions Committee, with four subcommittees responsible for interviewing, rating, and selecting students. In addition to academic records, the Admissions Committee required students to take the Medical Aptitude Test and submit five letters of reference. They also had to submit a photograph and undergo a physical examination to qualify.[38]

The new selection formula was to be based 70 percent on the student's scholarship as reflected in undergraduate grades, 15 percent on personality and aptitude, and 15 percent on intelligence. The committee judged applicants based on "personality, as shown by his manners, care of his personal appearance, ability to get along with others, ability to take criticism, industry, and steadfastness of purpose." The committee cited as evidence of its impartiality the fact that it refused to admit the son of one of the medical school department chairs. In the 1941 application round, the school received more than 1,000 inquiries, with 278 finishing applications and an acceptance rate of 50 percent, down considerably from a decade earlier. The 140 students accepted included two African American students and five candidates from out of state. The latter were capped at five and only admitted if they showed exceptional qualifications. Due to the war, the committee had the chance to use this new formula just once before adopting accelerated admissions and degree requirements to meet wartime demands for physicians.[39]

One consequence of the university's efforts to restrict admissions was a reduction in the number of women who entered the medical school. Just as the elimination of the proprietary medical schools after 1903 reduced opportunities for women to enter medicine, the constraints of the 1930s erected new barriers and further marginalized women. For example, in 1935 the IUSM Medical Council recommended, "in consideration of the difficulty of securing internships for women," women who did not hold a bachelor's degree and who were less than twenty-one years of age "should only very exceptionally be admitted to the School of Medicine."[40] Thus, discrimination in medical school admissions actually increased during the interwar period against not only women but also African Americans and other minorities. Although from the beginning, the Indiana University School of Medicine had been a pioneer in graduating African American physicians, second to only the University of Michigan among predominantly white medical schools, the numbers were small because official and unofficial medical quotas against minorities, cultural groups, and women were common across the United States. In addition, other factors such as premedical training requirements, high tuition, and lack of scholarships acted to limit admission of minorities and women. Women faced the additional stereotype, which continued to be widely held well into the second half of the twentieth century, that medical training was "wasted" on women who would likely marry and drop out of practice to raise a family.[41]

The small number of women who were admitted at IUSM in the 1930s and 1940s, like the women admitted earlier in the twentieth century, continued to face great pressure from male students and faculty to excel in medical school and prove their worth as doctors. In addition, as mentioned in the previous chapter, these women also faced harassment, teasing, and discrimination from men in medical school. Several men bore witness to the process, such as Herbert Chattin, who began medical school in 1937 and recalled, "It used to be hell for a woman." He explained, "The amount of harassment, they wouldn't let us get by [now]. And we would be harassing them now, I guess." When asked if men questioned whether women should be doctors, Chattin replied, "Well I think a lot of the men did."[42] Byron Kilgore enrolled from 1934–39 and recalled that two of the four women in his class dropped out in the first year, and only one "durable" woman survived. Although the dropout "rate" could be seen as higher for women, the small number of women in the program makes it difficult to draw conclusions about underlying reasons.[43]

This process was exacerbated by the trend toward specialization and the rise of graduate medical education. As will be discussed later, by the late 1930s, the path to practicing medicine increasingly required access to an internship or residency, and this became another barrier to the entry of women and minorities to the medical profession in addition to admission to medical school. For example, although there was a "colored wing" of the City Hospital where the first black intern (Sumner Furniss, a graduate of Indiana Medical College) was allowed to train in 1894, neither black patients nor black interns were allowed in any of the university hospitals.[44] In 1933, this prompted F. Katherine Bailey, president of the Indiana Branch of the NAACP, to send a letter to Governor McNutt indicating, "Applications have been repeatedly made for the admittance of colored people to the [Robert Long] Hospital and we have received on two occasions letters from the trustees board of the hospital saying that there is absolutely no provision for Negro patients there." She went on to indicate, "This not only creates extreme suffering and neglect in cases requiring hospitalization, but also serves as a bar to Negro students of medicine in Indiana University for clinical practice."[45] She concluded with a call to end "this un-American situation." McNutt referred the letter to the hospital trustees, who referred it to President Bryan. The university president submitted the following carefully constructed response to the university trustees and Gatch for approval.

> With regard to the admission of medical students to the service of patients; the University will not undertake to compel any patient to accept the service of any physician or medical student against the patient's will. The number of beds available for clinical use by the University School of Medicine is so large that no medical student lacks adequate opportunity for clinical study.
>
> With regard to the admissions of patients to the hospitals under the control of the university: It is unavoidable that selections must be made among applicants for admission to the hospitals so long as the facilities are limited. The Board of Trustees maintains the right, under the law, to make those selections through its agents in the School of medicine. As facilities increase wider selection will be possible.[46]

It took another ten years before African American patients and interns used university hospitals.

In a larger sense, the marginalization of women and minorities reflected the continuation of teaching medical students much as had been done since the beginning of reforms twenty-five years before. Cadaver dissection in gross anatomy was still a rite of passage for students and typified the hard work and long hours they put into school.[47] Faculty expected students to memorize and learn a great deal of information in their first two years, mostly basic scientific knowledge they would need to know during their clinical experiences. Fortunately, there are firsthand recollections from students that describe this experience thanks to a series of oral histories of Indiana physicians educated in the 1930s. For example, William Sholty, who was enrolled from 1938 to 1942, said of the first two years of medical school, "You worked your fannies off."[48] Future Indiana Governor Otis Bowen, who also graduated in 1942, described much of the work in the first year: "It's just downright memorizing."[49] Bowen recalled often studying until three in the morning to prepare for exams.[50] George Compton recalled that the resulting atmosphere among students was "tense and all work" but still congenial. Students felt they were all in the same boat, so they studied together and shared their notes.[51] Still, that tension took its toll. Charles Fisch, who graduated in 1944, remembered that the "attrition rate after the first year was horrendous." Fisch also recalled, "Lectures were a bore." In fact, he claimed, "I remember listening to a lecture and a professor who shall remain nameless but he put everybody to sleep. And one of the students suddenly couldn't take it any longer and jumped out the window—fortunately it was the first floor of Emerson Hall."[52]

In the 1930s and 1940s, the third and fourth years of medical school were still a mix of classroom education and practical experience despite the expanded clinical facilities. Bowen also commented that he continued to feel like a student for the first two years of medical school due to all the courses and memorizing work; he only felt like a doctor during his last years of medical school because then he gained clinical experience.[53] However, Fisch, who graduated in 1944, recalled getting to see patients only during his last year of medical school.[54]

Exams and finals were an equally stressful time. Victor Vollrath, who graduated in May 1942, recalled a final exam where the professor placed the 1,600-page *Gray's Anatomy* on the table. "Then he'd take a pocketknife and hand it to us, and we'd have to open that book with a pocketknife and then he expected us to discuss anything that we opened the page to. Theoretically, we had to memorize the book. That was our final exam." He continued, "And we'd even go home and we'd try to practice hitting certain pages so we would know what to talk about."[55]

George Compton, who graduated in 1942, recalled a similar although more positive final exam experience for Frank Forry's class on microscopic pathology, which consisted of ten slides that students had to identify.

Compton made his way through seven of the slides. However, when he got to the eighth one, he recalled that what he "thought it was, wasn't supposed to be on this test." He continued, "Well, I knew the tissue and the disease process," and Forry "jumped clear across the room" and looked in the microscope and said, 'How did this get in here?' . . . That sure made my day [and my grade in the class]."[56] Compton also recalled a dermatology clinic at the City Hospital that illustrated the gap between students' classroom knowledge and their need for real clinical experience. Students observed a skin case and were to identify the skin disease, but none could correctly identify the disease by actual observation and examination of the patient. However, when a doctor described the symptoms in medical jargon, every student recognized the condition from the medical description they had read in their medical books.[57]

As mentioned in the previous chapter, the Great Depression added significantly to the financial stress faced by medical students, many of whom could not afford the cost of tuition. To his credit, Gatch granted them extra time to pay their fees, and trustee Fesler and local philanthropist Hugh McK. Landon each donated $2,000 for a student loan fund. When requests from students exceeded the amount deposited in the fund, Landon also offered to permit the use of unexpended research income for this purpose. Gatch, however, thought it best to "get the necessary money from other sources if possible."[58] In 1933, the Federal Emergency Relief Administration (FERA) made some assistance available to students at the Medical Center. During the summer of 1934, forty medical students were assigned to Civil Works Administration jobs. They received thirty-five cents an hour from FERA doing this work until the program was disbanded in 1935.[59]

Despite the stress of medical school, or because of it, the students used humor as a way of coping, such as the anecdote recalled by Herbert Chattin (entering medical school class of 1937) of how he and classmates found ways to enjoy anatomy class. They played a joke by putting an ear from a cadaver in the janitor's pocket, but it was the janitor's wife who found the ear, and he angrily told Chattin and other students that his wife was not amused.[60] Naomi Dalton, who enrolled in the early 1930s, recalled that students could take bones home to study, but Dalton's father owned a restaurant and was "quite put out" when she would spread out the bones on the restaurant counter to study.[61] Brice Fitzgerald recalled unexpected humor during one of his outdoor obstetric cases, where third- and fourth-year students went into the community to see low-income obstetric patients. "And when I was a junior, I went with a senior, and he had been trying to place a catheter before the delivery. And he couldn't do it, and so I pressed on the belly and

I said, 'There must be some urine here somewhere.' And as I pressed, the urine hit him in the face. And he didn't like that very well."[62]

Faculty did their part to motivate students to work hard to master needed medical knowledge. Brice Fitzgerald, who enrolled from 1935 to 1939, recalled that before his interview, Burton Myers asked him and others in his group, "How many of you have had Latin?" Fitzgerald recalled that only about one-third raised their hands, and he was not one of them. Myers then reportedly responded, "The rest of you [who have not had Latin] are going to flunk." Fitzgerald concluded, "So that made us study pretty hard."[63] L. B. Miller, a classmate of Fitzgerald, felt as if medical school was very autocratic—the administration could expel students on any pretext, so students were always studying.[64]

Other Health Education and Internships

Training in other health fields continued to grow at the medical center, especially the Training School for Nurses. By the late 1920s, however, Emerson and others had begun to view the curriculum of the nursing school that was developed by Ethel P. Clarke as having "swung too far toward the general cultural and theoretical subjects and . . . too far away from the practical work necessary in the training of a nurse." In response, Clarke surveyed nursing education across the country for comparison to the experience at IU. Her 1929 report found that as the clinical load increased, the nursing staff struggled to meet the growing patient load. The result, as shown in table 6.1, was that the majority of the nurses hired to staff the hospital expansion were student nurses and not graduate nurses.[65]

Clarke also discovered why there was a shortage of degreed nurses in the hospitals. As table 6.2 indicates, her graduates went on to a wide variety of fields including public health, education, and institutional, with less than half choosing to do private patient care.[66]

Clarke's vision for the nursing school differed greatly from that of the deans and male physicians in the medical school who held the reins of control. Emerson believed this curriculum had inculcated in the minds of nursing students "false ideas as to their relation to doctor and patient." The result was to hinder "the hard work which good nursing requir[ed]." In fact, Clarke was attempting to mold a professional curriculum and rename the institution the Indiana University School of Nursing, but to no avail. Convinced that Clarke was incapable of effecting "any satisfactory reorganization" of the school, Emerson asked her to resign at the end of 1930.[67] No one was immediately named as Clarke's permanent replacement, and

Table 6.1. IUSM Patient and Nursing Levels, 1914–1929

Year	Daily Average Patient Census	Nursing Students	Graduate Nurses	Nurse Supervisors	Instructors	Graduates
1914	—	8	10	5	1	19
1915	69	20	11	5	1	19
1916	—	35	7	5	1	16
1917	—	39	5	5	1	14
1918	98.5	56	5	5	1	13
1919	108	56	0	5	2	9
1920	108	59	0	5	2	10
1921	108	60	0	5	2	10
1922	116	72	0	5	2	10
1923	116	72	0	5	2	10
1924	120	94	0	14	3	20
1925	248.33	118	18	14	3	38
1926	240.39	150	8	14	3	28
1927	218	178	1	21	3	29
1928	317.69	185	7	21	3	35
1929	365	162	9	25	3	41

Source: "Correspondence of Ethel P. Clarke," Box 1, IU School of Nursing, UA25, InUI-Ar.

Table 6.2. Career after Leaving IU Training School for Nurses, 1926–1929

Year	Total	Housewife	Instructor	Institutional	Public Health	Private	Ill
1926	17	3	2	5	5	2	0
1927	29	4	1	14	3	7	0
1928	47	3	0	15	9	17	3
1929	19	1	0	8	4	6	0

Source: "Correspondence of Ethel P. Clarke," Box 1, IU School of Nursing, UA25, InUI-Ar.

the 1931 survey of the Medical Center reported that problems still existed, including insubordination and a lack of proper supervision for nursing students.[68]

Upon his appointment as interim dean, Gatch arranged for the former assistant superintendent of Riley Hospital from 1928 to 1930, Cordelia Hoeflin, to become head of the training school. She had experience as an operating scrub nurse and in X-ray departments, which were increasingly important to hospital operations. To rectify the nursing and staff shortages at the Medical Center, Gatch advocated a "Back to Fundamentals"

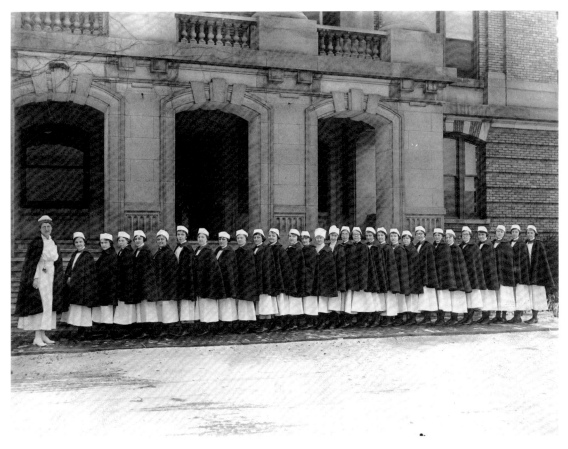

Figure 6.3. Nursing class of 1925 (with director Ethel Clarke), criticized by Emerson for straying too far "from the hard work which good nursing required." IUPUI image UA024_004913. Description on back of photo: "Class of 1925, Mrs. Ethel P. Clarke Supt. of Nursing School with 29 nurses in uniforms and caps, standing in front of Long Hospital."

movement that identified the nurse's prime duty as "the care of the sick room and the patient under the direction of the physician."[69] One of the underappreciated challenges with the rapid expansion of the hospitals was the need for student and graduate nurses to take care of the services. As Clarke's report found, students did the bulk of the nursing because graduate nurses received job offers from other hospitals and private services. The hospitals were also hindered by "a lack of cooperation between nursing and housekeeping departments." A specific bone of contention was the bedbug problem that had plagued Long Hospital for years. Gatch ordered a vigilant inspection of beds twice daily "to discover infested beds early and to remove and sterilize them at once" to make sure that all bedbugs

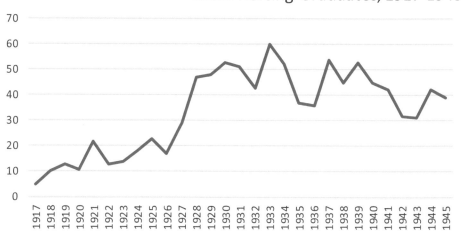

Figure 6.4. IU School of Nursing Graduates, 1917–1945. "Lists of Students," "SON- #of Graduates," Ethel Clarke Correspondence, Box 1, IU School of Nursing, UA25; Rock, *A History of the Indiana University Training School for Nurses*, 127–38.

were destroyed. He also insisted that "orderlies and maids be kept busy scrubbing, scouring, washing and painting at all times" when they were not working with patients.[70]

Despite these difficulties, as shown in figure 6.4 the graduates of the nursing program grew to meet these challenges and, under the leadership of Hoeflin, total enrollment reached over 175 students.

In part, this was because difficulties in finding candidates eased during the Great Depression as families attempted to find employment for their daughters. Nonetheless, by the 1930s, IU graduates were especially in demand for public health and administrative positions, and this was even before the war greatly exacerbated the problem. Gatch found that nursing shortages as much as space limitations restricted his ability to expand clinical operations.[71] One way to gain additional staffing was through an affiliation program, whereby six other nursing schools sent students for three- to six-month rotations in pediatrics, communicable disease, and obstetrics. By 1945, this program expanded to include over ninety students. In addition, Riley Hospital hosted one to four students in postgraduate training courses in pediatrics.[72] As the Great Depression ended, the nursing school attempted to raise its minimum educational requirements. Beginning with the spring class of 1939, the Training School for Nurses required entering students to have at least one year of college preparation.[73] The crisis of

World War II and the drastic need for nurses in military service quickly rescinded the change in admission requirements before this new class could complete the program.

In addition to the nursing school and the dental school, education in allied health professions increased in importance on the IU School of Medicine campus by the end of the 1930s. As was the case elsewhere in the United States, the dietary department at the IU Medical Center evolved into a School of Dietetics. It had begun as a small program with five or fewer students in the mid-1920s; but by 1937, it was rated one of the three best schools in the United States. Directed by Lute Troutt, the School of Dietetics was affiliated with the IU Graduate School and offered formal classes in nutrition and practical experience in all of the activities involved in running a large dietary department. Students who completed the program received graduate credit toward a master's degree.[74] Another allied health field that achieved national recognition in the 1930s was the Department of Occupational Therapy. Headed by Winifred C. Kahmann, a pioneer in the field, this department attracted students from professional schools in Milwaukee, Philadelphia, and St. Louis for three-month internships. In addition, other new allied health programs were developed. For example, in 1939 Clyde Culbertson, who headed the laboratories for the State Board of Health, organized a School for Laboratory Technicians to meet an increasing demand for well-trained laboratory assistants. During its first year, five women enrolled in this program. With the increasing complexity of hospital-based medical care, a new range of technical and support positions were being created and occupied primarily by women.[75]

As mentioned earlier, Gatch, like Emerson before him, continued to devote increasing time to graduate and postgraduate medical instruction. Before the 1930s, multiple paths toward specialization had been acceptable, but the residency system, which involved a lengthy period of hospital service after internship, became more and more widespread. Taking a residency in a hospital approved by the Council on Medical Education and Hospitals of the AMA soon became the only acceptable way to specialize in any medical field. Rather than the universities, the medical profession through its various regulatory boards was gaining more control over graduate medical education. The agencies initiated these measures to prevent "the entry . . . of ill equipped and incompetent men" into the specialties.[76] They created formal curriculum guidelines that included both clinical experience and didactics for interns and residents in such subjects as anatomy, applied physiology, pathology, and research. Students were divided into groups for their clinical rotations and didactics in order to give them more personalized

Table 6.3. 1931 and 1940 IUSM Graduating Class Internship Placement

Placement	1931	1940
Methodist Hospital, Indianapolis	7	13
Indiana Medical Center	15	21
Indianapolis City Hospital (Eskenazi)	24	21
St. Vincent, Indianapolis	7	8
Indianapolis sub-total	53	63
Other, Indiana	10	11
Other United States & international	33	26
Other, none	4	1
Other sub-total	100	101

Source: School of Medicine, Indiana University, Bulletin, 1930–31, 1939–40.

attention. "Since the examinations of the National Examining Boards are very difficult and since these Boards require in general about four years of postgraduate work as interne and resident," Gatch explained to Wells soon after he officially became the university's president in 1938, "it has been necessary for Medical Schools to make provision for the training of men who seek them." By 1940, the school was able to achieve this goal.[77]

Table 6.3 shows that almost all graduates were placed in internships, but it also indicates two problems that persisted in subsequent decades. First was the placement of significant numbers of graduates at sites outside of Indiana. This reduced the likelihood that they would practice in the state, because residency location has always been a key determinant of where physicians eventually work. Although the number of in-state placements increased by 1940, over one-quarter were outside the state. The second feature is the very high number (85 percent) of the Indiana internships in Indianapolis. This was a logical consequence of the development of hospitals in the city appropriate for graduate medical education, but for the same reasons as applied to out-state internships, this concentration of placements worked against IU-trained physicians practicing around the state.

Gatch was intent on making the internship and residency program at IU of the highest quality. At IU's hospitals, residencies were reserved for the best students and were prized positions. One important consequence of the increased importance of residency, as mentioned earlier, was that it increasingly became another barrier to women and minority medical school graduates who wished to enter medical practice. Few women were admitted to internship, and Riley Hospital was the only university hospital that accepted African American patients. Their numbers were small, and no

African Americans served on the house staff. As a result, until the 1950s, City Hospital remained the only hospital in Indianapolis where African Americans could serve their residencies.[78]

"Low Prices . . . Increased Demand": The Hospitals in the 1930s

Beyond teaching, the expanding Medical Center and especially the hospitals required much attention to finances and administration. It was primarily for this work that Dean Gatch was handed the reins of the school, and the new dean immediately demonstrated his ability to impose new economies on the school and hospitals. For example, one of the first and most important steps he took to improve efficiency was to establish a central clinical laboratory, the lack of which he considered "a great handicap to the hospitals and school." According to Gatch, the many smaller laboratories that Emerson had put into place not only hampered the treatment of patients and the instruction of students but also put the IU Medical Center at a competitive disadvantage. Because it took so long to process laboratory work and no controls existed to ensure its accuracy, some doctors were reluctant to bring their private patients to the university hospitals. In contrast, other health-care facilities in Indianapolis, such as Methodist Hospital, already had central laboratories. By combining the six decentralized laboratory units into one, Gatch hoped to provide prompt and reliable service and predicted that the initial expense of setting up a central laboratory would be easily offset by its ability to bring in new revenue. That prediction was fulfilled in 1933 when the McNutt administration agreed to unify the state labs with those at the medical school.[79]

Gatch inherited a medical school far larger than his predecessor and one also with much larger problems. Although greatly expanded under Emerson, the IUSM physical plant was insufficient to meet the even greater demands it had engendered. For example, despite increases in faculty, the Bloomington staff remained seriously undermanned, and part-time faculty continued to make up a majority of the teaching staff. At the Medical Center in Indianapolis, the physical plant was insufficient to accommodate the school's operations. Plans for a much-needed psychiatric unit had been on hold since 1919, Long Hospital was overcrowded and in need of maintenance, and defects in the construction of Coleman Hospital and the Ball Residence for Nurses caused leaks that resulted in extensive water damage. Although quite functional, the Medical Center certainly had its deficiencies. Much of the campus had not yet been landscaped, streets and sidewalks remained unpaved, and everything was covered in dust during dry weather. After it rained, mud and water made the campus difficult to navigate. Students named "one noteworthy puddle" between the medical school building and Riley Hospital "Lake Neff" after the institution's former hospital administrator.[80]

In addition to the facilities and teaching staff, the clinical departments also suffered growing pains. With Emerson's departure, Gatch temporarily assumed the chairmanship of the Department of Medicine, which needed to be reorganized to meet the growing clinical demands.[81] In Orthopedic Surgery, Gatch proposed an arrangement to bring peace to a division of the medical school he claimed had long been "handicapped by violent internal animosities."[82] Gatch found the X-ray department (the most common reference to this service until the Radiology Department was created in 1947) in a complete state of disorganization. By the time he became acting dean, it had no personnel except students and technicians. In fall 1931, he carried out a complete reorganization whereby radiology became a division of the Department of Medicine, and Cecil S. Wright was appointed the first full-time roentgenologist at the IU Medical Center. Radiographic training was integrated into all four years of medical school, with additional elective training for those interested. Radiology teaching continued to be done by local physicians on the faculty, but the full-time clinical staff conducted the clinical film reading and therapy procedures. Although Gatch recommended delaying purchase of any new equipment until the personnel could be moved from its quarters in the basement of Long Hospital. An apparatus for deep therapy treatments was acquired by 1932 which enlarged the department's scope to include the care of cancer patients.[83]

Gatch's close relationship with Indianapolis physicians allowed him to expand medical school services for private patients and avoid charges of "socialism" by private practitioners. This was of crucial importance because without maintaining an income from private beds, he predicted that the hospitals would quickly go into debt. His strategy of attracting private patients to the university hospitals through the improvement of services worked. By improving the Laboratory and X-ray departments and by paying "close attention to the private patient wards," Gatch brought an increased number of paying patients to the Medical Center. For example, in 1930, the X-ray department saw just over four thousand patients, but by 1942, its patients numbered over fifteen thousand.[84]

The new dean also made economies in the purchase of supplies and took advantage of funds that had been unexpended before his appointment. Because overhead administrative costs had "increased beyond the proportionate rate of increases in patient volume and administrative responsibility,"

Gatch eliminated several positions from the Medical Center's payroll, including custodians and clerical workers. By taking all of these measures, at the end of 1931, Gatch was able to accumulate a reserve fund of $30,000, helped in addition by the Depression-era reductions in the cost of food and other basic commodities.[85] Lute Troutt, head of the Dietetics Department, was able to lower the cost of serving a meal to such a degree that she saved the school thousands of dollars. It was one example of the large number of "shop floor" improvements, such as rigid economy in the use of drugs and other supplies throughout the hospitals, that helped the school contain its costs.

Gatch also initiated the first measures to prevent conflict of interest. For several years, because of the low salaries they were paid, some members of the full-time, preclinical faculty had engaged in outside work for fees. Myers in particular was concerned that this practice endangered the school's ranking with the American Association of Medical Colleges, and it troubled Gatch because university personnel and supplies were used "without any record or payment." To put a stop to this, Gatch established rules that full-time faculty had to report any work done outside their positions within the school. The work could not interfere with their official duties, it could only be of small amount, and any university supplies used had to be purchased.[86]

Yet even with these measures and a reserve fund in hand, the financial acumen of the medical school leaders continued to be tested as state finances deteriorated further. In 1932 and 1933, the state legislature cut the School of Medicine's budget from $425,000 to $350,000, forcing medical school officials to find ways to economize even further without jeopardizing the quality of instruction and patient care.[87] This budget was a bit above the minimum amount that Gatch estimated the medical school and hospitals needed to remain in operation, not counting income from other sources,[88] but the next state budget brought further bad news. For the 1933–35 biennium, Gatch had to reduce the budget by an additional 15 percent. To accomplish this, the dean eliminated more positions and cut all salaries by 1 percent. Through these methods, Gatch again balanced the budget and worked to ensure that the medical school and hospitals always had a surplus of $10,000 "to take care of emergency demands."[89]

However, no amount of economizing could overcome the reality that demands for services were exceeding the physical capacity of all the hospitals. As Gatch summed up the cause of the dilemma, "While the depression brought low prices, it also gave rise to increased demand for services." In the early 1930s, the waiting list for Long Hospital seldom counted less than six hundred patients, and at Coleman Hospital, waiting lists rarely dipped below three hundred women. Later in the decade, this problem became even worse. At one point in 1938, the waiting list for Long Hospital reached almost two thousand patients, and in 1936, nearly one thousand children waited to receive care at Riley Hospital. Because of this situation, these hospitals had to admit patients with the greatest need. There was little room for patients who suffered from chronic conditions. Patients with mental illnesses continued to be cared for in state psychiatric facilities.[90]

Despite frequent fear that the medical school would run out of money during the 1930s, Gatch's cautious approach soon netted surpluses. Because of the continued uncertainty of the financial situation, the dean deferred expenditures for equipment replacements or any improvements until he was certain that he had adequate funds to keep the school and hospitals operating. By June 1934, the medical school's surpluses totaled over $115,000, and Gatch finally believed that there was enough money in the school's coffers to cover any emergency. He therefore asked permission to use $50,000 to retire much of what the school still owed in bonds from construction projects undertaken in the 1910s and 1920s. The surplus accumulated from Riley Hospital was used to reduce the institution's patient per diem charges. The dean also authorized the purchase of new beds, mattresses, and operating room equipment for Long Hospital and appropriated money for repairs to Ball Residence and Coleman Hospital.[91]

Calls for austerity obscured the tremendous growth of the school operations in the preceding decades. Despite cuts in appropriations, the school's budget was more than three times greater than it had been just one generation earlier. At the time of the Flexner Report, the medical school had operated with a budget of less than $100,000. Although the school did not compare with the nation's leading medical institutions whose annual budgets surpassed $1 million, by the mid-1930s, net expenditures for the IUMS, excluding the hospitals, reached about $230,000. By the end of the decade, expenditures exceeded the national median of $244,350.[92]

One reason for this growth was philanthropic donations, which had been crucial for hospital facilities from the start. They now helped resolve some of the fiscal and physical constraints that were limiting the ability of the medical school to respond to the increasing demand for clinical services. The best example is support for Riley Hospital, which in 1931 received a $75,000 donation from Psi Iota Xi sorority "for the complete equipment of an oxygen treatment room" at the hospital. In 1935, the women's organization equipped a light therapy department in the pediatric facility. Earlier, prominent businessman and School of Medicine Research Committee member Peter C. Reilly gave $21,000 "for better facilities for

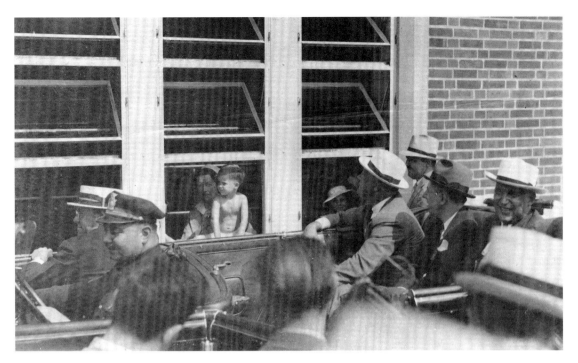

Figure 6.5. Roosevelt visit to new Riley swimming pool, September 5, 1936. IUPUI image UA024_001775.

the treatment of . . . infantile paralysis and other [orthopedic] difficulties" at Riley Hospital. Medical school officials and the Riley Memorial Association (RMA) ascertained that "chief among the services needed was a therapeutic pool." Although Reilly's donation was made in 1931, because of economic circumstances, construction of the pool did not begin immediately. In August 1934, the FERA joined with the RMA and the university to finance its construction. Fashioned after the one used by President Franklin Delano Roosevelt in Warm Springs, Georgia, it was dedicated in October 1935 and acclaimed as one of the most complete therapeutic pools for the treatment of polio in the United States. Roosevelt himself visited the Riley Pool in September 1936.[93]

By far the most important capital investment during the interwar period was the construction of the Clinical Building that was added to the back of Long Hospital in early 1938. Thanks to funding from the Public Works Administration (PWA), the addition included six modern operating rooms, new facilities for occupational and physical therapy, and space for an increased number of hospital inpatients. One floor was designed as a dormitory for residents who moved from space in Riley Hospital that was

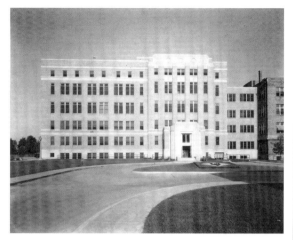

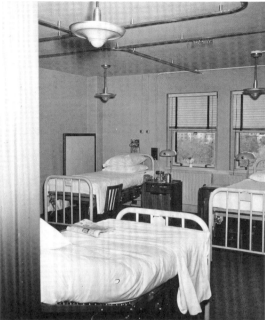

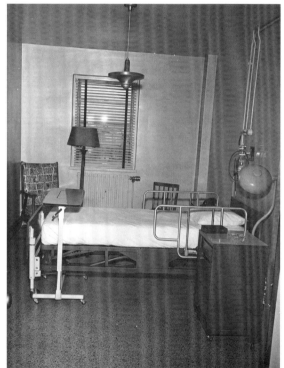

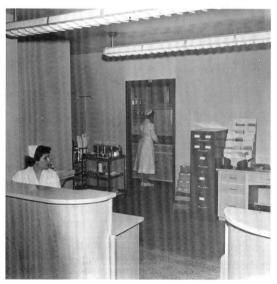

Figure 6.6a, b, c, & d. Clinical Building attached to rear of Long Hospital, published in *IUMC Quarterly Bulletin* 1, no. 1 (January 1939): (*clockwise from top left*) exterior view, IUPUI image UA024_002580; four-bed ward, IUPUI image UA024_003684n; private bed important for additional hospital income, IUPUI image UA024_003685n; nursing station, IUPUI image UA024_003683n.

made available for nurses to use as housing.[94] The new building allowed the clinical departments to move from Long, Coleman, and Riley Hospitals to the new six-story structure. One of the most important departments that relocated to the Clinical Building was the cancer clinic, which took up a large part of one floor in which radium and X-ray treatments were provided to aid the many patients who suffered from the disease. The building's formal dedication was on May 14, 1938, at which Gatch declared that "this department alone [was] worth to the people of Indiana far more than the dollar and cents cost of the whole building in the alleviation of pain and suffering."[95]

By concentrating various activities in one central location, the Clinical Building became the "nerve center" of the Indianapolis campus as soon as it opened. Gatch explained the improvement it brought to the Medical Center's functions in a number of different ways: "Broad extension of facilities for teaching students of medicine; greatly increased patient capacity; a speeding up of all clinical and technical services and, most important, a greater economy of operation have been the ends sought by the university . . . in this splendid addition to the [medical] school." Gatch added, "The state will benefit largely throughout the years as we put our new facilities to good use."[96] Whereas the Medical Center formerly had three admitting rooms, now it only had one. About twenty outpatient clinics had been held on various parts of the campus, "often in very crowded conditions." The Clinical Building permitted the centralization of all of these clinics in one modern facility. In addition, the X-ray and laboratory services were now much closer to the departments they served.[97]

With the opening of the Clinical Building, Gatch hoped that the establishment "of an efficient out-patient service in the new building would diminish . . . waiting lists." Instead, any shift to outpatient care was more than exceeded by an increasing number of patients who sought admission to the hospitals. In fall 1938, the waiting list for the beds in Long Hospital reached over 1,900 people. Newspapers and local physicians across the state heaped criticism on the medical school because its hospitals could not admit patients. The tremendous demand for the services of Long Hospital had created "a dangerous situation" because "the need of many of these patients for medical and surgical care [was] so urgent that death or great suffering result[ed] from their not receiving it."[98]

Although sufficient clinical facilities were provided for children, the adult hospital beds available at the Medical Center were grossly inadequate, "both to meet the needs for service and for purposes of instruction." Medical Center officials had boasted about their ability to care for an increased number of cancer patients in the Clinical Building's new radiology facilities, but there were no beds for cancer patients. Therefore, radium and deep therapy "X-ray apparatus [lay] idle while patients suffer[ed] from the lack of their use." Gatch told President Wells that these were powerful arguments "for the necessary money to open the unused part of the new building and even to erect another hospital."[99]

Wells understood that these circumstances had broader implications for Indiana University as a whole. The costs of medical education were much higher than in any other field of instruction. During 1937–38, $430,000 out of a total state appropriation of $1,890,000 for the university (almost 23 percent) was allocated to the operation of the Medical Center. Yet the medical and nursing schools had an enrollment of 498 students, "as compared with a total university enrollment of 7,085," or just a little over 7 percent of total enrollment. In addition, almost $60,000 was appropriated for the medical school in Bloomington. The high percentage was not unusual for university medical education, and Wells admitted that the IU School of Medicine received less money "in proportion than other state-supported medical schools comparable in rating." But he pointed out, "Surely, fairness to the remainder of the departments of the University would not allow us to go further than we have already gone in support of medical education."[100]

The solution Wells proposed grew out of his previous experience in state government and financial institutions. First, he recognized "that the larger part of the money allocated to the Medical Center ha[d] to be spent for direct assistance to indigents." These were patients from across the state who, according to the agreement of the state to support the construction and maintenance of Long Hospital, could be referred to the hospitals in Indianapolis if they were unable to pay for their care. Otherwise, they would become patients at a county institution. Second, he realized that a large proportion of the state's funding for the School of Medicine in Indianapolis was being applied to the costs of caring for these indigent patients, and this in turn limited the amount of money left to spend directly on educating medical students. Therefore, instead of asking for increases in special appropriations, Wells proposed legislation "to enable the actual cost of charity work to be charged to the county from which the patient comes." Wells warned, "Unless some such plan is followed . . . charity hospitalization and medical treatment threaten not only to engulf medical education itself, but also to engulf and destroy the entire University."[101]

Heeding Wells's warning, a bill was introduced to the 1939 General Assembly that empowered state circuit judges to commit adult indigent patients to the IU Medical Center and required county authorities to pay for their care. This bill followed model guidelines that were similar to those contained in the law respecting admissions for Riley Hospital. Gatch asserted that the university hospitals provided better medical care for the indigent than elsewhere. Moreover, with the Medical Center's new and stronger infrastructure of administrative and medical facilities, he told legislators that implementing the new law would represent a saving to the state. Throughout the Great Depression, the school had "practiced the most drastic economies," the dean told legislators, but the time had come when these were no longer possible. With the strong support of the Indiana State Medical Association, the General Assembly passed the legislation in February 1939, which relieved the university from paying for the care of the sick poor and restored the institution's budget to the level at which it stood before Depression-era cuts.[102] Specifically, it also provided a means of defraying the cost of operating the new charity wards on the fourth floor of the Clinical Building.[103]

Gatch called 1939 the "most eventful" year "in the entire history of the Medical Center." He praised the passage of the law-making counties responsible for paying for the care and treatment of indigent adult patients because it made possible the completion of plans for the Clinical Building, including opening the new hospital wards and increasing the number of patient beds for the establishment of an isolation ward in Long Hospital. Relief from the burden of paying for charity care and the increase in the budget also enabled the school to occupy the operating rooms on the fifth floor. In turn, the old Long Hospital operating room suite was renovated into a central sterilizing room that served the entire campus.[104]

Other Program and Administrative Changes

In December 1939, the State Board of Health moved into another new structure at the Medical Center built with PWA funds and a state appropriation. This was the culmination of years of lobbying by IU professor of bacteriology Thurman B. Rice, who also held an appointment with the Indiana State Board of Health. Although resisted by McNutt, Rice ultimately was successful in convincing his successor, Governor M. Clifford Townsend, that a separate building for the agency was needed and that it belonged on the IU School of Medicine campus. Rice was "very anxious to have the building *right in the middle of the campus*" because it would be more convenient for them and "for the students who might use the building." More importantly, he felt this location, immediately northwest of the Clinical Building, "would insure freedom from political influence." Rice had trained with Emerson and John Hurty in the 1920s and hoped for the establishment of a public health program in the medical school that would serve the same purpose

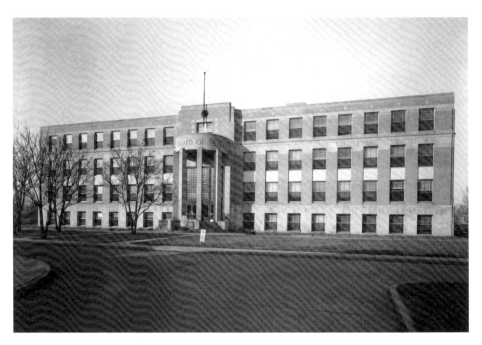

Figure 6.7. Board of Health Building, 1939 (now Fesler Hall). IUPUI image UA024_003765.

as Emerson's Social Service Department. In 1937–38, he became chairman of a new Department of Bacteriology and Public Health that split off from the Pathology Department. This allowed Rice and the new department to work more closely with the State Board of Health, which was relocated to the medical campus. It was housed there for the next ten years and was named Hurty Hall after Rice's mentor and the first secretary of the Board of Health. When the Board of Health needed more space and moved into a new building west of the campus on Michigan Street in 1949, IU obtained the old facility and renamed it Fesler Hall.[105]

As mentioned earlier, at the end of the 1940 spring semester, Burton D. Myers announced his retirement from the School of Medicine after thirty-seven years, thus marking the end of an era and prompting a major change for the institution. In 1903, Myers had been the first person Bryan hired to be a member of the school's faculty, and he had played a critical role in almost every step of the institution's development.[106] Since 1927, Myers had the title of dean of the School of Medicine for Bloomington as well as chairman of the Department of Anatomy. This meant that administration of the two medical school campuses were separate, and Myers submitted separate budgets and annual reports for the first year of the medical course. Because the two campuses did not function administratively as one unified school, this situation heightened the division between the preclinical and clinical departments that resulted from their geographic separation and differences in their culture.[107] As mentioned earlier, this was also the source of criticism by the Weiskotten Report and the AMA Medical Education Council.

Myers's retirement permitted Wells to correct this situation. He suggested integrating the work of the School of Medicine on both campuses by the appointment of a single dean. Wells was advised that unifying the school's administration would "be beneficial and [would] go a long way toward overcoming any objections" that had been made by the Rockefeller Foundation and the AMA Council on Medical Education in the past about the school's divided organization. The university president recommended that Gatch assume the deanship of the school for the two campuses on condition that he spend one day a week in Bloomington. Gatch agreed to work out the details of this arrangement with Wells and officially became dean for all medical education on July 1, 1940.[108]

Making Gatch dean for both campuses also had the effect of giving the medical school more autonomy. Myers had always exercised a strong influence on medical school policy, which acted as a check on the power of the Medical Center in Indianapolis. He represented the portion of the faculty that had more in common with professors in the Arts and Sciences in Bloomington than with the clinical faculty in Indianapolis. Gatch's expanded authority moved the medical school's center of power completely away from the Bloomington campus, and despite "gradually consolidating [the School of Medicine's] forces for a more concerted development in the field of research," Gatch leaned more toward the clinical and fought to maintain as much independence as possible for the medical school within the university. This stance soon pitted him against Wells and continued the rift between Bloomington and Indianapolis, albeit in a somewhat different form.[109]

One final administrative change came in an effort to alleviate problems of waiting lists at the hospitals. In June 1940, John D. Van Nuys, a 1936 IU School of Medicine graduate who had also served his internship and residency at the Medical Center, became director of all hospital admissions. The appointment of such a junior person to a position with this scope of responsibility is explained by his strong ties to the local medical establishment. Van Nuys was a third-generation physician whose father, W. C. Van Nuys, had served as head of the Indiana Epileptic Village since its creation in 1907, the year of his birth.[110]

The responsibilities of the Van Nuys position involved everything connected to the admission and discharge of patients, including "the most important relations of the Medical Center with the public, physicians, judges and public welfare workers." As director of hospital admissions, Van Nuys kept a waiting list of hospital patients, saw that patients were admitted as promptly as possible, gave preference to those most in need, and eliminated from the list patients who could be cared for at home. He also carried out the critical duty of making sure that patients were not kept in the hospital an unnecessary length of time.[111]

Despite Van Nuys's efforts to reduce the hospital stay of each patient, waiting lists continued to exceed one thousand patients. Only two years after the Clinical Building opened, all space on the IU Medical Center campus was occupied. The school still lacked a psychiatric unit, and isolation wards in Riley and Long Hospitals were inadequate. Although the medical school entered into a contract with City Hospital to treat African American patients from outside Indianapolis, the university hospitals continued to refuse admission of local African American patients. This prompted the City Hospital's assistant superintendent to complain that these patients from outside Indianapolis kept city residents from receiving care in his institution. Gatch responded by proposing the creation of a "temporary" African American facility, but the war crises prevented the proposal from being acted on. In addition, Gatch was concerned that admission of black patients to the Medical Center would increase the demand to train African American interns and nurses in these facilities, a step that he viewed as unnecessary and further complicating graduate medical education.[112]

The Clinical Building provided genuine relief to the physical strains on clinical services, but once again, the possibility of building substantial space for medical research was pushed off into the future. This was another deficiency that reflected poorly on a school that was eager to enhance its national reputation. Increasingly, research was becoming "a prime requirement of any school which hope[d] to maintain a good national standing." Gatch noted in his 1931 annual report on the school that a 1930 White House Conference on Child Health and Protection reported that the Department of Pediatrics "was without provision for research."[113] For the school to remain competitive, Gatch argued, he needed to stimulate research activity within the institution. Even if he could not obtain new facilities, he wanted at least to rationalize existing research policies. Although the School of Medicine now had over $10,000 available annually for research, it had not established a mechanism to administer funds or to review the conduct of research. By creating a Research Division for the School of Medicine in December 1931, Gatch recognized that research would "no longer be regarded as an incidental matter" in medical education.

In connection with the establishment of the Research Division, Gatch appointed a committee of faculty and donors to make the best possible use of research funds in the future. This committee first met at the end of 1931 and included Gatch, Myers, Robert E. Lyons, Hugh McK. Landon, Eli Lilly, and Peter C. Reilly. Although neither a physician nor researcher, Landon was appointed not only because his deceased wife had been responsible for providing the school with its largest research fund but also because of his position in the RMA and his expertise in banking. The other two laymen on this committee, Eli Lilly and Peter C. Reilly, each had extensive experience supervising research within their respective corporations: Eli Lilly and Company and Reilly Tar and Chemical Corporation.[114] Following the establishment of the Research Division in 1931, Gatch worked toward the creation of a research institute. Unfortunately, as late as 1939, IU's small amount of research funds made this impossible. The School of Medicine had available a sum approaching only $18,000 each year for research, whereas the annual research expenditures of some of the leading medical schools, such as Harvard, approached $1 million.[115]

Despite the ad hoc and underfunded world of research at the school, the work of the Research Division included both clinical and laboratory success. Laboratories for investigative work had been set up in the medical school building under the direction of Harold M. Trusler. In 1939, Trusler received national attention for his pioneering work on the treatment of burns. In Bloomington, Sid Robinson, a former Indiana University track coach who earned a PhD "under the direction of David Bruce Dill at the Harvard Fatigue Laboratory," began important "studies in the physiology of exercise and temperature regulation."[116] In addition, the School of Medicine was involved in research on acute intestinal obstruction and related physiologic disturbances, bacterial flora of the liver and other tissues, liver and bile peritonitis, studies on the nutritional elements contained in liver and other tissues, circulatory shock, and shock syndrome in peritonitis. Clinical research "included studies on wound healing . . . vascular disturbances of the extremities, and the therapeutic value of pectin in the treatment of diarrhea in infants." Hiring as chairman of the Department of Mental and Nervous Diseases someone like David A. Boyd Jr., a graduate of the Jefferson Medical College in Philadelphia who had been a professor at the University of Michigan School of Medicine, finally gave the IU School of Medicine the opportunity to extend its research into psychiatry. When he arrived in Indianapolis in 1939, Boyd immediately began a study of psychiatric behavior problems in children.[117]

Louis Mazzini in the Serology Department and Rolla N. Harger of the Biochemistry and Toxicology Department also brought national attention to the School of Medicine. Mazzini developed a new test for syphilis, and Harger developed the "Drunk-O-Meter," predecessor to the modern

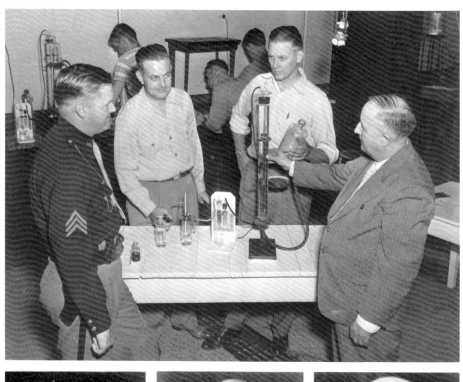

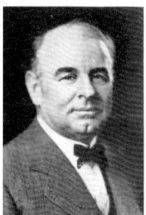 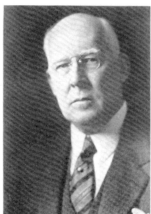 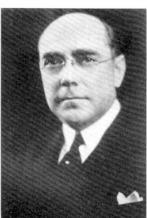

Figure 6.8a & b. IUSM Research in 1930s: (*top*) Rolla Harger, professor of toxicology and pharmacology, demonstrating his Drunk-O-Meter (precursor to breathalyzer) to Indiana State Police Trooper, n.d., IUPUI image UA024_000485; (*bottom*) IUSM Research Committee, 1939, whose members (*left to right* P. C. Reilly, Hugh McK. Landon, and Eli Lilly) helped provide $18,000 annually for research, *Quarterly Bulletin Medical Center* 1 (January 1939): 2.

Breathalyzer, which was developed by his collaborator at the Indiana State Police, Robert F. Borkenstein. In 1937, Harger donated the patent for the Drunk-O-Meter to the IU Foundation, the first ever held by this organization, and Mazzini followed his example. The medical school expanded its work in the study of forensic medicine and toxicology in conjunction with Harger's research. Robert B. Forney was appointed chemist in the Department of Biochemistry and Pharmacology to assist Harger "in doing analysis for poison." He became state toxicologist when the state legislature created the position in 1948, taking over work that Harger had done in an unofficial capacity since 1924.[118]

Gatch wanted to expand the school's research into "matters of hospital administration, nurses training, dietetics and medical pedagogy." He told the trustees at the end of 1939, "the spirit of research should permeate every activity of the Medical Center." Essential for medical schools "to be a genuine part of the university," research had become so central to their mission that it was a commonly held belief that "a faculty which [was] not constantly eager to improve its knowledge and practice [would] soon perish intellectually."[119] When Wells received the annual report on research from Gatch in 1939, it was an easy read of five pages. That same year the school began publishing its *Indiana University Medical Center Quarterly Bulletin* with articles on faculty research and clinical cases.[120] Nonetheless, by the end of the 1930s, the School of Medicine remained severely limited in the resources necessary to engage in advanced medical research. In addition, developments in the rest of the world made planning for the future very difficult.

Conclusion

The uncertain years of the 1930s were a test for the IUSM and the changing leadership of the university and the medical school. On the eve of the much greater trials of the war years, the school had shown a remarkable ability to adapt and even grow in response to the underlying and relentless demands on its training of doctors and other health professionals, as well as care for patients at its hospitals. Gatch, who was dean during most of these years, was well suited to the task, but his record can be better assessed after examining the medical school during the Second World War.

7

The Medical Center at War and After, 1941–1946

When the United States entered the Second World War, Willis Gatch had been dean of the IUSM for ten years. He had proven himself, under dire circumstances, to be an able administrator of a medical center that, in addition to a large medical school, included university hospitals, growing programs for nursing and other health-related fields, plus a relocated dental school and state Department of Health. His influence and the autonomy of the school had increased with the retirements of Bryan and Myers, architects of the beginning of the school. The demands of the war added to this trend, in the sense that the IUSM responded directly to outside demands, often bypassing the university administration in Bloomington.

Other trends affected by the war most obviously included a dramatic increase in enrollment of medical students, a long-standing demand of the state legislature, but this was recognized by all as only a temporary arrangement. Other wartime developments were more indirect or delayed in their impact on the IUSM. One example was support for research, which the school took advantage of only after the war. Nonetheless, American researchers made breakthroughs during the war, which dramatically affected medical practice and training, but this also came more gradually after the war to places like IUSM. Examples of these included the development of penicillin and other antibiotics, simpler transfusion techniques and blood fractionation, and a device put together by an isolated doctor in the German-occupied Dutch countryside to remove waste products in the blood of people with kidney failure.[1]

The impact of these developments took time, but the immediate challenges of the Second World War were formidable. Although the earlier world war was well within memory, this time the United States was involved much longer, thus greatly increasing the impact of the conflict on places like the IUSM. The state government expected the medical school to provide specific support for the war effort while maintaining its public services for the duration. Over eighty medical professors from the school eventually enlisted in the military, and the Indiana University School of Medicine instituted an accelerated education program allowing the school to teach more students within a calendar year than ever before, despite the strain on facilities, faculty, and staff.[2] Although the school took little advantage of research support offered by the federal government, throughout this period and continuing after World War II, Gatch articulated a vision for new investments in research. The dean had little idea, however, just how dramatically medical research would change after the war.

Well before December 1941, the Indiana University School of Medicine, like many American institutions, was planning for the conflict. As early as August 1938, Wilson von Kessler was appointed to the first full-time ROTC medical unit faculty post. By 1940, after the outbreak of hostilities in East Asia and Europe, many at IUSM felt that it was only a matter of time before the United States entered into another world war, and the medical school's executive committee stated with confidence that the Indiana University Medical Center was "prepared to meet any demand which the Government [might] make upon it." For example, by mid-1940, the Medical Center established a blood bank to meet any emergency, and in addition to training nurses and physicians, the school expected to help fulfill the US Army and Navy's demand for laboratory technicians. The medical school was also ready to expand its training, particularly to prepare men and women to be orderlies and ward helpers in case of a possible nursing shortage. Based on the experience of World War I, when Indianapolis physicians had organized an army hospital funded by J. K. Lilly, the School of Medicine also expected to be asked to plan to activate a general hospital unit. In the fall of 1940, the Army Medical Department made such a request.[3] There was little expectation of substantial increases in funding or the means to expand, so the coming of war prompted the medical school to brace itself for even more stress on its already severely strained budget and physical plant.[4]

War Comes to the Medical Center

In spite of this increased preparation, the attack on Pearl Harbor on December 7, 1941, both surprised and devastated the IU School of Medicine students and faculty. On Monday following the attack, they gathered in the auditorium of the Medical Building to hear President Franklin Roosevelt's message to Congress announcing that there was a state of war between the United States, Japan, Germany, and Italy. "For a time, the students and faculty seemed stupefied by the catastrophe," Gatch informed Wells. "It was hard for the students to study, and hard for the faculty to teach. There was a general feeling that 'nothing matters now.'"[5] After the attack, the "National Emergency" came to dominate all aspects of the activities of the medical school and the hospitals. The Medical Center provided extra community war services such as blood collection for the Red Cross, and the administration developed war precautions to protect the Medical Center from the possibility of air raids.[6]

In addition to concerns about the broader war effort, Gatch looked ahead and worried about struggling "to keep together a faculty able to instruct the students." Before national authorities issued definite orders to the nation's medical schools, Gatch feared that the school might "lose some irreplaceable men because of their determination to enlist." For example, in January 1942, Robert Glass, the school's neurosurgeon, applied for a commission in the navy, thus leaving the Medical Center without a neurosurgeon or neurologist. Gatch encouraged all essential faculty members to refrain from enlisting and warned Wells that the loss of Culbertson, the director of the school's laboratories, and Van Nuys, the director of hospital admissions, "would make it extremely difficult to operate the Medical Center."[7]

To prevent this, Gatch prepared a list of all essential teachers and staff and submitted them to the American Medical Association (AMA), the American Association of Medical Colleges (AAMC), and the Procurement Committee in Washington, DC. Gatch was advised that the Procurement Committee would deny commissions to all essential medical school personnel. He was also assured that the Medical Center would be allowed to keep "a skeleton staff of residents" in addition to a staff of interns; but he was told that he should "reserve as few men less than 36 years of age as possible." Demonstrating how much the Medical Center depended on residents as a labor pool for teaching and service, Gatch nevertheless placed all of the resident staff on the list of essential personnel. "It will be almost impossible," the dean said, "to carry our patient and teaching load if we lose them."[8]

As soon as war was declared, plans were quickly made to follow the recommendation of the Executive Council of the AAMC that member schools adopt "accelerated programs of instruction" to meet the anticipated increase in wartime demand for physicians.[9] On January 16, 1942, the Indiana University Board of Trustees adopted a "War Service Plan," and three days later, the Medical Advisory Council unanimously agreed to implement immediately a new three-semester-per-year schedule that would permit graduation in three years. Each semester included seventy-seven teaching days and six days for examinations, "making use of enough Saturdays to make the plan workable." The accelerated program was initiated with the January 1942 spring semester, which was followed by semesters that began in May and September. The three-semester plan required more teaching from a faculty that was greatly reduced in number. Students and faculty worked twelve months without breaks.[10]

Medical students faced new realities as the government ordered all third- and fourth-year medical students to apply "at once for a commission under pain of being subject to the draft." During World War II, medical students could enlist in the armed forces but still finish medical school. Once enrolled, they joined the Enlisted Reserve Corps so that they would not be drafted and sent to the front, and the army paid for medical school. Alternatively, if a medical student had already enlisted or been drafted, he could apply to be discharged from that service and immediately join the Enlisted Reserve Corps. After graduating from medical school, the newly minted doctors served as needed in the military.[11] Harold M. Manifold was one student who enrolled in this program. While in school, he was considered a private until he finished medical school, after which he became an officer while he completed two years of service.[12] Otis Bowen recalled that during the summer between his junior and senior year, he spent six weeks at Camp Carlisle in a medical officer training school. Once he graduated and completed a one-year internship, Bowen was commissioned as a first lieutenant in the medical corps.[13]

Because each commissioned student would be called to active duty in the medical corps, physical training was important at the Medical Center, and students reported for fifteen minutes of calisthenics each morning and forty-five minutes in team sports in the afternoon. Military discipline was enforced, with medical school officials informing the draft board about students who had unexcused absences or committed other infractions. These students could be declared "unfit for a position in the Medical Corps of the Army."[14]

The most visible contribution of the IU Medical School to the war effort was the Thirty-Second General Hospital Unit. As had been the case in the First World War, the US military once again encouraged medical schools and larger hospitals to organize medical units with staff who already had experience working together, so that they could be sent to war zones overseas and immediately be ready to function.[15] Cyrus J. Clark, son of Edmund D. Clark, who had led the medical school's World War I hospital base, was commissioned as a lieutenant colonel to serve in the newly created

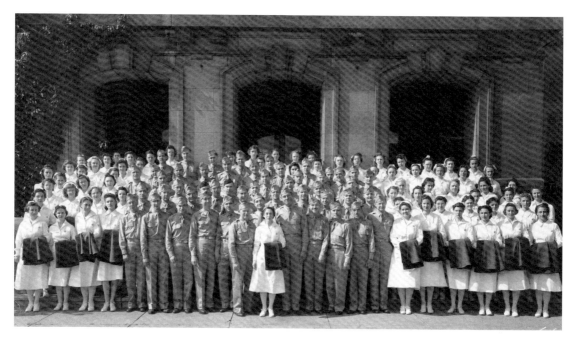

Figure 7.1. Induction ceremonies for 32nd General Hospital, May 13, 1942. Most of the doctors were either alumni or faculty members at the medical school, and most of the nurses were either graduates of the IU Training School for Nurses or on the nursing staffs connected with the IU Medical Center. *Quarterly Bulletin of IUSM* 5 (January 1943): 12–13. Also appeared in *Indianapolis Star*, May 14, 1942.

Thirty-Second General Hospital, and Charles F. Thompson became chief of the unit's surgical section. More than three thousand people attended induction ceremonies for the forty-seven doctors and dentists and seventy-two nurses at the IU Medical Center campus in May 1942. "The staff of the General Hospital 32," Gatch proudly declared during this ceremony, "is a contribution of Indiana University to the national cause and to the fighting forces of the nation. . . . We know that wherever they are they will acquit themselves in a way which will bring lasting credit to the university which sends them forth."[16]

The Thirty-Second General Hospital prepared for service at Camp Bowie near Brownwood, Texas, from March until August 1943, when it received orders to move to England. The unit was under the command of Lt. Col. Frank Alexander, a career army officer, and Cyrus Clark was named chief of medical service. Lt. Col. Charles Thompson became chief of surgical service, and 1st Lt. (later Maj.) Aurelia Willers served as chief nurse. The medical officers and enlisted men sailed from New York to Swansea (in Wales), and the nurses sailed from New York to Halifax, Nova Scotia, and

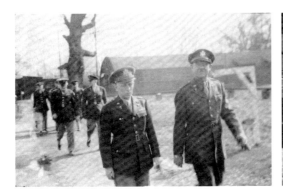
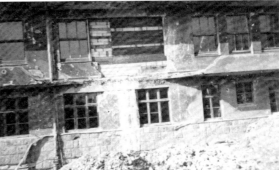

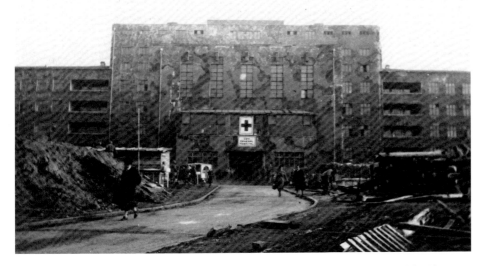

Figure 7.2a, b, & c. Thirty-Second Base Hospital: (*clockwise from top left*): "Cyrus Clark (*right*) with Surgeon General of the U. S. Army Norman T. Kirk, during an inspection, March 15, 1944," in Fairfield, England; Goering Hospital before repair; hospital after repair, Remagen, Germany, 1945. IUPUI archives, US Army Base Hospital No. 32 Mss 015. Clark, son of Edmund D. Clark, who headed Base Hospital 32 in WWI, helped organize the WWII hospital and was chief of medical service.

then to Scotland and reassembled at Fairford, Gloucestshire. The Thirty-Second General Hospital remained at Fairford from September 1943 to May 1944, and then after a brief stay at Minchinhampton, Gloucester, they shipped across the English Channel in July 1944 as the first Allied general hospital to arrive in France after the D-Day landings.

While stationed at La Haye du Puits in Normandy, the hospital unit handled 12,400 patients between August and November 1944. After this critical service, the Thirty-Second was transferred to a recently liberated area of Belgium before moving back toward the front as the Allies approached Germany. The unit then went to Aachen, Germany, early in 1945, where it was the first US Army general hospital stationed in Germany at a former thousand-bed hospital that had "suffered only minor bomb damage." The slight damages were repaired, and from March to July 1945, it became "one of the busiest general hospitals in Europe, handling 10,700 cases in the first ten days of operation." The IUSM staffed hospital treated a total of 53,820 patients before moving to Mourmelon, France, in August 1945, from whence most of the personnel left for New York in October 1945.[17] In late October 1945, the army officially deactivated the Thirty-Second General Hospital, and the officers and enlisted men were discharged at Camp Atterbury near Edinburgh, Indiana. "I find myself at a loss for words to describe the superb quality of medical personnel that came with this unit," proclaimed Major General Paul R. Hawley, a 1912 Indiana graduate who was chief surgeon of the European Theater of Operations. In particular, he commended Clark "for his inspiring leadership."[18]

Including the faculty who staffed the Thirty-Second General Hospital, eighty-three IU School of Medicine professors joined the armed forces during World War II. Defending the service of those that remained behind, Gatch asserted that "the patriotism and devotion of the members of the faculty" who stayed at home and bore "the load of teaching and medical service" at the Medical Center made the achievements of the Thirty-Second General Hospital possible. In cooperation with the Procurement and Assignment Agency, Gatch was able to keep his key personnel at the School of Medicine, including David Boyd in Psychiatry, Lyman Meiks in Pediatrics, Carl P. Huber in Obstetrics, and Robert Vandiever in Internal Medicine, in addition to Culbertson in Clinical Pathology and Van Nuys, who had become the Medical Center's director. All of the preclinical departments were adequately staffed except for the Department of Pathology, where Gatch lost the chair, and the Public Health Department, which Thurman Rice left to serve as acting state health commissioner from 1943 to 1945.

The Home Front

During the war emergency, part-time faculty, mostly over the age of fifty, taught the majority of the courses in the clinical departments. Because of increased patient loads, due to a general physician shortage on the home front, these part-time faculty members devoted much more time to teaching

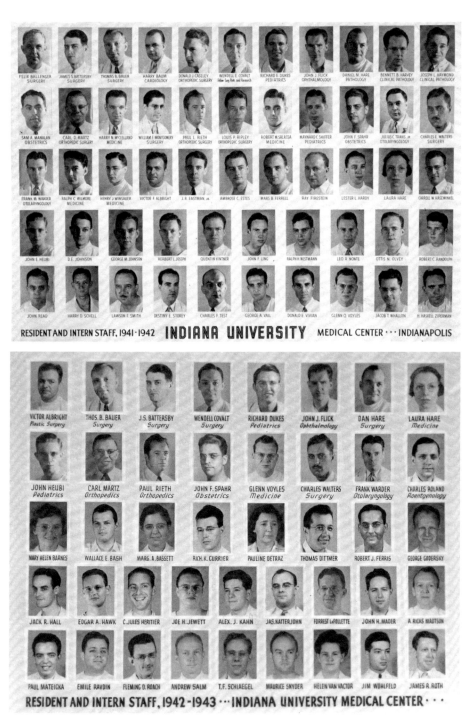

Figure 7.3a & b. Residents at IUMC during wartime: (*top*) 1941–42, typical in number and rare (one) female members, IUPUI image UA024_001008; (*bottom*) 1942–43, significantly smaller number in total and includes five women, IUPUI image UA024_001009.

than they had before the war. In fact, Gatch feared that "some of these men [would] break under the heavy strain of teaching and other work which they [were] doing."[19] The war also exacted a heavy toll on all graduate programs and research fellowships throughout the nation. The lack of residents added to the duties of the faculty who remained on the home front and soon created a shortage of young teachers and scientific investigators. In addition, internships were reduced from one year to nine months. Like other medical educators, Gatch was not pleased with the shortened internship period, and he recognized that at best, IU's hospitals would be able to retain only half of the normal quota of residents. By June 1942, seven residents had already left the Medical Center for military duty, leaving only one resident, a woman in internal medicine. The latter is an example of one of the results of war: previously marginalized women finally enjoyed opportunities on the teaching hospital house staff. In fact, the government urged medical schools to appoint women as residents so that men could be released for military service. As a result, the School of Medicine added three more females to the house staff. Gatch complained that the army even tried to pressure women into taking military commissions.[20]

The demand for nurses was even greater. Within nine months after the war began, the IU Medical Center lost nearly half of its graduate nursing staff, and the national nursing shortage made it impossible to replace the personnel who left. Therefore, IU hospitals could maintain only a skeleton staff of nurses to supervise trained nurses' aides; Cordelia Hoeflin, director of the nursing school, and the rest of her instructors had to take over a considerable amount of the duties ordinarily carried out by head nurses on the university hospital wards.[21]

In addition to the professional personnel lost to the war effort, the Medical Center experienced a large turnover of nonprofessional staff due to competition from private industry, a dramatic shift from the Depression years. Gatch admitted that without them, even "the lighting plants and elevators would have been out of service." So many employees left the laundry, housekeeping, and maintenance departments that it was necessary to drop all but the most essential work and services. "At one time the laundry was so behind with its work that even the operating rooms and nurseries did not have sufficient clean linen," and for much of the war, "painting, plastering, and care of the buildings had to go undone."[22]

Medical students also faced new problems. Deprived of the opportunity to work during the summer to earn money for tuition and expenses, the three-semesters-per-year schedule caused many medical students financial hardship, especially for nearly half of the students on the Indianapolis

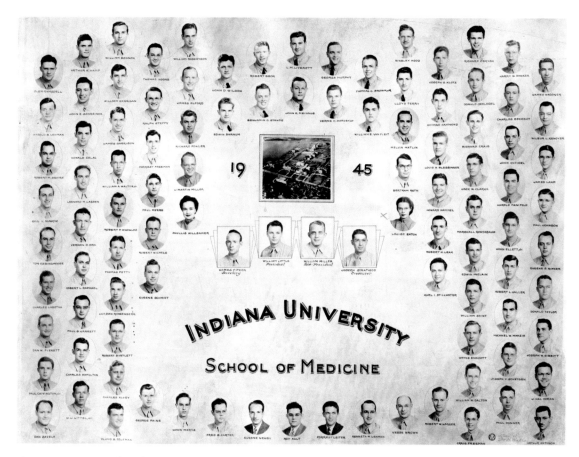

Figure 7.4. IUSM MD class of 1945, IUSM Alumni Association, IUPUI archives (cataloging in process).

campus who received financial aid. In response, at the beginning of the war, the Kellogg Foundation provided $10,000 to the IU School of Medicine as part of a national program to supply financial assistance to medical students. In addition, the School of Medicine received a private donation and transferred money from the Landon Research Fund for use as student financial aid. These funds enabled many medical students to remain in school until the fall of 1942, when $61,000 in federal loans became available.[23]

In late June 1943, all medical students with reserve commissions were inducted into the armed forces. A majority participated in the US Army Specialized Training Program (ASTP); and a smaller number entered the Navy V-12 Program. This was in keeping with national trends, where 55 percent entered the army, 25 percent the navy, and the remaining 20 percent went into civilian service.[24] The army and navy established these programs for officers in specialized fields, including medicine and dentistry, to absorb the increase in medical personnel produced by the accelerated pace of medical training. In all fields, from July 1943 to June 1946, IU trained more than three thousand men in the ASTP program, for whom the military helped to pay tuition as well as improve infrastructure. Among them was Charles Fisch, who earned his medical degree in two years and eight months and later became head of a heart institute at IUSM.[25]

Federal support for the accelerated teaching program was crucial. For Indiana alone, the added public expense for educating medical students the first year was estimated at a minimum of $1 million. In fact, Gatch was concerned that the army and navy would take control of the admissions process, whereas others feared even more that "Washington would get a permanent foothold in this field of education," as part of a scheme to socialize medicine.[26] The military initially planned to run the program, but it was turned over to the colleges for administration.[27] There was some basis to Gatch's concern about admission, however, because the accelerated program reduced the premedical requirement to two years of college preparation, thus making it "possible to graduate in twelve semesters [and only 5 years] above high school graduation." By January 1943, Gatch also received directives that current students would be inducted into the army but would be allowed to remain in school on inactive duty. Once they completed school, they would be called to active duty. Only those with aptitude would be allowed to stay in the army on active reserve to continue their studies; hence, the military now exerted influence on the critical matter of retention of students.[28]

With the shortened degree plan, the tempo of instruction accelerated at medical schools throughout the war. At the IU School of Medicine, the schedule required students to put in ten hours a day, six days a week and pushed them to the limits of their physical endurance. In addition, those in the army were required to drill five to seven hours a week. This prompted Gatch to complain, "The Medical School curriculum ha[d] been cut to the bone." As a result, he appealed to the registrar, "We need every hour of class work we can possibly get . . . to give the students the information they must have." At the same time that some material was eliminated, the military plan required the addition of instruction in military science and tactics. The IU School of Medicine, along with other medical schools, also had to increase instruction in such areas as tropical medicine and parasitology because of their relevance for some anticipated battlefield locations.[29]

The new enrollment challenges were of great concern to the dean, faculty, and students alike. Because admissions requirements were shortened at medical schools across the country, students "were younger, less mature, and not as thoroughly prepared." During this period, many individuals earned medical degrees by the time they were twenty-two. As Thurman Rice put it, "It is possible to teach the student that fast, but it must be admitted that he doesn't have much chance to 'grow up' during the process."[30] It was no surprise that problems appeared from the outset. In 1942, eleven members of the new accelerated freshman class failed. Although the Bloomington faculty offered to develop summer makeup courses, the student names were turned over to the draft board.[31] One of these students was Walter Tinsley, who enrolled in the Navy V-12 military program but lost his deferment after failing neuroanatomy. He was immediately activated, went on active duty, and worked in various navy hospitals during the war. For Tinsley, this was only a temporary setback. After the war, he took additional courses at IU to receive his BA prior to reapplying to the medical school. He was accepted, passed his neuroanatomy class (with a new instructor), and graduated in 1952.[32]

Due to wartime shortages of house staff, clinical experience increased for senior medical students. In 1943, for the first time, the School of Medicine gave fourth-year students the opportunity to have direct contact with patients when the institution "experimented on a limited scale with resident clerkships." At this time, the same kind of advanced clinical electives were developed, as was the case at other American medical schools. Senior medical students were "placed in the hospitals for a short period on all-time duty . . . under the direction of the resident staff." The following year, these senior clerkships were extended from six weeks to one full semester.[33]

The accelerated system was effective in increasing the number of graduates during the wartime years, although with a slight delay.

As table 7.1 indicates, for the four years from 1942 through 1945, the IUSM graduated 662 MDs, which was much more than the one hundred graduates per year before and after the war.

Table 7.1. IUSM Graduates, 1930–1950

Year	Graduates
1930	107
1931	108
1932	106
1933	115
1934	122
1935	100
1936	108
1937	101
1938	86
1939	104
1940	106
1941	97
May 1942	107
Dec 1942	104
1943	124
Apr 1944	116
Dec 1944	110
1945	101
1946	82
1947	101
1948	84
1949	81
1950	93

Source: Van Nuys to Wells, January 18, 1951, C213, InU-Ar.

One example of the impact of the war on the daily life of the Medical Center was the feeding of all the patients, students, and staff at the medical school. This became increasingly difficult with war shortages and rationing. Table service was discontinued in the nursing dining hall, but the university opened a canteen to help feed the workers who needed lunch at the Medical Center. Due to tight rations and budgets, even the serving of refreshments at a meeting could lead to heated discussions.[34]

By the beginning of 1941, nursing education had evolved to where one semester of college was required to begin programs offered at colleges and universities. In addition, more attention was focused on ward teaching, following the recommendations of the National League of Nursing Education. To handle the training of these increased numbers, the Medical Center was fortunate to have Ball Nursing Residence, which could house larger class sizes.[35] After Pearl Harbor, however, the system of nursing education faced severe challenges. Many graduate nurses at Medical Center hospitals entered military service and could not be replaced, and for similar reasons, students left the program before graduation. Out of a total of 135 beginning nurses, ninety resigned between July 1942 and March 1943. In addition to personnel, there were shortages in linen, medicines, and other supplies—and personnel in other support positions from kitchens to laboratory technicians.[36]

To meet the growing needs at the hospital and at the front, the nursing school also adopted an accelerated, yearlong program. In addition, the school conducted refresher courses for fifteen alumni on surgical and obstetrical nursing, and the school worked with the Red Cross Volunteer Nurses to train eighteen aides to help serve in the hospital. The Kellogg Foundation also gave a $4,000 grant for loans and scholarships. In 1943, the federal government stepped in and passed the Nurses Training Act to provide federal funds for student nursing training. Despite these efforts, nursing schools had a difficult time simply retaining the number of personnel to continue teaching, let alone recruiting and retaining students in the programs. As a result, the school waived the preparatory requirement of one year of college education, and with Riley Memorial Association support, the program recruited 103 freshman nurses in the fall of 1943. The response was so strong that Ball Residence threatened to burst at the seams, with nurses sleeping in the gymnasium to accommodate the incoming class.[37] The wartime exigencies also led to the entry of married women into nursing training for the first time, but they were still required to live on campus. Some of the clothing restrictions were relaxed, and for the first time, students were responsible for their own laundry.[38]

The federal government's involvement in the training of nurses was less direct than with medical students. The United States Cadet Nursing Corps program was operated by the United States Public Health Service to train nurses for a variety of government services. Unlike the military medical school program, there was no outside pressure on entrance requirements or operation of the school, nor did the government draft women into service. The Indiana Training School for Nurses was approved as part of the US Nursing Corps in September 1943. In the fall 1943 freshman class of 103, only seven did not join the Corps program. The federal government helped with financial support by providing stipends, uniforms, and money to pay for instruction. The Corps had a somewhat different system of labels for the various training periods. In their last phase of training, so-called senior cadets could go into federal military service, public health service, or other approved hospital settings. Those students electing to remain in their home school served at the IU Medical Center. Although the government asserted that it was not involved in changing the curriculum, those in the senior cadet program had to complete coursework in new areas of ward management within thirty months instead of thirty-six. The program ended in October 1945. Of the 107 IU School of Nursing graduates who saw actual military service during the war, twenty-one were with the Thirty-Second General Hospital Unit sent from the medical school. The school was able to recruit more students and move them more quickly through the program, but because of difficulty in retaining students, there was no dramatic increase in the total number of nurses who graduated during the war era.[39] As the previous chapter indicated (fig. 6.4), from a high of sixty in 1934, the annual number of nursing who actually graduated during the war was rarely more than forty.

In addition to medical education and clinical care, the war brought changes to the school's research mission. The government ordered that research should be limited "to projects of military importance" in the fight to conquer the soldier's greatest enemy, disease. As Gatch explained to the Research Committee in April 1942, this kind of research "covered a wide field," so that nearly every medical specialty could contribute to wartime research in some fashion. Although heavy teaching loads curtailed the opportunity to do much research, between July 1942 and August 1944, IU School of Medicine faculty published ninety-one scientific articles, more than doubling the number produced a decade earlier. Their research included studies of wound healing, gas gangrene, shock, and streptococcus infections. Harold Trusler continued his work on burns in plastic surgery, and in the cancer clinic, Arthur P. Echternacht did research on radiation therapy. In collaboration with K. K. Chen, chief pharmacologist for Eli Lilly and Company, IU School of Medicine faculty members Thomas B. Bauer and Harry Baum participated in clinical trials for sulfa drugs and for "certain synthetic digitalis-like drugs."[40]

In biochemistry, Donald E. Bowman made important discoveries about amylase and protease inhibitors contained in beans. When Bowman first arrived at the IU Medical Center, Gatch questioned him relentlessly about "the disturbances of digestion following the ingestion of beans." Bowman later explained that "the Dean meant to leave no stone unturned in his search for a better understanding of postoperative gas pains." Finally taking up Gatch's questions, Bowman's research resulted in the discovery of the Bowman-Birk protease inhibitor, a substance in soybeans, which was later found to have "the ability to suppress the carcinogenic process" and therefore potentially be an agent in the treatment of cancer and other diseases.[41]

During World War II, medical faculty sought research contracts for the first time from federal agencies, thus taking advantage of greatly expanded opportunities and setting important precedents for the postwar period. To this end, Washington established the Committee on Medical Research (CMR) in June 1941 as part of the Office of Scientific Research and Development (OSRD), which coordinated all defense-related scientific investigations. In addition to well-known projects such as production of penicillin and blood fractionation, the CMR funded projects of more limited scope in aviation medicine and infectious disease. In all, 591 research contracts were given to 135 universities, hospitals, and research institutes.[42]

Examples of faculty receiving federal funding include Rolla Harger of the Biochemistry and Toxicology Department in Indianapolis, who prepared manuals at the request of the government on the detection of poison in water supplies and on the identification of gases. Sid Robinson in the Department of Physiology in Bloomington, after a leave of absence at the Harvard Fatigue Laboratory, received a contract for over $34,000 to study physiological reactions to the exigencies of war from the Committee on Medical Research. Although this direct federal involvement in funding research at the School of Medicine was new, the relative paucity of contracts from the CMR indicated once again that compared to other medical schools, Indiana was a minor player in the growing fields of biomedical research.[43]

The Postwar Agenda

By 1944, the leadership of the university and the IU medical school began to plan in earnest for changes to the school after the end of the war. This was in keeping with a national recognition of the issue. Although helping the United States and its allies to win the war remained the immediate goal of medical schools, the AAMC advised that plans should be made "to handle intelligently many perplexing problems which [would] certainly arise for solution during the postwar period."[44] Much was uncertain, but some continuities and changes appeared obvious. For example, medical schools and the universities expected that the federal government would continue to fund scientific and medical research after the war. Although by statute the Office of Scientific Research and Development (OSRD) was to end when the war concluded, other federal agencies (both military and civilian ones like NIH) were making plans to continue to support research. Medical schools, which had received the bulk of research contracts from the Committee for Medical Research, shared a belief in the effectiveness and importance of federal involvement in the advancement of science and medicine. The ability to mobilize science to solve medical problems in the war was widely recognized as transferable to diagnosing chronic and degenerative disorders of civilian life. As stated by OSRD director Vannevar Bush in his widely influential book *Science, the Endless Frontier*, the American scientific effort that helped win the war need not and should not come to an end. Rather, "New frontiers of the mind are before us, and if they are pioneered with the same vision, boldness, and drive with which we have waged this war we can create a fuller and more fruitful employment and a fuller and more fruitful life."[45]

A second continuity that the IU medical school anticipated after the war was increasing demand from the state legislature to provide adequate numbers of qualified physicians to serve the people of Indiana. This was hardly a new issue because the fulfillment of the educational mission was continually a question among legislators. In January 1945, this took the form of a joint resolution introduced by State Senator C. Omer Free of Vincennes, claiming that "even before the war," by "maintaining too high standards," the Indiana University School of Medicine was responsible for "a scarcity of medical doctors in the State of Indiana." Free believed that the medical school should have been graduating more students considering "the total appropriations [it received] from the State . . . [had] been so great." A special legislative commission was soon appointed "to make a thorough investigation . . . to see if more students [could] be graduated."[46]

Senator Free complained specifically that the School of Medicine had not increased admissions either in proportion to Indiana's population growth or to replace physicians who died. Although it is difficult to determine how many physicians died each year, in fact the increase of Indiana's population from 1920 to 1940 was 17 percent, whereas the annual number of IU Medical school graduates increased from forty-eight to ninety-three (94 percent). The response of Indiana University officials was that the policy of the School of Medicine had been "to graduate as many Medical Doctors [*sic*] as possible without lowering the standards of [the] school with regard to the facilities available." According to John Hastings, an attorney who represented the board of trustees during legislative hearings, "if we rank sixth in out-put and we don't rank sixth in facilities," then legislators had to agree that "we have been strained to our limits."

Although it proposed no new legislation, the Free Commission raised two issues that have remained continuing subjects of concern ever since. The first was whether to establish a second medical school in the state. Despite the data supplied by the medical school, the commission's determination was that Indiana had "not increased the number of medical students graduated in proportion to the increase in population, probably because Indiana ha[d] only one Medical School . . . and further because . . . the facilities at the Indiana Medical Center [had] not been expanded within the last ten years." However, because of the continued national emergency, the commission agreed that it was not an expedient time to enlarge facilities. Its report concluded by commending Gatch and all of his personnel for their "splendid record of service in maintaining . . . [the IU School of Medicine] upon a high standard."[47]

Although not featured prominently in the debates, the second issue besides the number of graduates was where they practiced, and more specifically how many stayed in Indiana and whether they practiced outside the urban areas of the state. As shown in the previous chapter (table 6.3), according to a 1940 study, nearly one-third of the students did their internships outside of the state of Indiana, which made them much less likely to return. And of those internships in the state, only a small percentage (15–16 percent) were outside of Indianapolis, which made the students less likely to practice where most people lived.[48] Moreover, according to the medical school's placement of graduates in 1940, there were ten more internships in the state capital than in 1931, whereas only one more internship was added outside of Indianapolis.[49]

When the Free Commission made its report in February 1945, it was not clear when World War II would be over. The previous September the IU Board of Trustees passed a resolution stating that "the progress of the war" made it imperative for the university to prepare "to meet its postwar responsibilities and obligations." The School of Medicine responded to this resolution by appointing special committees to study various aspects of the institution's future needs, including education and administration, research, postgraduate study, public health, Riley Hospital, and the physical plant.[50]

In June 1945, just weeks after victory was secured in Europe, the School of Medicine delivered its report on postwar plans to the board of trustees. From the beginning of this document, it was clear that the faculty members who remained on the campus and served on the special postwar planning committees took their assignment very seriously. They stated that they had promised their colleagues who had left to serve in the armed forces that they would maintain and preserve the school of medicine until they came home. Committee members had, "a deep sense of responsibility in making . . . plans for its development" and understood that the school's future depended upon the decisions they made. Although the IU School of Medicine was in urgent need of new buildings, the postwar planning committees regarded "as more important than any material improvement, the adoption of proper and better plans for its educational, scientific, and administrative work."[51]

Nevertheless, much of what these special committees envisioned hinged on the physical expansion of the Medical Center campus because little could be done to improve the school of medicine's programs and services without new construction. As facilities were filled to capacity and pressure was again building to produce more physicians and care for more patients, the Committee on Plans for New Buildings turned to ideas that had been on hold since before the war. The need for research facilities and classrooms had become so critical that the building committee concluded that the first structure erected as an addition to the Indianapolis campus should be a medical science building, which would include laboratories, departmental offices, recitation rooms, and amphitheaters. In addition, the committee contended that space in this building should be provided for expanded instruction in the School of Medical Technologists and a proposed School for Physical Therapists.[52]

Another committee on Plans for Research, directed by Gatch, concluded that the school had always had a sound research policy and that these same principles should be followed in future plans for its promotion. Therefore, it recommended that the existing school Research Committee (established in 1931) should continue its work but that a new research director should be hired to serve "as general adviser to all research workers, evaluate research problems and stimulate research workers to continued effort both in the conduct of research and in the publication of its result." The postwar research planning committee assumed that ample space would be provided for laboratories in the new medical science building, and it recommended strengthening the staff of both preclinical and clinical departments to give faculty sufficient time to carry out important investigative studies. Because it was not yet clear what form future government funding would take, the committee report merely suggested that the Research Committee "should co-operate with the Indiana [University] Foundation in the solicitation of gifts for research and in the provision of grants for research." Nevertheless, the goal was to make the school's program "elastic enough to make use of any promising opportunities for research and for any activity which [would] directly or indirectly help research." Similarly, the committee encouraged investigators to cooperate across preclinical and clinical departments and directed special attention toward clinical research, "especially in the determination of end results of treatment."[53]

Finally, the report to the trustees again raised the matter of the geographic separation of the first year of instruction in Bloomington from the rest of the school in Indianapolis as standing in the way of meeting many of these goals. It argued that as long as the departments of anatomy and physiology were in Bloomington, it would be impossible for the School of Medicine to reach its potential in terms of cooperative research in the preclinical and clinical departments. Moreover, the institutional split made it difficult to give proper emphasis to the basic sciences beyond the first year of the medical course. The postwar planning committees concluded that the consolidation of the school in Indianapolis had become critical to the School of Medicine's reputation.[54]

Another Change of Dean

The issue of consolidation was not new, but it quickly and unexpectedly flared up into a major personal confrontation between Gatch, the longserving medical school dean, and University President Wells. The postwar planning committees were dominated by Indianapolis medical faculty, and their recommendations were met with anger and disbelief by medical faculty in Bloomington. It was easier, however, for Wells to appreciate the benefits of consolidation in Indianapolis. Unlike Bryan forty years earlier, Wells had no need to rely on the medical school to ensure there were enough students in Bloomington (in 1903 Bloomington had 790 students, and in 1945 there were 4,498).[55] In fact, the criticisms from the AAMC regarding the split campus further encouraged Wells to plan for medical education on a single campus in Indianapolis. Given the push for consolidation, however, Wells sought to guard against the possibility of demands for more autonomy at a unified medical campus by implementing new policies that would make financial affairs at Indianapolis subject to additional control from Bloomington. Gatch, who had labored through economic depression and war for the opportunity to expand research and modernize the school, chose to focus on what he saw as the president's new meddling in the affairs of the medical school. The stage was set for another confrontation between the university president and the medical school dean over the direction of the school, but in the end the bone of contention was retirement.

From his perspective, Wells anticipated that Gatch would soon retire, which would give him the opportunity for the balanced plan he desired. According to the rules that the board of trustees had adopted following the establishment of a university retirement plan for deans in 1943, the medical school dean would reach retirement age in July 1946. When Gatch was informed of this in fall 1945, he claimed that he had never been notified and declared that these rules for retirement did not apply to him or anyone else at the Medical Center. He told Wells that he would be able to "carry on" as dean until he was eighty. Later in this conversation, Gatch asserted that the new retirement provisions had been passed to oust him and "to prevent the first year of medicine from being moved." A very embittered Gatch made it clear to the board of trustees that if forced to choose, the president should go. In other words, he asked them to be "willing to sacrifice the presidency [for him] to stay on as dean of the Medical School."[56]

The board of trustees thought that the matter of Gatch's retirement was something that the two men should work out themselves, instead of forcing its members to choose between them. In part, because Gatch had provided medical advice to almost everyone on the board, some trustees were just as devoted to him as they were to Wells. Therefore, according to Wells, the president attempted to find a compromise solution. Accordingly, Gatch would turn sixty-eight in July 1946, and Wells indicated that the dean might be permitted to continue until he reached the age of seventy, after which Wells could start to implement his program for the medical school. Gatch stood firm, however, telling the university president that he would retire only when he was ready.[57]

The situation dragged on for several months, and it became obvious to the board of trustees "that Wells and Gatch were more and more at swords' point." Although Wells acknowledged that Gatch deserved the opportunity to discuss his retirement with the board, the president decided to remain just as obstinate as the medical school dean. He therefore declared that Gatch had to retire on July 1, 1946, unless either the trustees repealed the university's retirement policy or an exception was made in his case.

At the same time, Wells stated that in his opinion, any proposal to extend Gatch's tenure was unwise. Demonstrating that their differences were not based solely on a conflict of personalities, Wells divulged that he opposed some of the principles Gatch wanted to employ in the School of Medicine's postwar plans. "The University must present critical problems to the next session of the Legislature," Wells said to the board of trustees. "I cannot accept responsibility for our legislative program if Dr. Gatch has any administrative position with the University." If Gatch were retained as dean, Wells informed the board that he would "no longer be useful as President." Wells offered his resignation to "provide the University with the maximum protection" against claims Gatch might make that his termination was due exclusively to irresolvable personality issues.[58]

As July 1946 drew near, an executive meeting of the board was called at the Columbia Club in Indianapolis with the purpose of coming to some agreement about the situation. Because some trustees still wanted to find a peaceable resolution to the problem, this board session "lasted quite some time." However, because both Wells and Gatch had issued ultimatums, the board finally concluded that Gatch should resign. Following this meeting, IU Board of Trustee members Ora L. Wildermuth, C. Walter McCarty, and George W. Henley reported that they "had an extended conference with Dean Gatch . . . and that . . . Gatch tendered to the committee his resignation both as Dean of the IU School of Medicine and as a member of the faculty." The Indiana University School of Medicine was ready to stake a claim on the "endless frontier" and confront the rising expectations of medical science, but after more than forty years of service to the school and fifteen arduous years as dean through the Depression and war, Willis Gatch would not lead the school to that frontier.[59]

Following Gatch's resignation in 1946, the Indiana University Board of Trustees appointed John D. Van Nuys, J. O. Ritchey, Matthew Winters, and Frank Forry to an interim committee to discharge the duties and responsibilities of the dean until a new one could be selected. Van Nuys accepted the position of executive secretary of this committee "with real reluctance."[60] In the dean search, the enduring tensions between the Bloomington and Indianapolis perspectives made finding consensus difficult, however there was enough agreement to begin a national search for the new dean. Even so, Thurman Rice spoke for many faculty members in suggesting to President Wells that Van Nuys was "the best person that could be found to be the permanent dean."[61]

As mentioned in the previous chapter, John D. Van Nuys was a third-generation physician whose father, W. C. Van Nuys, had been a prominent

Indiana physician. John graduated from the IU medical school in 1936 and completed his residency at the Medical Center in 1939. The following year, with the war looming, Van Nuys was appointed director of hospital admissions. Despite the fact that he had no faculty appointment, he quickly demonstrated his practical management skills, such that Gatch kept him from military service and appointed him director of the Medical Center. Van Nuys impressed faculty with his quick transition to planning for the future of the school on the Interim Committee. In the fall of 1946, Van Nuys emerged as the leading internal candidate for the position of dean.[62]

Although held in high regard, Van Nuys was a questionable choice for some who thought him to be too young and too parochial. These concerns, however, were *prima facie* unlikely to be viewed as a problem by President Wells, who was a native Hoosier and Indiana University graduate, and who became president at the age of thirty-five.[63] In June 1947, Wells reported to the trustees that he had narrowed the choices down to Van Nuys and an outside candidate, Irvine McQuarrie, professor of pediatrics at the University of Minnesota.[64] Some trustees felt that Wells's preference for Van Nuys recast the young physician as a latter day version of himself. He was known to favor youth as being helpful in adapting to changing conditions, and being local was valuable in understanding Indiana medical politics. For the record, Wells said of Van Nuys that he had demonstrated "the ability to get along with various groups and factions of doctors."[65] Responding to the criticism that Van Nuys had never been in private practice, Wells argued that the physician's loyalty was to the university and maintained that the dean must be a full-time administrative position to properly serve the school.[66] Announcing the decision to appoint Van Nuys as the dean of the School of Medicine on June 5, 1947, Board President Ora L. Wildermuth echoed Wells's perspective. "I liken the situation somewhat to the position the Board was in when we were looking for a president. We have always been very happy that we chose, in that instance, to stay within our own family." As a result, Wells now felt he had his man at the head of the medical school in a way that was never true with Dean Gatch.[67]

Conclusion

The fifteen years of Willis Gatch's tenure as dean of the IUSM were dominated by the need to respond to the cataclysmic events of the Great Depression and the Second World War. The initial years also were ones of transition in university and school leadership, but by the 1930s, the medical school was well established, and Gatch became dean after extensive experience in the important Department of Surgery, eventually serving as chair. The response of the school to these challenges was mixed. For example, Gatch and Wells were quite successful in fiscal affairs, trimming the budget without major cuts in services and even managing to secure increased support from the state and private philanthropy for patients in the hospitals. In addition, after a slow start, both the medical campus in Indianapolis and the first-year program in Bloomington obtained funds for new construction from the New Deal Public Works Administration. One of the buildings at the medical center was for the State Department of Health, but despite obtaining more laboratory facilities, the medical school missed another opportunity to develop an expanded program in public health.

The medical school's response to the war was also rapid and extensive but with a mixed record of results. Most immediate and impressive was the stepped-up pace of training doctors, and the service of graduates and faculty in the war effort. Especially noteworthy was the service of the reactivated Base Hospital 32 in the European Theater. One missed wartime opportunity was taking advantage of greatly increased research support offered by Vannevar Bush's Committee on Medical Research. This is understandable, however, given the much stronger emphasis at the IUSM on teaching and clinical care.

The dramatic events of the 1930s and world war masked some slower evolving developments that shaped the nature of the medical school since its beginning. The power and control of the dean clearly grew to what was probably its strongest point in the school's history. This was marked by confirmation of his control of medical teaching in Bloomington when Myers retired, as well as the continuing growth of the medical center in Indianapolis. The limits of Gatch's influence were found, however, when he challenged the president of the university and failed to secure his demands about retirement. This was more pointed but similar to the Emerson/Bryan disagreements, which also ended in the medical dean's departure, but there were other reasons for the decline of the influence of the dean after the war despite an even greater growth of the medical center. In fact, the increase in resources and responsibilities of the medical center made it more and more difficult for the medical dean to exercise control.

One important feature of the medical school that was called into question by the increased influence of the dean and the medical center was the division of instruction between Indianapolis and Bloomington. Discontent with the 1911 compromise simmered at first but grew along with the medical campus and drew much greater attention when the Weiskotten Report was issued at the end of the 1930s. Even though the events of the war interrupted the movement to consolidate, it was picked up shortly after the conflict came to a close, with every indication it would be a major part of postwar plans.

Overall, the IUSM emerged from the Depression and the Second World War not just as an institution that had survived but one with a stronger base, a record of resilience, and the ability to take advantage of some, if not all, opportunities. The most important new opportunities were offered by the federal government in matters of health. In the postwar years, after some internal, university, and statewide rebuilding and expansion, the IUSM was well prepared to take advantage of these national and global opportunities.

8

Crossing the New Frontier, 1946–1963

*A*fter 1945, while the conflict between Dean Gatch and President Wells was coming to a head, it was clear to the faculty and administration at Indiana University School of Medicine, as well as the rest of the world, that great changes were at hand. Although few anticipated just how extensively the world would be transformed, no one expected a return to the status quo antebellum. As to the field of medicine, it was approaching the peak of its "golden age," as some historians have dubbed the post-1945 period.[1] The major features of modern medicine had been emerging since the nineteenth century, and twentieth-century education reforms were part of the professionalization that ensured training in the new discoveries and practices. The world wars accelerated the application of this knowledge, and following the Second World War, it was soon clear that the federal government would dramatically increase support for medical research and hospital construction, two of the driving forces in modern medicine.

At the local level, the faculty and staff of IUSM who had served in the war returned with a sense of confidence that looked with optimism toward a new era, although from top to bottom, there was anxiety about exactly how things would work out. To the leadership of the medical school, the evidence was inescapable that the new dean of an expanding institution would confront growing responsibilities, albeit with possibly diminished control and resources. Likewise, students at the bottom of the medical school hierarchy were anxious about completing their degree and residency and then practicing their profession in these changing times.

The same underlying dynamics that exercised their influence on the medical school since its beginning were even more evident after both the war and economic depression had muted and diverted their impact. As mentioned in the previous chapter, at the close of the war, Gatch and his school (which had a monopoly on medical education in the state) were faced with demands from the Indiana legislature for increasing the number of physicians they trained. The returning veterans added significantly to that pressure. Shortly thereafter, Gatch and others revived the call for moving the first year of instruction from Bloomington to the Indianapolis campus. As to matters of hospitals and clinical care, any increase in enrollment would require additional clinical instruction, but the demand for more hospital facilities was also fed by the overall increase in medical diagnoses and treatments that were developed in the postwar period as well as the immediate need to expand services for returning veterans.

The medical school was eager to meet these demands, and the record clearly shows its success. Between 1946 and 1963, the School of Medicine faculty trained more doctors who saw more patients than ever before. In operational and funding terms, however, this growth in education was dwarfed by the growth in research. The story of this postwar period was deciding on requests and obtaining the additional resources to respond.[2] When John D. Van Nuys was named as dean in 1947, these changes were already taking place at other medical schools, where there was significantly more support from private philanthropies. Van Nuys was forced to confront the challenge of training more doctors without a faculty or facilities large enough for either classroom or clinical teaching or the laboratory facilities necessary to recruit the researchers who were expected to form the foundation of an enlarged faculty.

Given the growing size and complexity of each aspect of the school's teaching, research, and clinical care missions, their development during this period is best understood by examining the history of each in turn while identifying the ways they affected one another.[3] Before doing so, it is worth noting that all three were immediately affected by two broader developments in medicine at midcentury: specialization and growth of facilities. Specialization expanded after the war at every level of American medicine: training, clinical practice, and research. Physicians promised progress in clinical care as one argument for specialization. Accordingly, the growth in knowledge, techniques, tools, and therapies required specialization to provide the best diagnosis and treatment for each disease. In addition to this broad rationale, other forces influenced the transformation of medical practice toward specialist domination, such as compensation, professional rewards, and acclaim, plus regulation and licensure. The experience of many physicians during the war, where the military differentiated salary and gave higher rank to certified specialists, offered further evidence that

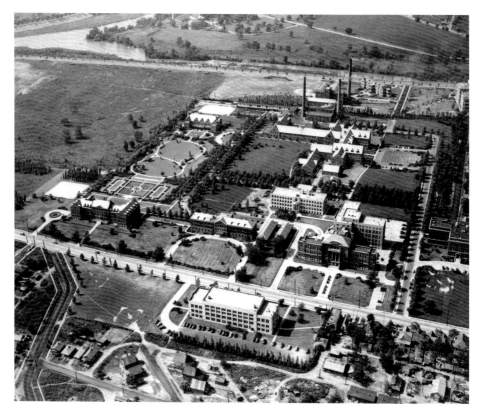

Figure 8.1a & b. Aerial view of medical center in 1946, IUB Archive photo collection P0035506; and in 1954 (*facing*) including addition of Union building plus VA and Larue Carter hospitals to the west and north, IUPUI image UA024_002492.

specialization carried benefits and rewards for the physician as well as the patient.

The result of these changes brought an end to the era dominated by the general practitioner.[4] In 1950, according to one analysis, 69 percent of active physicians were in primary care, but by 1980, that had dropped to 37 percent.[5] Within the medical schools, the increasing trend toward specialization was accommodated by the largest department (Medicine) by allowing autonomy within divisions while providing a base of support to foster research growth and remain primus inter pares of departments that followed suit.[6] In the process, most departments grew stronger, richer, and more independent of the dean's control. Whereas in the past the deans had to contend with part-time community faculty, they now faced the internal challenge of new, full-time faculty in departments supported by external research funding and eventually practice plans that allowed them to run

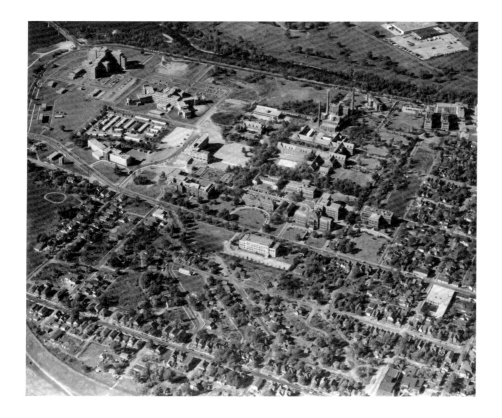

laboratories and offer services to private patients as a way to supplement income.[7]

As to facilities, the IUSM was constrained by the underinvestment during economic depression and war that made it ill prepared to respond to the pressures of rapid growth in all aspects of the school's mission. More than anything else, questions over what to build, where to build it, and how to pay for it resulted in conflicts during planning for the development of the medical school. The growing competition between responsibilities for training doctors as the only state-supported medical school, and the ambition to be a national biomedical research center, heightened tension between full-time and part-time faculty and produced clashes between the interests of the university and those of the medical school.

Most of the major conflicts of the era were fought out in bricks and mortar that can be summarized as follows. The school shifted the uses of space while new facilities were obtained first for the Riley Hospital expansion, which had its own source of philanthropic support, and a new Veterans Administration hospital, which was an obvious national funding priority. A mental hospital followed soon thereafter. The solution to the consolidation of medical teaching, as well as the expansion of research facilities necessary to recruit new full-time faculty, was a new Medical Sciences building in Indianapolis, but it took ten years to obtain the funding from the state legislature. Once completed, the consolidated medical school and expanded medical center truly entered a new postwar era.

Van Nuys's Postwar Medical School Reorganization

Van Nuys's plans for the IU School of Medicine emphasized reorganization for future growth. For example, very soon after his appointment, he requested eight additional clinical instructors, and over the longer term, he advocated replacing part-time department heads with full-time faculty as vacancies occurred through retirement or resignation. This gradual approach mitigated conflict with the part-time faculty, but Van Nuys also understood that to attract "top-flight" physicians to full-time positions, they required space as much as salary. Hence, a viable plan for expanding laboratory facilities was a minimum requirement in the short term.[8] Van Nuys also appointed John J. Mahoney, formerly a member of the University of Illinois School of Medicine teaching staff who had served as an executive officer for Base Hospital 32 during the war, to be assistant to the dean and assistant professor of experimental medicine. In this capacity, Mahoney played a key role in Van Nuys's administration, participating in essentially all of the School of Medicine's functions.[9]

The Interim Committee and Van Nuys hoped that the transition to a "peacetime operating basis" for IUSM would allow for regular operation as well as the integration of returning faculty before an expected surge in medical students in 1949. Thanks to returning veterans and the GI Bill, however, the increase came early, beginning with applications for the 1947 academic year. This created an immediate problem because the medical school had not requested funds for increasing class size in the 1946–47 legislative biennium.[10] The resolution to the problem will be discussed in more detail later, but to put it in perspective, before 1942, when the school committed to a wartime goal of admitting 140 students, it had been averaging about one hundred per year. The rapid and exceptional wartime increase was done by speeding up education, not by adding space or medical instructors. In fact, the IUSM had difficulty even before the war in teaching so many students, and the new dean expressed his frustration during the 1947 legislative session as the number of applicants grew: "Most medical schools of the standard of this one have greater budgets, larger plants and fewer students."

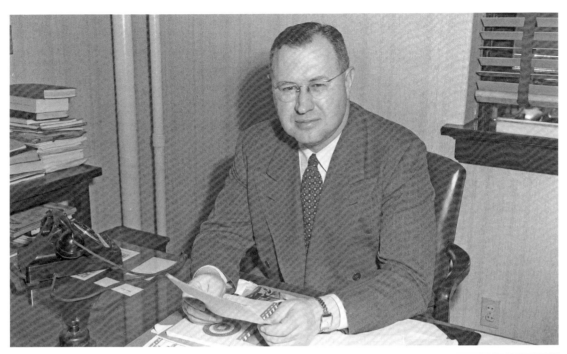

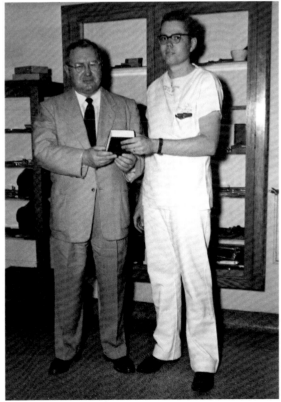

Figure 8.2a & b. John D. Van Nuys (IUSM dean, 1946–64) at his desk, 1948. IUB Archive photo collection P0072858. Van Nuys presenting Merck Manual Award to top medical school graduate and future dean Walter J. Daly. IUPUI image UA024_002285.

The medical school growth was part of a challenge to the broader university presented by the dramatic increase of returning veterans. Wells, who saw enrollment more than double at Bloomington from 4,498 in 1945 to 10,345 in 1946, told the Indiana Senate Budget Committee of the need "for unprecedented expansion to meet the needs of large numbers of additional students, increased research, graduate and professional training, and new sciences." In addition to the demands of expanded teaching and research, the medical school also faced the challenge of maintaining clinical services.[11]

Van Nuys's goal of increasing the number of full-time faculty continued an effort that began with the establishment of the medical school fifty years before.[12] Even before the recommendations of the Flexner Report in 1910, most medical schools in the United States had sought to create more full-time faculty positions. As opposed to the proprietary schools whose faculty were mostly concerned with their private practice, full-time faculty were expected to devote all of their energies to improving the quality of medical education by putting students in touch with new research and new knowledge in medicine. By 1950, the most highly regarded medical schools pursued this agenda, usually thanks to large endowments often helped by substantial Rockefeller Foundation funding. The latter always required as a condition that the school promote the hiring of full-time faculty.[13] The IUSM now had a full-time dean, but in 1946, only thirty-seven out of the more than three hundred faculty members held full-time positions. To be sure, the school had grown and flourished with some extraordinary part-time faculty, perhaps the best example of which was James O. Ritchie. His exceptional story includes graduating from IUSM at the top of his class in 1918, joining the faculty the following year, and eventually chairing the Department of Medicine from 1931 to 1956, all without drawing a salary.[14] The obvious rationale for more full-time faculty was that as teachers, these fully dedicated clinicians would better train new doctors. The expansion of research was expected to strengthen teaching by placing medical students in closer contact with the rapidly expanding new discoveries of medical research. Little thought was given to the possibility that the pursuit of research funding might compete with the time and attention to undergraduate medical teaching.[15]

Because securing funding and hiring new faculty would take time, Van Nuys reorganized departments and restructured the school into divisions to foster research growth and improve teaching. Emblematic of the change was the division and renaming of the old Department of Bacteriology and Public Health into a separate Department of Public Health and a Department of Microbiology. The change from bacteriology to microbiology, defined as "the study of all microbial organisms," focused particularly on microbial physiology and genetics. Thurman Rice, who had headed the old Department of Bacteriology and Public Health since 1938, became chair of the new Department of Public Health. and Randall L. Thompson, a graduate of the University of Chicago School of Medicine and Johns Hopkins School of Hygiene and Public Health, came from the Medical College of Virginia to head the Department of Microbiology.[16]

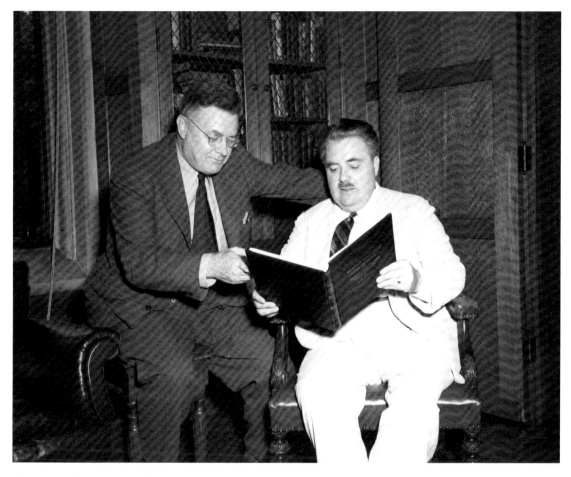

Figure 8.3. Thurman B. Rice (*left*) presenting a copy of his book, *The Hoosier Health Officer*, to Herman B Wells, July 14, 1947, IUB Archive photo collection P0047832.

Rice hoped that his new department would be a major step in his on-going efforts to establish a school of public health and fulfill the goals of his mentors John Hurty and Charles Emerson. In the 1930s, as has been mentioned, he served as assistant secretary of the State Board of Health and successfully lobbied to move the state agency into a new building on the medical campus in 1939.[17] During the war, he served as acting State Health commissioner. Rice proposed a new school in 1947 that included instruction not only in relevant disciplines of medicine but also public health administration, education, epidemiology, and nutrition.[18] The ambitious plan called for cooperation with the State Board of Health, as well as

Indianapolis City Hospital and Purdue University's rural health initiative under dean of Agriculture Harry J. Reed. Wells and Van Nuys endorsed the plans, but in just a few years, the proposal for a School of Public Health ended in failure. Despite Rice's campaigns in the media and at the Statehouse, the IU trustees supported instead a competing proposal for a BS in public health in the new School of Health, Physical Education and Recreation at Bloomington.[19] In addition to internal debate, another reason for Rice's failure is that public attention generally shifted away from the prevention of disease to the quest for discovery of "miracle" cures. Other medical schools continued to develop their public health programs, yet in 1960, there were still only twelve accredited public health schools in the United States, and as late as 1999, there were only twenty-nine.[20]

Although the public health school initiative was unsuccessful, the medical school was more successful in managing the complex challenge of the nursing program. A graduate nurse diploma was first issued in 1917, but beginning in 1932, the university established a bachelor of science degree in Bloomington that was placed in the School of Education in 1945. At Indianapolis, the bachelor of science in nursing (BSN) program was first offered in 1951 and led to confusion and disagreement over the role of "diploma" nurses (those taking a three-year, nonuniversity program) and those with a university degree. The problems were resolved in July 1956, when the Indiana University Training School for Nurses became independent from the School of Medicine and was renamed the Indiana University School of Nursing. In 1957, Emily Holmquist was hired from the University of Pittsburgh to be the nursing school's first dean. She faced a tough job to develop a separate budget for Nursing, combine the programs at Indianapolis and Bloomington, and discontinue the traditional three-year diploma program in favor of developing a four-year, full collegiate course leading to a bachelor of science degree.[21]

At the same time, the overlapping, multidisciplinary, health-related degrees that had developed over the years were studied by a special committee led by Aaron Andrews in the IUSM Department of Public Health, and it proposed moving six health-based programs from the College of Arts and Sciences into the control of the IUSM, within a division of Allied Health Sciences. Then in 1956, the trustees approved two new degree programs in occupational and physical therapy, which raised the total number of allied health programs at the medical center to eight. The new division established a framework that not only enabled more effective administration and coordination of education in these various fields but also allowed continued growth.[22]

The reorganization of departments under Van Nuys also created one of the nation's first Departments of Anesthesiology, moved gynecological surgery into a new Department of Obstetrics and Gynecology, and created departments for Radiology and Orthopedic Surgery. In addition, the trustees approved Van Nuys's plan to reorganize school functions into larger divisions with the intent of developing a more cohesive curriculum. This followed the dean's assertion that "closer cooperation in determining the content of courses, areas of teaching responsibility, and uniformity of thought on teaching objectives" were prerequisites for improving medical education. Van Nuys also stressed the importance of better integration of preclinical and clinical subjects, such as the curriculum committee's recommendation to introduce certain clinical subjects to freshmen. Van Nuys was quite aware that this recommendation reinforced his advocacy to unify all four years of the medical school at Indianapolis.[23]

One feature of Van Nuys's new emphasis on full-time teaching ran into a familiar obstacle. The "rather serious limitations of facilities for private patients" in Long, Coleman, and Riley Hospitals hindered opportunities for full-time faculty to practice inside the university hospitals. Even though at first it seemed to contradict the principle of full-time faculty, the need for limited private practice was soon recognized by the university as necessary in order to attract and keep its teaching faculty "in more intimate contact with private patients." As a result, along with the other elements of the reorganization by Van Nuys, the board of trustees approved, with little discussion or debate, a practice plan for full-time physicians following the example of Chicago, Iowa, Michigan, Minnesota, and the University of Pennsylvania. Details will be examined in the next chapter, but the budgetary terms set by the trustees fixed the salary at $8,000 for a full-time clinical chair and then limited to $18,000 the total income of a chair, with the addition of fees earned through private consultation. The practice plan was viewed as a small convenience to attract and retain quality full-time faculty. Like the unforeseen consequences of increased external research funding, the potential was not seen of the practice plan to grow and alter the economic structure of the school, including the balance of power between the faculty and administration.[24]

Postwar Student Growth

Whether in response to the pressure of the legislature or the postwar flood of veterans returning to college, the number of students at IUSM grew dramatically at midcentury. This in turn added to other changes in medical training, including expansion of the basic sciences, specialization, and growth of graduate training.[25] From the end of the war to the early 1950s, the school rose in the rankings of the medical schools in the United States, with the largest enrollments from twenty-fourth in 1945–46 to fifth in 1951–52, when it had a total of 577 students.[26]

As mentioned earlier, the medical school responded positively to the legislature's call to train more doctors because, as Van Nuys agreed, of the need "to replace those who . . . died, retired or discontinued practice, as well as to meet any of the more critical shortages such as those that ha[d] developed in rural communities during the war years." In their reports and testimony, however, the plan of Van Nuys and the Interim Committees repeatedly contrasted the resources available to the Indiana University School of Medicine with those available to its peers in the Midwest. For example, they pointed out that not many schools had larger enrollments than Indiana University, but those with more students had larger facilities and more faculty members.[27] The dean estimated that 170 new physicians were required each year to meet the needs of the state, but that was far more than the prewar level of one hundred graduates per year.

Wells discussed at length the matter of increasing medical school admissions with the board of trustees. In the end, he and Van Nuys agreed that the governor's request "should be considered as an emergency measure." As a result, and in spite of the physical constraints, a record of 141 students were admitted in the 1947 entering class.[28] When William Paynter began medical school in 1948, he recalled the medical building in Bloomington was "bursting" while accommodating 140 students.[29] The following year, with additional funding from the legislature, the school accepted an entering medical school class of 150 students. As indicated in table 8.1, the number steadily increased thereafter.

This increase in postwar medical school admissions in Indiana was typical, but whereas other schools experienced a

Table 8.1. IUSM Entering Class Size, Selected Years, 1931–1965

Year	Number
1931	126
1936	110
1947	141
1948	142
1949	150
1953	150
1954	154
1955	155
1956	159
1957	158
1958	160
1959	183
1960	188
1961	196
1962	202
1963	216
1964	216
1965	215

Source: Gatch, Report to the IU Board of Trustees, June 14, 1935, Bryan Papers, InU-Ar; *QB*, 1948–1965; LCME Report, 1963.

leveling off of applicants in the 1950s, the number of students who applied to ISUM increased, as did legislative demands on the medical school. This led the dean to insist, as had been the case since Van Nuys took over, that further expansion of freshman enrollment would be possible only if a new Medical Science Building was built and fully staffed. Because this required funding, the School of Medicine thus shifted the solution to the problem of increasing the number of doctors back to the legislature. As indicated in table 8.1 and explained below, this was eventually agreed to, and after the new building opened in 1958, the entering class size quickly rose to over two hundred.

There were some out-of-state and foreign students accepted into each freshman class, although the numbers were quite small by today's standards. For example, in 1955, IUSM accepted four out-of-state students and four foreign students in a freshman class of 150. The *Quarterly Bulletin* of the medical center was very careful in describing the practice: "Four students have been accepted from other states as reciprocity for acceptance of Hoosier applicants by medical schools outside Indiana, and four foreign students selected to carry out Indiana's obligation to aid in building up medical practice abroad."[30]

After the initial influx of returning veterans, thanks to the GI Bill, the nature of the entering medical students was influenced in part by the lack of scholarship funds. As a result, the school attracted students of above-average affluence, which admittedly was in line with national statistics. The median income of the families of medical students graduating in 1959 was $8,375, at a time when the mean annual income for white urban families in the United States was $5,557. The difference had grown since the end of the war. According to a 1960 financial survey conducted by the IU medical school, a little over 25 percent of IU senior medical students had parents who fell into a middle-income category, and about 20 percent were from families with incomes under $5,000. Despite medical education at Indiana University being more affordable than at many other institutions, physicians everywhere were becoming increasingly exclusionary and homogeneous in terms of social class.[31]

The school had a long practice of admitting only a few women and African Americans to each class. In 1949, approximately 95 percent of the students accepted were white males and predominantly Protestant. Not surprisingly, many of these students were veterans. As had been the case from its beginning, the school's entering classes, with a handful of exceptions, were from inside the state, with a large proportion having received their premedical education at Indiana University. This demographic profile remained unchanged throughout the decade. In 1956, men outnumbered women in the entering class thirty-eight to one, well below the national average of female matriculants. By the early 1960s, this began to change, with women making up 8.5 percent of the class entering in 1963. Through the 1950s, an average of only two African American physicians graduated per year. Nonetheless, outside of historically black medical schools, Indiana University had a reputation as one of the leading institutions for graduating black physicians.[32]

Women continued to face pressure and harassment in medical school at midcentury. Elsie Meyers, who enrolled in 1947, recalled that the female students were ignored in class, faculty addressed their classes as "You men," and professors told "raunchy" jokes in class.[33] When Meyers was enrolled in medical school, only 5 percent of the IUSM students were women, compared to the national average of 10 percent. To make matters worse, eight of fifteen women in Meyers's class dropped out, compared to twenty-two of 105 men.[34] Many of the men were not aware of the struggles of their female colleagues. Robert F. Reed, a fellow medical student, felt that female students were "accepted real well" in medical school in 1948. No doubt some were, but other women still faced harassment and discrimination from faculty and students.[35]

This ethnic, gender, regional, and economic homogeneity of the IUSM fostered a sense of being close-knit, in spite of the growing size and complexity of the medical school. For example, future dean Robert W. Holden, a member of the 1963 graduating class, recalled, "We knew the good and the bad of each of us; and, basically, we were under a fair amount of pressure to behave and to perform. But people were very supportive of each other." There were many fewer electives, and most had to be specially arranged. "So as a result," Holden later explained, "life was much more corralled for medical students of my era than currently. We were much more contained within this campus. We didn't migrate all over the state."[36]

The norms and values of student life in the 1950s reflected a sense of undergraduate bonhomie that was sometimes decadent, tawdry, and excessive. All medical students still faced a great deal of hard work in medical school. Elsie Meyers recalled, "The amount of materials that we had thrown at us was awesome." William Paynter, who began medical school in 1948, commented that his first two years were "an exercise in qualifying yourself to get to the next year."[37] Some students felt that the atmosphere of the first year was not so much educational but sorting the wheat from the chaff, which served to create a tense atmosphere of medical training. Robert Reed, who began medical school in 1948, described the first year in Bloomington as a weed-out year and stated, "I tell you, I equate the first year of medical school at the time with boot camp in the marine corps. You're just scared all the time. I mean, they just had you in a constant state of fear." He felt the faculty created that pressure and not the students.[38] Charles Bonsett, who graduated in 1952 and later became a professor of neurology, called medical school a "traumatic experience." He considered the first year in Bloomington a hard year, saying, "They flunked out a good portion of the class back in those days." As examples, Bonsett recalled two professors in particular, Anatomy professor Edwin Kime and Physiology professor Paul Harmon. "These two men were responsible for decimating the class." Both received their training at IU and continued the type of training they'd received in the early days of the school.[39] That said, students did recognize and appreciate the professors who cared, professors such as Ritchie mentioned earlier. Reed recalled Pathology professor Frank Furry fondly after fifty years because he took a "genuine interest" in his students.[40]

One common complaint from former students that continued from previous years was the amount of classroom learning versus clinical experience during medical school. The result, students claimed, was that they often found themselves quickly thrust into situations in which they were called on to treat a patient but had to move on because of insufficient training. William Paynter said of the first two years, "You were totally divorced from anything that looked like a patient."[41] Some felt the clinical experience was not enough to prepare them thoroughly for the medical field. Bonsett said of his clinical experience, "Well at the time I finished, at the time I got my MD degree, I didn't feel like I was trained adequate to be a physician."[42]

Reorganizing Clinical Instruction

As had been the case throughout the 1930s and 1940s, the hospitals in the Medical Center—Coleman, Long, Riley, and City Hospital (after 1951 renamed Marion County General Hospital)—were the primary locations for clinical teaching. Before the reorganization of the medical school's curriculum, Van Nuys acknowledged the complaints raised by students that they "spent very little time in clinics or on the ward service and had . . . limited contact with patients. . . . Juniors and seniors were given lectures and occasional case demonstrations throughout most of the day." Although the dean maintained that "the university hospitals . . . provided [a] fairly adequate source of teaching material [patients]," the increased number of students after the war created a need for additional hospital beds and patients for clinical instruction.

With the expanding need for clinical teaching, the arrangement with Marion County General became increasingly dysfunctional. The medical staff of the municipal hospital was self-governing, electing departmental officers annually. The result was that many members of its clinical departments were not part of the university faculty because they either lacked qualifications or did not desire to make "the time sacrifices involved." To clerkships on the floors, it was not always clear to students which physicians were certified for teaching. In 1949, Van Nuys warned Wells, "the plan as it now operates is not one that would stand careful scrutiny by an accrediting body."[43] The opening of the new West Tenth Street Veterans Administration Hospital in 1952 alleviated some of the clinical teaching shortages in the short term, but it did not solve the problems of governance and faculty oversight.

The lack of patients for medical education was exacerbated by changes in the clinical cases at the hospitals run by the university. As the former director of Hospital Admissions, Van Nuys understood that in the 1930s, the Medical Center had accepted "a fairly satisfactory volume of patients suffering from rather common illnesses or ailments." Since then, however, because the practice of medicine continued to specialize, the university hospitals were developing into referral centers treating problem cases sent from other hospitals in the community. This left the university hospitals increasingly treating "rare and difficult conditions out of all proportion to the experiences of most hospitals." For this reason, maintaining a close relationship with Marion County General Hospital, which continued to serve the broad medical needs of a large metropolitan area, was more crucial than ever to the school. Medical students needed to see simple fractures, common childhood problems, appendicitis, strangulated hernia, viral pneumonia, and mild diabetes because that was what most would encounter in their practices.[44]

Therefore, already by the late 1940s, "a very fine balance" of cooperation was needed between the medical school and the General Hospital to help expose medical students "to all possible clinical conditions." Consequently, to strengthen the School of Medicine's association with the hospital, in 1949 Van Nuys proposed the following to Wells: "In the expansion program of the school of medicine, I feel that it is extremely essential that we allocate substantial funds to the teaching program at the General Hospital and that[,] in any new agreements between the institutions . . . the complete direction of all student teaching programs in that hospital be made a responsibility of the school."[45]

As clinical and research activity grew, graduate medical education also became not only a bigger physical presence in the university but also a growing focus of concern. This reflected a national trend as the growth of specialization and new hospital construction resulted in rotating internships being replaced by specialty-defined residencies. In addition, residencies helped staff the postwar hospital expansion; by 1955, 80 percent of residencies nationwide were at community hospitals unaffiliated with medical schools.[46] At IUSM, prewar levels of staffing were quickly restored, but the school's residency programs needed expansion and improvement because they were unable to match this growth in the number of MD graduates, the number of departments, and the expansion of medical subspecialties. In 1946–47, twenty-eight interns and twenty-nine residents were employed at medical school hospitals for a graduating class of eighty-two, with the result (as will be shown in the next chapter) that less than half of IUSM graduates did their residencies in the state. In response, Van Nuys worked with departments and hospitals to increase the residency positions at Long, Riley, and Coleman Hospitals as well as the new West Tenth Street VA facility. In addition, changes were made to provide residents with better instruction, such as the establishment of a graduate anatomy laboratory, and development of advanced courses in psychology and pathology. Further, the Departments of Medicine, General Surgery, Orthopedic Surgery, Otolaryngology, Neuropsychiatry, Obstetrics and Gynecology, and Pediatrics initiated either weekly or monthly teaching staff conferences.[47]

In the end, individual departments took the lead in developing and strengthening residency programs while at the same time helping to build the relationships between the medical school and local medical facilities. One of the earliest was in the anesthesia department where Vergil K. Stoelting was appointed the first department chair in 1947. Stoelting pushed to develop the educational program, improve patient care, adopt the latest techniques, and promote research. The residency training program he started was one of the first in the country, and by the time Stoelting retired in 1977, the program had trained 275 residents, many of whom went on to be leaders in the field.[48] Somewhat later, John Hickam developed internal medicine residencies soon after he was appointed chair of Medicine in 1958, beginning at the Veterans Administration, Marion County, and University Hospitals, which allowed students to receive a broad set of experiences. This effort also helped standardize training across the campus facilities, such as in the IU surgical training program that combined the Marion County General Hospital's surgical training program into a unified resident training program that was lengthened from four to five years. Beyond surgery, in 1964, the department began its first respiratory therapy program, then called inhalation therapy. By 1972, the Surgery Department had fifty-four residents, one of the largest programs in the country. Residents in psychiatry not only enjoyed an expanded opportunity for postgraduate training in child psychiatry but also benefited by clinical rotation at Marion County General Hospital and Long Hospital, in addition to Larue D. Carter Psychiatric Hospital, a state facility that opened in the 1950s.[49]

Driven by demand from returning veterans and growing specialization, Van Nuys also worked to improve and coordinate continuing medical education. For example, the Department of Radiology increased participation by giving "joint seminars for the major clinical departments." Outside Indianapolis, the School of Medicine expanded its postgraduate offerings by conducting courses in Fort Wayne, Evansville, Terre Haute, and Lafayette. The faculty also provided scientific programs for county, district, and state medical society meetings. In May 1948, the first Alumni Day program included a series of medical discussions led by prominent graduates. Medical seminars became a regular feature of this annual event.[50]

Although related more to research than clinical teaching, Van Nuys worked with the University Graduate School to organize graduate training programs in the increasingly important basic science departments of anatomy, physiology, biochemistry, microbiology, and pharmacology. Just as efforts to expand research and hire more investigators were constrained by a lack of space, inadequate facilities continued to hamper growth in these basic science graduate programs. For example, microbiology had early success in winning research funds, but the department could only handle fifteen to twenty graduate students. As a result, in 1949 it accepted just four new students, although almost seventy applied.[51]

Teaching facilities and faculty in Indianapolis were the most challenging problems, but there were also problems in Bloomington. Myers Hall in Bloomington had been built in 1937 "in accordance with recognized standards of medical education for a maximum class of 128 freshman medical students." With a larger medical school class size, plus first-year dental students and anatomy and physiology graduate students sharing the building, it was continually used beyond capacity. The space problem in Indianapolis was even worse because the laboratory, classroom, and departmental office sections of the Medical Building, which opened in 1919, had been designed for only sixty medical students. At the end of 1950, Alan Gregg, the director of the Rockefeller Foundation's Division of Medical Sciences, which was supporting Alfred Kinsey's research on human sexuality, criticized IUSM for teaching more than twice as many students as the campus accommodated. "I do not believe that 150 students is the right number per class," Gregg concluded in a letter to Wells. "It seems to me that 100 is the maximum; that with 125 the effects of over-size begin to show, and that with 150 there is a definite and steady handicap to the efficiency of the teaching—a handicap that cannot entirely be offset by mere increase in the number of other teachers."[52]

By 1950, the medical school's response to a variety of demands had reorganized the postwar medical school for the transition to the "golden age" of medical research. Van Nuys had assembled the core of a new generation of faculty leaders such as Harris Shumacker, Lyman Meiks, Virgil Stoelting, John Mahoney, and Randall Thompson.[53] The medical school had taken the first steps toward new expansion and reorganization in response to the acute pressure of rising public expectations and inadequate facilities for patient care and research. In the process, the school increasingly realized that building construction was needed to take full advantage of these changes.

The New Frontier of Research

The US government's support of medical research during the Second World War promoted unprecedented optimism about the ability of the nation to improve health and cure disease, and this continued after the war especially thanks to funding from the National Institutes of Health (NIH) and the new National Science Foundation (NSF).[54] By 1963, the median amount of external research funds for each medical school in the United States exceeded $5 million, with the top ten medical schools averaging $11.3 million. Although the IU medical school was significantly below this ($2 million in extramural research grants in 1960), it was a dramatic increase from prewar levels and moved the school into the mainstream of American biomedical research.[55] Understandably, leaders of the school often felt as if they were running faster only to stand still; nonetheless, the ever-growing quest for heroic cures contributed to an expansion of its research mission and expectations. President Wells was quick to recognize that expanding research could change the scale of legislative support for the school, which he continually hoped would extend to the university as a whole. In a 1961 talk to alumni, he stressed that the federal grants of the previous years were "a tremendous breakthrough putting the Center in medical research among the top institutions in the United States."[56]

The growth of medical research at IUSM was not quick or easy; in fact, it started slowly in the 1920s and 1930s thanks mostly to private funds, which had seeded investigators and facilities, but only to a limited extent ($15,000 annually as of 1939) compared to other medical schools.[57] The relative weakness of medical research at Indiana made the opportunity to pursue new federal research funds provided by NIH and NSF compelling to the leaders of the medical school. This was possible because policy makers and the public saw the lessons of medical research in the Second World War and were optimistic about the continuing benefits of medical research. As mentioned in the previous chapter, Vannevar Bush, head of the federal government's wartime research efforts, made the connection explicit in *Science: The Endless Frontier* when he declared that victory in the "war against disease" required greater federal support for basic medical research.[58] Van Nuys embraced this military metaphor even as he articulated the importance of full-time faculty in all aspects of the medical school's mission.[59]

The connection was obvious. To establish a wider claim on the new frontier of medical research, the school needed to recruit and retain more full-time faculty. That need in turn drove calls for expanding labs and fostered changes to the role of clinical practice at the school.[60] Given the scant resources of money and space available at the medical center, Van Nuys initially turned to existing contacts with local philanthropic supporters to meet these needs. In 1947, he quickly responded to the James Whitcomb Riley Memorial Association (RMA) Board of Governors' request that the medical school outline "a comprehensive program for research within the limitations of the financial resources that the association could make available." This quickly led to a $50,000 grant to support John J. Mahoney's studies on the endocrine system and Dwain N. Walcher's work on infectious disease. In addition, such groups as the Indiana Elks Association, the Indiana Cancer Society, the Junior League of Indiana, and the Indiana Lions Clubs made significant contributions that accelerated the growth of research at the medical school.[61] By turning to local philanthropies, Van Nuys increased research funding tenfold between 1945 and 1948 without having to compete for federal grants against other schools whose research facilities were larger and more modern. In turn, these local philanthropic funds helped establish a research record and open up opportunities with industry and government, including projects with Burroughs Wellcome Company, Eli Lilly and Company, and the National Research Council.[62]

Van Nuys's efforts made him an important liaison between funder and researcher, as well as allowing him to coordinate new research initiatives with a broad plan for the development of the medical school, a rare accomplishment in the individualistic culture of research funding. For example, Van Nuys realized that pediatric medicine was moving away from contagious diseases thanks to discoveries of "miracle drugs" and breakthroughs in surgery and neonatology. He also knew that he had an unusual resource available locally in the Riley Memorial Association. As a result, he followed up on the grant in 1947 from the RMA by bringing to their attention the work of Shumacker and Meiks on heart disease while the association prepared for its campaign to mark the twenty-fifth anniversary of Riley Hospital and the centennial of the birth of James Whitcomb Riley. The researchers' interests in diagnosis and treatment of congenital heart disease matched the interests of the RMA, and Van Nuys identified the field as one with "great opportunity for improvement of knowledge."[63] Another example of recruiting dynamic faculty to the campus to work in targeted growing fields was the appointment of Edwin A. Lawrence in the fall of 1949 to expand the school's cancer research effort. Attracting Lawrence from the University of Utah's cancer center, one of the earliest recipients of NIH funding, was, according to Van Nuys, "another step in the school's integration of medical education, research, and patient care, into a more effective campaign against cancer."[64] The move paid off quickly when Lawrence received a teaching grant from the National Cancer Institute (NCI) shortly after he arrived on campus, which permitted the further enlargement of the teaching staff. In March 1950, the *Indiana Alumni Magazine* announced that "development of the Indiana University Medical Center as one of the most important teaching and research centers for the expanding battle against cancer [was] continuing steadily."[65]

In recruiting new faculty, the medical school faced the problem that space for research was equally as important as salary for attracting quality physicians and scientists. The local foundation support allowed the school to expand its faculty and support staff, but without a major expansion of facilities, the limits to that growth were obvious. Van Nuys insisted that no medical school could succeed in the new age of research without substantial investments in larger, more modern facilities.[66] In 1948, he therefore requested additional help from the RMA to build on its support for research on heart disease, but in this case, it was the need for "a particular type of building to house all research activity associated with Riley Hospital." Despite the awkward timing so quickly following a major fund-raising effort, the association board embraced the idea as part of its anniversary and Riley centennial fund raising.[67] Additional funding was needed from the state, and in 1949, Governor Henry Schricker endorsed the plan. The legislature allocated the medical school $400,000 to build a new Riley Research Wing, and in turn the RMA agreed to equip the new facility at a cost of $100,000. The Riley Centennial Campaign eventually raised $1 million, part of which helped ensure that the facility had sufficient funds for ongoing operations.[68]

The Riley Research Wing provided not only a home for pediatric research but also a platform for expansion through new funding opportunities. For example, encouraged by the success of new faculty member

Lawrence, in 1950 the medical school requested a $500,000 grant from the National Cancer Institute (NCI) for the construction of a research facility deemed "essential to the advancement of Cancer teaching and research in the State of Indiana." When the NCI approved only $126,000, a state appropriation for $500,000 allowed the project to proceed, and it was added to the Riley Research Wing. By 1952, the school claimed it had placed "all the large research facilities together."[69]

Psychiatry was another field with opportunities for national research funding. Early efforts had been limited, as seen in the work of Larue Carter, a professor of neuropsychiatry and neurology at IUSM who also had a clinical practice across the state. A veteran of World War I, he knew the importance of mental health in demobilization, and in 1945, he chaired a study committee that recommended to Governor Ralph Gates the building of a new mental screening hospital at IUSM, part of a shift in mindset from custodial care to treatment. Carter, who died in 1946, did not live to see the facility, which was named for him and opened in 1952.[70]

Another significant milestone was reached in 1952 when the Rockefeller Foundation awarded a three-year grant of $56,500 to the School of Medicine for research on psychotherapy. Although the foundation had supported several Indiana University researchers in the past, most notably Alfred Kinsey's research on human sexuality, the medical center had been unsuccessful in obtaining Rockefeller funding. This was the first funding from the foundation to the medical center in Indianapolis despite requests dating back to Bryan's efforts when the school was first established. Under the direction of neurologists Herbert S. Gaskill and Philip F. D. Seitz, the grant funded research "to compare the effectiveness of methods of treating emotionally ill persons," including psychoanalysis and new psychotropic medications.[71] This research fostered the transformation of a program with a long clinical and teaching history into an important center for research. Even after the creation of separate departments for neurology and psychiatry, the research program at the Department of Psychiatry, now with Gaskill as chairman, reflected close ties to neurology through its early and persistent interest in the physiological foundations of psychiatric illness. Gaskill and Alexander T. Ross, chair of the Department of Neurology, transformed the investigation of mental health and neurological disease into an integrated research program more typical of midwestern medical schools.[72] The rapid success of the psychiatry department in attracting new support also exposed the IUSM to the new world of competition for academic researchers. Unfortunately, just one year after securing the Rockefeller grant, Gaskill accepted a position at the University of Colorado,

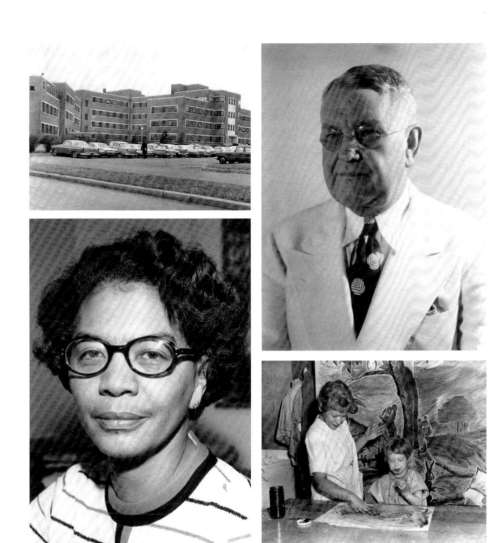

Figure 8.4a, b, c, & d. Larue D. Carter Memorial Hospital (*clockwise from upper left*): Larue Carter Mental Hospital, opened 1952, 235 beds, IUPUI image UA024_003920; Larue D. Carter, professor of neuropsychiatry, IUSM, d. 1946, IUPUI image UA024_005639; occupational therapy at Larue Carter Hospital, 1962, IUPUI image UA024_001964; Clare D. Assue, staff physician 1958–89, director 1981–89, IUPUI image UA024_005261

taking his grant with him. Dissatisfaction with the process of selecting the next chair led to the resignation of Seitz and two other colleagues.

By 1954, the development of the Psychiatry Department that once looked so promising had stagnated, but its revitalization soon came from a combination of local initiative and new faculty recruited to Indiana.[73] Locally, research in psychiatry had been largely neglected in Indiana despite

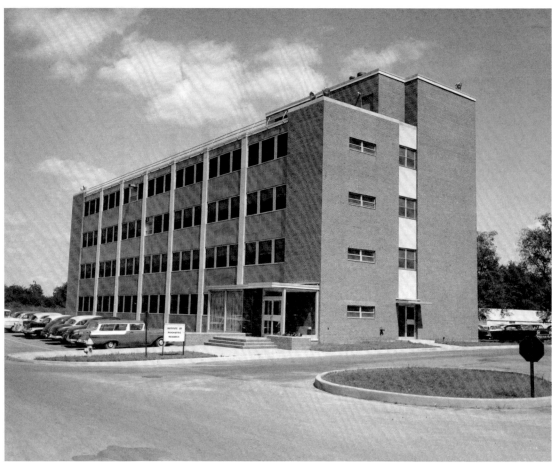

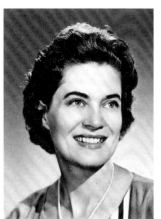

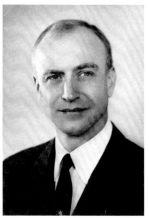

Figure 8.5a, b, & c. Psychiatric research (*clockwise from top*): Institute for Psychiatric Research, est. 1957, IUPUI image UA024_004002; John I. Nurnberger Sr., IUSM 1956–1974, IUPUI image UA024_007931; Marian DeMeyer, MD IUSM alumna, 1961 NIH grantee, IUPUI image UA024_006059.

the fact that one out of every sixteen Americans suffered from some form of mental illness whose care cost the taxpayers $1 million per year. Beginning in 1953, Margaret Morgan, who was then state commissioner of mental health, convinced Indiana Governor Gordon N. Craig to support the construction of an Institute for Psychiatric Research, incorporated as a nonprofit organization using private donations as well as a state appropriation of $1 million for construction to house a full psychiatric research program.

Demonstrating again the importance of facilities, the institute helped attract John I. Nurnberger Sr. to the medical school as chairman of the Department of Psychiatry. "We feel, that Dr. Nurnberger has the specialized qualifications and experience necessary to develop an outstanding department of psychiatry in the School of Medicine," Van Nuys said when he announced the Yale psychiatrist's appointment. By the time the institute's building was ready for occupancy in September 1957, Nurnberger had attracted a diverse group of investigators to the department, including A. Lester Drew, the chief of Pediatric Neurology who also served as associate director. The institute's staff was drawn from psychiatry, psychology, neurology, and biochemistry, which reinforced the strong and distinctive emphasis on interdisciplinary neurobiology and neurochemistry in psychiatric research throughout the decade.[74]

Even as community and state mental health professionals lobbied for support of the Institute for Psychiatric Research, the medical school's leaders continued their push for a new medical science building to house researchers in numerous other fields on the Indianapolis campus. The result was a request for the largest single expenditure at that time by the medical school, testing the limits of public commitment to medical research and innovation. This building proved to be equally as critical to the teaching goals of the school as it was to the new research agenda. Drawing from the recommendations of the Interim Committee plan, Van Nuys called for coordinated development of a new medical science building for teaching and research as well as hospital expansion to relieve pressure on antiquated clinical facilities. With Van Nuys and Wells lobbying the General Assembly and John Mahoney developing detailed implementation plans, the legislature in 1953 approved $4.5 million for the construction of the Medical Science Building; this also coincided with the fiftieth anniversary of the school. No funds for hospital expansion were approved, but in return, the medical school agreed to increase enrollment to two hundred students per year within the decade.[75]

In 1958, the year before the Medical Science Building was dedicated, the Department of Medicine belatedly started to emphasize research, thanks to its newly appointed chair John B. Hickam. Hickam was not the first choice as successor to J. O. Ritchey, who had retired the year before after four decades in the Department of Medicine. At first, William M. M. Kirby was recruited from the University of Washington to be the new chair, but his ambitious plans exceeded the resources available, and he resigned a few months after taking the position.[76] Unlike pediatrics, which benefited from the support of the RMA, medicine could not easily turn to a dedicated local funding source.[77]

Hickam was a transformational figure, very much representing the new generation of medical school faculty recruited nationally like Nurnberger and fully engaged in research, yet like Gatch, he had Indiana roots. His father, Horace Hickam, an aviation pioneer for whom Hickam Field in Hawaii was named, was born in Spencer, Indiana.[78] John was born while his father served in the US Army in the Philippines, and he was raised at various military posts before attending Harvard for undergraduate and medical school. The new chairman had been "chief resident and star pupil" of Eugene A. Stead Jr. at Emory University and had followed his mentor to Duke University, where Stead not only developed one of the nation's premier Departments of Medicine but also created an organizational culture that produced large numbers of physicians who, like Hickam, became "prominent department chairs." In many ways, Stead demonstrated that "research scientists could be produced as the by-product of the education of physicians." Hickam inspired his residents and faculty. "Hickam was a wondrous man, a very warm, personable individual who somehow was able to spot talent in a simply amazing way," his former resident Charles Clark Jr. once stated. "He made you feel like he was your friend and confidant, and somehow he got the best out of people."[79]

Hickam's work on cardiovascular research reveals the way he expanded the existing research capabilities, coordinated them, and strengthened the Department of Medicine at IUSM. Before Hickam arrived, the department had taken several promising steps but failed to build on its research success. An example was the field of cardiac research, which included the work of Shumacker and Meiks on congenital heart disease, Lurie on cardiac catheterization, Lurie and Campbell on cineradiography, and George T. Lukemeyer and Hunter Soper, who received a $20,000 grant from the Indiana Heart Association for work on artificial blood vessel grafts, the use of the artificial kidney, and the study of hypertension. Hickam brought the heart researchers together and organized their efforts into a coherent and comprehensive research program. In fact, the integration of efforts in heart research within and around the Department of Medicine became a

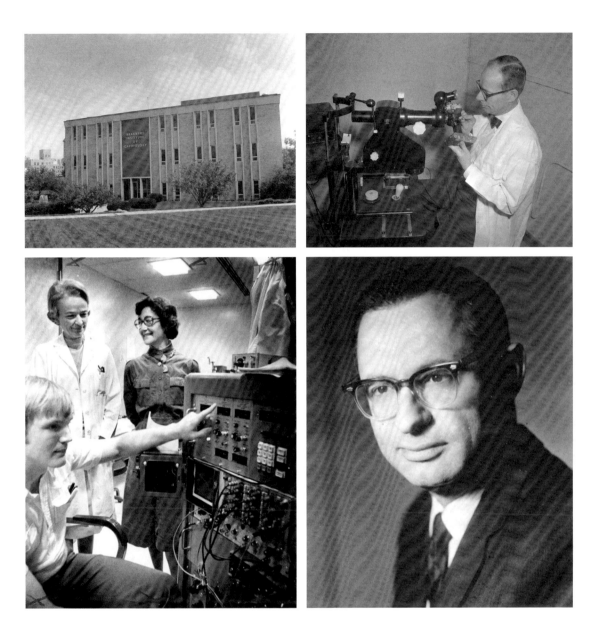

Figure 8.6a, b, c, & d. Krannert Heart Research Institute (*clockwise from upper left*): Krannert Institute of Cardiology, est. 1963, IUPUI image UA24–003917; John Hickam in laboratory, IUPUI image UA024_000522N; Charles Fisch 1965, IUPUI image UA024_006292; Suzanne Knoebel and Doris Merritt, IUPUI image UA024_000362.

major goal for the department and established the model for attracting more outside resources to the medical school. As was the case with other research, the department was helped by a donation from local philanthropist Herman Krannert, who funded a heart research institute headed by Charles Fisch that combined research at City and Methodist Hospitals.[80] Cardiologist Fisch emphasized that Hickam "made us look out instead of in" when considering the possibilities for support and that the chairman was instrumental in building personal and institutional connections with NIH and the American Heart Association.[81]

Before dying unexpectedly in 1970, Hickam became an international figure during his twelve-year tenure at the School of Medicine, particularly recognized for his research in the areas of lung, heart, and circulatory diseases and as one of the authors of the landmark Surgeon General's *Report on Smoking and Health*, which was a turning point in offering evidence of the statistical link between smoking and cancer and lung disease. His recognized leadership as "the kind of person that NIH or other chairmen of medicine across the country would turn to for the solution of problems" made it possible for members of the Department of Medicine to work on projects with the NIH and assume roles on various national committees.[82]

In April 1959, when the university dedicated the $7.5 million Medical Science Building, its boosters claimed that it was the most modern structure of its type in the United States. Its role in medical education is examined below, but the more explicit purpose of the Medical Science Building was to support research, and as mentioned earlier, within two years after its dedication, annual extramural research grants awarded to the IUSM surpassed $2 million, twenty times more than in 1950. Van Nuys's commitment to enlarging the full-time faculty, his creative use of local funding sources, and patience in the face of inadequate facilities yielded a school that was a viable candidate for larger and continued federal support for medical research. To many, by this time, there was no doubt that research was the material and intellectual heart of the school. "Research is as imperative to higher education as food is to life," Van Nuys said in reiterating the importance of the university research ideal in the modern medical school. Moreover, research funds played a major role in the rapidly growing medical school budget, whose total in 1960 was $3.9 million. In addition to being almost a dozen times greater than it had been at the end of the war ($346,000 in 1946), over half of the operating budget ($2 million) came from outside sources and were intended primarily for research purposes. Now the largest recipient of extramural research dollars in the university, the school was truly a research institution, and its potential for autonomy from the larger university had greatly increased.[83]

External funding growth and the new Medical Science Building allowed transformation of existing departments as well as the development of new ones. In 1958, the newly created Department of Biochemistry, under Donald Bowman, moved into the building. Among his early recruits was James E. Ashmore, who became chairman of the Department of Pharmacology in 1960. While he was in the Department of Biochemistry, Ashmore developed a productive program in experimental diabetes and introduced the department to new methods for studying the metabolism of isolated tissues. In 1959, he invited George Weber, one of his Harvard colleagues, to join his research group. Weber eventually created an independent Laboratory for Experimental Oncology.[84]

Ashmore and Weber are examples of faculty recruited from the top schools in the country. Warren Andrew came to the School of Medicine from Wake Forest Medical School to head the Department of Anatomy and oversee electron microscopy on the campus. Ewald E. Selkurt came from Western Reserve University School of Medicine to become chairman of the Department of Physiology. J. J. Friedman, Paul C. Johnson, Sidney Ochs, and Carl F. Rothe joined the Department of Physiology at the same time Selkurt did, and Ward W. Moore, Leon K. Knoebel, and Robert W. Bullard moved from the Department of Physiology in Bloomington to Indianapolis to consolidate the four-year curriculum. "All the same age, all with somewhat different backgrounds," Moore later said, describing himself and his colleagues from this time. "We just fit together like a glove."[85]

Although research had long played some part of the medical school activity, only in the past decade had it materially altered the life of the school. No longer just a future promise in public pronouncements, research now played a major role in budgets and payables. According to the chief financial officer and assistant to the dean, Arthur D. Lautzenheiser, "The emphasis on research is a fairly new attitude. We used to spend nearly all our money on teaching and teachers. Investigative work was incidental. However, that was ten years ago. Today the emphasis is on large, formal research projects." The search for new medical knowledge was no longer an ideal; it was a quantifiable, bill-paying way of life.[86]

Three major grant awards received by the School of Medicine within three weeks in the summer of 1961 totaling over $5.8 million illustrate how important research had become to the school, and Van Nuys believed that finally made the school a major player in national medical research.

The first grant was the result of American post-Sputnik investment in science to develop the space program. A collaborative effort between the IU School of Medicine and the Air Force, this $200,000-a-year government contract permitted the establishment of a specialized cardiopulmonary laboratory for use by School of Medicine faculty at Wright-Patterson Air Force Base in Dayton, Ohio. Hickam and Joseph C. Ross undertook studies at this specialized laboratory and at the medical center in Indianapolis to observe and measure the cardiopulmonary system's reactions to aerospace conditions. In addition, Robert W. Bullard did physiological research on "the problems of breathing encountered in space." These grants diversified the federal funding sources and expanded fields of research at the medical school.[87]

The other two grants clearly built on the groundwork laid in the previous decade. In June 1961, the School of Medicine received $4.3 million, the largest federal grant the institution had ever received, from the National Heart Institute to establish a heart research center. This built on the earlier work of the Krannert Heart Institute and institutionalized interdepartmental cooperation around a major disease process on an unprecedented scale. The new center's purpose was "to improve heart disease prevention and diagnosis and treatment of major types of heart diseases as well as the related disorders of the circulatory system, lungs and kidneys." Involving members of Medicine, Surgery, and eight other departments, the heart center was designed to "stimulate cross-disciplinary interests and communication among the investigators to accomplish more critical research." The grant, which was spread over seven years, quadrupled the extramural research funds available for the school's heart research program, enabling laboratory expansion and acquisition of specialized equipment. Within a year after the grant for the heart program was awarded, Van Nuys stated, "The meticulous administration of this program is resulting in the technical strengthening of the medical school faculty . . . [and] producing a cohesiveness of effort which is bound to establish the reputation of this Medical Center as a genuine leader in the field of cardiovascular research."[88]

The third major grant also built on the locally funded efforts of the previous decade that were crucial in making the school more competitive for large federal grants. The National Institute for Mental Health awarded $800,000 to establish a center for the study of childhood schizophrenia. The director of the project, Marian DeMyer, worked with many staff members of the Institute for Psychiatric Research, including Charles B. Ferster, whose appointment was at the Bloomington campus. DeMyer explored the effects of operant conditioning on these children and did experimental analyses of their behavior. The institute itself was awarded additional outside funding the following year, bringing the total of extramural support in neurology and mental health to over $1.4 million by 1962.[89]

A large portion of the other research in the Department of Medicine developed around cancer, with $750,000 available for cancer research across the medical school in 1962. Following the model of Hickam and heart research, Van Nuys developed a Cancer Committee to help basic and clinical researchers work more closely together, use resources efficiently, and seek additional outside support across the multiple departments. Like the Heart Research Center, establishing a coordinated cancer program was the new goal in changing the scale of biomedical research at the medical school in the next decades.[90]

Behind the headlines, Van Nuys and Hickam understood that the big awards in 1961 also heralded a shift of funding toward the "big diseases" like cancer and heart disease, but not without some potential risks. As was the case at many other schools, this reliance on research-based, soft money bought future growth but required continual renewal and reinvestment to attract subsequent grants.[91] Although this emphasis on research permitted expansion of the number of full-time faculty, as well as physical plant, graduate training programs, and overall operating budget, it also threatened to divert attention and drain resources away from the teaching of medical students, which until then had been the central part of the school's mission. This raised a legitimate question about how much actual medical instruction benefitted from this approach of pursuing research to attract more full-time faculty. The Indiana University School of Medicine, like medical schools elsewhere, was far from alone in this regard. In 1963, Clark Kerr, the chancellor of the University of California at Berkeley, named this new phenomenon in higher education the "multiversity." He did not, however, see this as an entirely positive development. Neglect of undergraduate education permeated American universities as they became preoccupied "with research, consulting, government service, and graduate training." In the largest US research medical schools, power was slipping away from deans toward department chairmen awash in research dollars. These chairmen filled the role of the professional administrators in the medical branch of the multiversity. Although IUSM participated in this, Van Nuys carefully cultivated new chairmen and maintained an unusual degree of control and coordination. Nonetheless, the distance between the physician leaders of the medical school and the medical student grew even as the state and community practitioners demanded expansion of the medical school class.[92]

With the growth of full-time faculty, the part-time faculty who were more important to teaching held fewer of the more prestigious and administrative positions in the clinical departments. As a result, some part-timers were critical of Van Nuys, and the situation became serious enough for Thurman Rice to inform President Wells that "deliberate untruths" about the dean were being told and that there were disturbing parallels to faculty attacks on Dean Emerson in the 1920s. Although the complaints were similar about part-time faculty being overshadowed by newly hired faculty trained elsewhere, the expansion of extramural research funds provided Van Nuys with resources Emerson never possessed.[93]

One other federal program provided funds for the Medical Center in the early postwar period, which although not directly for research did benefit the whole medical campus and offers another example of how the medical school took advantage of these new funding opportunities. The Hospital Survey and Construction Act (more commonly called Hill-Burton after its congressional sponsors) was passed in 1946, and in June 1950, the university received approval from the program for a grant of over $800,000 for part of the cost of the Indianapolis food services building to serve the Medical Center. Estimated at a total cost at least $2.5 million, the building was allocated matching funds in 1951 for the project from the State Budget Committee. In the end, the US Public Health Service contributed almost $1.5 million of what eventually was $4 million in total construction costs. Although it did not directly create new clinical, let alone instructional or research space, the Student Union and Food Services Building improved the quality of life for students on the campus and allowed space in the hospitals to be repurposed. The *Monthly Bulletin of the Indiana State Board of Health* described the eight-story building as "a major addition to the campus," which provided a solution to the pressing problems of food service and housing, of recreational facilities for the growing number of students, and as an important factor in expansion of postgraduate education programs in the Medical, Dental, Nursing, and auxiliary schools on the campus.[94]

In the two decades following the Second World War, research at the IUSM underwent a major transformation in securing external funding, hiring new full-time faculty, and expanding research facilities. In this sense, the school followed a national pattern, but two features of these changes are worth noting. First was the crucial availability of local philanthropic support that greatly helped in securing external funding. In addition, the resulting change was all the more dramatic because the medical school was staring from such a low level of research activity. The second change was recruiting strong chairs and other researchers with established national reputations and external funding. The dean could identify a field and find the resources for recruitment, but once hired, these faculty and chairs enjoyed an independence that gave the dean less control over the school. At the same time, ironically, the growth and success of these researchers enhanced the school's position and independence from the rest of the university.

The Medical Center

The postwar era of expanding medical research and education also changed the clinic. Not only did medical innovation and an affluent society increase the number and kinds of patients coming to the medical center, but the hiring of more full-time faculty also required changes in university-based clinical practice. At Riley and Long Hospitals, physicians complained that the facilities were inadequate, inefficient, incomplete, and increasingly out of date. There were too few beds at Long, particularly for private patients, and there were the wrong kind of beds at Riley, built at a time when most inpatient pediatric diseases required long convalescence. In addition, the medical school's growing involvement with Marion County General Hospital and the new Veterans Administration Hospital made clinical affairs increasingly complicated. Beyond the campus, as innovative medical practices became more widespread, many of the cases that had previously been referred to the medical center were now being treated in local community hospitals. In order to create attractive opportunities for the best faculty, and despite its contradictory implications for the goal of increasing "full-time" faculty, the board of trustees followed a national trend and approved creation of a practice plan that allowed university faculty to devote more time to patient care.[95]

Overall limits on physical space often made decisions about facilities for research or patient beds a zero-sum game. In response, as early as 1947, Van Nuys argued for a new hospital at the Medical Center. He pointed out that the "rather serious limitation of facilities for private patients" in Long, Coleman, and Riley Hospitals made it difficult to recruit physicians on a full-time basis if they expected to practice in these university-run hospitals. As a concrete and immediate example, Van Nuys complained to Wells that he needed to appoint eight to ten heads of clinical departments, but there was sufficient space to offer private practice privileges for only three or four of these department chairmen. To add more physicians in this category, he told Wells that more private patient accommodations were needed, even suggesting that to meet this goal, the university could enter into a partnership with a private, nonprofit organization to build a hospital on land immediately east of the Medical Building. Wells listened but was not converted to the cause. The university president was not willing to accept the resources from collaboration at the expense of giving up the university's control of the hospitals.[96]

In the meantime, Van Nuys took advantage of fortuitous opportunities as they arose, such as the national reform of medical services by the Veterans Administration after World War II that substantially expanded the clinical operations. In 1946, the new Department of Medicine and Surgery in the federal Veterans Administration promulgated a policy that its hospitals should, wherever possible, be affiliated with schools of medicine. The liaison committee created under Dean Gatch had studied the possibilities for closer ties, but Gatch's view was that work with the VA would be "a tremendous burden for the Medical School to carry." In contrast, as soon as Van Nuys was named dean, he aggressively pursued closer ties with the VA, which, the same year he took over, announced that the VA would build a new hospital on city-owned land at the west end of the Medical Center.[97]

As Gatch feared, by assuming duties in VA hospitals, medical schools undertook a formidable professional and administrative responsibility. However, the relationship had many benefits. The first five-hundred-bed unit of the Indianapolis facility was part of "a 1000-bed chassis" plan designed for several VA hospitals across the country. This large facility with likely "broad medical and surgical coverage" offered significant opportunities for medical education and research. When it opened in 1952, the West Tenth Street Veterans Administration Hospital, renamed the Richard L. Roudebush Medical Center thirty years later, had some of the best new medical equipment available. Designated a center for tumor, chest, and neurosurgery, the nine-story hospital had seven operating rooms and fourteen standard wards designed to give veterans "the maximum in nursing service."[98]

Van Nuys also worked to strengthen the relationship with Marion County General Hospital to provide more opportunities for clinical services. For example, when the chief of pathology position became vacant at the General Hospital in 1949, Van Nuys worked out a plan whereby the School of Medicine "would appoint both the chief pathologist and a clinical pathologist," with the understanding that "both of these appointees would hold faculty rank and be regarded as members of the medical school pathology department." In addition, he proposed that they "would be responsible for teaching duties at the Medical Center as well as at the General Hospital and would agree to contribute to the total research effort and to [the] expanded program of postgraduate education." The dean foresaw that a similar program could be instituted in radiology.[99]

In return for receiving this staffing of its departments, the General Hospital "agreed to maintain a minimum of 175 beds on medicine, surgery, obstetrics and gynecology, and orthopedic surgery wards and to permit an even greater participation in out-patient services." As a result, the IU School of Medicine would secure "complete control of the full-time and visiting staffs for these in-patient services, would appoint the resident physicians, and rotate university appointees through these services when their training demanded it." Van Nuys pointed out that the relationship of Harvard University Medical School with Massachusetts General Hospital operated exactly in this fashion and was a great success.[100]

These steps were important because increasing specialization presented training problems for students as well as the growing number of full-time faculty at the university hospitals, because it reduced the total number of beds and kinds of patient illnesses. Despite the fact that referral patients at the university hospitals allowed them to work near the leading edge of their subspecialties, only by taking advantage of the new VA Hospital along with Marion County General Hospital could the university offer a satisfactory range of clinical opportunities to keep faculty members and their students familiar with the routine details of medical practice.[101]

In order to solve these and other problems in the future, the board of trustees hired New York architects Eggers and Higgins in 1951 to prepare a master site plan for the overall development of the medical center campus. The plan they developed proposed new buildings to replace Long and Coleman Hospitals, both of which were being considered for demolition due to their inadequate space and expensive upkeep. Once completed, the plan was presented by Van Nuys to President Wells and the trustees, who, though generally supportive of the ideas, were "reluctant to commit."[102]

Despite this hesitation, there was outside assistance available at the national level for expansion of the Medical Center. In the same year of the Master Plan (1951), the Indiana Hospital Development Association (IHDA) commissioned a study by James H. Hamilton and Associates of Minneapolis to fulfill the survey requirements for Indiana's participation in programs authorized by the Hill-Burton Act.[103] "A Hospital Plan for the Indianapolis Area" recommended that by 1953, the IU Medical Center should add two hundred hospital beds for chronic diseases such as arthritis, rheumatic fever, heart disease, cancer, and diabetes that were "rapidly becoming the foremost problems in medicine." After these beds were added, this report stated, IUSM should add expanded training and residency programs in geriatrics. Finally, the authors concluded that an additional 550 beds for chronic and general acute care should be constructed at the IU Medical Center by

1975. Following these recommendations, as consulting architects for the university, Eggers and Higgins sketched a two-hundred-bed addition to Long Hospital; and the IHDA proposed a program to apply for Hill-Burton funds, which included $1 million to cover an additional one hundred beds at the Medical Center with the hope that the Indiana General Assembly would provide supplemental monies.[104]

These recommendations were difficult to defend, however, based on census statistics from the university hospitals, which showed that recently (as of late in 1951), two hundred beds were regularly empty in these facilities. Few private patients wanted to go to the medical school hospitals because most of the beds in them were still in large wards, and many of these patients did not want medical students to treat them. In addition, laws that had required the state's welfare agencies to send indigent patients to IU were rescinded in 1949. Moreover, the university hospitals also faced growing competition from local hospitals for charity patients who just a few years earlier had crowded Long, Coleman, and Riley Hospitals' wards beyond capacity. This included the long-established St. Vincent and Methodist Hospitals, which rapidly expanded after the war, and they were joined in the early 1950s by a new three-hundred-bed Community Hospital on the underserved eastside of Indianapolis.[105] Relief agencies around the state reported that their clients were "getting care for much less at local institutions." Ironically, these developments were somewhat the result of the medical school's own success. Most of these hospitals were staffed by the growing number of physicians who had trained at the School of Medicine and could handle many complicated cases that previously had been sent to the Medical Center in Indianapolis.[106]

A large part of the vacant bed problem was at Riley Hospital thanks to dramatic changes in the prevention and treatment of childhood illness after the war. "While both Coleman and Long Hospitals are operating as well as can be expected under existing conditions," Wells told the board of trustees, "Riley Hospital has been showing a steady and serious decline over a period of ten years." Leaders of the school of medicine had long recognized that "an imperfect balance" of services existed at the Medical Center. In 1950, Van Nuys claimed that the institution could use two or three times the number of beds for adults in medicine and surgery; but because at times one hundred beds were vacant in the children's hospital and in the Rotary Convalescent Home, he calculated that the capacity of the children's service was "at least twice greater" than what the university could "operate on an economical basis except during epidemics."[107]

The Rotary Building exemplified the root of the problem. When it was dedicated in 1932, the facility added sixty beds to Riley Hospital thanks to $276,000 raised over ten years by the Rotary Clubs of Indiana. Its initial purpose was to serve "sick, crippled under-privileged children" in need of convalescence after treatment in the hospital.[108] By July 1951, however, the census of the Rotary building was critically low, with only sixteen patients in the unit. One big reason for this change was the dramatic advance in medicine that practically eliminated the need for long convalescence. For example, the availability of penicillin and other antibiotics allowed for quick recoveries from tuberculosis, rheumatic heart fever, and other diseases whose treatment previously included bed rest, fresh air, and exercise. In addition, there soon followed equally dramatic advances in prevention, such as with polio. During the last years of its operation as a convalescent unit, the Rotary Building had been used for the overflow of polio cases during summertime epidemics, offsetting low occupancy rates throughout the rest of the year. Twenty ventilators frequently ran simultaneously in Riley Hospital to keep children with polio alive. With Jonas Salk's discovery of a polio vaccine in 1955, this situation also "changed in a minute's notice." Because of these changes, the type of patient that Rotary had served became rare.[109]

Further analysis by Van Nuys of the problem indicated that the actual decrease in occupancy throughout Riley Hospital "resulted primarily from the rapid processing of patients rather than from a reduction in numbers of patients coming to the hospital." More patients were being treated more quickly at the hospital than ever before. By May 1952, this otherwise good news had resulted in such a decline in the hospital's average census that there was "a very serious financial problem" for the IU Medical Center. During that fiscal year, university officials expected an overall loss of $400,000, and Wells concluded that it was impossible "to increase facilities in any way." Moreover, this was not the only problem of the Medical Center's clinical facilities. Services in Long and Coleman Hospitals, as well as Riley Hospital, needed to be brought up to new standards required by changes in medical practice, especially for the patients increasingly referred for specialty diagnosis and treatment.

Using the children's hospital as an example, Van Nuys explained to the trustees, "We will undoubtedly continue to receive children for neurosurgical work, complicated orthopedics, congenital ailments, and a few for highly technical pediatric management." Nonetheless, Van Nuys went on, "Should we receive all of such cases from the state of Indiana, it is inconceivable that this would guarantee satisfactory operation of a unit of 276 beds." With well-established children's hospitals associated with the University of Chicago, Washington University at St. Louis, Western Reserve in Cleveland, and the University of Cincinnati that "had long held an impressive lead over . . . [Indiana University's] institution in the matter of professional services and research," the Medical Center was not very well situated to expand geographically beyond its Indiana market.[110]

These changes in the medical marketplace and medical practice made reorganization and further development of outpatient services at the medical center mandatory. Again, Riley Hospital offers an example of how adaptations were made even while planning for a new facility. In the early 1950s, the children's hospital had only five examining rooms designated for outpatient use in the pediatric facility. The underused space in the Rotary Building and areas vacated by the Dietary Department made it possible to temporarily relocate and convert space to accommodate a variety of patient services and clinics. This included "a redesign of the building to provide more operating rooms, a recovery ward, a diagnostic X-ray department, enlargement of admitting facilities, and provision for specialty clinics on the main floor." In addition, the hospital's staff recommended that several outpatient clinics, including the Cerebral Palsy Clinic and the Audiology and Speech Clinic, be moved to the Rotary Building. Early in 1952, the Well Baby Clinic was transferred to the Rotary Building from Coleman Hospital; and in 1953, the clinic sponsored by the Department of Ophthalmology also moved into the structure. Within two years, after all of these clinics were established at this location, the Rotary Building had already served nearly as many children in its new capacity as it had in twenty years as a convalescent home. From a teaching standpoint, the Rotary clinics were invaluable; medical students could observe firsthand many of the pediatric medical problems they would encounter in general practice.[111]

As part of these ongoing renovation plans, in 1956, RMA and the Indiana Kiwanis Clubs pledged their support to convert Riley Hospital's dining facilities into a well-coordinated outpatient facility, and in 1957, the state allocated funds for part of the renovations. The cost of this expansion program to RMA and the Medical Center totaled over $500,000.[112] The new Kiwanis Diagnostic and Outpatient Clinic for Children was designed to contain three times the number of examining rooms that had been available before, making "far more efficient use of equipment" and enabling hospital personnel "to treat more individuals for more ailments at one time." In addition, as with the Psychiatric Research Institute and the Medical Science Building, new facilities helped in the effort to attract new full-time faculty talent. Lyman T. Meiks asked Indiana University School of Medicine graduate Morris Green to return to Indianapolis from Yale University to run the new clinic. "It is always a distinction to return to one's Alma Mater," Green later said. "It is a further privilege to be associated with Riley Hospital. But beyond these very personal considerations, I had the conviction that this was the time and place for a fresh look at programming services for children."[113] Among other things, the new clinic also enhanced teaching in pediatrics. Before the unit opened, medical students "seldom had an opportunity to follow patients through an entire work-up."[114]

In 1960, with these modifications done, President Wells addressed the Riley Memorial Association in a request for its financial support for a complete package of building modifications that involved constructing new surgery facilities, transforming space to create a modern and complete department of radiology, and remodeling the existing operating rooms after they were vacated to meet long-range goals for outpatient departments. He summarized the reason quite simply: "We are having an explosion of knowledge." As a consequence, he went on, "At the university level almost everything is having to be redone in order to bring it up to date and make it possible to proceed with what we know. It means radical revision of space, as well as other facets of learning."[115]

The plans for the new Riley surgery addition fit Wells's qualifications perfectly because they incorporated advanced operating room design ideas. Instead of being constructed along L-shaped corridors, as operating rooms were traditionally oriented, Riley's new surgery suites were arranged "as an octagonal around a central work area." As Harris Shumacker, chair of the Surgery Department, explained,

> Those who render service to all of the operating rooms, for example, the nurses and anesthesiologists, have their equipment and work space more or less in the center of this area so they can supervise what is going on in each of the operating rooms with a few steps rather than by walking long distances down a corridor.
>
> This octagonal organization of the operating rooms also reduced the possibility of contamination. No one could get into an operating room without being properly clothed or having proper masks and shoes. Therefore, they were "purely isolated from the rest of the hospital." The innovative design received a special grant from the National Institutes of Health, and when Riley Hospital's new surgeries opened in 1965, they drew national attention.[116]

The reorganization of hospitals also extended to Coleman Hospital, where the removal of the Well Baby Clinic from the basement made other remodeling possible at the obstetric and gynecological hospital. Some ward space had already been converted to private and semiprivate rooms for these patients, and in addition to making more facilities available for the nursing and housekeeping departments, part of the basement and first floor of the building were reconfigured to provide outpatient departments. Despite making renovations after World War II, the women's hospital experienced a decline in its average daily census over the course of the next decade. In 1950, the Department of Obstetrics and Gynecology experimented with a rooming-in concept, which allowed newborn babies to remain in hospital rooms with their mothers. Van Nuys soon eliminated the program, however, because he felt it was ill suited and too expensive for the space Coleman Hospital provided. "The [women's] hospital will continue to be an expensive operation," Arthur D. Lautzenheiser, chief accountant at the Medical Center, explained to the university treasurer Joseph A. Franklin, "because of the small number of beds over which the supervision, admitting room and other expenses must be spread. It is unfortunate that the feeling that beds are not available in Coleman is so widespread."[117] The situation at Coleman continued to worsen while the university waited to construct new clinical facilities. The result was a failure to modernize its women's hospital to keep pace with current demands, and during this period, women in Indianapolis increasingly chose to go to community hospitals for their deliveries.[118] In the larger picture, these efforts at reallocation and renovation from the late 1940s to the early 1960s were only temporary solutions while the IUSM awaited the opportunity to break through the bottleneck in providing the much-needed, modern clinical care by building a new university hospital.

The Move to One Campus

After the war, there were once again proposals from the political establishment and the Indiana State Medical Association to consolidate the medical school in Indianapolis. By 1949, for the first time in the university's history, there was an internal consensus that the university would benefit from all four years of medical school on one campus. The Indiana University School of Medicine was one of only four medical schools in the nation that did not offer a four-year program on one campus. The Indiana State Medical Association had demanded it for decades, and outside reviewers noted the split as a deficiency. When Indiana University started its medical school, a main reason for teaching the first year in Bloomington was in response to the university's concern about sufficient enrollment on that campus, but increased enrollments there over the years plus new concerns regarding the structure of undergraduate medical education combined to make consolidation a university goal.[119]

Two new developments in teaching the undergraduate medical curriculum reinforced the push toward unification. First, the faculty for preclinical training was increasingly expected to take part in the expansion of research work in the medical school. One reflection of this was the increased use of the term "basic sciences" to describe these departments and faculty instead of "preclinical." These disciplines (anatomy and physiology, etc.) were no longer considered simply building blocks for clinicians but ongoing subjects for scientific research and discovery. Second, given concerns that the growing size of individual departments was "likely to produce graduates well drilled in facts and incapable of practical application of this knowledge in the practice of medicine," Van Nuys pushed for curriculum reorganization to integrate teaching objectives and responsibilities across departments, both clinical and basic science. To this end, the school's curriculum committee also recommended introducing certain clinical subjects to freshmen and integrating basic sciences into the entire curriculum, presenting advanced and applied units of these subjects beyond the first year.[120]

The catalyst that eventually brought consolidation in Indianapolis was not this concern with the quality of medical instruction but rather, as mentioned above, the renewed demand by the legislature to educate more doctors. Despite already operating at overcapacity in aging and inadequate facilities, the School of Medicine continued to be criticized for not just too few graduates but also inefficient use of resources. One physician complained directly to Indiana Governor Henry F. Schricker "about the organization of the Medical School and claimed great waste in operation." Many private practitioners argued that in contradiction to statements of school of medicine leaders, creating more full-time faculty impeded the ability to train more doctors. Among their complaints was that some departments were "overstaffed with highly specialized instructors," that the "application of everyday medicine in teaching [had] been changed to specialties and research," that too many part-time faculty members had been replaced by instructors who had never engaged in private practice, and that treatment costs in the university hospitals were too high. Collectively, this was an attack on the medical school's professionalism and long-range plan for improvement and expansion. In response to these criticisms, a resolution was introduced in the 1951 legislative session to authorize the governor to appoint a committee to investigate possibilities for increasing enrollment. The resolution directed this special committee to report back during the next General Assembly.[121]

Wells, the IU Board of Trustees, and other allies immediately mobilized to amend the "extremely unfriendly" proposal so that the resolution could be perceived as "helpful rather than harmful." Van Nuys feared that the

Indiana General Assembly might do what the state legislatures in Iowa and Michigan had done: "direct the school to expand but not make adequate budgetary provisions." Wells hoped that this committee with its amended charge could work to the institution's advantage.[122]

The governor appointed the Indiana University School of Medicine Expansion Study Committee, which was chaired by Merrill S. Davis, a Marion, Indiana, surgeon and IU Board of Trustees member. The committee included Eli Lilly and Company executive vice president Carl F. Eveleigh among its members. The committee members worked throughout 1951 and most of 1952, and they made their recommendations in October 1952. These were quite comprehensive in identifying the size of the physical plant, availability of full-time teaching staff, supply of clinical patients, and the number of qualified applicants for admission as the reasons the school could not expand enrollment.

To the great relief of medical school leaders, the inadequacy of the physical plant even for existing enrollment was chief among the Expansion Committee's findings, just as it had been for the medical school's postwar planning committee. As a result, the committee supported the construction of the Medical Science Building at Indianapolis to allow for increased enrollment and "possible removal of the first year of medicine from Bloomington to Indianapolis." The committee's report pointed out that a closer integration of students and staff on one campus would result in a more efficient program "in accordance with current practices in medical education." In addition, due to a shortage of space for teaching in adult medicine and surgery, the Expansion Committee concluded that at least one hundred additional beds were needed at Long Hospital to ensure a sufficient adult patient supply for clinical instruction. At the same time, the committee concluded that immediate provisions were needed "for alterations and modernization necessary to bring the existing, old University hospital structures into acceptable condition to meet present-day requirements."[123]

Beyond the general, and now inevitable, recommendation for more faculty members in preclinical and clinical area, the committee singled out instruction in the second year as being especially in need of improvement. "The ratio of teachers to students . . . was far below that generally accepted by national accrediting agencies." The Expansion Committee recognized that facilities in Bloomington did not have either offices or laboratories to accommodate medical faculty. Moving them to a consolidated school in Indianapolis would further justify the need to build a new medical science building and increase the ability to recruit a sufficient number of strong basic science faculty members, although the latter was expected to be difficult because of fierce competition with other expanding medical schools attempting to attract such individuals. The Expansion Committee also determined that any augmentation in enrollment would require additions to the clinical staff. At the end of 1952, there were sixty-two full-time faculty members at the IU School of Medicine out of a total of 387, or approximately 16 percent. For the most part, full-time faculty members had taken over administration of the clinical departments, but "by far the greater portion of the teaching load" continued to be carried by part-time faculty who included, according to the report, one-third of the physicians practicing in Indianapolis at the time. The Expansion Committee concluded, "Any substantial increase in enrollment would necessitate the employment of more full-time clinicians to afford adequate staff coverage."[124]

The call to expand the medical school classes was predicated on the belief that there was a large pool of well-qualified potential in-state applicants. The committee found, however, that the number of qualified Hoosier applications for admission to IUSM was "a critical problem" whether or not capacity was expanded. After the inundation of veterans who clamored for admission following World War II, the number of applicants to medical schools across the United States fell. Medical schools had to compete with other fields, including science, education, law, government, and business for the best college graduates. In 1951, the Indiana University School of Medicine already "ranked fifth in the nation in order of size of enrollment, with 542 medical students, having advanced from twelfth place in 1948–1949 when enrollment was 438." Only the University of Illinois, the University of Tennessee, Jefferson Medical College, and the University of Michigan exceeded IU in enrollment. The expectation of maintaining high standards for the growing number of entering students was a "matter for serious concern." Nonetheless, the Expansion Committee hoped that in time, there would be an increase in qualified medical school applicants that would keep pace with plans for expansion, "because of the time necessary to construct buildings, add staff, assure the patient supply, and attract a larger number of well-qualified applicants."[125]

The Expansion Committee also noted that a large number of School of Medicine graduates left the state to practice elsewhere, and thus attention was needed to ensure adequate residency opportunities. To summarize, the final report of the committee served to reinforce the school's long-held view that any solution required more facilities and funds for full-time faculty. It also found that two important constraints to increasing physician supply in Indiana—undergraduate preparation and residency positions—were beyond the medical school's control.

In 1954, the medical school received a welcome if unexpected endorsement of its plans for the Medical Sciences Building when it had its first evaluation visit in twenty years from the Committee on Medical Education of the Association of American Medical Colleges (AAMC). This committee was the result of the decision by the AAMC and the AMA in 1942 to cooperate in monitoring compliance with the standards for their membership. The immediate reason was concern about the quality of the accelerated programs adopted to produce more physicians during the Second World War, but soon it was decided to find a more systematic practice than responding to individual problems or new applications for membership. In the following years, the Liaison Committee on Medical Education (LCME) became the accrediting organization for educating physicians, including the system of visiting all approved medical schools every ten years.[126] Although this and the revised standards (*Functions and Structure of a Modern Medical School*) were not formally adopted until 1956, Indiana University's turn came up in fall 1954 for a customary, less formal visit.

The report on the IU School of Medicine was sent November 18, 1954, and was based on a three-day visit (October 21–23).[127] It was quite positive about the "many advancements and readjustments [that] have been made in finances, facilities, personnel, and curriculum" since the last "official survey" in November 1934. Noting especially the "sound leadership, wisdom and foresight of the incumbent dean," the report mentioned the growth in budget as well as building construction in Bloomington and Indianapolis, including expansion to existing hospitals and the new VA facility. There were somewhat equivocal comments about the number of part-time and full-time faculty, which "should be carefully evaluated," but an explicit warning was given about the growth of student enrollment, which the report stated "would appear to be the maximum consistent with present and planned facility expansion." On the latter point, the report was equally as explicit about the role of the planned medical science building. "The construction and equipment of the new medical science building on the Indianapolis campus will play a very important role in meeting some of the current needs for teaching and research in the basic medical sciences. It will facilitate the long delayed and long needed consolidation of the undergraduate medical school and should mutually be of great advantage to the departments of anatomy and physiology as well as to all the other basic medical science and the clinical departments in the institution."[128]

With the endorsement of the Expansion Committee appointed by the governor and representatives of what was becoming the accrediting body for medical schools in the United States, the construction of the Medical

Sciences Building moved ahead in order to eliminate the bottleneck restricting medical research and enable the medical school to make the changes necessary for growing enrollment and consolidated instruction. As the building in Indianapolis neared completion, the 1957 entering class was the last to spend the first year of medical school in Bloomington. Except for a few transition years at the very beginning of the school when the first two years of instruction were offered at both campuses, since 1911, the first year of coursework had only been offered at Bloomington. Along with this change, however, an exception was made with the establishment of a pilot combined degree program whereby a small number of entering students took their first two years of coursework at Bloomington plus an additional year of courses for an MS degree before transferring to Indianapolis to complete their MD. More will be said in a subsequent chapter about this program, which by 1963 admitted fifteen students and part of which unexpectedly became a model for its much wider adoption.

As medical students participated for the final time in traditions that had been developed by previous classes of freshman on the university's main campus, it was the end of an era in which undergraduate campus culture still shaped medical student attitudes and behavior.[129] The last class to enter medical school in Bloomington numbered 158 students, making it the largest class ever admitted to the School of Medicine at the time. As the Expansion Committee had hoped, the quality of the students who applied for entrance had improved since the beginning of the decade. Van Nuys reported that all but a very few members of the 1957 entering class presented academic records with a grade point average of B or above. A greater proportion also matriculated already possessing a college degree, which was still not a requirement.[130]

After consolidating in Indianapolis, the School of Medicine was finally able to make the other curriculum changes it had planned, including incorporating biochemistry into the freshman schedule. In 1957–58, Curriculum Committee members discussed plans to implement changes to better orient beginning students for the study and practice of medicine. With geographic barriers removed, the curriculum finally could be organized so that clinical departments could take a more active role in the instruction of first- and second-year medical students. In turn, the activities of the basic sciences departments could be extended into the instruction of advanced students. Even so, there were limits to these changes. The first two years were still devoted primarily to the basic sciences, which included massive amounts of information presented to the students in the classroom. This meant working as hard as ever to learn the information, so from their viewpoint, the student experience had not changed much from what it had been since the early twentieth century.[131]

The Curriculum Committee recognized some new problems that arose independent from but exacerbated by the increased enrollments. The most significant was ensuring the instruction of an increasing amount of medical knowledge to larger class sizes. Committee members acknowledged that with 150 students or more in each entering class, the medical curriculum risked being too mechanical, focusing too much on rote memorization rather than on reasoning and analysis. One result was that the brightest students "tended to be neglected" and were not given the opportunity to realize their full potential. In addition, with new departments and sections reflecting specialization, the school could not give all students instruction in all the new specialties. In an attempt to remedy this problem, the medical school adopted a program, beginning in 1956–57, which permitted senior students in the top third of the class to elect one to three months of special study instead of the routine clerkships in medicine and surgery. The inauguration of these special electives proved "a stimulus to the departments involved," and in 1957–58, the Department of Microbiology adopted a similar elective honor program for sophomores.[132] This later became the widely adopted practice of all students choosing electives in their fourth year.

The new Medical Science Building was dedicated in April 1959, with construction and equipment costs for the building totaling over $7 million. The USPHS contributed $109,500 for research facilities, the third major grant from this government agency, and the balance came from state allocations as part of the effort to expand enrollment. The building included carefully planned laboratory and office space for faculty and graduate students, an impressive library with a capacity of seventy-five thousand volumes, and a pair of two-story amphitheater lecture halls. During the dedication, President Wells emphasized how the building strengthened the public mission of the school: "This structure with its superb facilities for scholarly work will further contribute to the reputation of our state as a center for education, culture, and science, thus enriching the life of every Hoosier and helping us to achieve an unexcelled standard of health and physical well-being."[133]

It took fifty years to fulfill again the promise that William Lowe Bryan had made to Henry Jameson and other members of the Indiana Medical College faculty to provide all four years of medical education in Indianapolis. Early in the century, Bryan had viewed the presence of the medical school in Bloomington as essential to the survival of the university, but by

1957, both the university and the medical school had developed in ways that made the continued division irrelevant to the university's survival and detrimental to the medical school. "Bringing . . . the freshman class to Indianapolis has been quite an occasion for this campus," Van Nuys said. "It has made a complete change in the atmosphere of this campus in a variety of ways. . . . The transfer of the faculties of anatomy and physiology and the addition of new faculty in the basic science and clinical departments has also been one of the factors that have changed the character of our living here at the Medical Center."

Quite appropriately, in 1998 after a major renovation, the Medical Science building was renamed Van Nuys Medical Science Building.[134]

Toward the New University Hospital

As often happens, the relief of a bottleneck one place creates a new one elsewhere. In this case, relieving the pressure on classrooms and laboratories by building more space for first- and second-year students increased the need for clinical training opportunities, especially residency. The solution was the long-proposed construction of a new university hospital, and as soon as the Medical Sciences Building opened the hospital became the highest priority of Van Nuys and Wells. Planning and advocacy had begun long before, even though there were higher priorities immediately after the war. In addition to the Indiana Hospital Development Plan recommendations of 1951, there was a major step taken in the 1955 Indiana General Assembly when legislators approved $200,000 for planning a new hospital along with some additional appropriations for the Medical Science Building that was under construction. This permitted the administration and medical staff to begin studies for the proposed new hospital facility as well as remodeling Long Hospital and the Clinical Building for ambulatory care and renovating Coleman Hospital "to provide a teaching area for allied medical courses."[135]

In 1958, after two years of study, medical center department heads issued a report stating their consensus about programming for a new hospital. Since 1952, when Eggers and Higgins had sketched plans for an addition to Long Hospital, the number of beds at the Medical Center had decreased, and demand for additional outpatient activities in the Clinical Building had grown. By the late 1950s, the outpatient situation was such that the center was "under constant pressure to accept patients for whom there [was] no accommodation." The hospital planning committee concluded that, as soon as possible, the fifth-floor surgeries and some inpatient wards should be removed from the Clinical Building, and four hundred beds should be added to the Medical Center's facilities. This committee suggested that these four hundred beds should be built as a first stage of construction of a new university hospital. All central services would also be included in stage one. According to the committee's plan, three hundred to four hundred beds would replace all inpatient services in Long and Coleman Hospitals in a second stage. The committee's proposal met the guidelines of the 1951 IHDA survey for hospital development in Indianapolis and followed the recommendations of the 1951–52 governor-appointed Medical School Expansion Committee. Following release of the report on programming for the new university hospital, the IU Board of Trustees approved a formal contract with Higgins and Eggers to develop architectural plans.[136]

The hospital planning committee identified the area east of the Clinical and Medical Buildings facing West Michigan Street as the site for the new hospital. The university worked in cooperation with the Indianapolis Redevelopment Commission, as part of the general urban renewal plans in the area, to acquire the houses south of Marion County General Hospital to Michigan Street in preparation for construction.[137] Despite this preparation and support, the 1959 General Assembly turned down Indiana University's request for an appropriation for the project, and in 1961, it allocated only a little over half of the university's $4 million request for this purpose.[138] Despite the legislature's rejection, as they had done so many times in the past, university administrators did everything possible to prepare to build once funding was secured. Indeed, by the end of the 1960 academic year, the university had obtained the land, and the hospital site had been partially cleared for construction.[139]

University officials were determined to find sufficient funds, so they decided during a meeting with architects from Eggers and Higgins in early 1962 "to proceed with the development of plans for the *entire hospital* (approx. 800 beds)." Over the course of the next several months, Eggers and Higgins worked intensively with Fleck, Quebe & Reid Associates, an Indianapolis architecture firm, and the IU Medical Center staff so that working drawings and specifications could be ready by the opening of the next legislative session in January 1963. When plans for the hospital were reviewed at a board of trustees meeting in September 1962, these architects revealed that the cost of the initial phase of the hospital would total approximately $12 million. Construction expenses for phases two and three were estimated at over $5 million each, raising the anticipated outlay for the entire project to over $20 million. Despite these unprecedented sums, after a decade of partial efforts, the trustees and Wells finally decided to proceed with the new university hospital, much to Van Nuys's great relief. The promise of federal Hill-Burton funds plus lack of opposition from the other public universities raised Wells's confidence in obtaining funding during the 1963 legislative session.[140]

Indiana University requested $7,990,000 from the state for construction, rehabilitation, and repair at the School of Medicine for the 1963–65 biennium. Elvis J. Stahr Jr., who replaced Wells as Indiana University president in July 1962, called the upcoming 1963 legislative session "the most crucial for higher education of any session since the War." Although he left the office of president, Wells accepted the title of chancellor and effectively used his decades of contacts and reserve of esteem in the General Assembly to tip the scales in favor of the new president and the request for the new hospital. He still had "a knack for getting what he wanted from the Legislature during his years as president," quipped Stahr, who had served as president of West Virginia University and was no stranger to dealing with state lawmakers. He also had experience dealing with issues that pertained to medical education, having expanded the two-year medical program to four years during his tenure as president at West Virginia.[141]

University officials stressed the exceptional need for a new hospital. Stahr called Long Hospital "about as obsolete [a facility] as one could find." Because the Medical Center lacked a modern hospital, the quality of the institution's clinical teaching was deteriorating rapidly. A new university hospital would "be much more attractive to patients and [would] allow . . . much better care." Van Nuys added that it was "absolutely imperative that this facility be provided as quickly as possible before the reputation as a teaching Medical Center [was] irretrievably damaged."[142]

Ten years after first receiving recommendations that additional clinical facilities should be built at the Medical Center, the state legislature made an appropriation that provided funding for a new hospital during the 1963–65 biennium. Much to the disappointment of the university and in spite of the budget agreement, the legislature cut the request in half to $4 million. One reason was a reaction to overall rise in expenditures on higher education that alarmed legislators. Thus, despite the university's claim of having "fallen well below the national average in academic space per student," state lawmakers and members of the public had a different view, as expressed in an editorial in the *Indianapolis Star* that claimed the facilities of public universities like Indiana University were "luxurious," because they spent "lavishly." The editorial went on, "As for the huge new increases asked by the state supported colleges and universities" at the beginning of the 1963 legislative session, "we are not convinced that it is really necessary

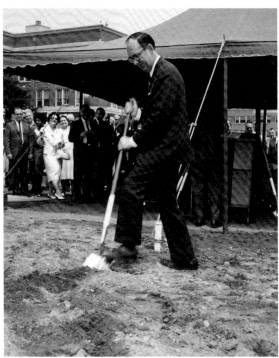

Figure 8.7a & b. University Hospital: Glenn W. Irwin Jr. (IUSM dean, 1964–75), ground-breaking ceremony, June 10, 1965, IUPUI image UA024_000878; (*below*) University Hospital in 1970, IUPUI image UA024_002627.

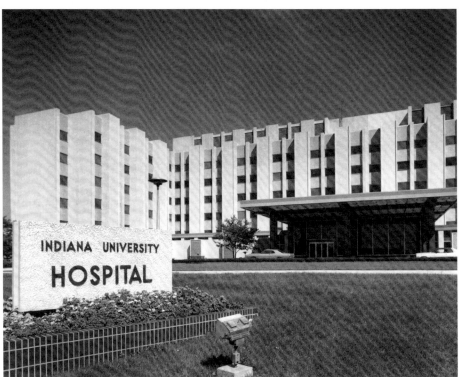

to virtually double their expenses in the next two years." The General Assembly reduced Indiana University's original capital budget request by over $20 million, including the separate request for the Medical Center, which was cut nearly in half to $4 million.[143]

In the larger picture, even cut in half, the hospital appropriation was one of the few encouraging items in the state budget for the next biennium. As a result, despite this disappointment, the board of trustees agreed that the university should take bids on the project by mid-May 1963 with the anticipation of federal funds. Again, complications arose, first over negotiations for Hill-Burton funds and then because of a delay in collection of new Indiana sales tax revenues upon which capital appropriations of the 1963 General Assembly depended. This caused further postponement of the hospital groundbreaking, which took place in June 1965, and the hospital was dedicated in 1970.[144]

Conclusion

In 1963, the IU School of Medicine was larger and more influential within Indiana than ever before, but the medical school still struggled to overcome disadvantages compared to other medical schools. Leaders understood the national picture that suggested their school was running faster just to stay in place. No one could deny that the IU School of Medicine had become a serious research institution; in the previous seventeen years, annual extramural research funding rose from $11,000 to $5 million. Nonetheless, this placed it only in the middle of the national average of medical school research funding. Intensifying the school's research program coincided with the employment of more full-time clinicians and substantial additions to the basic science faculty. In 1946, the school had 337 faculty members, thirty-seven of whom worked full-time. By the time that the LCME visited the institution in December 1963, the number of faculty had almost doubled, but even more significant, of the 607 faculty members who worked for the school, the number of full-time professors had grown to 173, an almost fivefold increase.[145]

With 216 students in the fall of 1963, the IUSM admitted the largest entering medical school class in the United States.[146] Those students confronted a student-teacher ratio that the school viewed as barely defensible, but the growing role of the School of Medicine at Marion County General Hospital, the VA Hospital, and Larue Carter Hospital created a range of clerkship opportunities unimaginable in 1950. Joint residency training programs were available in almost all of the clinical specialties in these affiliated hospitals. In addition, Van Nuys also instituted postgraduate and continuing medical education programs that attracted approximately one thousand physicians a year. The missing piece in the program, however, was the need for a new university hospital, which remained little more than a hole in the ground.[147]

In the middle of addressing these concerns and developments, John Van Nuys unexpectedly died early in 1964 at the age of 56. As the school prepared to find a new leader, all involved inevitably reviewed the almost twenty years of service of Van Nuys as dean, during which time the school had undergone dramatic changes that were part of the transformation of all medical education, research, and health care in the United States since the end of the Second World War. To be sure, Dean Emerson and Dean Gatch before him had also overseen crucial periods in the school's history as it was transformed from a proprietary to a public university institution with major hospitals, and as it responded to the unprecedented challenges of economic depression and world war. In the decades after 1945, however, the addition of research as a core feature of the school's mission, plus the shift to more full-time faculty and consolidation of the school in Indianapolis, both expanded the school and defined its character for the remainder of the twentieth century. What was not expected was the accelerated pace and extent of change after the early 1960s, beginning less than a decade after unifying instruction on one campus, with the medical school spreading education to more than a half dozen new locations in the state.

PART III
SERVING INDIANA AND THE WORLD

By the mid-1960s, the IUSM had grown to a size and complexity that established its main features in subsequent decades to meet its obligations in education, patient care, and research. Immediate and broader changes in circumstances soon resulted in significant new developments that extended the contributions of the school to the state, the nation, and the world. First was the creation of IUPUI, a home campus that added several schools (e.g., law, art, science, social work, and liberal arts) to the medical school and other health schools already part of the medical center (dental and nursing). Then shortly after consolidating medical teaching in Indianapolis, the school's monopoly on medical education was challenged by proposals to establish a second medical school to increase training of physicians. In response, the IUSM secured agreement for it to create a statewide system of eight centers where the first two years of medical school were taught. Thirty-five years later, this was expanded to all four years. Similarly, concern about admitting enough patients and receiving sufficient referrals for teaching and clinical income prompted the school to combine its hospitals with the largest private hospital in the state (Methodist) into a joint institution that eventually added hospitals around Indiana.

Underlying these changes were broader demands for access to health care and increased government programs to fund patient care (e.g., Medicare and Medicaid). In addition, research opportunities continued to grow thanks to both local philanthropy and federal programs. The school added numerous specialty institutes and research centers, staffed with researchers of national and international renown. Their work took them around the state, country, and world, and it included research at the medical center (the university and affiliated city, VA, and mental hospitals), whose clinical staffing the school had long provided.

9

The Indiana Plan: Statewide Medical Education, 1964–1974

The term of Glenn Irwin, who succeeded John Van Nuys as dean of the IU Medical School, was shorter than his predecessors and in many ways was a transition between the postwar period and the last quarter of the twentieth century that brought unprecedented diversity in students and even more dramatic increases in research and changes in clinical care and hospital funding. Yet there were four presidents of Indiana University between 1963 and 1974, after having just two for the previous sixty years. During these eleven years, the IU School of Medicine built a new hospital, greatly expanded a second, and fundamentally altered the operation of a third. The medical school also found itself—along with other schools and programs of higher education at Indiana and Purdue Universities as well as some private schools—as the major component of a new urban university that was created in 1969 in the capital city. Its awkward name reflected its hybrid nature: Indiana University–Purdue University at Indianapolis (IUPUI).

Despite the inclusion of the medical school in the new urban campus, the developments of the twenty-five years before Irwin became dean increased the independence of the school from the rest of Indiana University as well as many of its components from control by a dean or university president. In other words, the institution had taken on a life of its own. This was first and foremost because of its size and complexity but also because of its responsibilities to entities outside the university. These are easy to list and include teaching to meet requirements for professional licensing, increasing enrollments to satisfy the legislature (and federal government during WWII), caring for patients in its hospitals, and conducting medical research in exchange for funding from the federal government and private philanthropists.

Although most of these specific and general changes were welcome, there were some causes for concern. From the mid-1960s to the mid-1970s, after having just achieved its fifty-year goal of consolidating medical education at Indianapolis, the medical school committed itself to a new model of expanded undergraduate medical education to be taught at seven other sites across the state. In addition, at the end of a decade of hospital building, the Medical Center found it necessary to reform and expand its ambulatory care program to maintain its financial viability. There were important changes of personnel during this period of continued growth of the IU School of Medicine, but even more significant was the establishment of a new academic governance unit, IUPUI, that linked the school to the university in a very different way than the relationship to the main campus fifty miles away that had existed for sixty years. The reformed administration was essential for managing the tremendous growth during this decade in all aspects of its mission: teaching, research, and clinical care.

The Consolidated Medical School

In December 1963, a survey team from the AMA Liaison Committee on Medical Education (LCME) visited the medical school campus, and its subsequent report was highly anticipated by IUSM administrators. LCME accreditation was essential to the continuation of the medical school whose leadership hoped for a validation of the progress that had been achieved over the past decade. The school's first LCME report in 1954 had been laudatory but pointed out the inadequate resources for its increased teaching and research as reflected by the low faculty-to-student ratio and inadequate laboratory facilities. On the other hand, it welcomed the plans to move the first year of instruction from Bloomington to Indianapolis in a new building that would also provide more research space. That plan having been achieved, the department chairmen, six of thirteen of whom remained from 1954, were anxious to see whether the second LCME report would recognize the progress made at the medical school.[1]

The numerical growth of undergraduate medical students had continued during the past decade. From 1954 to 1963, the first-year class increased its size from 154 to 201 students at Indianapolis, plus fifteen in a new program at Bloomington that allowed students to take two years of coursework for the MD plus a related master's degree before transferring to Indianapolis.[2]

Those 216 students were the largest entering medical school class in the United States that year. The total student population also grew during Van Nuys's tenure from 437 students to 737 students by the 1963–64 term . The medical school classes remained overwhelmingly Hoosier, male, and white. The entering class in 1963 had 189 students from Indiana (87.5 percent), and although the number of women and black students had slowly increased in recent years, it remained low (5.4 percent women, 4.1 percent black). This was progress over past ratios, and it was better than the national percentage of black medical students enrolled at predominately white medical schools, which remained steadily around 2 percent.[3]

This growth also involved attempts to place graduates in residency positions, which proved more difficult than increasing the size of the undergraduate medical class. In addition to the residencies at the IU Medical Center facilities, over the past decade, Van Nuys developed clerkships for advanced medical students at Marion County General Hospital, the Veterans Administration Hospital, and Larue D. Carter Memorial Psychiatric Hospital. Joint residency training programs were available in almost all of the clinical specialties in these affiliated hospitals. As will be seen below, even though the number of students who continued their medical education through hospital residency programs supervised by faculty of the School of Medicine had grown since 1946, the school was unable to keep up with the increased number of its MD graduates.[4]

These developments in undergraduate and graduate education improved the quality and reputation of the School of Medicine, but this remained uneven because it depended on the strengths of a particular department or chairman. Most important for Van Nuys had been the overall progress since the last LCME visit in increasing the size of the faculty and the proportion of those who were full-time, which had risen from 16 to 28 percent, with the greatest increases in Medicine, Psychiatry, Pharmacology, and Biochemistry. The last two had split to form two separate departments, and each now had more full-time faculty than the parent department in 1954. These four departments also had the most faculty with research grant funding.[5]

The opening of the Medical Science Building provided vital space for the establishment of more robust research activities. The establishment of the Heart Research Center in 1961 showed the possibility of conducting research on a new scale within the school. In contrast to the Liaison Committee report of 1954, which found the research facilities inadequate, the 1963 survey found the laboratory spaces "conveniently arranged and well maintained," but it also recognized the need to move quickly to keep up

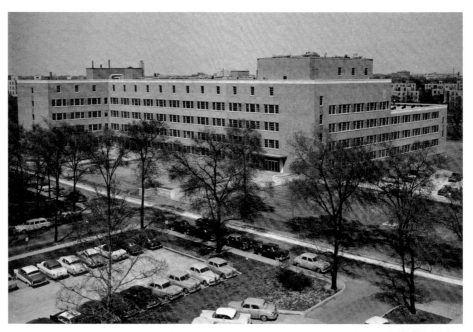

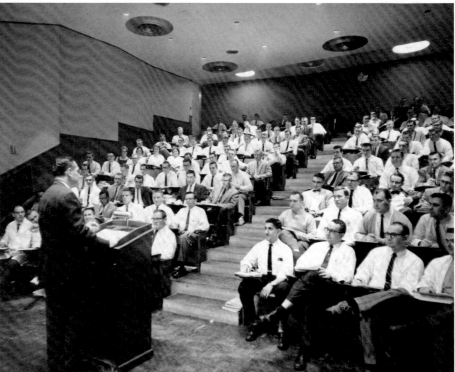

Figure 9.1a, b, c, & d. Medical Sciences Building, 1958 (*top to bottom*): Medical Sciences Building, exterior, 1958, IUPUI image UA024_004615; lecture hall, IUPUI image UA024_000863; library, IUPUI image UA024_004621; "Medical students working in laboratory," IUB Archive photo collection P0051335.

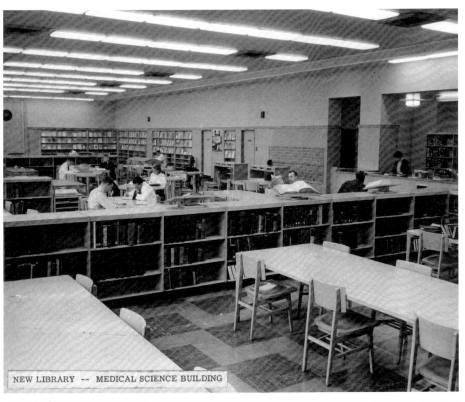

NEW LIBRARY -- MEDICAL SCIENCE BUILDING

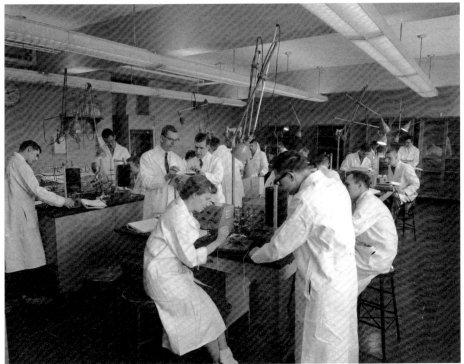

with the growth of research at the school. Outside research funding had increased ninefold since the last report, and within the four largest research departments, the increase had been even greater.[6]

Overall, the much-anticipated Liaison Committee report affirmed that the last decade had been one of "distinct progress" for the medical school. In particular, the transfer of first-year instruction to Indianapolis allowed for better undergraduate medical education through "the highly desireable consolidation of all four years of instruction on one campus." It also enabled creation of the new Combined Degree Program in Bloomington, which received particular commendation. The committee understood these outcomes to be the result of stable, thoughtful leadership, but it also noted, "While the present administrative staff and organization appear to be sufficient for routine functions," there was concern about the ability of the school administration to develop a cohesive policy for the school's continued growth.[7]

The committee recommended that "sufficient time and help" be provided to the dean's office to faciliate such planning and policy development. They particularly noted that Van Nuys, as dean, seemed "to carry an extremely heavy administrative burden." It was often through personal relationships and diligence that he maintained important institutional realtionships in an environment where he had "insufficient or no authority in his dealings with some of the institutions that comprise the medical center." He had direct charge of the university hospitals and did his best to promote a supportive atmosphere for faculty and students. He was a member of the Dean's Committee for the VA Hospital, dealt directly with the administration of the Marion County General Hospital, and met frequently with deans of the Schools of Dentistry and Nursing. Although the school's alumni association helped "to develop better relationships with organized medicine," VanNuys personally met regularly with members of local and state medical societies. In addition, he fostered relationships with such organizations as the Riley Memorial Association, which continued to make vital contributions to the medical school and hospitals.[8]

On February 15, 1964, before the Liaison Committee report was completed, VanNuys died unexpectedly at his home, apparently of a heart attack. He was only fifty-seven years old. Ironically and tragically, this seemed to confirm the LCME's observations about the burdens of the office. In fact, it was the prevalence of heart disease in increasingly affluent American society that prompted the United States Public Health Service to fund major research grants such as the one the School of Medicine received for its Heart Research Center. Especially after World War II, being dean of an American medical school became more demanding. Whereas Emerson and Gatch had time to do research, teach, and even head major departments while serving as dean, VanNuys had to dedicate all of his efforts toward the institution's administration. As dean of the medical school, Van Nuys had much more in common with the men who succeeded him than with those who preceded him, thanks to the size and complexity of the institution now requiring such extensive attention.[9]

The combination of growth and consolidation of centralized authority that demanded increased operational knowledge was not matched by increased administrative support staff in the dean's office. This in turn created a major challenge for a smooth transition following Van Nuys's death.[10] In addition, ground had not yet been broken for the new hospital, and calls for medical education reform suddenly arose, which meant that the dean's death came at a most inopportune time. "His great fund of common sense, his friendly manner and his extraordinary competence and experience in the vital field of medical education will make him not only sorely missed as a human being and friend, but well nigh irreplaceable as dean," IU President Elvis Stahr declared in homage to Van Nuys.[11]

As the initial shock and grief of Van Nuys's death began to subside, the university's board of trustees turned to the issue of who would now lead the medical school. After almost eighteen years as the dean of medicine, Van Nuys had put his personal stamp on the office. Most of the department chairmen had served at least eight years, all of whom were appointed by John Van Nuys. The trustees moved quickly to unanimously name John Nurnberger as acting dean upon the recommendation of President Stahr at the February 21, 1964, meeting. Nurnberger had been at the medical school since 1955, and as chairman of the Department of Psychiatry and director of the Institute for Psychiatric Research, he had overseen one of the school's most successful research programs and increased the department to twenty-two full-time faculty members. Nurnberger reluctantly agreed to serve but only temporarily, and he relied heavily on the few administrative officers in the dean's office. John Mahoney became associate dean in 1958 when the school was unified at Indianapolis. He oversaw the work of the admissions committee and had a good understanding of most of the office operations. Edmund Shea had been administrator of the Medical Center since 1953 and ensured continuity of operations at the hospitals.

Also noteworthy for a number of reasons was Doris Merritt, who as assistant dean had responsibility for grants and contracts. She was the youngest in the office and the first with specific responsibility for coordinating grant activity at the medical school. Merritt earned her MD from George Washington University School of Medicine in 1952, one of three women in a class of eighty. She completed a residency at Duke in pediatrics and moved to the NIH Division of Research Grants in 1957; in 1961 she came to IUSM with her husband Donald who helped organize the new medical genetics department. During the following seventeen years, she oversaw more than $55 million in successful external grant funding for the growing campus. That included assistance in the development of the Heart Research Center, and she was commended by the 1963 Liaison Committee report for providing "guidance and supervision for the entire research program."[12] In an era when much of the power of the dean's office was control of access to space, Van Nuys had also entrusted Merritt with research space allocation. Nurnberger relied on Merritt, an assistant professor of pediatrics, as a liaison to the Riley Memorial Association. In addition to attending meetings both formal and informal, she wrote the Dean and Provost Reports for the Riley Memorial Association.[13]

In the summer of 1964, Stahr and Nurnberger convened a search and screen committee to make recommendations for the next dean of medicine. There was support internally and among the board of trustees for Nurnberger to continue as dean, but he was adamant that he was not interested in the position. The committee then narrowed the list to ten candidates and ultimately recommended Dr. Glenn Irwin in January 1965. Stahr presented Irwin's name at the next trustees meeting, at which he was unanimously approved. At the same meeting, the trustees also approved the appointment of Kenneth Penrod, the vice president for Medical Education at the University of West Virginia, to the newly created position of provost for the Medical Center at Indiana University.[14]

The appointment of Irwin showed that the university administration viewed continuity as essential for the medical school following Van Nuys's death. Irwin had been at the school for twenty years as a student, resident, and faculty member in the Department of Medicine. He received his MD in spring 1944, one of the school's two wartime classes that year, and after serving at the Schofield Barracks Hospital in Hawaii, he joined the faculty at the School of Medicine in 1950. Irwin worked closely with both J. O. Ritchey, previous chairman of the Department of Medicine, and John Hickam, the current chairman, who was very supportive of the recommendation of Irwin as dean. The two appointments showed Stahr's desire to reassure the medical school that programs would proceed as planned, whereas in the case of Penrod, a trusted friend from Stahr's days at West

Virginia, where they'd worked together in creating a new medical school, the university president made it clear that he planned for management and oversight to be more robust and closely aligned with the president's office.[15]

A Statewide Medical Education Plan

Throughout its history, the effectiveness of the Indiana University School of Medicine in fulfilling its public trust had been most frequently measured by the number of doctors the school graduated. In 1952, the Indiana University Expansion Committee report called for increased medical school enrollments in Indianapolis, and the postwar growth of undergraduate bachelor graduates provided an ample supply of prepared applicants. The opening of the Medical Sciences Building at Indianapolis in 1958 was the culmination of a decade-long process of responding to the reported shortage of physicians in Indiana as well as consolidation of instruction on one campus. When the new building opened, the Indianapolis campus welcomed an entering class of 160, a number that steadily rose for the next decade. The medical school thus claimed to have met the goal of increased undergraduate medical enrollment that was unified at Indianapolis.[16]

Nonetheless, within a decade, the School of Medicine relinquished the one-campus model at Indianapolis that had been a stated goal for decades. The reason for this dramatic change was a continuing concern with physician supply combined with political circumstances that fundamentally altered the School of Medicine's model of how best to fulfill its educational mission to the people of Indiana. Although there were numerous constituencies proposing different solutions, the evolving politics of public medical education put the medical school on the defensive in its response to these demands. The school's proposed solution was to distribute medical education across multiple campuses in Indiana, and after several years and numerous study committees, the school was eventually successful in achieving a broad consensus for this approach. The resulting statewide system, however, placed the medical school under even more public scrutiny as the sole provider of medical education in the state. This change also reopened the school to charges from national accrediting boards of spreading rather than effectively concentrating its resources.

In October 1959, at the start of the second year of the unified medical school program at Indianapolis, the US Surgeon General's Consultant Group on Medical Education, chaired by Frank Bane, published its report, *Physicians for a Growing America*. The report sparked a national discussion about the future supply of physicians in the United States. The immediate inspiration for the report was a speech in 1957 by President Dwight Eisenhower that identified a looming physician shortage as a major problem facing the nation in the coming decade. In its simplest form, American medical schools were projected to graduate 7,900 doctors per year by 1965. To maintain the ratio of 140 physicians per 100,000 population, viewed as a minimally adequate supply, these medical schools would need to increase the total number of annual graduates to 11,000 by 1975.[17] For Indiana, this required 274 MDs each year to reach the guideline of 140 physicians per 100,000 population.

It should be noted that there were some errors and omissions in the Bane Report's methodology, from incorrect estimates of population growth to focusing on physician distribution on the national and state level, and not within states.[18] The latter would have shown the great urban/rural differences in access to doctors. The biggest omission was ignoring the role that residency plays in determining the location of practice—it is at least as important as where a doctor attends medical school. Finally, although a lesser criticism, was underestimating the ability of existing medical schools to increase enrollment, especially with increased federal funding, plus the increase of the number of women and to a lesser extent minorities entering medical school. As will be seen in the next chapter, by the end of the 1970s, the medical professions and schools were most concerned about a glut of MDs[19]

Initially, the Bane Report was received by the IUSM and the broader medical establishment in Indiana as recognition of the foresight of consolidating and expanding the medical school at Indianapolis. The report's recommendation for the development of new public medical schools received little discussion in Indiana before 1962, in spite of the fact that Indiana was cited as one of seven states that "might be warranted in establishing new medical schools" to create "equitable opportunity for medical education" and increase the number of physicians.[20] As the previous chapter has shown, throughout Van Nuys's tenure, the consensus remained in favor of centralizing in order to expand medical education at Indianapolis. The results were highly visible: from 1958 to 1963, the number of students admitted to IUSM grew from 160 to 216, a 35 percent increase

Having successfully increased enrollment, during the fall of 1962, Van Nuys began meeting with senior faculty members to address an equally important but publicly neglected problem: the persistence of a significantly high percentage of IU School of Medicine graduates practicing outside of Indiana. Although the Bane Commission had identified the relative decline in physicians for the overall population, in Indiana the physician supply varied widely, with by far the highest density in Marion County and the

Table 9.1. Residency Placement of IUSM Graduates, Selected Years, 1931–1963

Year	Total	Indianapolis	Other IN	Placement	
				IN subtotal (%)	Out-state (%)
1931	96	53	10	63 (66%)	33 (37%)
1939	103	63	11	74 (72%)	27 (28%)
1940	101	63	11	74 (73%)	26 (27%)
1950	93	39	3	42 (45%)	51 (55%)
1951	106	45	9	54 (51%)	52 (49%)
1952*	135	47	8	56 (41%)	80 (59%)
1953	134	52	13	65 (49%)	69 (51%)
1954	137	35	20	55 (40%)	82 (60%)
1957	138	44	8	52 (38%)	86 (62%)
1958	139	44	20	64 (46%)	75 (54%)
1959	139	39	27	66 (47%)	73 (53%)
1963	153	52	16	68 (44%)	85 (56%)
1964	160	58	14	72 (45%)	88 (55%)
1965	152	64	11	75 (49%)	77 (51%)

*Beginning of National Residency Match Program
Source: School of Medicine, Indiana University, Bulletin, 1930–31, 1939–40, 1952, 1958–59; Quarterly Bulletin IUMC, 1939–65.

lowest in rural counties in the southwestern part of the state. In addition, although the medical school expanded its enrollment and graduates, the number of residency slots remained stagnant. The state's only medical school was graduating over 150 students per year in the early 1960s, but the state had just over one hundred internship slots. In addition, whereas almost 75 percent of MDs produced by IUSM took residencies in Indiana in 1940, as table 9.1 shows, since the late 1940s, less than half of IU's medical school graduates took residencies in-state. Moreover, the overwhelming majority of those residencies were in Indianapolis. There were rarely fewer than forty IUSM graduates who did their residency in the capital city, and rarely more than twenty in the rest of the state. At the end of this period, from 1963 to 1965, the number of IU graduates doing residencies in Indianapolis rose from fifty-two to sixty-four, whereas the total for the rest of the state declined from sixteen to eleven.

Looking at these figures in another way, the increase in class size at IUSM was most successful in providing a greater opportunity for Hoosiers to become doctors because they always represented a very high proportion of the entering class, and the medical school was always quick to point this out. As mentioned in the last chapter, not more than a handful of students came from out of state, and by the 1960s, the school also admitted about a half a dozen foreign students. As table 9.1 shows, however, most of the additional graduates of the medical school could not be accommodated by residencies in Indiana. Because location of residency has long been identified as the most significant factor determining where a physician would later practice, if the increased number of medical graduates left the state to pursue their careers, they would not help the need for physicians in Indiana generally and outside of Indianapolis specifically. Therefore, Van Nuys increasingly viewed creating more residencies in more parts of Indiana as the highest priority of the medical school.[21]

Throughout 1963, Van Nuys cultivated support for expansion of graduate medical education first through promoting the building of the new Indiana University Hospital and subsequently through increased support for residency opportunities in the other metropolitan areas. The planning process was informal and included Van Nuys, Harris Shumacker, John Hickam, and John Nurnberger. Their goal was to find ways to expand graduate medical education to meet the immediate needs of the School of Medicine and the long-term need for physicians in the state. One useful document was a study for the Indianapolis Hospital Redevelopment Association that had recently called for 2,123 additional beds in the Indianapolis area by 1975. Those beds could form the foundation for expanding graduate medical opportunities in and around the Medical Center.[22]

Outside of Indianapolis the subtle relationship between medical graduates, residencies, and medical practice was not well understood. Instead, following Governor Welsh's call in August 1963 for a second medical school Indiana,[23] by the end of the year, community leaders in Indiana cities such as Muncie, South Bend, and Gary were less interested in graduate medical education and much more eager to see the expansion of medical education in their regions through establishment of a new medical school. From their perspective, the consolidation and growth of the medical school at Indianapolis had done little to expand the number of physicians in their communities. Ignoring the simpler strategy of building hospitals and residencies to attract doctors, business and political leaders were much more transfixed by the potential of federal funding and the economic benefits of a medical school, like that in Indianapolis, which brought new revenue and jobs into a community for medical research as well as hospital construction. Common wisdom at the time maintained that a major medical center could employ six thousand or more people.[24] Nor were these Indiana proponents alone; seventeen new medical schools (excluding osteopathic) were established in the United States from 1960 to 1970, and another twenty-three in the next ten years.[25]

Most of those concerned about the number and distribution of physicians in Indiana ignored the role of residencies and concentrated instead on whether and where to build another medical school in order to produce more MD graduates. The resulting rise in calls from regional newspapers and within the General Assembly for an additional medical school in Indiana were often justified by the simple observation that the state had a physician ratio that was well below the national and regional average and that multiple medical schools were the norm even in states with smaller populations.[26] In response, the IU Board of Trustees moved quickly to defend its "statutory responsibility for medical education" in Indiana. While directing the "University administration to continue with the plans which have been underway for several years to continually enlarge the admissions to medicine," in November 1963, the trustees also commissioned a study by the firm of Booz, Allen and Hamilton to examine the development of medical education in Indiana.[27] The firm had already worked with the School of Medicine on studies prompted by the Hill-Burton federal legislation on hospital construction, and this study was about options for medical education expansion, including "further expansion of the present medical school, increased reliance on medical schools in other states, establishment of another medical school by Indiana University," and establishment of a new medical school by another university. The Booz, Allen and Hamilton team consisted of H. Lawrence Wilsey, a vice president at Booz, Allen and Hamilton; Rockwell Schulz, a senior consultant in health and medical administration; and Lowell Coggeshall, a special consultant who was vice president of the University of Chicago and past president of the Association of American Medical Colleges.[28]

Coggeshall, who was born in Saratoga, Indiana, a small town north of Richmond, attended Indiana University and its medical school, graduating in 1928. He thus was an example of the medical brain drain from Indiana when he left to do his graduate medical education at the University of Chicago, where he remained and pursued a distinguished career in tropical medicine. He then moved into administration, and because of his work with foundations and the federal government, Coggeshall became a recognized expert in government and medical school relations. At the time of his work for the IU trustees, Coggeshall was in the midst of writing the book, *Planning for Medical Progress through Education*, eventually published by the AAMC in 1965. Hence, his views played a decisive role in shaping the study of medical education in Indiana.

Coggeshall was sensitive to the larger forces influencing medical schools such as the changing patient demographics, medical specialization, advancing technologies, rising health care costs, the expanding role of government in health care, and the emerging team approach to patient care. He was also sympathetic to the institutional needs of IUSM, aware of the vital role

Table 9.2 Entering Classes at Selected Medical Schools, 1932, 1964, and 2015

	1932–33	1964–65	2015–16
Private			
Harvard	125	116	165
Johns Hopkins	71	88	120
Pennsylvania	131	126	156
Stanford	52	68	90
State			
UCSF	63	128	165
Illinois	178	200	315
Ohio State	100	150	191
Michigan	131	203	170
Minnesota	121	151	230
Washington		76	245
Wisconsin	120	99	176
Indiana	123	211	355

Sources: Fred C. Zapffe, "Study of Student Accomplishment in Seventy-nine Medical Schools in the United States," *Journal of the Association of American Medical Colleges*, 8 (1933): 331–46; Davis G. Johnson, "The Study of Applicants," *Journal of Medical Education*, (1965): 11:1017–30; AAMC, "FACTS: Applicants, Matriculants, Enrollment, Graduates, MD/PhD, and Residency Applicants Data—Data and Analysis—AAMC." Accessed December 16, 2015, https://www.aamc.org/data/facts.

federal support played in the development of the modern medical school, and supportive of medical schools playing a more active role in the development of health policy. Overall, Coggeshall was acutely aware that the increasingly complex missions of medical schools and their associated hospitals required ever-greater resources and managerial competence. He was therefore concerned that small institutions could not accommodate the ever-expanding demands of research and the resulting expansion in medical knowledge.[29]

During the summer of 1964, the committee conducted interviews and corresponded with faculty, which revealed problems with simply expanding the size of the medical school at Indianapolis. For example, there was still no solution for the shortage of residency slots in the state, nor was there any obvious evidence of a connection between more students in Indianapolis and more doctors in rural Indiana. IUSM had just admitted the largest class in its history and was already one of the largest medical schools by enrollment in the country. In addition, many faculty members didn't equate bigger with better for undergraduate medical education.[30]

As table 9.2 shows, most of the elite medical schools at the time had between 100 and 125 students in their entering classes, and to this day they have not much exceeded 150. State medical schools had generally larger entering classes, some of which were close to the size of Indiana, which was the largest, but most have remained closer to two hundred matriculants, except for Indiana and Illinois.

Harris Shumacker, who trained with Alfred Blalock at Johns Hopkins and had been chair of surgery at IUSM since 1948, was representative of faculty who supported the idea of "splitting the faculty and student body into smaller school units." One idea was for the students to be placed in one of three "schools" within the medical school at Indianapolis, where students would attend classes and training with the same cohort throughout.

Large departments would assign faculty to each "school" as a way of fostering closer mentoring relationships between faculty and students. In the LCME survey in late 1963, students had identified a major problem stemming from a feeling of anonymity and lack of close advising relationships. The LCME site committee linked this concern to the large class size and the higher than average student attrition rate from 1958 to 1963, going so far as to advise "that the class at Indianapolis should not be expanded further, even upon completion of the additional facilities proposed and with the additions to the faculty contemplated."[31] Under this "schools-within-a-school" plan, the students would still benefit from access to the full range of subspecialties available only at a large academic medical center, which would create a better environment for retention. The supporters believed the plan combined the best of the intimate teaching relationships of a small school with the breadth of resources of a large school. This plan reflected the views of an internal constituency against simple expansion but still in favor of a centralized School of Medicine at Indianapolis.[32]

When the final Booz, Allen and Hamilton report was released on December 8, 1964, its findings were very sympathetic to the position of the IU School of Medicine. After evaluating several options, the report found that expansion of the current medical school offered the best chance to meet the need for physicians while maintaining educational quality. It did, however, report in favor of a substantial reorganization of the medical school that would divide the classes into smaller organizational units, reflecting the position of many faculty members who thought that students needed to work in smaller groups within a large school. This approach was scalable. New modular divisions could simply be added to the school once enrollment crossed a certain threshold. With this reorganization, the report concluded that the first-year total enrollment of the "schools" within the School of Medicine could increase to four hundred at Indianapolis by around 1975, before considering expansion to another location. Phase I of the plan would entail reorganization and expansion of the Indianapolis campus, as well as the much smaller combined degree program in Bloomington and a concerted effort to expand the number of internships and residencies.[33]

The most important consequence of the Booz, Allen and Hamilton report was its argument against creation of a new medical school. The report repeatedly stressed that increasing the size of the School of Medicine would be cheaper and quicker than development of a second medical school. Citing the high cost and slow development, the report estimated development of a new medical school would take a decade or more. Moreover, each of the suggested sites for the new medical school had a major documented

Table 9.3. Study Committees and Commissions on Medical Education in Indiana, 1964–1969

Date	Committee	Appointed By	Notes
1964 (report filed Dec. 1964)	Booz, Allen and Hamilton Inc.	IU trustees	"A Plan for the Development of Medical Education in Indiana"
1965 (report filed July 1966)	Legislative Committee to Study Medical Education in Indiana	Indiana legislature	Recommended funding to Ball State to plan new medical school
1965	Committee on Medical Education	Indiana University School of Medicine	
1965	Medical Education Board	Indiana legislature	Charged to implement a plan for (mostly graduate) medical education
1967 (report filed Dec. 1968)	State Policy (Stoner) Commission on Post High School Education	Indiana legislature, Richard Stoner Chair	Medical education included in charge
1969	Commission on Medical Education	Governor Whitcomb	Beurt SerVaas, chair

shortcoming that would make development of a new school difficult. For example, in the case of South Bend, it was the lack of a public university with a strong graduate program; in Muncie, it was the lack of a strong graduate program in the sciences.[34]

The reaction to the Booz, Allen and Hamilton report was swift. The South Bend advocates published "A Commentary on Medical Education in Indiana," which went back to the findings of *Physicians for a Growing America* to argue for a second medical school at South Bend. Evansville advocates lobbied legislators. Muncie advocates not only published a report on the advantages of their site but also submitted legislation to fund planning and construction of a new medical school there. Hearings on Senate Bill 336 in January 1965 brought out advocates for a new medical school both in Muncie and elsewhere, while Lawrence Wilsey, presented the findings of the Booz, Allen and Hamilton report. The disagreement among the advocates for a new medical school about a specific location prevented passage of any bill to fund a school. Instead, the legislature created a study commission on medical education.[35] This was the second of what was to be six committees or commissions and boards to examine the question between 1964 and 1969, as indicated in table 9.3.

During the spring of 1965, senior faculty and administrators at the medical school continued to explore options for a statewide "Medical University" to accommodate planning for future growth of the School of Medicine. In May 1965, President Stahr asked Dean Irwin to appoint a committee to formulate a plan for the university, based on the several studies developed in the past few years and anchored by the Booz, Allen and Hamilton report. That June, Provost Kenneth Penrod of the medical school distributed a draft discussion paper that connected the recommendations of the Booz, Allen and Hamilton report with the earlier concerns about the quantity and quality of graduate medical education in Indiana and proposed the notion of distributed instruction. He pointed out, "Much of the thinking and discussion generated by the Booz, Allen and Hamilton proposal for a medical university under the aegis of Indiana University has been of an institution confined to the geographic boundaries of the present Medical Center campus in Indianapolis." He suggested instead that the medical university could extend to off-campus sites, thus proposing the basis of what later grew to become the current system of multiple medical school campuses around the state. Penrod argued that with support from a telecommunications network, "much of the instruction of the first two years of medicine can be provided in a setting apart from patients and clinical medicine and it makes little difference whether this classroom is one block or fifty miles from the teaching hospital."[36]

In subsequent testimony before the Legislative Committee to Study Medical Education in Indiana, Dean Irwin, Wilsey, and Penrod emphasized the medical university as a statewide concept that went well beyond just graduate and continuing education. They also claimed that "basic medical education can take place at selected places" across Indiana. They envisioned the medical university shaped like an hourglass with diverse premed settings, giving way to a smaller set of basic medical education settings, then through the single site of clinical education at Indianapolis, expanding out again for graduate medical education, and even more so for continuing medical education.[37]

When the Committee on Medical Education appointed by Irwin, chaired by George Lukemeyer, and including Associate Dean John Mahoney plus departmental chairs such as Hickam and Shumacker, reported to the dean in March 1966, the concept of the statewide dispersed and multifaceted plan had matured. The summary began, "The concept of a medical school and medical center as a discrete geographic entity should be abandoned." The medical school leadership had digested the lessons of the 1964 Booz, Allen and Hamilton study calling for the development of the "Medical University" concept, and it emerged with a "medical school without walls." It wedded the Booz, Allen and Hamilton calls for expansion and improvement in Indianapolis with a concrete plan for supporting graduate and continuing medical education with additional but limited financial support and a new statewide telecommunications system. That system could also support subsequent development of multiple sites for the first two years of medical school. To be administered by the IUSM, the plan sought to increase retention of physicians throughout the state rather than simply increase the spaces in the medical school classes.[38]

During this same period, the legislative response to the Booz, Allen and Hamilton report continued. The Legislative Committee to Study Medical Education in Indiana, created in 1965, sought to balance the interests of the School of Medicine with the desire of several communities to become home to a new medical school. Dean Irwin tried to steer the committee to the medical school's new proposal. He presented the committee with an initial report on the "Indiana Plan," as the medical university plan was now called, in April and updated committee members regularly throughout the summer as they developed a budget for the telecommunications network and payments to support interns and residents in approved nonuniversity hospitals. The final version of the budget developed by Penrod requested $2.7 million during the 1967–69 biennium.[39]

In its final report, the state committee provided some support for the Indiana Plan, including both the Indianapolis component and the state-wide network, while also seeking to settle the contentious issue of which city would host a new medical school. After hearing testimony from all the universities and communities with proposals for expanding medical education, the committee recommended that the General Assembly "properly fund" the medical center and appropriate $2.5 million to the medical school for development of a regional internship-residency program. It also recommended, however, $300,000 to Ball State to begin work on a new medical center in Muncie. The study committee had thus declared Ball State the winner of the new medical school competition. The strident dissent by State senator Elmo Holder, committee co-chair from Evansville, indicated clearly that the issue had not been settled.[40]

Throughout 1965 and 1966, the university and the School of Medicine laid the groundwork for legislative action on the medical university concept. IU president Stahr traveled across the state speaking to medical societies and chambers of commerce about Indiana's medical education needs and the growth of the university, emphasizing the need to support "opportunities for internships, residencies, and continuing medical education." His remarks frequently pointed out that "producing, at great expense, more new doctors to promptly leave us is surely not the smartest way to start off." Indiana had a doctor shortage because it had an internship and residency shortage, and more of those residencies needed to be outside of Indianapolis.

The Indiana Plan, as presented publicly across the state, contained four elements: additional support for the medical school, curricular reform for undergraduate medical education, improved and expanded opportunities for graduate medical education throughout the state, and expanded continuing medical education. The last item was essential for any statewide plan, Stahr argued, because "technological advances which would have been thought 'far out' only a decade ago" enabled a "broadening of the geographical base of instruction" through a statewide educational and communication network. The communication network would provide support for the new residencies and help the physicians in all parts of Indiana stay informed through higher quality and more frequent continuing medical education.[41]

As the 1967 legislative session approached, the advocates of a second medical school remained divided by regional allegiances to one location or another. In contrast, the Indiana Plan had been backed by the Booz, Allen and Hamilton report, reiterated by the medical school study committee, and supported by the legislative study committee. It is therefore not surprising that the part of the Indiana Plan addressing graduate and continuing medical education, plus the telecommunications network, was passed by the legislature, and the still controversial new medical school proposals spawned another committee. SB 359 called for creation of a Medical Education Board, but fortunately for the medical school, it was chaired by the dean of the school and instructed to oversee implementation of a "plan for state-wide medical education" that would include supplemental income for interns and residents, a telecommunications network, and coordination of efforts to develop "formal teaching opportunities for intern and resident training" throughout the state. The Medical Education Board could also make recommendations regarding development of other medical programs, but most important, it was Indiana University that would receive $2.5 million in the biennium for development of the statewide program.[42]

Given the action of the 1967 legislative session, the efforts to promote a second medical school subsided. The new Medical Education Board began discussions with hospitals and colleges across the state about developing graduate medical education. Almost as quickly, plans were developed for basic medical education outside of Indianapolis. With an increased pool of well-qualified applicants in 1968 for only 220 slots, Irwin wrote to Stahr informing him that Indianapolis could not absorb another enrollment increase. "It seems appropriate to explore the possibility of assigning a limited number of medical students this fall at the three other state universities (Indiana State, Ball State and Purdue Universities) and Notre Dame," for basic science coursework. Presented as a choice between working with other institutions or denying students access to medical school, Stahr supported the proposal to the board of trustees in August of 1968.[43] Even on a small, contingent basis, this action ended the ten-year experiment of unifying undergraduate medical education in Indianapolis.

Meanwhile, yet another study group, focused more generally on higher education, was created by the General Assembly in 1967: the State Policy Commission on Post-High School Education, often called the Stoner Commission after its chairman, Richard Stoner, Cummins vice president and IU alumnus (and future IU trustee). The Stoner Commission's mandate included medical education as part of higher education, and testimony before the commission included arguments again for creation of a new medical school. For example, while noting the progress on improving graduate medical education, Thomas Stewart from the Committee on Higher Education in Northern Indiana testified, "For the foreseeable future, Indiana University at Indianapolis, will be turning away fully qualified students because there is no room for them." Citing the Bane Report, Stewart urged the commission to support reintroduction of the 1967 House bill to create a new medical school in the next legislative session. Eight years after the Bane Report, he argued, the supply of undergraduate medical education had not significantly increased. The solution, though expensive, "is to do what every other state faced with this problem has done. And that is to establish new medical schools prepared to meet the challenge facing our state." That new medical school must be "linked to the research and development of modern science and engineering," and be located in a major population center, which made South Bend and the University of Notre Dame the obvious option.[44]

The Stoner Commission reported its findings to Governor Roger D. Branigan in December 1968, just shy of eighteen months after the Indiana Plan received approval. It was also right after the 1969 general election that saw Indiana Democrats swept out of the governor's office and the legislative majority. The findings of the Stoner Commission centered on its recommendation for a strong board of regents with responsibility for all public post–high school education in the state. These findings were politely received by the new General Assembly in January 1969 and ignored.[45]

The Stoner Report's discussion of medical education did not ignore the Indiana Plan and its new Clinical Teaching Centers established under the Board of Medical Education and the concomitant expansion of internship programs "in six major population centers in Indiana." In fact, the commission called this "a truly significant development." In the program's first year, the number of intern positions rose from 117 to 139, though questions lingered about the quality of some of the positions. Overall, the Stoner Commission offered an endorsement of the distributed medical university model. The report also included a proposal in an appendix for a statewide plan, presented by commission member and Marion County councilor Beurt SerVaas, that seemed to follow the same logic as the earlier work of Lukemeyer, Penrod, and Irwin in extending the idea of regional programs from graduate medical education to basic medical education.[46]

With the funding for the Indiana Plan already in place and the possibility of a board of regents defeated, the advocates of the second medical school began another round of lobbying in 1969. In response, Governor Edgar Whitcomb appointed another committee to put the issue back on the legislative agenda, with Beurt SerVaas as chairman of the new Commission on Medical Education. SerVaas had been a member of the Stoner Commission, and his new charge was to complete an inventory of all medical education resources and make recommendations for the organization and administration of those resources. Perhaps most relevant, SerVaas was an outspoken supporter of creating an independent state university at Indianapolis that would have the medical school as its core, a proposal that ultimately took shape in a slightly different IUPUI, as explained later.[47]

At the first meeting of the commission, "Mr. SerVaas pointed out that as member of the Stoner Commission he had recommended that a modification of the Indiana Plan be put into effect." At the same meeting, Dean Irwin reported to the commission that the School of Medicine was implementing its first basic science programs at the regional sites, with three first-year students at Purdue and two at Notre Dame. Thus, even before the commission reported, one could argue that the statewide system was starting. The commission echoed SerVaas's earlier ideas and adopted a resolution in support of a Statewide Medical Education Program that was almost identical to the Indiana Plan. The commission work was also important for allowing proponents of the new medical schools to enter into discussions and planning about eventual expansion of clinical teaching centers at other communities that led to the "Seven Center" Program: Lake County, South Bend, Fort Wayne, Muncie, Lafayette, Terre Haute, and Evansville.[48]

This proposal became HB 1439, and when it passed in 1971, the School of Medicine became responsible for the orderly development and expansion of a medical education program in cooperation with the host institutions of the seven centers. An appropriation of $1.75 million was made for the 1971–72 academic year to allow the centers to begin operation. Steven Beering was appointed as associate dean with responsibility for coordinating the implementation of the system. When the Liaison Committee on

Medical Education reported on the IU School of Medicine in 1971, the scope of change and the remaining challenges presented by the Indiana Plan were clear. Between 1967 and 1971, the General Assembly appropriated $5.5 million to support aspects of the plan. According to the 1971 LCME accreditation report, "These funds have been used for the support of salaries of community Directors of Medical Education, stipend supplements for interns and residents, the creation and maintenance of a medical telecommunications system, a program of visiting professorships and joint clinics, and a large number of individual grants in aid for community hospital education programs." From 1967 to 1971 the number of interns and residents increased by 42 percent. Previously only located in Indianapolis and South Bend, graduate medical opportunities now also existed in Evansville, Fort Wayne, Gary, and Muncie. The committee found the program uneven at the various centers, with the deepest concern about the Muncie center at Ball State, where "there seems to be uncertainty in the faculty and administration regarding the significance of the medical student program." This uncertainty was compounded by Ball State's continued references to starting an independent program. The committee applauded the effort to implement such an innovative program but reserved judgment until better faculty supervision and control, akin to Indianapolis, were in place. Given the medical school's opposition to a creating a second medical school, even the qualified endorsement by the LCME report was a major victory.[49]

Internally, the medical school very quickly recognized the difficulty of creating the statewide system. Although the total number of internships had grown by 53 percent, the percentage outside Indianapolis had decreased slightly from 18.6 percent to 17.8 percent. For residencies, the only hospitals in the state with an increase of more than ten positions were all in Indianapolis: university hospitals, Marion County General Hospital, and Methodist Hospital. Initial undergraduate growth (first-year enrollment from 227 to 250) came through a US Department of Health, Education, and Welfare grant of $1.6 million in April 1970 that allowed expansion of the pilot programs at Notre Dame and Purdue and establishment of the program at Ball State. Greater growth was anticipated in the coming academic year with the "Seven Center" Program, now funded under House Act 1430, providing $1.75 million in operating support for the new centers' increasing enrollment.[50]

The single medical university without walls had yet to be achieved, but the medical school's altered view and governance of statewide medical education had won the day. The Indiana Plan officially became the Indiana

Figure 9.2a & b. Statewide medical education system: (*right*) "Statewide Medical Education System," *Your University* (September–October 1971), Box146, UA 073, InUI-Ar; (*below*) Glen Irwin with George Lukemeyer, two of the main architects of the statewide plan, 1970, IUPUI image UA024_002209.

Statewide medical education system

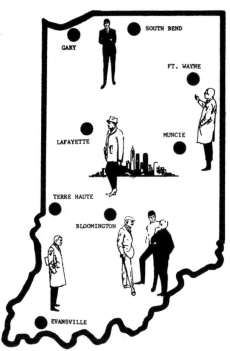

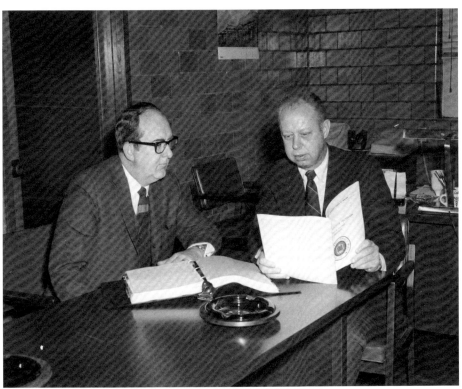

Program in 1967 and then the Indiana Statewide Medical Education System in 1971. The goal of the system was now explicitly "to increase medical school enrollment by establishing health education centers in multiple communities" for instructing medical students. In its first year of operation at six of the seven sites, the undergraduate portion of the program was already receiving $3.25 million in state and federal funds compared to just over $2 million for the graduate and continuing medical education portion of the system. Over $1 million of this funding went to altering, renovating, and equipping the new Centers for Medical Education outside of Indianapolis and Bloomington.[51]

The next chapter will examine the implementation of the statewide plan, but how did this Indiana response to the national call for more doctors compare to that of other states? The Bane Report singled out seven states in 1959, including Indiana, "that might be warranted in establishing new medical schools." An article in 1980 on the responses to the report indicated that since the Bane Report, Florida added a medical school at the University of South Florida. In addition, Michigan added a school at Michigan State, New Jersey added two, Ohio added three, and Texas added four new medical schools.[52] The only other state besides Indiana not creating a new medical school was Washington, whose WWAMI program was established in 1971 to serve the surrounding states of Wyoming, Alaska, Montana, and Idaho. Students attended their first year at a campus in their home state, then the second year in Seattle at the University of Washington, and the third and fourth years at regional sites across the four states for clinical education.[53] A few other states established sites for the first two years, but they were usually a transition to building four-year medical schools. Perhaps most significant is that twenty-six other states not judged in the Bane Report to be in need of additional schools established at least one more medical school by 1980.[54]

The Local Friends of Research

Even though dramatic and highly public decisions were being made about statewide medical education, other transformations of the IU medical school continued, especially in the areas of research and medical specialization. In research, thanks to the changes begun in the 1950s and early 1960s the IUSM now benefitted from a nationwide expansion of activities supported by the dramatic increase of federal support for biomedical research since the end of the Second World War. Congressional allocations to the National Institutes for Health, for example, grew from just under $900 million in 1964 to approximately $1.8 billion in 1974.[55] Yet this expansion did not necessarily make it easier for institutions like the Indiana University School of Medicine to develop and expand their research programs. As available federal dollars increased, so too did both the competition for these resources and the cost and complexity of providing the facilities, talent, and proof-of-concept data needed to secure grants in a competitive and increasingly specialized market place. It took time, therefore, for IUSM faculty to be competitive, and in the interim, the school's researchers were assisted through an unusual windfall of philanthropy.

These donations followed a tradition that had earlier been crucial in building the hospital infrastructure of the medical center, such as the gifts from Long, Coleman, and the friends of Riley. But there were some important differences in this new philanthropy. As before, the donors were local residents, often with little personal connection to medical research, but this new generation of donors elected to dedicate a substantial portion of their personal wealth not to building construction but to supporting medical research in Indiana. Through their family foundations, these philanthropists offered the School of Medicine a new and flexible source of funding that could be used to build the research infrastructure, engage in innovative work, and then leverage that work to secure larger federal funding. The example of the Krannerts, mentioned in the previous chapter, proved to be a model for others, and medical school leaders like Glenn Irwin and John Hickam recognized and seized the opportunities.

Two examples will illustrate how local philanthropy supported medical research.[56] In 1967, Sam Regenstrief, the founder and majority shareholder of Design and Manufacturing Corporation (D&M), the world's largest manufacturer of residential dishwashers, faced the problem of having no direct descendants. The Connersville, Indiana, resident and his wife did not wish to leave their multimillion-dollar estate to more distant relatives but instead hoped to use their fortune to benefit a local cause. The Regenstriefs' legal advisors suggested that a nonprofit foundation would solve their problems.[57]

Choosing the foundation as a legal vehicle meant that some portion of the assets would need to be given out as philanthropic gifts, and Sam Regenstrief wanted to create a fund large enough to provide a budget of $1 million a year. Although he did not initially have a specific cause in mind, he wanted to target his money toward one objective rather than creating a general-purpose fund, and this meant identifying a cause.[58] Initially Regenstrief, who enjoyed productive working relationships with Purdue faculty, leaned toward dedicating his foundation to support the engineering school at Purdue, but Harvey Feigenbaum, a faculty member at IUSM and the husband of the Regenstriefs' niece, had another idea.

Feigenbaum joined the IU faculty in 1962 and began working with Charles Fisch, the first director of the Krannert Institute of Cardiology, the research center described in the previous chapter that had opened in 1963 thanks to the gift of Indiana businessman Herman Krannert and his wife, Elnora. The Krannerts' endowed gift allowed the school to create a cardiology research institute, which in turn was crucial in obtaining additional federal funding. Fisch, a prominent expert in electrophysiology, received NIH funding through the Department of Medicine for some of the institute's expenses. He also had an eye for talent and successfully recruited and trained young faculty, including Feigenbaum, whose pioneer work in echocardiography beginning in the 1960s and 1970s will be described in the next chapter.[59]

Feigenbaum often discussed the health-care system with Regenstrief during family gatherings.[60] The manufacturer's business had been built on his talent for identifying and eliminating manufacturing inefficiencies, and he was troubled by significant problems he noticed in the provision of health care.[61] Feigenbaum rightly suspected that Regenstrief would be attracted to the opportunity to improve an inefficient health delivery system, and he encouraged his uncle to consider directing his philanthropy toward that cause.[62]

To help persuade Regenstrief, Feigenbaum enlisted the help of John Hickam, the chairman of the Department of Medicine who not only oversaw the Krannert Institute but also had developed a national reputation for, among other things, his work on the analysis and improvement of healthcare delivery and medical education. Not surprisingly, when Feigenbaum introduced Hickam to Regenstrief, the two men developed a quick rapport.[63] Regenstrief sat on the board of the small hospital that served the workers of his Connersville plant and was particularly sensitive to the challenges of ensuring access to quality medical care in smaller communities. Through their conversations, Hickam helped Regenstrief settle on a focus. Regenstrief would devote the charitable efforts of his foundation to finding and nurturing improvements in the way that care was delivered. This choice of focus on applied rather than on bench medical research was well timed to take advantage of the expansion in access to health care following the passage of Medicare and Medicaid in 1965.[64]

Regenstrief and several of his advisors met with representatives of the Indiana University School of Medicine through the winter of 1966–67. Given the breadth of the agreement they reached, it is clear that the school intended to build a long-term collaborative partnership with the donor.[65]

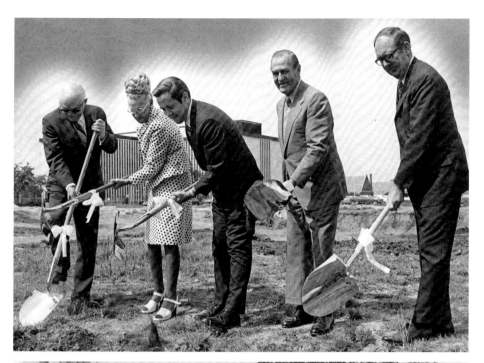

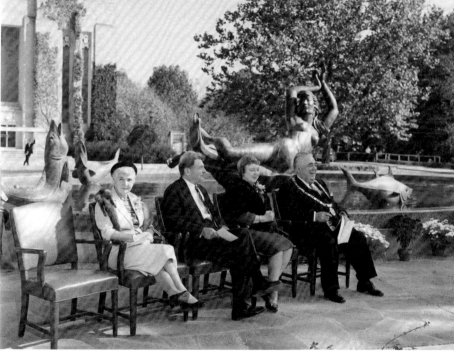

Figure 9.3a & b. Local research philanthropists: (*top*) Regenstrief Center Groundbreaking, 1971, Sam and Myrtie Regenstrief on left, IUPUI image UA024_002255; (*bottom*) Grace Showalter, second from right, seated next to President Wells, far right, in front of Showalter Fountain in Bloomington, 1961, Archive photos IUB P0029549.

The Regenstrief Foundation was incorporated in April 1967, and the Regenstrief Institute was formally chartered in 1969 with Raymond Murray as director and Joe Mamlin as the institute's first researcher.[66] The purpose of the institute was to be a working clinic and a laboratory to test ways to improve the health-care system. The foundation trustees expected regular reports on the productivity and impact of sponsored research as measured by the number of publications generated and the amount of extramural funding that Regenstrief-supported projects attracted from other funders, including the federal government.[67]

Hickam's unexpected death in 1970 delayed the work of the institute, but successors established other clinics around the state to collect data for analysis. More will be said about this work in the next chapter, but one of the key values of the Regenstrief Foundation's contribution was its willingness from its inception to provide sustained funding for work that was novel and had a potential for making a widespread impact. The primary example of this willingness to support improvement of healthcare delivery was the institute's support for a young researcher attracted by the promise of computer technology to improve medical care. Clem McDonald, a medical doctor who also held a degree in biomechanical engineering, hit upon the idea that hospital care could be dramatically improved if doctors did not need to depend on paper charts. This was a radical idea in 1970 when these charts, battered scrapbooks of notes, and orders were transported by hand and filed in large basement storage rooms. Locating charts was time-consuming, and records were often incomplete and illegible, all of which impeded the speed and quality of care.[68]

McDonald, an early advocate for expanded use of computers, envisioned a system built around standardized and computerized order sheets that would be immediately created in an electronic file available to everyone on the system regardless of their location in the hospital or clinic. He and his colleagues also understood that an electronic chart repository could constitute a rich vein of thousands of individual data points that could be mined by researchers working on more traditional medical questions. In 1972, McDonald and his team began work on an integrated computerized system that eventually grew to link inpatient and outpatient information at Marion County General Hospital. The project started in the diabetes clinic, and although it made steady progress, this was a long-term effort that required over a decade of support before it was complete. By 1986, the "Medical Gopher" system housed records for 140,000 patients and was hailed as one of the first such computerized systems in the world.[69]

In 1968, one year after the Regenstrief Foundation was incorporated, Grace Showalter began discussions with her lawyer about the formation of her own charitable trust. She and her husband, Ralph, a former senior executive at Eli Lilly & Company, had no children, and after Ralph died, Grace explored opportunities to support research efforts at both Purdue and the Indiana University School of Medicine. Her choices regarding the fields to be supported and the potential beneficiaries came as a surprise to some, particularly the Indiana University Foundation. It was not surprising for her to support IU because she and her late husband had already given generously to the university. Grace was the first woman to serve as a trustee on the Indiana University Foundation Board, and the foundation building bears her name. Many students and alumni are familiar with the Showalter name because Grace, a devoted art collector, provided the funds in 1961 for a fountain portraying the birth of Venus outside the school's performing arts center.

In the fall of 1967, the Showalter Fountain was a hub of student activities, including student protests over civil rights and the Vietnam War, but those antiwar protests caused Grace, a political and social conservative, to look north for new beneficiaries of her estate. Although she had made charitable gifts in Indianapolis, including to the Indianapolis Museum of Art, Grace Showalter chose to create a charitable foundation. She selected Purdue, her husband's alma mater, as one recipient of the proceeds from her proposed trust and the IU School of Medicine as the other. Showalter made clear that she had no interest in financing the construction of a building, laboratory, or clinic. Instead, she wanted to support research. She therefore left her trustees with a significant task after her death in 1972. Her estate closed with a payment of approximately $15 million into the new trust, which allowed the trustees to distribute $369,102 in the first year.[70] Yet she armed them with only the most general guidance regarding her philanthropic goals and preferences, including that the proceeds be split and allocated roughly evenly each year between the two universities and that endowed chairs in pharmacology or biochemistry be created at each institution. Moreover, only one of the four people she originally selected as a trustee had a medical or scientific background.

When the Showalter trustees met for the first time in 1973, they decided on grant-making policies and procedures for the trust. They established a date to submit requests in advance of the single grant-making meeting, and they capped the amount of money that schools could request for overhead but placed no other restrictions on funding requests.[71] Both the IU School of Medicine and Purdue recognized that Showalter's lack of specificity and the appointment of trustees with limited technical knowledge created an opportunity to exercise significant influence over the direction of the funds. As will be shown in the next chapter, during the following decades, Dean Glenn Irwin and his successors developed a sound partnership with the Showalter trustees to strategically grow research in selected departments of the school.

These and other philanthropic donations for research at the medical school during this period, notably from Joseph E. Walther,[72] reflect the continuing high regard in which the medical school was held both locally and statewide, but the amount of the support was hardly adequate compared to the amount of medical research and scale that was being supported by the NIH, NSF, and other government agencies and national foundations. The importance of the local funding was greatly magnified, however, because it made support available immediately to new researchers desperately in need of seed money to start projects and demonstrate some results in order to be competitive in larger national grants programs. This bore fruit in subsequent decades and will be described in more detail in the next chapter.

Teaching and New Departments

As was the case with research, there were important changes in teaching and the administration of the medical school during the time that the statewide teaching plan was developed. Some were immediate and necessary to implement the reorganization of teaching statewide, but most of those and related changes came later and took several years. On the other hand, the reorganization and introduction of new departments, divisions, and research centers continued the longer term changes in medicine since the Second World War, particularly the acceleration of new medical specialties. As a result, the number, size, and complexity of departments and divisions in the medical school were greatly increased. While the dean's office grew in administrative complexity, individual departments began pursuing their own strategic agendas in response to these developments. For example, the growth of clinical care and insurance requirements led to the development of practice plans, but at the same time advancing costs of graduate research programs continued to be critical for the future direction of the departments. Many of these programs stemmed from residency programs, uniting the growing number of hospitals and clinics, as well as the rapidly expanding research centers and institutes that required new administrative

Table 9.4. IU School of Medicine: Examples of New Departments, Divisions, and Centers, 1958–1977

Year	Name	Notes
1958	Physiology	new department in Indianapolis
1961	General Clinical Research Center	
1962	Heart Research Center	later Krannert
1962	Center for the Study of Childhood Autism	in Dept. of Psychiatry
1963	Dermatology	
1966	Orthopedic Surgery	
1966	Medical Genetics	
1967	Nephrology Division	division in Dept. of Medicine
1970	Radiation Therapy	previously part of Radiology
1971	Specialized Center for Research in Hypertension	
1971	Pediatric Surgery	division in Surgery
1974	Transplant Surgery	division in Surgery
1974	Family Medicine	
1975	Rheumatology Division	division in Dept. of Medicine
1977	Diabetes Research and Training Center	

relationships. Space does not permit a description of all these changes, but table 9.4 provides a representative list of new units in the school, and a number of examples will illustrate what happened.[73]

The changes undertaken by Hickam in the Department of Medicine illustrate the pattern for the rest of the school. From the time he was recruited as chair in 1958 until his death in 1970, Hickam was involved with medical education and research at the university. Hickam's training at Harvard and Duke also helped him connect Indiana to some of the leading physicians and researchers across the country. As mentioned above, Hickman was a consultant for the US Air Force, participating in aviation medicine research at Wright-Patterson Air Base in Dayton (his father was a military pilot), and he also conducted research on the pathology of cardiovascular disease in relation to smoking. One indication of Hickam's national reputation came when he was named a member of the 1964 Advisory Committee to the Surgeon General that issued the report on smoking and health. He became perhaps best known, however, for "Hickam's dictum," a counterargument to the application of Occam's razor to medicine often referred to as the concept of diagnostic parsimony. As opposed to Occam's philosophical principle that "the simplest solution is usually the correct one," Hickam is commonly quoted as saying, "Patients can have as many diseases as they damn well please." Reflecting this same pragmatism and experience, Hickam published nationally on medical education and licensing.[74]

The Department of Medicine grew steadily under Hickam's leadership, focusing on centralizing department administration, building research activities, revising the medical school's curriculum, and integrating educational experiences at the IUSM clinical facilities.[75] During his tenure from 1958 to 1970, the department grew from fewer than ten full-time faculty members to almost seventy. Likewise, grant funding was negligible in 1958, but research expanded when the General Clinical Research center was established on the top floor of Long Hospital in 1961 and when the Heart Research Center began the following year. The divisions within the department were not yet formally established, but Hickam recruited outside experts to lead new specialty areas. By 1970, the department's grants totaled approximately $2.3 million.[76]

Hickam negotiated the education and service affiliation between the IUSM and the new Veterans Administration Hospital, as well as the new contracts with Marion County General Hospital that facilitated the formation of the Regenstrief Clinic.[77] Although the Veterans Hospital was very important to education at IUSM, federal control of the facility, he noted, was a bit like dealing with an absentee property owner, with personnel changes in Washington producing new relationships that required renegotiating budgets and programs. Hickam's untimely death in 1970 prevented him from seeing the new university hospital completed on campus; the fulfillment of his vision of the department was thus left to the new chair of Medicine and later IUSM dean, Walter Daly.[78]

Daly served as department chair from 1970 until he became dean of the school in 1983. Under his leadership, the faculty grew from approximately seventy full-time faculty members to 130, and the house staff and fellows from ninety-five to 140. Research funding grew to approximately $8.1 million. Daly had a long-term, broad agenda and recruited major national researchers in critical areas of internal medicine by offering them research space and the freedom to pursue their own research agenda. Some of his recruits included C. Conrad Johnston in the field of metabolism and D. Craig Brater in clinical pharmacology. Future chair Augustus Wantanabe recalled that when he first was hired in 1971, he had only a closet as an office and gradually built his team and laboratories at IUSM.[79]

As the number of faculty and staff increased, Daly accelerated the process of separating the management of each division, which began the process of decentralizing many functions from the chairman's office to the divisions. He also published national articles on hospital and medical education reform based on IUSM research with the Regenstrief Institute on health economics. New federal legislation and restrictions meant developing new accreditation polices for the hospitals and research facilities. As will be seen in a later chapter, Daly worked to negotiate the first Department of Medicine Practice Plan, an important part of the administration of care that was based on an executive physical program set up by Hickam at the Regenstrief Institute in 1971.[80]

For some departments, the reorganization surrounding the Indiana Plan for statewide medical education caused them to immediately implement substantial reorganization. First were the basic science departments, which had responsibility for providing most of the coursework at the regional campuses. Among other things, this entailed moving staff and identifying local physicians for affiliation with the IUSM. Earlier, the move of the first-year medical student classes to Indianapolis in 1958 meant that some of the Bloomington faculty moved there, although others remained as members of an Anatomy and Physiology Department under Sid Robinson as chair. In 1963, the Bloomington department opened the Human Physiology Laboratory to conduct applied physiology research. In Indianapolis, a new Physiology Department was established under the leadership of Ewald E. Selkurt, and in 1959, it started accepting PhD students as well as teaching MD students. Then in 1976, as a part of the Indiana Plan reorganization, Bloomington's Anatomy and Physiology department was merged with the IUSM department in Indianapolis.[81]

Other new departments and divisions (as well as research centers and institutes) that were established included new subspecialties in the Pediatrics Department, reflecting rapid growth in the field.[82] The department's offerings in turn became a catalyst for other departments and sections to grow and recruit physicians and surgeons who were primarily interested in the care of children, along with developing residency and fellowship programs for training of pediatric surgical and medical subspecialists.[83] Another example of collaboration and specialization was in the Department of Urology, where Robert Garrett became the first full-time chair from 1953 to 1972 and built the department through growth of the residency program. John Donahue, the IUSM professor leading the renal transplant efforts at IUSM, then took over as chair and worked to create the Nephrology Division of the Department of Medicine to assist with donor kidney harvesting.[84]

The subspecialties in surgery also grew at a rapid rate. In 1966, James B. Wray became the first full-time chairman of the Department of Orthopedic Surgery, joining Robert Palmer as another full-time faculty member. With the retirement in 1971 of Harris Shumacker as chair in the Surgery Department, his replacement, John E. Jesseph, was typical of the new generation of chairmen trained in the postwar environment who encouraged a strong focus on specialization and research. After Jesseph returned from

World War II, he completed his undergraduate and medical school training in Seattle and served as a resident and faculty member in general surgery at the University of Washington. In 1971, he was appointed the fourth chairman of the Department of Surgery at IUSM. Under his leadership, the department expanded through the recruitment of specialists from across the country to head up services for Pediatric Surgery (Jay Grosfeld) and Transplant Surgery (Ronald Filo). Jesseph's tenure marked a significant step in improving relations between the practicing surgeons in the state and the Department of Surgery which in turn helped build relationships with surgeons when the statewide program for medical education was developed.[85]

Radiology is an example of a department that expanded thanks to new technology. In addition to improving body imaging, nuclear medicine became increasingly important during the postwar period as a new treatment offered initially by Radiology until 1970, when the Radiation Oncology Department split from Radiology to become a new Department of Radiation Therapy. Ned Hornback was the first chair, and the department was housed in a new facility with support from the Indiana Lions Club.[86] Beyond physicians, advances in radiologic technologies required the development of training in new ancillary medical fields. For example, the department developed a radiation technologist program, for many years under the supervision of Roscoe Miller, that combined one year of coursework with an additional year of clinical experience to pass the national examination. This served as a pipeline of trained and experienced technicians to help staff the expanding department.[87]

In addition to the Department of Radiation Therapy, other new technologies and medical practices made medical care more complex and prompted creation of new departments. In 1963, Dermatology split from Internal Medicine to become a separate department, with Victor Hackney recruited from Stanford University to be the first chairman. Hackney brought additional staff from Stanford, including Arthur Norins in 1964 and Walter Epinette in 1971.[88] The increase in medical specialties was coupled with a decline in general practitioners, to which one response was the emergence of family medicine as a field separate from pediatrics, internal medicine, and obstetrics-gynecology. At IUSM, in 1971, A. Alan Fischer, a nationally known family physician, developed the medical school's first Family Medicine residency program and was appointed the first director, with the department being established in 1974.[89]

With rapid advances in understanding the human genome, Medical Genetics began in 1961 as an interdepartmental committee directed by A. Donald Merritt, the husband of Doris Merritt. The primary goal of this committee was to establish a graduate training program in medical genetics. This was different from other fields because it resulted from both large clinical advances and the emergence of a new interdisciplinary basic science, as increasing numbers of scientists and physicians from various basic science and clinical departments studied genetic diseases. At IUSM, graduate training began in 1962, with the help of an NIH training grant, and the success of the interdepartmental program led to the formation of the Department of Medical Genetics in 1966 and the appointment of Merritt as chairman. It was one of the first independent genetics departments in the nation.[90]

In addition to research institutes such as Krannert and Regenstrief that started with philanthropic support, other new institutes and centers were established on campus, supported primarily through grants. Within the Department of Medicine, a Specialized Center of Research (SCOR) in Hypertension was established by James T. Higgins in 1971—the first of four established with funding from the NIH. In similar fashion, the Diabetes Research and Training Center was funded in 1977, one of five such centers in the nation.[91] In the research field of child psychiatry and development, Marian DeMyer established the first research center for the study of childhood autism at Larue Carter Hospital with the strong support of the medical director of Carter Hospital, Donald Moore, who played a continuing strong role in the development of not only research facilities but also research staff recruitment and training.[92]

Medical Students

The impact of these changes was much less noticed by the average medical student than the faculty or administrators. To be sure, medical students were aware of the dramatic changes in medicine after the Second World War, such as new medical discoveries that made the headlines from the birth control pill to heart transplants. But the administrative and organizational changes in the medical school in the late 1960s and early 1970s hardly affected their intense undergraduate medical instruction. Moreover, they were in between the major changes in demographic composition of medical students, with the postwar boom of students having finished and the dramatic entry in unprecedented numbers of women and ethnic groups to American medical schools just beginning in the early 1970s.[93]

Medical students were also affected differently by the social ferment on college campuses during the 1960s and 1970s, and this included the medical school in Indianapolis. The impact was much more limited than, for example, at the Bloomington campus fifty miles away, or even at other medical schools. At IUSM, some campus activism was focused on student organization, social justice, and civil rights, but medical students were viewed as being more conservative than students in other schools who organized civil rights and Vietnam War protests in the 1960s and 1970s. When Robert Kennedy spoke in Indianapolis on April 24, 1968, some IUSM students spoke critically of Kennedy's plans during the question-and-answer session.[94]

Because of policies established by Selective Service, deferments for induction to serve in the Vietnam War were eliminated for all but medical, dental, and veterinary students. Medical schools and hospitals did not organize medical units as in the world wars. After internship, most medical students were drafted into one of the military services. They could also apply to become a commissioned officer in the Public Health Service, although only a small percentage was accepted. One of those was the future chair of the Department of Medicine Gus Watanabe, who attended IUSM from 1964 to 1967. He lived with his wife in campus housing on the south side of Michigan Street, and he remembered the medical school as a "small oasis" where people were isolated from the surrounding "rough area." After graduation, he elected to accept a medical internship at IUSM, thereby avoiding the draft during the escalation of the Vietnam conflict, but this placed him in the Commissioned Officers Residency Deferment (CORD) program. He was to go into the air force but also applied to the program with the Public Health Service. He was accepted into a position at the National Institutes of Health at Bethesda, which gave him formal training in research that led him to stay in the field of academic medicine.[95]

Although most students focused on their studies, the largest of student organizations, the Student American Medical Association (SAMA), played an important role in the lives of IUSM medical students through the 1960s. SAMA was a national organization with branches at various medical schools, and early on, the Indiana students distinguished themselves. In 1960, they attended the annual SAMA scientific sessions and won first- and second-place awards for their original research exhibits, as well as third place for a paper on original research. One IUSM student was elected vice president of SAMA. It was described as "the most sweeping victory ever scored by students from a single medical school and drew many favorable comments from medical educators attending the sessions as reflecting the quality of teaching and encouragement of student research by the school and its faculty."[96]

SAMA bought uniforms, sold them to interns and medical doctors at the hospitals, and bought doctor's coats for each incoming first- and second-year class. SAMA offered a range of programming during the academic year, including noontime educational films, a student-faculty acquaintance coffee hour for freshmen, a Christmas party, and presentations by pharmaceutical representatives. SAMA also helped coordinate Alumni Day, sold used textbooks to students, and gave regular talks to high school students (a total of 145 during the 1964–65 academic year). The group gave a best professor award, helped with a scout program, and offered fifty-dollar loans—without interest for thirty days—to students. Medical students paid a nominal fee to join, and during the 1964–65 academic year, Indiana University was the largest SAMA chapter of all medical schools.[97]

In the late 1960s, the SAMA chapter at IUSM began the Southside Community Health Clinic Corp., an outpatient clinic in an area of Indianapolis where health services were not available. The two students who started the clinic raised the initial capital by selling $1,300 worth of their own blood to IUSM hospitals. The empty parsonage of the Mayer Presbyterian Church at 234 Morris Street served as the first location for the clinic. Students wrote to drug companies and asked them to supply the clinic; in response, they received $23,000 worth of medicine. They also asked for, and received, donations and financing from local individuals and organizations in Indianapolis, such as the Sertoma Club. The clinic was run by a board and staffed by community members, IU faculty, and medical students. In 1968, staff included 175 medical students, twenty-nine doctors, and nine nurses.[98] Third- and fourth-year medical students staffed the clinic and were supervised by doctors. Forty-two doctors and two hundred medical students donated their time in 1969.[99] The clinic was originally scheduled to be open two nights a week, and on the first day, eight patients came. That grew to twenty-two patients the following Saturday, and from there the clinic continued to grow and serve the community. Membership cards cost patients one dollar, and each visit cost fifty cents, but family income could affect the cost that patients would pay.[100] The program attracted national attention, and in 1969, the national SAMA awarded the IUSM chapter $1,000 for the clinic.[101]

This period saw the beginning of major changes in the demographic makeup of the medical student body. More will be said about female and African American medical students in a later chapter, but as an indication of the low starting point, since its beginning, most incoming classes of the medical school had at least one but rarely more than two black students. In the late 1960s and 1970s, however, this began to change. In 1969, for example, IUSM received eleven applications from African Americans. Six were offered admission, and four accepted the offer. The remaining five applicants were rejected as "not competitive on the basis of their overall applications."[102] By 1970–71, the number of African American applicants

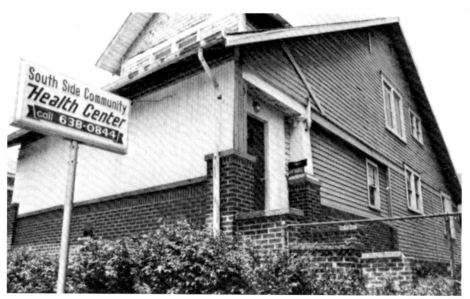

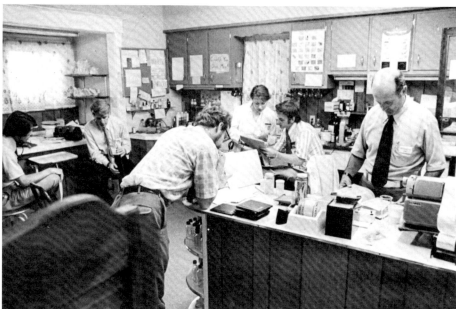

Figure 9.4a & b. "The South Side Health Clinic, a nonprofit free clinic staffed by students and faculty of I.U.M.C.," exterior view, *Retrospectroscope* (1975): 6; and interior view, Class of 1971 Yearbook.

had increased to forty, with fifteen accepted and ten who ultimately enrolled in the 1971 freshman class.[103]

On May 12, 1970, IUPUI chancellor Maynard K. Hine met with the newly established Black Health Student Association. The students stated that current black students were not provided as much financial aid as other students, and they also wanted a black recruiting officer who could help with financial aid. Hine agreed to develop a list of financial aid options that would be given to all students when they were accepted, and to discuss the feasibility of hiring a black recruiting officer.[104]

The Indianapolis University

The consolidation of the IU School of Medicine in Indianapolis as a result of opening the Medical Sciences Building in 1958 reinforced the view, often expressed by President Wells, that Indiana University's facilities and programs in Indianapolis should all be moved to the area near the medical school north of Michigan Street. Of the numerous programs in the state capital, the medical school and hospitals were by far the largest part of Indiana University's presence, which since the early 1900s included extension services of numerous departments at the Bloomington campus.[105] In addition, Wells continued the policy first established by the Bloomington campus decades earlier of buying available land near the medical campus without immediate need for a specific project. This policy became a program in July 1962 when Charles O. Hardy was hired to oversee Indiana University's real estate operations in Indianapolis from an office in Fesler Hall. In the master plans of both the City of Indianapolis and Indiana University in the early 1960s, there was an expanded medical center plus consolidated Indiana University programs located in the area between downtown and the White River.[106]

The medical school understood the plan in 1963 to entail creation of a University Quarter that would be home to a campus for graduate and professional education. The already confused nomenclature for the university hospitals, medical center (including the VA, MCGH, and Larue Carter), and medical school facilities were about to be compounded by the expected move there of several schools in Indianapolis that eventually joined IU (see table 9.5), such as a local proprietary law school that became part of IU in 1944 and an expanded business school.[107] From 1963 to 1965, there was growing convergence between the visions of the city and the university. The university began to formally plan for an Indiana University at Indianapolis campus, and in 1964, in conjunction with the Indianapolis Metropolitan Plan Committee, the university released a proposal for a three-hundred-acre

Table 9.5. Pre-Existing Schools in Indianapolis That Became Part of Indiana University

School	Predecessor	Became Part of IU	Originally Founded
School of Medicine	Indiana Medical College, College of Physicians and Surgeons	1908	1869
School of Social Work	Department of Social Service	1911	1911
School of Nursing	IU Training School for Nurses	1914	1914
School of Dentistry	Indiana Dental College	1925	1879
Robert H. McKinney School of Law	Indiana/Benjamin Harrison Law School	1936	1894
School of Health and Human Sciences	Turnlehrerseminar [Gymnastic Teachers Seminary]	1941	1866
Herron School of Art and Design	John Herron Art Institute	1967	1902

urban renewal project to the southeast of the Medical Center. Not only would the University Quarter be developed, but there would also be a civic center, hotel, and stadium. All of this would be part of the larger process of transforming the street grid and neighborhoods for more effective filtering and distribution of traffic pouring into downtown with the construction of the new Interstate Highway system. In November 1965, the IU Board of Trustees reviewed a Campus Master Plan for Indianapolis developed by Smith and Eggers, the university's architects and planners, which envisioned a medical campus stretching north of Michigan Street and west from West Street to the White River, to be complemented by an undergraduate, graduate, and professional campus for Indiana University south of Michigan with the same east-west boundaries.[108] (See figure 9.5.)

The sheer size of the medical center and the perception among Indianapolis leaders that the distressed, predominately black residential neighborhoods at its boundaries were in need of "renewal" combined to push the idea to the center of broader plans for urban higher education in Indianapolis. From 1966 to 1968, Indiana University continued to develop its proposal for a consolidated campus around the Medical Center. This quickly attracted the support of many Indianapolis community leaders such as Beurt SerVaas, who advocated for a new independent public university to serve the capital's need for higher education. Beginning in 1966, Indiana University president Elvis Stahr began discussions with Frederick Hovde, president of Purdue University, about possibly moving all Indianapolis area programs for both universities into facilities in the proposed University Quarter. The talks continued between the two university presidents without much tangible progress for two years.[109] Then in April 1968, Indiana University

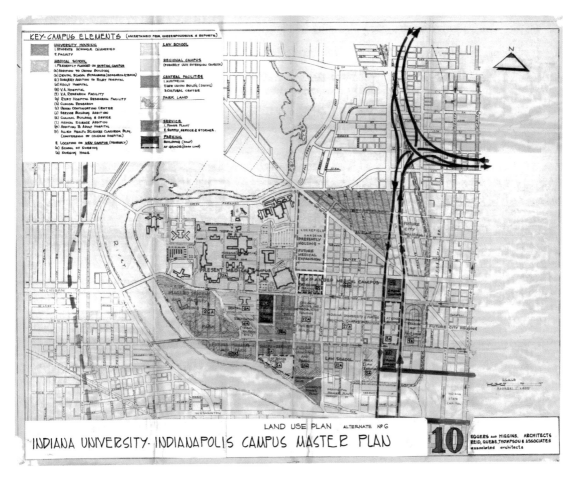

Figure 9.5. IU-Indianapolis Plan. Well before the call for IUPUI, Indiana University planned consolidation of its Indianapolis programs around the medical center. UA 073, InUI-Ar, cataloguing in process.

revealed an updated version of its plan for the Indianapolis campus, initially a three-building complex to be built on Michigan Street. Purdue had not committed to joining, and on September 4, 1968, Indiana University broke ground on its new downtown campus adjacent to the medical center.[110]

The election of 1968 changed the political landscape in Indianapolis, and high on the list for the new Republican regime at city hall and the statehouse was creation of a new university in Indianapolis. Richard Lugar, who had been elected mayor of Indianapolis the previous year, spoke on December 14, 1968, in favor of a new public university for the city, encouraging the General Assembly to pass a bill to be submitted in January for "the creation of a State University to be independent of all other state universities

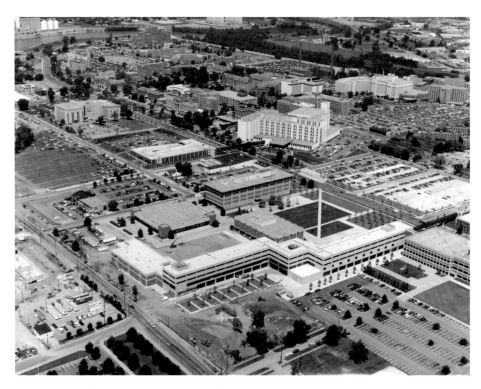

Figure 9.6. Aerial view of IUPUI campus, 1982, showing addition of library and classroom buildings to the south and east of the medical school and center. IUPUI image UA024_002558.

and to be located in Indianapolis." Republican leaders in the General Assembly were briefed throughout the process by those who developed the proposed legislation, including Beurt Servaas, president of the Marion County Council; Thomas Hasbrook, president of Common Council; John Burkhart, president of the Metropolitan Capital Improvements Board; and Charles Whistler, chairman of the Metropolitan Planning Commission.[111]

The reaction from Indiana University and Purdue University to the proposal for a new university was swift. In quick succession in January 1969, the boards of trustees of each school adopted almost identical resolutions committing to a merger of their respective programs at one site at the new downtown campus to be managed by Indiana University. Maynard Hine, longtime dean of the Dental School, who only three months before was named as the first chancellor of Indiana University–Indianapolis, was now to be the chancellor of the newly created Indiana University–Purdue University at Indianapolis (IUPUI).[112]

Aware or not of the 1905–1908 struggle over the medical school, leaders of Indiana and Purdue universities were able to rapidly find common ground when an external mutual threat was perceived. In 1908, it had been the risk of losing General Assembly support for higher education. In 1969, it was the risk of losing the capital city to a new university. By committing to work together to transform the new Downtown Campus into a robust urban university, negotiating with Indianapolis leaders to better meet their concerns, and lobbying the General Assembly to wait on action as it had with the recently received Stoner Commission report, Indiana University in alliance with Purdue was able to implement its plans before the alternatives were fully articulated or funded.[113]

At the time of IUPUI's creation, the School of Medicine was dominant, most obviously as a physical presence as well as research center. In July 1969, the sponsored program support at IUPUI totaled $13.7 million dollars, $11.5 million of which was at the School of Medicine. On the other hand, the arrival of IUPUI brought thousands of undergraduate and graduate students (thirteen thousand students including the medical school) that gave the School of Medicine at Indianapolis further stability as part of a broader university community.[114]

Conclusion: Bigger, with Accompanying Problems

Between 1963 and 1974, Indiana University and its School of Medicine continued to react to the ongoing impact of specialization in medicine, the demand for training more doctors, and the provision of more patient care. Research also continued to grow, and the resulting increase in the size and complexity of the school and its hospitals made it even more difficult for a dean or university president to control it. Adding to this were three major changes that expanded the statewide presence of the medical school and placed it at the heart of the "new" state university. The Statewide Medical Education System created by the Indiana Plan ensured that the Indiana University School of Medicine would remain the sole provider of medical education in Indiana for the foreseeable future. Rather than face the competition for research as well as education funds from an independent second medical school, the School of Medicine was now present on the campuses of former rivals in medical education. The particular configuration of the plan by 1974 ensured that the demand for teaching and clinical services in Indianapolis would remain strong, an outcome even more desirable as clinical income became a large part of faculty salaries and medical school revenue. Nonetheless, graduate medical education remained concentrated in Indianapolis, leaving a basic goal of the Indiana Plan unfulfilled.

The second change was to make the medical school part of Indiana University–Indianapolis, a change from the original plans for a graduate center that eventually became the practical compromise of IUPUI. The third change—the rapid expansion of the hospital system and operating agreements with Marion County General and the VA Hospital—ensured that the medical center could continue its growth as a specialized referral center while still serving a more general patient population, which was necessary for training doctors and fulfilling its clinical service mission.

In all three of these areas, the university and the medical school had risked losing control of its immediate future. That it managed to emerge from all of these opportunities and threats stronger and bigger than ever, locally and statewide, is a testament to a resilient and distinctive culture. During the tenure of Dean Irwin, the Indiana University School of Medicine was remarkably adept at working in the political and social culture of Indiana that valued consensus over conflict, reaching out over hunkering down. Although the school had dispersed its presence to all corners of the state, it found itself now as an even stronger influence on Indiana medicine than it had been in the preceding era of consolidation, although with equally increased responsibilities to its outside constituencies.

10

The Medical Center, 1975–1995:
Administration and
Medical Education

*I*n 1975, former associate dean for State Partnerships Steven Beering became head of a medical school experiencing growth with a complex set
of partnerships in nearly every area. His responsibilities included managing
the six hospitals of the medical center, the thirteen research institutes and
centers, the nine medical education centers, and the numerous programs
of the Division of Allied Health Sciences across the IU system. This is a
reminder that neither deans nor university presidents in the last decades of
the twentieth century could control medical schools like their predecessors
in the first half of the 1900s. In fact, some departments had larger faculty
and budgets than the entire medical school just two decades earlier.

The history of the IU School of Medicine in the years after the mid-
1970s in many ways continued changes set in motion during the previous
decade. This included implementation of the statewide medical education
plan and integration into the new IUPUI campus. Other circumstances
fostered continuity. For example, Beering replaced Dean Glenn Irwin because Irwin had been appointed chancellor of the IUPUI campus, and he
was thus very much connected to developments at the medical school. In
addition, Beering and his successor, Walter Daly, were selected following
the practice of promoting from within, which made them quite familiar
with school practices and policies. As a result of these circumstances, from
the start of Beering's time as dean (1975–83) to the end of Daly's tenure in
1995, the IUSM continued to function in the institutional framework created during the 1960s.

Broadly speaking, Beering was head of the IU Medical Center, a term
increasingly used to describe the complex of hospitals and research centers

that had grown up around the medical school, and with which it established long-standing working relationships based on formal agreements. The medical school was the center of the state medical establishment, enjoying an unparalleled combination of political power, medical education monopoly, and economic success. Not surprisingly, these growing resources, including those of the faculty practice plans and increased expectations for research funding, placed new strains on the dean's office, which in the postwar years was more preoccupied with managing than controlling the changes. For example, by 1991, budget shortfalls plus talk of physician surpluses and changes in health care brought a serious reexamination of the system of regional medical education centers. Ultimately, the statewide model survived the challenge as it continued to spread academic and economic benefits across the state. Yet despite the national fear of oversupply of doctors and the expansion of the statewide system in Indiana, there continued to be a lack of physicians in more rural areas of the state.

Another general concern for the dean's office was the tension produced by rising expectations from the university and state leadership that coincided with increasing independence of researchers and clinical faculty who were able to secure their own resources for support. The dean and other administrators therefore had larger but more restricted budgets to meet the growing demands. This dilemma was sharpened by the continuation of the medical school's strategy, which had been followed since its creation, that the optimal size of the school was the maximal size—all while the school was expected to follow the IU tradition of consensus decision making. Accordingly, the expanded statewide education system, growing clinical practice, and a plethora of new research centers thanks to NIH grants—plus additional private and state dollars—produced a complex ecosystem of teaching, research, and clinical practice.

In sum, the local events and decisions of 1964–74 created a new organizational model and culture at the medical school, but it was subject to the same national trends that shaped medical research, clinical care, and medical education. The very scope and nature of health and medicine changed dramatically after the 1970s both nationally and locally, and they were reflected in developments at the IU Medical Center. The interaction of these local and national influences determined the nature of the IUSM as it completed its first century of operation. This chapter first outlines changes in the school administration and then examines in more detail the teaching and students of the medical school, the main features of which were the implementation of the statewide plan (a local development) and the accommodation to new medical students (women and minorities) that were part of a broad national trend. The next chapter will look at the accelerated growth of research and clinical activities at the medical school during this same time period.

Beering as Medical School Dean

In addition to these broad concerns raised by the evolution of modern medicine in the last decades of the twentieth century, Beering faced some pressing tasks when he took office, the most immediate of which was the implementation of the Indiana Plan and the related growth in the number of medical students admitted each year. In addition, the management of university hospitals and agreements with the affiliated hospitals required changes in order to work better with the medical school, including achieving parity in wages, working conditions, and hiring standards at all facilities. The need for ever-increasing research dollars also led to pressures for more laboratory space and the growth of new institutes. Finally, alongside the medical campus, the growth of IUPUI required negotiating the relationships with both Bloomington and Indianapolis administrators.

The administrative issues growing out of this increasing complexity, particularly in research and clinical affairs, will be dealt with in the next chapter, but an example is useful in showing how these collaborations, such as the operation of the newly renamed Wishard Memorial Hospital, could lead to changes across the school. Beginning in the 1960s, John Hickam had recognized the critical potential of what was then Marion County General Hospital for developing a robust program of research through the new Department of Community Health services and the Regenstrief Institute.[1] Therefore, the IUSM, and particularly the Department of Medicine, assumed responsibility for and fostered reform at Wishard, thanks to the operating agreements of 1975 and 1983.[2] The result of the collaboration with Wishard Hospital plus the Regenstrief Institute, helped make the Department of Medicine's Division of General Internal Medicine an increasingly powerful research engine while simultaneously extending the service culture of academic medicine into the county hospital.

Steven Beering was familiar with many of these pressing needs of the medical school, but his appointment as dean was not expected. It was prompted when Maynard Hine, the first chancellor of IUPUI, retired in 1973 and was replaced by then dean of the Medical School Glenn Irwin, who, in a reorganization the following year, also became IU vice president. The appointment of a new IUPUI chancellor was at a tense time on the campus. The medical school was in the midst of a radical expansion and reorganization, but the Indianapolis campus was also establishing its own identity, with many new faculty members in programs and schools that joined the campus. As a result, the nonmedical faculty pushed for what they thought was an appropriate say in the future of the campus. For example, many of the IUPUI Liberal Arts faculty were "disappointed" in Irwin's promotion because they saw it as a slight to the growing list of non-health-related academic programs.[3]

The appointment also initially went against the desires of the new IU president, John Ryan, who preferred his own candidate, Edward C. Moore, associate dean for Academic Affairs at the Bloomington campus. Ryan came to IU as vice president for Regional Campuses in 1968 and then took the helm of IU during the pivotal period from 1971 to 1987. Ryan went so far as to delay the acceptance of the IUPUI Chancellor Search Committee recommendation but eventually appointed Irwin, according to Daly, "because Glenn had so many friends and was well known and was an excellent administrator and brought so much to the institution." Irwin and his experienced staff worked to win over the doubters and the faculty whom Irwin did not already count as friends with adroit management. His close colleague and successor, Beering, agreed with those who pronounced Irwin the "kindest and most wonderful person . . . and a caring great doctor, teacher."[4] One of the key administrative figures originally appointed by Irwin who remained through Beering's tenure was Associate Dean George T. Lukemeyer, who provided continuity through the end of the 1980s (1972–90), especially in administrative areas such as admissions, student affairs, and budgeting.[5]

Beering had worked closely with Irwin on the planning and implementation of the Statewide Medical Education Plan, so his choice as Irwin's successor was not a complete surprise, although the historical record is largely silent about the deliberations.[6] For his part, Beering was not anxious to take the position. He felt he was just settling into his research and teaching roles when he was asked by IU President Ryan to consider becoming dean. Beering later recalled that he was persuaded to advance his candidacy because of his close relationship with Ryan and by the promise he would still be able to continue seeing patients and conduct research. He soon found there was little time for his role as a researcher or physician. The time for a part-time dean had passed.[7]

Although Beering was promoted from within the school, he had only joined it in 1969, and his background was quite different from the tradition of appointing deans of IUSM with roots in Indiana. Beering was born in Berlin in 1932, just before the Nazis came to power, and he grew up in a merchant family that tried unsuccessfully to flee Hitler's Germany in 1938. The war split the family, and afterward they tried to rebuild their lives in Hamburg. Soon afterward, the Beering family moved to Pittsburgh, where Steven graduated from the University of Pittsburgh in 1954 with a BS and a medical degree in 1958. Beering joined the US Air Force Medical Corps, where he remained until he was recruited by IU in 1969. During his time with the military, he became director of the internal medicine program at the Wilford Hall Medical Center in San Antonio, Texas, and at the national level, he served concurrently as chair of the Council of Deans for the Association of Medical Colleges and as a leader in the College of Physicians.[8]

Even after the appointment of Beering as dean, Irwin continued to influence the direction of the medical school from his position as IUPUI chancellor. In part, this followed from providing campus services as well as other administrative practices, including approval of faculty appointments and reviews. However, Irwin opposed integrating the Medical Center too closely as part of IUPUI, arguing that as a statewide medical education system IUSM needed an "all university designation." This was reinforced, perhaps most importantly, by keeping the budget of the school separate from the rest of the new university campus. Nonetheless, this was a major change for the medical school to be part of a university campus close at hand and not fifty miles away. The health programs initially dominated IUPUI, but as new schools were added and grew, the campus quickly took on the features of the comprehensive urban university its promoters desired. By 1973, IUPUI included schools of dentistry, nursing, law, social work, the Herron School of Art, plus a School of Engineering that granted Purdue degrees. Schools of Science and Liberal Arts were also established with faculty who had been teaching for Purdue and Indiana in programs in Indianapolis. Across campus, Irwin promoted the strategy that each program should retain the name of the university (Purdue or Indiana University) that had charge of the academic program, hence the name Indiana University of School of Medicine.

Despite his caution about IUPUI, Irwin encouraged the IUSM faculty to participate in both the IU and IUPUI campus governance including the Faculty Council. This presented quite an opportunity for change, in the opinion of Hugh Headlee, professor of parasitic diseases and one of the senior medical school faculty, who recalled in 1973 that when he started at the school in 1943, "authoritarian administration" of the medical school was "accentuated by the exigencies imposed by World War II."[9] The main administrative unit, he recalled, was the Dean's Executive Committee, "consisting primarily of the departmental chairmen," which along with the dean appointed standing and ad hoc committees as needed. He admitted that the school "theoretically" came under the policies and procedures of the Indiana University Faculty Council and Faculty Handbook, but practically the medical school faculty was "neither very aware of or alert to these provisions for democratic governance."

The reason for Headlee's observations was that that the establishment of IUPUI required the medical school faculty "to write a constitution by which it would govern itself," and it was also "obligated to participate in the activities of other governing bodies, such as the IUPUI Faculty Council, by providing Unit Representation." Each of the schools had at least one elected representative on the council (Law, Physical Education, Social Work, and Art) except Dentistry and Nursing with two, Purdue science and Indiana liberal arts faculty with three each, and the School of Medicine with five.[10] Headlee was skeptical about how well the medical faculty would take advantage of the opportunity to formulate "policies and procedure of governance," but the school did participate in campus governance, eventually developing the practice that the president of the Faculty Council was alternately held by a faculty member from the nonhealth and health schools.[11]

The 1979 Liaison Committee for Medical Education (LCME) report provided a snapshot of the medical school in the middle of Beering's tenure, viewed from the perspective of national practices. These visits and reports had become much more important than the first visits to Indiana in 1954 and 1963 because after 1972, the LCME became the official accrediting agency for medical schools. The LCME accreditation focused specifically on the educational mission of the school by measuring the school's achievements against national standards. In addition, because these were closely tied to clinical practice and research, the accreditation served as a check on these other forces pressuring the school's teaching priorities. The visits were taken seriously because they could have important ramifications for the school. For example, only students and graduates of accredited schools could sit for state licensing examinations. Any deficiencies or areas found in need of growth could result in the committee recommending a probationary status.[12]

Not surprisingly, of special interest to the LCME report in 1979 was the multicampus model in Indiana, which among other things was the main reason IUSM had the largest medical school entering class in the country (305 students admitted in 1978). As will be seen, this number proved to be unsustainable because a significant drop in medical school applicants soon followed, but one result of this large size, the LCME noted, was that IUSM had one of the lowest faculty/student ratios and smallest spending per student in the country. On the positive side, the committee cited the "magnitude of the financial support given by the state legislature," as well as the "statesman-like manner in which the funds were used." They also commented on Irwin's campaign of building renovations on the Indianapolis campus.[13]

Viewed from the outside, the web of relations between the school and the other components of the medical center were seen to be "ambiguous and rather puzzling." This meant not only the relationships outside the school but also the organic development of the department system, which led to an unwieldy structure with considerable power at the department level and a resultant reduction in the attention to faculty governance (confirming Headlee's fears). The report noted that many department chairs had been appointed since the new statewide plan was introduced, and some formerly strong departments, such as Anatomy and Otolaryngology, struggled for leadership. The regional centers were run by young faculty who took on heavy teaching and administrative roles, which limited the time and resources for their own research.[14]

Another problem mentioned in the LCME report was in the area of preventive and public health, as well as coordination of teaching and research in this area. This was the legacy of earlier failed attempts by Charles Emerson and Thurman Rice to establish a department or school of public health. On the other hand, the report endorsed the new system of senior electives that allowed for more geographically and thematically diverse experiences. More than 45 percent of the students took electives off campus, but the LCME report suggested that the system needed more coordination, development, and standards for evaluation. In addition, following national priorities, the LCME found IUSM needed more attention paid to student involvement in curricular changes, student governance, and diversity. Perhaps the most difficult challenge noted by the LCME was to prevent the school from becoming insular, with more than half of the faculty and resident spots going to its own graduates, while the multicampus model isolated students and faculty working in outposts across the state.[15]

Of assistance in managing the increasingly complex components of the medical school for both Beering as well as his successor, Daly, were new administrative appointments beginning in 1976 that reorganized and expanded the dean's office. For example, in recognition of the importance of the affiliated hospitals, William Jenkins was named administrator of Wishard Memorial Hospital in 1976. His appointment was also noteworthy as part of an effort to increase African American administrators at higher levels during the period, but because he also came from both hospital and

Table 10.1. Example of Degrees Granted by Division of Allied Health Sciences, 1971–1987

Bachelors	1970–71	1987
Cytotechnology		6
Medical Record Administration	19	13
Medical Technology		35
Occupational Therapy	60	73
Physical Therapy	76	84
Public Health—Dental Hygiene		12
Public Health—Environmental Health	6	8
Radiological Technology	117	9
Respiratory Therapy	6	14
Masters		
Health Administration Program	44	46
Anesthesiology Graduate Program	17	29
Dietetics	50	28

Sources: IUSM Annual Report 1970–71; LCME Self-Study and Final Report, 1987, Box 233, UA 073, InUI-Ar.

governmental positions, Jenkins represented a shift away from hospitals being managed by physicians. This was a national trend as hospitals increasingly turned to professional health-care administrators to oversee the complex management difficulties of the modern hospital.[16]

Another example of administrative reorganization was the consolidation, upgrading, and standardization of the many health-related programs that had been established at Indianapolis and other regional campuses. These had grown especially during and after the Second World War in response to new specializations in the health field and included physical, occupational, and respiratory therapy, as well as nutrition and various other laboratory and medical technologies. All of these associate, bachelor, and graduate programs were placed in a Division of Allied Health Sciences in 1959, which was separately administered from the rest of the medical school although it remained under the IUSM budget and oversight. Table 10.1 gives some examples of the degrees offered.

The division encompassed allied health programming on five of the eight campuses of Indiana University and included twenty-one distinct allied health academic degree programs, making it the third largest unit in the school.[17]

Beering found an unexpected but welcome high-placed champion for his efforts in the person of Otis Bowen, an IUSM alumnus who had become Indiana governor just before Beering was named dean. Bowen received his BA from Indiana University in 1939 and an MD in 1942. On his return from World War II, he set up his medical practice in his hometown of Bremen, Indiana. Bowen approached political life as a "small time doc." With a focus on cultivating relationships, he decided to run for public office in 1957, quickly moving up through the state legislature to become the speaker of the Indiana House of Representatives in 1967. Bowen became governor in 1972 and was reelected in 1976. Friendly to physicians and his *alma mater*, Bowen implemented several important health-related measures during his political career in Indiana, including some of the nation's strictest limits on medical malpractice, the creation of a statewide emergency medical services system, and the repeal the Indiana eugenic sterilization law first passed in 1907.[18]

After two terms as governor, Bowen returned to IUSM in 1981 as a clinical professor in the new Department of Family Medicine. This appointment gave legitimacy to that emerging field and was crucial to integrating its pedagogical methods into the broader medical school. Bowen's work was cut short, however, in 1985 when President Ronald Reagan appointed him as Secretary of the Department of Health and Human Services, the first physician in the role, where Bowen served until 1989. Bowen attempted to bring more resources to address health issues such as disability, drug addiction, and health-care reform. He replaced Margaret Heckler as HHS secretary, who had been widely criticized for the government's slow response to the AIDS epidemic, and Bowen's physician credentials plus the eloquent advocacy of his surgeon general, Everett Koop, were crucial in making the case for more government support and financial resources.[19] Upon returning to Indiana in 1992 after his retirement, Bowen loaned his name to a new Family Medicine Research Center at IUSM, run by the chair of Family Medicine, Deborah Allen, and health economist Deborah Freund. The center was originally developed as a joint collaboration between the School of Public and Environmental Affairs and IUSM to explore the relationship between medicine and public policy.[20]

In addition to family medicine, Bowen also exercised influence on the IU Medical School through people who served under him. For example, one of Bowen's key advisors was attorney Daniel F. Evans, who eventually became head of the Clarian (later IU Health) system, which was created in 1997 by University, Riley, and Methodist Hospital.[21] Evans graduated from the IU School of Law at IUPUI and was hired as campaign manager for Bowen's gubernatorial reelection. Evans worked with the governor and then went to Washington with Bowen to help him set up his HHS office and staff. There, Evans had the opportunity to see the complexity of health-care administration, particularly in the area of insurance reimbursement, and he encountered firsthand the workings of Medicaid and Medicare, which were beginning to mature.

Beering drew praise for his response to many of the issues raised by the 1979 LCME visit and his general handling of the growing complexity of administering a large academic medical center, including construction, strategic partnerships, and fundraising. As a result, many believed he might follow in the steps of previous long-serving deans such as Van Nuys and Gatch, if he did not move up in the IU administration as Irwin had done. All were surprised, however, at Beering's February 1983 announcement that he would become president of Purdue University in July. Despite the deep rivalry between the two schools, at the IU trustees meeting a day after the public announcement, President Ryan and the trustees welcomed this "appropriate opportunity for the flowering of cooperation between our universities." In West Lafayette, many Purdue alumni were skeptical of this "strange medical creature from I.U." Longtime Purdue administrator John Hicks reassured them, as well as faculty, that Beering was an accomplished administrator and fundraiser. In addition to encouraging donations from grateful patients and family, Beering had increased the number of endowed chairs at IUSM from three to thirty-four. His work on the IUSM Statewide Centers plan gave Beering some familiarity with the regional program at Purdue, although the potential collaborations predicted by some never came to fruition.[22]

The Daly Years

When Steven Beering left in July 1983, Walter J. Daly replaced him as dean with the mission to continue the medical school's growth and further accelerate the progress in attracting research dollars. Writing just a year earlier, Daly had prophetically observed, "I believe we are again at a time of important transition. Really, change has occurred so continually over the past 10 years that our course has been more a curve than stair steps."[23] At times over the succeeding years, Daly departed from the boosterish IU tradition of growth by more openly acknowledging problems and trying to steer the school along a steady path. To support the facilities and additional infrastructure, Daly increased charitable gifts and endowments. He appointed additional full-time associate deans, to oversee research, graduate medical education, continuing education, and academic affairs. His most lasting legacy likely came at the end of his tenure when he negotiated the consolidation of Riley and University Hospitals with the private Methodist Hospital.[24]

Daly's appointment reflects the return to a familiar path to becoming dean. He received a BA in 1951 and an MD in 1955 from Indiana University, graduating first in his class. After a pulmonary disease fellowship, he joined the faculty of IUSM in 1962 and attained full professorship in 1968. He served as chairman of the Department of Medicine from 1970 to 1983, along with positions at some of the most important research centers of the medical school, such as the director of the Regenstrief Institute for Health Care Research. (See the next chapter for more on its operation.) As chair of Medicine, he worked closely with many of the residents, researchers, and junior faculty who later served as the nucleus of his team as dean. Based on his experience, Daly was less concerned with growth and more interested in strengthening departments. Though he denied having a specific personal vision, Daly nonetheless acted to make research a priority, raised funds to support the school's expansion, and reorganized clinical responsibilities. He generally let departments have administrative freedom in the area of research grants, faculty recruitment, and collaboration with hospitals and centers. However, this led some faculty in smaller departments to feel shut out from the working of the dean's office.[25]

Daly became dean after the main features of the statewide plan had been put in place, but as will be seen later, it was a complex system, and he still faced the critical eye of the LCME as well as statewide stakeholders. Following national trends, Daly reduced admissions in the 1980s, but by the end of his term they climbed back to record levels. He supported a new initiative to meet rising costs by raising funds to be invested in the infrastructure needs for the research mission and the clinical practice operations of the departments in the school, with expectations they would bring in even more funds. The most important investments were made in patient care facilities, such as the opening at Riley Hospital of a new $56 million addition in 1986 to meet growing specialty and ambulatory care demand. Another important project was the Library and Research Building that opened in 1989, which housed the long-awaited expanded library and the Department of Medical Genetics along with additional biomedical research laboratories.[26]

In contrast to Beering's more top-down approach, Daly can be seen as a consensus builder, delegator, and problem solver. Indicative of Daly's approach to the job, upon taking office, he commissioned a series of strategic reports by outside health-care experts to evaluate the future of the relationship between the city, the IUSM, and the university. These reports demonstrated that the needs at this time were not just increasing capital but rather the better distribution of income from the departments, particularly those with practice plans, to pay for increased administrative and education costs. He was sensitive to the inefficient and problematic spots in the IUMC that blocked the flow of resources. Freeing up these resources was critical to Daly, as was the growth of the educational mission, particularly in the area of graduate education. This required increasing access to patients for clinical training of residents at a time when inpatient hospital stays were declining. In addition, the medical center could no longer rely on coordinating and receiving referral patients from hospitals across Indiana. The strength of other health facilities in Indianapolis required rethinking of relationships with other hospitals in the region.[27]

IUSM operated in a shifting academic "marketplace," as well. Daly's term saw changes in the university administration with the retirement of IU president Ryan and IUPUI chancellor Irwin in 1986. Irwin's replacement was Gerald Bepko (1986–2003), who directed IUPUI through a period of rapid growth. Bepko was the first nonhealth chancellor—he had been Dean of the IU School of Law in Indianapolis—and he worked to strengthen IUPUI's position within Indiana's higher education system and to increase the independence of the campus. As far as the relationship of the campus with the medical school, Bepko promoted the idea of a "research corridor" in life sciences that included IU-Bloomington, IUPUI, and Purdue–West Lafayette, which would aid in the economic development of Indiana.[28] In 1987, Ryan was replaced by Thomas Ehrlich (1987–94) from the University of Pennsylvania. Like Bepko, Ehrlich had previously been a law school dean at Stanford before he served briefly as provost at Penn, and hence he had little experience with state-supported universities. After years of operating under the Wells model, Ehrlich proposed a new era of academic planning, which came to be known as the "One University" plan. Although many faculty members grumbled, particularly at the medical school, Ehrlich remained committed to the idea of a united university with "8 front doors" and rejected the faculty sentiment that "one part of the university was inferior and the other part was superior." Ehrlich worked closely with the state legislature to keep support for higher education, which meant close work with Daly and Bepko, as well as Beering now at Purdue. As Beering put it, although often rivals at the statehouse and on the athletic field, "in really important things we're collaborators and we're going to do everything together." Despite the united rhetoric, it confronted the reality of growing size and differences between the universities and placed departments, campuses, and programs in competition for a share of the static or at best slowly increasing support from the state.[29]

The competition within the university for scarce resources made Daly concerned about the new IU president, who had little experience with state-supported medical schools. Budgeting had always been complex, involving growing hospitals, research centers, and regional campuses, all of which had to go through the IU Board of Trustees, who were often unfamiliar with medical issues. On the other hand, the school was able to find new sources of external revenue from expansion of clinical and research income. This did not, however, directly benefit medical education, whose income was much more closely tied to state government support, which was growing at a much slower rate than expenses. One response was a sharp rise in tuition during the 1970s and 1980s. Although this had little impact on the overall budget, the repercussions were quite dramatic for students. Hence, the increased tuition continued to represent less than 6 percent of the school's total income compared to approximately 40 percent of the budget coming from state tax dollars in fiscal year 1984. Within ten years (FY 1993), however, these two sources together declined to less than a quarter of school income because of the growth in clinical and research funds. The overall result was that many departments received the majority of their income from external funding. From the perspective of the students, however, the increased cost of medical school education quite simply meant dramatically rising levels of student debt.[30]

More will be said in the next chapter about these financial matters, which reflected national trends seen at other medical schools, but one of Daly's most important legacies was the development of a fundraising infrastructure and an endowment to help support the recruitment and retention of faculty, capital improvements, and student scholarships. In an interview after retirement, Daly recalled that the idea for building the fund-raising infrastructure within the school came from Gene Tempel, an IUPUI and IU Foundation development officer. Daly was skeptical, and Tempel agreed to pay the cost of lending J. David Smith to the school for a year—a deal he could hardly refuse. As Daly remembered, "it worked beautifully."[31] At the beginning of Daly's term as dean, IUSM received less than $100,000 per year in foundation and charitable income. Ten years later in 1993, the school had increased this figure to $6 million. In addition, Daly and Smith launched the first ever capital campaign, with a goal to reach $130 million.

Based on longtime ties with Eli Lilly and Company, Daly persuaded its president to chair the efforts. It drew heavily on the legacy of achievements of the medical school, so as part of its work, the school, along with various departments and the John Shaw Billings History of Medicine Society, began to collect archival materials and publicize the school's history. The campaign took a look both backward and forward to the rich legacy of the physicians who built the institution, preserving this legacy and helping IU take a leading role in new fields of research. Within a decade, charitable gifts brought in almost as much funding as the income from tuition and fees. IUSM was successful in building a strong institutional profile, a necessity because the IU Foundation, IUPUI, the hospitals, research and medical education centers, and even individual faculty research projects began to actively compete for the dollars from grateful patients and corporate partners. IUSM Dean Daly invested in promoting the image of the medical school, and increasingly the medical center, through professional production of annual reports, newsletters, and media stories, thus reflecting the growing pressure to make the IUMC more competitive in the health-care marketplace.[32]

An example of the results obtained from the new fundraising efforts was the construction of the new Medical Research and Library Building in 1989. From its start, the IUSM had received generous support from private philanthropy that supplemented state funding for new facilities, but these had either been large single donor gifts (such as from Long and Coleman) or the Riley campaigns dedicated to the Children's Hospital. Fund-raising for the library and medical research building also included the need for more general infrastructure support, and it was the first focus of Daly's new strategy of greatly increasing fund-raising for the school. These efforts brought in more than $14 million of the $34 million construction cost. The members of the class of 1963 alone raised a $1.6 million endowment for acquisition of new materials, led by alumni William Moores, John Pless, and Robert Holden, future dean of IUSM and then director of radiology at Wishard Memorial Hospital.[33]

Despite the message in the glossy brochures and newsletters, there were some at the medical school with a growing sense of insecurity about these changes. In the administrative files, board and committee minutes, and physician writings, plus later oral histories, the faculty expressed concerns about pressures to increase clinical and research income as well as the growing complexity of working with the different hospitals and services. Many of the changes at IUSM reflected broader changes within the profession. Faculty felt that they were not in charge of their practice or medical care because of the growing influence of university officials, health maintenance organizations, lawyers, and hospital administrators. In response to this sentiment, the LCME increasingly looked to see evidence of faculty and student governance as a check on executive deans and health administrators who held an ever-growing role in decision making that limited the role of the IUSM faculty in planning.[34] Some students and faculty exercised their option of filing grievances against administrative actions, disciplinary measures, and tenure decisions, and although they found the complaints handled efficiently, the call for participation in making decisions on larger issues largely fell on deaf ears. This confirmed the observations by Hugh Headlee about the medical faculty failing to play an effective role in governance. The perception of limited power of the faculty committees outside the area of curriculum development led to low participation and confidence. In particular, women students and faculty felt that despite considerable attention officially paid to the issues of inequality by the school, there was a general reluctance to address the issues at the individual or departmental level.[35]

The latter concern was all the more important because in response to the insecurities and growing bureaucracy, the departments increasingly turned inward and began implementing their own administrative infrastructure. Daly was more aware of this than anyone, having served as chair of the Department of Medicine. He recalled that he resisted the rapid expansion of enrollment because he thought there were not enough resources or planning. He felt that it "would take a much, much larger faculty size and patient numbers to provide the proper educational experience for the huge increase in the number of medical students." Reflecting later on these changes, he still saw these advantages and disadvantages but conceded that it had "not been harmful to the educational program."[36]

Central to the new departmental model was the practice plan. Although this will be discussed in the next chapter as part of clinical operations, some of the main features of practice plans were their decentralization and lack of oversight, which left a great deal of freedom to the department chairs. An important effect was to hide the cumulative extent of clinical work, something Daly was quite aware of when he was chair of the Department of Medicine. He therefore shrewdly decided to take as a first step the requirement of departments to report practice plan income, both to provide an inventory and also to reflect more accurately the balance sheet of the school for purposes of LCME reporting. Accordingly, from FY 1988 to FY 1989 the category of practice plan and services in LCME reports jumped from $378,441 to $57,001,208. Because no other category of income reported for FY 1989 declined, it meant that almost $60 million in income of the school (about one-third of the total that year) had previously gone unreported.[37]

Regional Campuses

Notwithstanding such things as practice plans, relations with other hospitals, and the exploding growth of research, the most immediate task facing Steven Beering when he became dean in 1973 was implementing the statewide medical education plan. The IUSM system was a new form of distributed medical education—the first of its kind in the nation.[38] Implementing the plan was a daunting challenge because although politically popular and less expensive than creating a second medical school, the statewide medical education plan required establishing instruction at eight different locations with the promise that would meet the standards of what existed at the fully functioning and recently consolidated medical school in Indianapolis. Without a major increase in state funding, however, it took time to hire the faculty and establish the facilities to teach the full complement of two years of medical science courses at the new sites. The plan called for a gradual implementation, but as table 10.2 shows, no one foresaw that it would take ten years before the two-year medical school curriculum was being taught at all locations but one.

Departments were traditionally responsible for planning what was taught, with individual instructors afforded wide leeway in instruction. In the case of the statewide system, however, the departments had very little involvement in the initial planning or implementation. Daly, who later had to manage and defend the system, remembered knowing very little about the plans as a faculty member. He attended a faculty meeting—a somewhat rare experience, he recalled—and was presented with the plans for the statewide system. Then he was simply asked to vote aye. Although some specialties like medical genetics needed little equipment and shorter time in the curriculum, and hence the subject could be taught by visiting faculty from the Indianapolis campus, the laboratory courses, especially gross anatomy, were another matter. Moreover, the introduction of some clinical instruction during the second year took ten years to implement.[39]

The school was not without experience in teaching the initial years of medical school at a different place from the main medical school in Indianapolis. That had been the arrangement since the merger in 1907 that created the school, which allowed the first year of medical school to begin in Bloomington. As mentioned in chapter 8, by the 1950s this was seen as an impediment to expansion and integration of instruction, a problem solved by the construction of the Medical Sciences Building, which consolidated the four-year MD at Indianapolis in 1958.[40] The following year, a combined

Table 10.2. Implementation of the Indiana Statewide Medical Education System

Year Instruction Began	Center Location	Host Campus
1969 (First year added)	Bloomington	Indiana University
1970	Lafayette	Purdue
1970	South Bend	Notre Dame
1971	Muncie	Ball State
1971	Terre Haute	Indiana State
1972	Evansville	Univ. of Southern Indiana, Vincennes
1972	Gary	IU Northwest (in 1975)
1981	Ft. Wayne	Indiana-Purdue at Ft. Wayne
1980 (Second year added)	All but Ft. Wayne	
1990 (Second year added)	Ft. Wayne	Indiana-Purdue at Ft. Wayne

degree program was started in Bloomington with initial funding from the Commonwealth Fund, whereby the first two years of the medical sciences curriculum of the medical school were taught (anatomy and physiology, biochemistry, microbiology, pharmacology, pathology) followed by a third year of courses for a MS in certain science programs. When the statewide system began, this experience not only served as a model for the statewide program but also meant that for the Bloomington site, the statewide plan simply required an increase in the number of students enrolled in the first- and second-year courses.[41]

Table 10.3. Faculty at IUSM Regional Centers, 1977, 1987, and 1993

Center	Full-Time			Part-Time			Volunteer		
	1977	1987	1993	1977	1987	1993	1977	1987	1993
Bloomington	24		1 8			0			89
Evansville	6	8	7		7	3		69	101
Ft. Wayne		6	8		6	1		36	93
Northwest	9	17	21	2	5	233	6	66	105
Lafayette	0	1	1	22	20	34	35	25	0
Muncie	7	2	1 1	3	10	0	0	31	0
South Bend	4	6	7		6	4		34	62
Terre Haute	8	9	8	0	2	2	64	25	51
All of IUSM	555	730	902	27	101	80	105	1,228	1,968

*The large number of faculty at the Northwest Center was because it adopted an innovative, problem-based curriculum in 1990.
Sources: LCME Self-Study, 1994, annex XIII, p. 27, Box 233; LCME Self-Study, 1987, Box 233, UA 073, InUI-Ar.

Bloomington was obviously exceptional in the faculty available for medical instruction, but the resources varied greatly at the other locations. For example, because they were home to major research universities, Purdue (three students) and Notre Dame (two students) were allowed to do a pilot test in 1968 by offering existing classes in biochemistry, physiology, and the other medical sciences required for first-year medical students. Then in 1970, ten to twelve students were admitted at these sites, and two years later, a similar number was admitted at the other sites. Selection of faculty also varied considerably depending on local resources. The medical school paid for the time of some existing faculty at Purdue and Ball State, but new faculty had to be recruited and assigned by the medical school at the other sites. These differences continued as the second year of the curriculum was added in 1980, with some sites requiring extensive numbers of faculty who were part-time and volunteer (so called because many local practitioners offered services without compensation).[42] As table 10.3 shows, by 1993 there were eighty-one full-time, ten part-time, and 501 volunteer faculty at the eight sites.[43]

The faculty at the regional centers were in the fields of first-year instruction: biochemistry, microbiology, anatomy, histology, physiology, neurobiology, and introduction to clinical medicine. Even though, as table 10.4 shows, they taught half the undergraduate medical students, the disparity compared to faculty resources at Indianapolis was obvious from the total number of faculty, which in 1993 was ten times that number for all the other sites combined. As figure 10.1 shows, since the 1950s, the medical school had made great progress toward its goal of increasing full-time faculty, although as the next chapter will show, this was thanks to increases

Table 10.4. First- and Second-Year Medical Student Enrollment at IUSM, 1979, 1987, 1993

Center	1979	1987	1993
Bloomington	70	83	63
Evansville	20	30	32
Fort Wayne	—	16	48
Northwest	20	31	49
Lafayette	20	31	32
Muncie	20	32	32
South Bend	20	30	33
Terre Haute	20	30	32
Indianapolis	453	289	*280

*Estimate based on enrollment plan.
Sources: LCME, "Self-study Reports," 1979, 1987, 1993, UA 073, In-U-Ar.

in clinical and research support, not the legislature's increase in support for medical education.[44]

Once established, regional centers (except Bloomington) usually admitted classes of twenty after 1976, and the second year was added in 1980 (except for Ft. Wayne). Then for reasons explained later, entering classes were decreased to sixteen in 1983. Thereafter, the system remained stable, admitting roughly half the students (140) at the regional centers and an equal number at Indianapolis, with all 280 finishing their third and fourth years at Indianapolis.

The regional centers also hosted some junior clerkships, as well as senior electives that later were the basis of teaching full third- and fourth-year classes beginning in 2008 at the regional sites.[45]

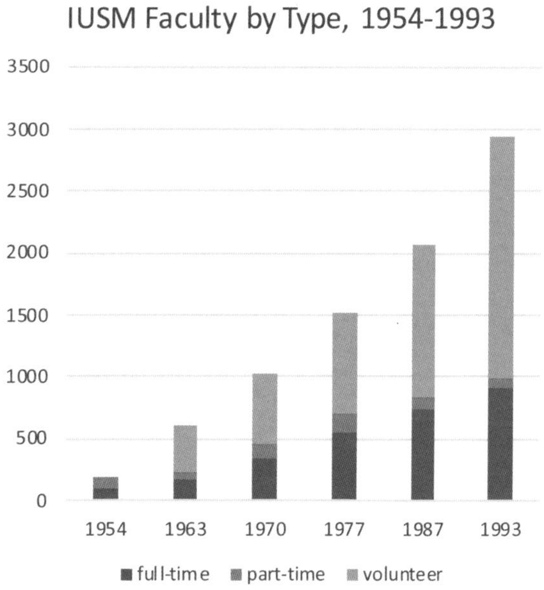

IUSM Faculty by Type, 1954-1993

Figure 10.1. Growth in IUSM Faculty, 1954–1993, LCME Self-Study, 1954–1994, UA 073, In-U-Ar.

The Nine Sites

As mentioned above, the Lafayette and South Bend sites began their programs first, thanks largely to the resources of the host Purdue and Notre Dame campuses. In the initial year at Lafayette, eleven of the twelve students had completed their undergraduate studies at Purdue, a pattern that continued. The number of students rose to sixteen, but the second year curriculum was added only in 1980.[46] The situation was similar in South Bend, the other initial pilot campus, although there were questions about the new program, according to the following quip attributed to Notre Dame President Theodore M. Hesburgh: "The question isn't what Indiana can do for Notre Dame, but what Notre Dame can do for Indiana." The South Bend entering class also reflected the demographics of the Notre Dame campus. IU officials commented, "The twelve I. U. students get Notre Dame football tickets at student prices, but the 11 men in the group find the dating situation almost impossible, even though Notre Dame is in the process of merging with St. Mary's College just across the highway."[47]

For the program sites located on smaller university campuses, the establishment of medical school instruction meant establishing relationships

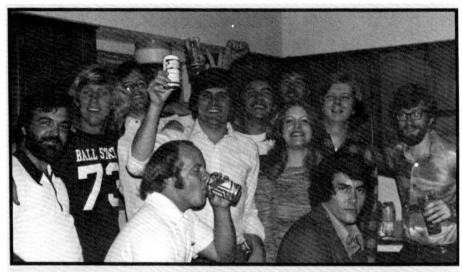

At Work

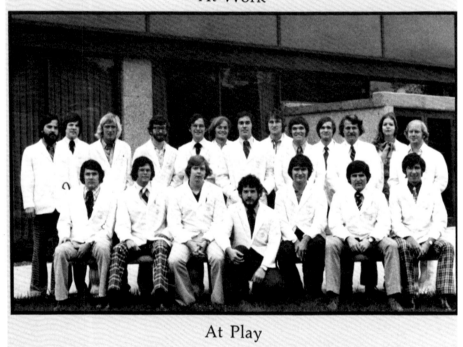

At Play

Figure 10.2. Evansville campus students, 1979, "At Work," "At Play," *Retrospectroscope* (1979): 19.

and finding resources that made the implementation process more gradual. The Evansville medical education center had small administrative offices and initially taught courses at the University of Southern Indiana (USI) and the University of Evansville. In 1994, the center moved to combined facilities at a newly constructed University of Southern Indiana Health Professions Center.[48] At Terre Haute, the medical courses were taught at the Indiana State University campus; at Muncie, the Ball State campus; and at Fort Wayne, the Indiana University-Purdue University Fort Wayne (IPFW) campus that was run by Purdue.[49]

In Gary, the medical education center was started from scratch in the daunting health-care landscape of the city, which at the time was facing the challenges of many rust belt municipalities during the industrial transition. In the area of medicine, there were critical physician shortages, and community leaders pushed for increased access to quality health care.[50] In 1972, the Gary Medical Education center opened in East Chicago with four students and five faculty members.[51] Three years later, the center relocated to the present campus of IU Northwest and was housed in trailers until new buildings were completed. Under the leadership of Panayotis Iatridis, the Gary center established an alternative curriculum in 1990, including Problem-Based Learning (PBL) and a didactic component called the Doctor/Patient Relationship.[52]

Bloomington was now viewed as the "oldest satellite program," as well as the largest in the system. As expected, those at the Bloomington medical education center saw themselves as having a different relationship with Indianapolis. Among the many obvious examples, the Bloomington campus had a much more developed research program than most other regional sites. Thus, IU-Bloomington established the Indiana Molecular Biology Institute in 1983, housed at Myers Hall, to create a campus-wide mechanism to foster research excellence in disciplines of the life sciences. Unfortunately, Myers Hall, originally constructed in the 1930s to house the anatomy program, was ill equipped to meet these growing research and teaching needs, but other priorities of the Bloomington campus delayed much-needed renovation until 2002.[53]

To first- and second-year medical students, Indianapolis was also technically a "regional" education center, albeit the largest of all. As a result, the students who completed their first two years at Indianapolis enjoyed the full complement of expertise in departments and subspecialties, as well as to the more mundane advantage that the campus had a paid note-taker system that made studying easier and classes occasionally unnecessary. The roughly 140 students per entering class in Indianapolis was a number close to the national average of US medical schools.[54]

From its start, the statewide system ran into numerous administrative problems. For example, faculty appointments and tenure, critical to the departments, were issues that proved continually difficult to solve. Initially at the Lafayette and Muncie centers, faculty from Purdue and Ball State were assigned on a part-time basis to instruct medical students, but when the second year of instruction began at Muncie, it was by IU medical school faculty and volunteer physicians in the local community.[55] From the perspective of Daly and the Department of Medicine, the problem with regional center faculty was not logistics but the challenges caused by the employment policies at the different universities that varied in terms of research resources and tenure policies.[56]

The numerous facilities for instruction were housed in buildings on the campuses that varied a great deal and required separate negotiations in order to keep facilities up-to-date.[57] The system required provision of comparable locker rooms, library access, committee meeting participation, computer access, and support services. To help counteract the isolation of the centers, the medical school provided a monthly newsletter as well as frequent "tele-meetings."[58]

At each accreditation by the LCME, the medical school took great pains to explain to the skeptical visitors how the regional centers, different even from each other, produced educational results similar to the Indianapolis campus. While admitting the obvious differences in research, clinical, and extra-curricular opportunities, the school relied on statewide curriculum committee work to ensure standards were met at all centers. In the beginning, this was measured in curriculum, facilities, overall grades, and national exam scores of the students attending the regional campuses, which were only slightly lower than the overall average. Increasingly, the medical school pointed to student performance on the Step I USMLE examinations taken in June of the second year as an indicator of the quality of teaching. By the time of the self-study for the 1993 reaccreditation, the school claimed that based on the exam results for the years 1991–93, there were "no statistically discernible difference from center to center."[59]

The LCME accreditation teams usually visited every site in the statewide system and interviewed both faculty and students. The findings and comments from these periodic assessments (1971, 1977, 1987, and 1994) have left a detailed record of the program viewed by knowledgeable, independent observers.[60] They describe the mechanics of a school hiring and securing teaching facilities but also persuading students and faculty to buy into the system. When students applied, they were able to express a campus preference for the first two years of instruction.[61] Admission officers then selected those to attend the regional centers based on a number of factors including early admission, demographic diversity, and performance, as well as preference. Not surprisingly, Indianapolis was the top choice of most because it was seen as the "main" campus, despite the marketing materials that described it as the "hub." As late as 1987, nearly 70 percent of students ranked Indianapolis as their top choice of sites for their first two years of instruction.[62]

As described in more detail below, once there, student responses to the instruction at the regional campuses were mixed. One benefit at the centers was the ease with which students formed close friendships with their fellow classmates. Evansville students recalled that "Because of the size of the class (16), we had no choice but to become a close-knit group."[63] On the other hand, many students' initial reactions expressed dismay at such placements. As late as 1991, members of the graduating class questioned, "Why was I stuck up here?" when speaking about their placement at Fort Wayne or Muncie. Some students who regretted missing opportunities only available at Indianapolis found the small class sizes made up for the lack of amenities.[64]

Part of the rationale for the statewide system was the need to develop more residency opportunities outside Indianapolis, where most had long been concentrated. The regional plan therefore charged centers to develop local clinical practice resources.

As table 10.5 indicates, all sites were able to find cooperating hospitals, but this did not necessarily result in more residencies. One exception was at Evansville, where by 1978, there were thirty-two interns thanks to the second director, Ray Newman, who worked with local physicians to expand the ranks of volunteer clinical faculty for undergraduate education.[65] Another goal of the statewide plan was to increase primary care specialization, and IUSM's longitudinal studies found an increase in total primary care specialization by the IUSM students, and more significantly on the

Table 10.5. IUSM Cooperating Hospital Programs, 1987

Location	Hospital
Evansville	Deaconess Hospital
	Saint Mary's Hospital
Ft. Wayne	Lutheran Hospital
	Parkview Memorial Hospital
Gary	Methodist Hospital
	St. Mary's Hospital
Hammond	Saint Margaret Hospital
Indianapolis	Community Hospital
	Methodist Hospital
	St. Francis Hospital
Lafayette	Home Hospital
	St. Elizabeth Hospital
Muncie	Ball Memorial Hospital
South Bend	Memorial Hospital
	St. Joseph Hospital
	South Bend Medical Foundation
	South Bend Osteopathic Hospital
Terre Haute	Terre Haute Regional Hospital
	Union Hospital

Source: LCME Self-Study, 1987, Box 233, UA 073, InUi-Ar.

regional campuses. In addition, the study found that during the time that the regional campus system was being established, there was an increase in primary care practice outside Indianapolis. This was encouraging because eight of the nine campuses were located in areas that qualified as being medically underserved, but the claim of a possible cause and effect relationship was difficult to substantiate.[66]

Enrollments and the Statewide System

The eyes of the Indiana statehouse and others from across the country were focused on the Indiana statewide medical education experiment to see whether it would be a viable solution to the issues of cost, physician shortage, brain drain, and coordination with regional hospitals. IUSM was one of the first to adopt the regional campus model; at most, only a few other medical schools used regional campuses in the 1970s and 1980s, and primarily for clinical experiences. Then, quite unexpectedly and soon after Indiana committed to this dramatic plan for increasing the training of physicians, the national call for growth of medical school admissions abruptly stopped. In 1976, after federal funding for medical education had tripled from the levels just a decade before, the federal government pronounced the end of the physician shortage and shifted its focus to primary care training, community-based clinical education, hospital reform, and containing rising health-care costs.[67]

Within the medical profession, these shifts created alarm but little disagreement. In 1981, the Graduate Medical Education National Advisory Committee (GMENAC), the Bureau of Health Professions, and the Council on Graduate Medical Education (CGME) predicted that the past decade of growth in the number of medical schools and class sizes would lead to massive physician surpluses. As a result, health planning shifted toward such goals as increasing the number of students going into primary care and meeting needs in underserved areas.[68] This move away from growth was dubbed by one observer as a form of "academic birth control," which was reflected in medical school admissions stagnating during the 1980s and 1990s. Nationally, the number of medical school applicants peaked in 1974–75 and

Table 10.6. Applicants from residents of Indiana to the IU School of Medicine, selected years, 1974–93

Academic Year	Number
1974–75	822
1976–77	743
1980–81	554
1984–85	650
1988–89	407
1992–93	587

Source: Indiana Commission on Higher Education, "Progress Report on State Policy Recommendations on Medical Education," May 4, 1994, UA 073, In-U-Ar, cataloging in progress.

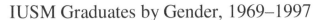

IUSM Graduates by Gender, 1969–1997

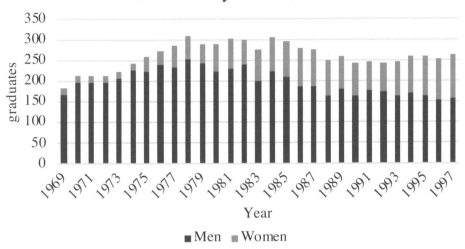

Figure 10.3. Total IUSM Admissions by Gender, 1969–1997, IUSM Annual Reports.

then declined 15 percent over the next decade. The top schools saw growing competition for the best applicants thanks to declining numbers of college graduates, increasing medical school costs, and limited financial aid options for graduate education. On the positive side, there was some evidence that the efforts to encourage the training of primary care physicians paid off, as reflected in the proportion of US medical graduates matching into primary care residency programs—internal medicine, family medicine, and pediatrics—which grew through the 1980s and 1990s, although falling sharply after 1998. There was much less success in channeling graduates into underserved rural and inner-city areas, which continued to see shortages of primary care physicians.[69]

Application patterns at IUSM largely followed these broader national trends, although initially thanks to the implementation of regional campuses, enrollments bucked the changing national pattern. After a peak of over 1,800 in 1976, the annual applications to the IU School of Medicine dramatically decreased by one-third to about 1,300 just two years later. As table 10.6 shows, the decline of applications from Indiana residents, the most likely to matriculate, was even more precipitous.

Despite Indiana government leaders continuing to talk about the "physician shortage," even as national sources predicted a "glut" of physicians, the IUSM followed the rest of the country in seeing a decline in enrollments, as shown in figure 10.3.[70]

Prior to the implementation of the Indiana Plan, admissions hovered around 225. After the plan, that number increased to a peak figure of 305 students in 1979, but this figure was difficult to sustain when applications declined. By the end of the 1980s, admissions stabilized near 265, higher than the level prior to the regional campus system but below the ambitious goals set at the beginning of the plan. During the 1990s, the number began slowly climbing, but graduates did not reach 300 again until 2008.[71] In a report given to the Central Association of Advisors for the Health Professions in 1979, George Lukemeyer concluded that the trends at IUSM mirrored the national patterns. Among the large number of factors, he pointed particularly to declining birth rates and availability of minority applicants, as well as the end of the "doctor draft"—that is, students applying to medical school to avoid or delay military service during the Vietnam War.[72] At IUSM and nationally, many applicants listed financial aid as a top consideration in deciding on medical school, and on a broader level, business and technical schools, as well as alternative careers in the sciences, attracted many potential applicants. Despite the decline in the number of applicants, however, Lukemeyer noted that the science GPA and MCAT scores of students admitted to IUSM actually improved during the period.

In 1991, there was a serious attempt at consolidation of the statewide system for a number of reasons. In addition to the fifteen-year decline in applications and campus competition, the more immediate precipitating events were state budget tensions and an increased operational deficit at the medical school. Moreover, new IU president Ehrlich had little personal investment in the regional centers system. When budget challenges combined with a desire to reprogram Myers Hall at Bloomington into a center of molecular biology, Ehrlich began discussions with Dean Daly over ways to close the budget shortfall. After limited informal discussion, Ehrlich proposed the closure of some medical centers and made this public without plans or details. The number of students had already been reduced due to budget and application reductions. Following this announcement, Daly was charged to find a way to balance the IUSM budget through the modification of the regional campus system.[74]

More than just a budget issue, the proposed changes, Daly feared, could reopen the old debate over of the creation of a second medical school. He later recalled that although he had been critical of the regional system in the past, in regard to making such changes, he "knew the misery it would cause me so I was highly ambivalent about it." The deliberation about plans for potential changes in the medical education system was done in public, with Daly crisscrossing the state to gather data and opinions on the system. After this study, Daly reported bluntly that in order to preserve the quality of the existing education programs, the state would need to cut some centers or provide additional funding to the medical school to continue all the centers.[75]

Similar to what happened in 1967, when a second medical school was proposed, the Indiana General Assembly commissioned a report, this time charging the Indiana Commission on Higher Education to investigate the status of medical education including the broader impact of the statewide system on the entire state. The final report, "The Future of IU System of Statewide Medical Education," laid out the arguments for and against the closures. Among reasons cited were student preference for the Indianapolis program ("normally oversubscribed" by students' choice of site for first two years) and AAMC exit surveys of students who studied at the regional sites which indicated "reports of weaknesses outnumber the strengths from 3:1 to 4:1 depending on the year of graduation." Student exit surveys also cited variation in course content and isolation "from the main stream of medical education and a sense of being second-class citizens." The medical school also claimed there was higher cost per student at regional centers: $38,033 average (as high as $47,729 at Terre Haute) versus $26,168 at Indianapolis.[76]

Strengths of the existing system mentioned in student survey included more personal attention because of small class size and good faculty/student ratio. In addition, a different method of accounting by the Higher Education Commission disagreed about the lower cost of educating students at Indianapolis. On the question about possible uneven quality of instruction raised during accreditation, supporters of the system argued that students from all the centers did equally well on exams and in clinical work, national exams, and fellowships. Likewise, in response to fear that the system had not significantly addressed the need for primary care physicians, especially in rural areas—because of the concentration of physicians in Indianapolis which was increasing—the medical education centers continued to be proposed by local communities as a promising way to attract and retain physicians, encourage high standards of practice, boost the local economy, and increase civic pride.[77] In the end, the legislature not only rejected the proposed changes in the statewide system but also covered the 1992–93 projected medical school budget shortfall of $2.5 million and added a further $1 million to enhance primary care education at sites across the state. The host cities were called on to seek local financial support for the centers and engage other statewide and national partners.[78]

This 1991–92 skirmish was the first and last major challenge to the statewide system. Since then, the medical school has defended the regional system in response to questions raised during the periodic accreditation visits. The results were more hopeful than conclusive. As will be seen in the next section, success in increasing the total number of graduates was uneven in the first twenty-five years, and despite the record of Step I scores, there was much duplication and inefficiency, as well as dependence on part-time and voluntary instruction. On the other hand, most local universities and communities heeded the call of the legislature in 1992 to raise funds to develop the centers further and integrate them into broader health science facilities. This local economic and political support was the most important reason for the defeat of the proposal to change the statewide system in 1991–92.

Training New Students in the Health Professions

While the IU medical school grappled with the challenge of providing medical education to the four-year medical school students across the state, the larger medical center on the IUPUI campus offered training in an expanding number of allied health fields. In 1975, IUSM faculty enrolled 8,169 students in degree programs, only 1,230 of whom were in MD training in 1977, as well as 2,758 students being taught through continuing medical education.[79] In the Division of Allied Health, there were 665 students including those in dietetics, occupational and physical therapy, and twelve other technical programs such as radiography. Dental student enrollment in 1975 was 789, although that number declined to just over three hundred in the 1980s and then rose gradually over the next decades. The IU School of Nursing, which had been established as an independent school in 1965, had over 1,500 nursing students. Despite the size, Nursing struggled to meet the diverse challenges in the expanding health-care field. In response to nursing becoming more specialized and requiring more educators, the school developed a Doctor of Nursing Science (DNS) degree, which was approved in 1976. Likewise, in response to the need for nursing graduates to fill rapidly expanding entry-level positions, the school developed distance education courses that were first offered in 1985 to meet needs on regional campuses. Another kind of training was taken by 130 students in either MS or MD/PhD programs in 1975, with that number climbing to 287 by 1995 in ten programs. Although Bloomington had collaborated in the MD/PhD program since 1959, there was now another opportunity in conjunction with the West Lafayette campus of Purdue, which offered combined degrees in medicinal chemistry, molecular biology, engineering, and neuroscience.[80]

The central focus of instruction by the medical school remained the preparation of physicians, and a great concern was to find ways to prepare students for clinical care. Some of this will be examined in the next chapter on research and practice, but as a result of expanding medical science teaching at the regional centers, the statewide plan also required additional clinical instruction for third- and fourth-year undergraduates, and graduate medical education. Into the 1990s, the majority of clinical instruction was still done on the inpatient ward services of hospitals. In addition, the state budget increases for the regional centers in the early 1990s explicitly targeted the need for primary care, particularly family medicine. As a result, a primary care initiative task force was established in 1994 to develop new approaches to primary care education, including a new family medicine clerkship, with time spent not only in the hospital but also in a family practitioner's office delivering care. Earlier in 1991, the Division of Internal Medicine added a one-month ambulatory care block within its three-month clerkships done in one of the primary care clinics within the IUMC and community outreach clinic—with two-thirds of medical students actually receiving this training. In addition, one of two months of pediatrics clerkship was spent in outpatient clinics. These initiatives soon paid off. By 1993, 59 percent of graduates chose primary care as specialty area, compared to 43 percent the year before. With the new family medicine clerkship, the percentage of students entering Family Medicine internships increased from 10 percent in 1992 to 22 percent in 1993. Despite the increases, Indiana still ranked only in the middle nationally of graduates choosing primary care fields, and longer term, these gains proved temporary.[81]

Table 10.7 All Interns and Residents in Indiana, 1967–1982

		All Interns and Residents in Indiana					
Year	Total	Indpls IUSM	%	Other Indpls	%	Other IN	%
1967	428	302	70.6	86	20.1	40	9.3
1971	609	416	68.3	111	18.2	82	13.5
1972	646	447	69.2	132	20.4	67	10.4
1973	697	454	65.1	145	20.8	98	14.1
1974	714	444	62.2	163	22.8	107	15.0
1975	732	455	62.2	177	24.2	100	13.7
1976	794	454	57.2	199	25.1	141	17.8
1977	862	485	56.3	219	25.4	158	18.3
1978	897	481	53.6	239	26.6	177	19.7
1979	927	510	55.0	236	25.5	181	19.5
1980	933	512	54.9	238	25.5	183	19.6
1981	953	520	54.6	250	26.2	183	19.2
1982	990	529	53.4	267	27.0	194	19.6

Source: Beering to James Scofield, Secretary, LCME, "5 Year Progress Report," January 3, 1983.

Another main goal of the regional campus expansion was to increase the number of physicians who practiced in the state, particularly outside of Indianapolis. As the last chapter showed, location of practice in Indiana was closely associated with place of residency, and Van Nuys worked hard to increase the number of first-year intern position in Indiana to one hundred by the early 1960s. The 1979 LCME reaccreditation self-study claimed that the number of graduating medical students who stayed in Indiana for residency increased each year after implementation of the statewide plan in 1971, and as table 10.7 shows, the total number of residencies grew significantly in the 1970s, albeit thanks as well to the expansion of funding from Medicaid reimbursement.[82]

The total number of residencies grew more than 50 percent in Indiana from 1971 to 1982, and the number of positions outside Indianapolis more than doubled. The increase slowed considerably, however, after the mid-1970s, and more significant, the vast majority of residents (over 80 percent) were still in Indianapolis. This trend continued in the 1980s, but the LCME reaccreditation for 1987 concluded that there was no need for any "immediate or dramatic change" in graduate medical education. Meanwhile, the state legislature added to the problem with its 1993 education plan, which recommended increasing admissions to the school without a clear mechanism for directing students into practice outside Indianapolis, such as creating the residencies needed for this physician training.[83]

These problems in the IUSM residency training were similar to the national trends in graduate medical education.[84] Periodic self-studies and reviews from the AAMC Graduate Medical Education Activity Report and National Resident Matching Program showed that IUSM graduates were typical in terms of placement, with no differences based on regional centers. Continuing the trend noted in the previous chapter, approximately half of graduates took Indiana positions (51 percent in 1990).[85]

Changes in the specialties of health care were one new development, but the nature of students in the MD program at the IUSM changed more dramatically in the last decades of the twentieth century than any time in the school's history. Although the size of the new entering class of students had grown through the 1960s, this had been very gradual. In contrast, the increase in female students after 1970, and to a lesser extent, the increase in minority students, was much more precipitous. There was also, for the first time, a significant fluctuation in the number of students as fears of a national oversupply of physicians conflicted with political demands in Indiana to increase students, all in the context of implementing the statewide plan. The only constant was the very high percentage of students admitted from in-state, which remained with few exceptions well above 90 percent each year.[86]

The resulting impact on students' experience was in part the result of long-term national changes in medical education over the course of the twentieth century. For example, with increasing specialization, students focused more on graduate medical training. Other new developments affecting students included the increased costs and need for financial aid, as well as the increase in the number of women and minorities admitted to medical school that literally changed the face of the profession. Medical schools strengthened polices limiting moonlighting, which increased because of the rise in tuition. The need for longer internships and residencies because of growing specialization also extended the period that students incurred debt. Student financial difficulties were not new, nor was the struggle to keep up with the vast amount of knowledge by an intense commitment of time to learn the information.[87]

Women in the Medical School

A dramatic new development for medical students was the growing number of female students admitted to the IUSM beginning in the 1970s. As mentioned earlier, there was a significant decline in applications to the medical school during implementation of the statewide plan, but it would have been more precipitous had it not been for the increase in women applying and being accepted. As figure 10.3 shows, during the 1970s the initial growth of the overall class size was accompanied by an increase in the number and percentage of women students. In fact, the proportion of female admissions and graduates at IUSM grew steadily through the 1970s and continued when enrollments declined in the 1980s. The IUSM increase was from 19.1 percent female admissions in 1974 to 35 percent a decade later, and it reached a high of 41 percent in 1993.

There were several reasons for the rise in female medical school admissions, most importantly the combination of the longer-term increase in the numbers of available medical school positions, coupled with the decline in male applicants and the rise in the number of women receiving undergraduate bachelor degrees. Although the Flexner Report reduced the total number of medical schools, and along with that the opportunities for women in the early twentieth century, the growth of medical schools in the 1960s resulted in an increase in the overall number of medical school admissions, with many of the new positions going to women.[88] Lukemeyer's analysis of the applications from 1972 to 1990 shows that female applicant GPA and MCAT scores did not vary greatly from the school average, however minority applicants were more likely to be from outside of Indiana and have lower GPA and MCAT scores.[89]

In some ways, the changes in the number of women presented an even bigger challenge than the statewide system in the functioning of the medical school. Women had attended IUSM in small numbers from its beginning, but they never threatened the gendered nature of the medical school.[90] The increase in female medical students in the 1970s therefore added to the breakdown of earlier social cohesion in medical training. The cultural power of physicians was under attack, and many male physicians resisted the changes. Admission to medical school was essential, but women's integration into academic medicine was slow as they struggled to see many issues addressed, from finding role models to participating in leadership decisions. This delay had consequences for the education of female physicians in future generations. For example, women in leadership positions at IUSM had to be recruited from other universities rather than their coming up through the ranks, as was the case with male leaders.[91]

Student yearbooks from the 1970s through the 1990s provide a window into other consequences of these changes for medical students: the sometimes hypersexualized and ribald atmosphere of gender relations that accompanied the increased number of women at the medical school. Prior to the 1960s, there was only one annual student yearbook, *The Arbutus*, for all of Indiana University. Then the medical school graduating class began producing its own yearbook each year—beginning with a seventy-page publication in the form of a patient's medical history that was labeled "Medical Class of [year of graduation]," followed in 1969 by the *Retrospectroscope* and then the *Caduceus*—which reflected the independence of the medical campus while helping to foster class identity. Until it was replaced by an administration-authored annual report in the 1990s, these student publications provided an opportunity for surprisingly honest and frank, if conflicting, views of medical school life from the students' perspective. Some of the pictures and cartoons were quite telling, such as an illustration of the overreliance on new drugs like thorazine at Larue Carter Mental Hospital, or the dragons to be slayed in the first years as opposed to clinical years of medical school (see figure 10.4).[92]

Much of the humor in the volumes of the late 1960s and 1970s was sophomorically sexual and sexist, as found in other male-dominated bastions such as fraternities, the army, construction sites, and locker rooms. The written columns provided more details and nuance about these experiences of some of the few females as well as the response of male students

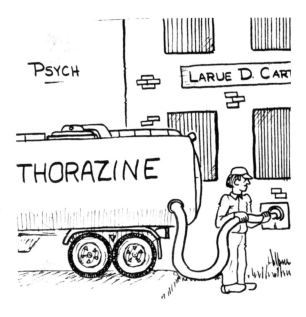

Figure 10.4a & b. Cartoons in medical student yearbooks: Thorazine at Larue Carter Hospital, IUSM Class of 1973 Yearbook; and anonymous "Cosmo" cartoon on first two years versus junior rotations in medical school, *Caduceus* (1981).

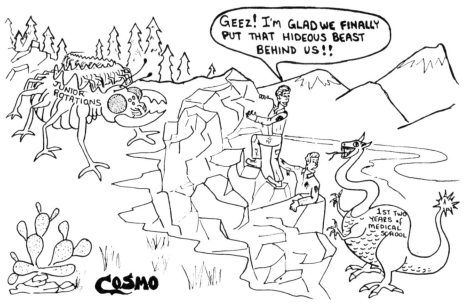

during this time of rapid demographic change in the student body. The following exchange in the 1979 *Retrospectroscope* volume to and from the so-called advice columnist "Ann Slanders" (a play on nationally syndicated columnist Ann Landers) illustrates some of the reaction to the growing number of female medical students.

Dear Ann Slanders, I am a medical student who has the terrible misfortune of being in a minority group in my class. I am a female. Now most people would assume that this is an enviable position since the ratio is in my favor, but let me tell you what it is really like. Imagine the cold stiff dismembered hand of a cadaver slinking up your thigh as you are industriously dissecting [an] eyeball. Or picture yourself being blamed by your resident for the spontaneous erection your comatose patient has during morning rounds. Or what do you say when your Psych resident is more interested in his student's than in his patient's sexual history? Or your surgery staff who feels that your grade is better correlated with your ability to flirt and bake cakes than with your suturing skills? Ann, how can I respond to these sexist pigs? Signed . . . Used and Abused in Indianapolis.[93]

Ann Slanders responded, "Dear Used: The only women who attract pigs are the ones who cry, 'Sooeee!' Read on as the pigs respond. (Oink, Oink)." The second letter read,

Dear Ann Slanders, I am a serious hard-working dedicated medical student with a problem—female medical students. I am sick and tired of spending 18 hours each day in the hospital providing superior care for my patients and barely getting a passing grade, while my female colleague spends one night 'on call' so to speak with the resident and receives 'honors.' I considered imitating my competition's strategy, but let's face it—I would look ridiculous in a short skirt and a tight white coat. Besides, Home Ec was not one of my Pre-Med courses and I had the embarrassing experience of having the one cake I baked refused by even the patients at the V. A. Hospital. The only one who gave me 'Honors' in a course was my Psych resident—and he was gay! How does one survive this reverse discrimination? Signed . . . Dedicated and Disgruntled.[94]

Ann Slander's response: "Dear Dedicated: Won't you also be a resident some day? Then maybe some disadvantages will become advantages."[95]

The IUSM Dean's Office was aware of some of these problems, and as early as 1972, it created an Affirmative Action Standing Committee as well as the position of associate dean for Student Affairs to help meet new accreditation requirements, national minority admissions, hiring targets, and Title IX of the Education Amendments.[96] IUSM appointed top faculty to the task force, although it did not escape notice that the majority were white men. The committee adopted a goal of slow, gradual increase to meet hiring and admissions needs over a decade (the ultimate target was 25 percent female admissions) and integrating diversity initiatives within the various departments, offices, and committees on campus. The number of female student admissions exceeded the 10 percent initial target each year after the new policy began in 1975, and because this coincided with the period of growth in admissions overall, it meant that admissions of men also grew. The 25 percent goal was reached the following decade, and in the 1990s, a third of the entering class was female. Some problems lingered; for example, treatment of women as well as mentorship opportunities varied widely. Hugh Hendrie, chair of the Affirmative Action Task Force, had a strong reputation of developing female leadership in the Psychiatry Department and was committed to making similar changes across the school. Other problems were more superficial. Although women began to appear in IUSM publications, they were most often featured in the library or classroom, making it unclear to outside observers whether women were in the physician program or in one of the allied health programs.[97]

Recruiting female faculty was another Affirmative Action goal of the medical school. Historically, women were presumed to be more likely to go into primary care or rural care and to stay in Indiana. This became less true as the number of female graduates increased. The Affirmative Action committee had greater difficulty increasing female hiring above the 25 percent goal for many years, falling consistently below the national average. For example, in the 1974–75 school year, although sixteen of the sixty-one new full-time hires were females, including two black women, a number of these were only part-time appointments. Part of the reason for this illusion of success, according to some critics, was the high turnover rate among female faculty. Some grumbled that this was proof that women were not meant to be physicians, as opposed to highlighting the immense systemic and cultural barriers facing women. The recruiting of women faculty was also influenced by the overall challenges of recruitment. The Affirmative Action Committee concluded that to meet its goal, the university needed to review and upgrade faculty salaries for both men and women, because both were in the lowest quartile in faculty compensation nationally. With such low pay, it was difficult to recruit top female and minority talent away from the urban centers on the East and West Coasts.[98]

Without a change, it would be difficult to create more diverse faculty role models. Women continued to be more prevalent in "female" areas of obstetrics and gynecology, pediatrics, and family medicine. An exception was Elizabeth Buchanan Solow, a professor of neurosurgery from 1962 to 1985 who worked through the various programs and committees to support students. At her retirement, she and her husband established a scholarship fund to help support medical students.[99] There were slow gains in adding female faculty, but by the 1990s, the medical school had only a limited record of placing women in key leadership positions. Noteworthy was Deborah Allen's appointment as chair of Family Medicine in 1989, the first female

Table 10.8. Enrollment of Blacks and Women at IUSM, 1970–1975

Year	All Yr 1 Students	Black Yr 1 Students		Blacks as % of Entering Class	Yr 1 Female Students	Females as % of Yr 1 Students
		Female	Male			
1970–71	250	5	0	2.0	26	10.4
1971–72	273	6	4	3.7	39	14.3
1972–73	290	10	2	4.2	39	13.4
1973–74	305	10	5	4.9	52	17.0
1974–75	305	10	3	4.3	62	20.3

Source: Jay M. Smith to Steven C. Beering, "Updated Statistics [to Report and Profile on the Academic Status of Minority Students]," May 7, 1975, Lukemeyer Papers, in process, UA 073, InUI-Ar.

chair in the school's history. Another exception was Doris Merritt, who, as mentioned in an earlier chapter, directed research for the medical school in the 1960s. In addition, Suzanne Knoebel was assistant dean for research in the 1970s and 1980s. She was a cardiologist who joined the faculty in the 1960s and was appointed associate director of the Krannert Institute in 1974. Among her honors was serving as the first female president of the American College of Cardiology.[100]

Women were not the only new group of medical students whose growing numbers faced challenges in the medical school. Nationally, the percentage of African Americans in the first-year classes of US medical schools rose from 2.7 percent in 1968–69 to 7.1 percent in 1971–72 but leveled off the next ten years (it was 6.6 percent in 1982–83).[101] As table 10.8 shows, the IUSM lagged behind the national trend, so in addition to other problems faced by the minority medical students, there was also the issue of pushing for higher black enrollments. The medical school established an Office for Minority Student Affairs in 1970, and a 1975 report described trends in enrollment of African Americans.

Although the very low numbers of black students increased as enrollments grew at the medical school, they quickly leveled off, unlike enrollment of female students, which continued to rise. In 1984, James Carter, the associate dean for Student and Curricular Affairs, wrote to IUSM Dean Daly indicating the situation had not improved. "It is my opinion that there is a problem and issue regarding the number of minority students in medical school. A 3 percent enrollment of black students in medical school today is a problem. Having a larger number of black physicians would be one factor that could help resolve some of the health care problems in the black community." This situation continued as late as a 1994 report by the

Indiana Commission for Higher Education, which indicated that from 1990 to 1994, the number of first-year black matriculants to the IUSM ranged between 9 and 11 students out of entering classes that rose from 265 to 280 (approximately 3.5%).[102]

An example of how the medical school was viewed can be found in an editorial of the black newspaper, the *Indianapolis Recorder*, the week following a January 30, 1977, feature article on allied health professions in the *Indianapolis Star Magazine*. Titled "The Gang behind Your Healthcare," the cover of the magazine article pictured fifteen representatives of the allied health fields taught at the medical school including medical technology, dietetics, cytotechnology, respiratory therapy, and radiologic technology. Although ten of those pictured were women, the op-ed writer pointedly noted,

> There isn't an Afro-American pictured anywhere. I proceeded to read through the article hoping to see or recognize at least one Afro-American, but to no avail . . . To me it is just another indication of the apartheid medical system Afro-Americans face here in Indianapolis . . . I think about all those Afro-Americans who are nurses, aides, environmental service engineers, but when it comes to showing who helps in health care, they are completely left out . . . They don't even train Afro-Americans to assume some of those roles pictured—at least not to my knowledge. Of course, what could one expect from I. U. Medical School?[103]

In the 1970s, IUPUI Chancellor Hine had met with African American students who voiced similar concerns, but the same issues still faced IUSM in the 1980s. As late as 1990–91 to 1994–95, there were between nine and eleven black first-year medical students out of a total that grew from 265 to 280 (approximately 3.6 percent).[104]

In Their Own Words: The Life of the Medical Students

It is one thing to describe statistically the demographic change in the students at IUSM, and it is another to understand the motivations, beliefs, and values of this new generation of medical students. Fortunately, there are some records by the medical students themselves during this period that show how these dramatic changes in the organization and delivery of instruction were viewed. An example of this was given earlier of reactions to the change in gender balance. These same sources—student yearbooks and other writings—also describe many other features of medical school students' experience, addressed to their peers. For example, despite the tremendous change in the broader practice of medicine, students' view

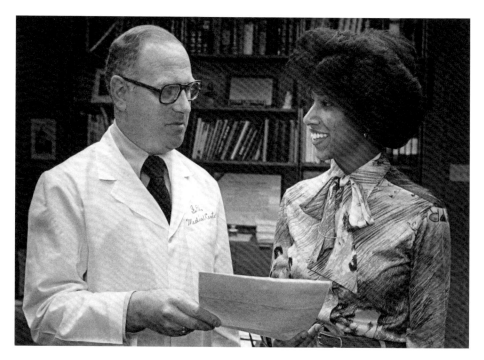

Figure 10.5. Alicia Monroe receiving the 1976 McLean Award from Steven Beering (IUSM deam, 1975–83) for the top graduating medical student from an underrepresented minority. After graduating from IUSM and doing a residency at Methodist Hospital, Monroe left and eventually became provost of Baylor College of Medicine. IUPUI image UA024_002166.

of the freshman year was similar to those from earlier generations. They struggled to manage the shock at the tremendous amount of information thrown at them, with the inevitable result of information overload, stress, and a struggle to cope. One student in the 1985 graduating class spoke for many in the following recollection.

> Freshman year began August 17, 1981 and the reality of Medical School hit fast. Class Notes were a saving grace to those at the Indy campus, but within two weeks we had a Biochem test and wondered how we got so far behind so quickly. . . . It was hard to believe, but in less than three months we learned multiple biochemical pathways and almost every bacterial, fungal and parasitic pathogen known to man . . . Dr. O'Connor introduced us to our cadavers (a tense moment for all medical students). . . . In just over one short year we were ready to learn MEDICINE.[105]

Stress and studying were constant themes during the freshman year throughout this period, as they had been during freshman year throughout the twentieth century. In recognition of the pressures facing medical students, especially freshmen, during the 1981–82 academic year, the school ran a program intended to address three key areas of student stress: starting medical school, mastering immense quantities of information, and adjusting personal and social lives to the rigors of medical school.[106]

Sophomore year quickly followed the welcome summer break. After surviving the challenge of the first year, sophomore students were disappointed to see more of the same, except for the first experiences with actual patients. This was a notable difference from students earlier in the twentieth century, who did not have direct patient experience until their junior or senior year. Because IUSM introduced some practical experience earlier in the curriculum, a 1994 graduate wrote that the sophomore year was "exciting as we donned the new white coats and went off to the hospital to learn how to use all the expensive equipment we now owned. We were seeing real live patients, learning real medicine, and taking a step closer to being real doctors. Nevertheless, we were put back in place each week by tests that remotely resembled what was talked about in class."[107]

After the pressure of the basic science years, students looked forward to the latter years of medical school when they had much greater opportunity for actual patient and clinical experience. That said, they quickly discovered the stress of assisting on clinical wards or rotations, which was just as taxing as the intense classroom learning of their first two years. A member of the graduating class of 1985 wrote, "Finally, after nineteen years of classrooms, lectures and tests, Junior year rescued us from those regurgitated phases and we were allowed on THE WARDS."[108]

Medical students recalled, "Without a doubt, the greatest transition from being a 'student' to becoming a 'doctor' occurred during the Junior year. And the transition was abrupt and sometimes cruel. Students discovered that they suddenly were not required to spend endless hours in a lecture room but were instead required to spend endless hours as a functioning member of a medical team. The vast amount of knowledge learned in two grueling years of basic sciences suddenly wasn't nearly as important as learning to start an I.V."[109]

Then came the blessed relief of senior year—choosing your own electives and schedule, having some vacation time, and knowing the end was in sight. But it also meant just as much stress from applying for internships and residencies. One representative of the graduating class of 1985 saw senior year as heaven. "We could actually think for ourselves, plan our schedules, and get out of Indiana if we chose to. India, Pakistan, Kenya, England, Ireland, Alaska, and Haiti were training and mission fields for our class. The decisions of specialty, residency, and the match loomed before us, with the added uncertainties of physician-surplus, HMO's, and decreasing numbers of residency spots; but, oh the freedom of senior year!"[110] Along with that freedom, senior year also brought additional obligations: "Responsibility increased as the senior was considered a 'Sub-Intern'; which means someone was always watching and hopefully protecting you. Now, you were really in charge of your patients—and sometimes a junior student too."[111]

The main goal of seniors, however, was to select their specialty, and medical students carefully selected electives in their chosen field to gain more experience.[112] One student compared this process to that of marriage. The summer preceding the senior year was the "scoping period," when seniors began to take electives to explore their chosen specialties and let those doctors check them out. Autumn was the "getting serious" stage, as seniors prepared applications and endured interviews. Winter brought the "commitment phase," as students ranked their preferred programs and finished up those final few requirements for graduation: "In medical school, the formality was known as the X802 research paper. After receiving numerous 'death threats' about not being able to graduate if not completed, many seniors began to work on their paper in December—two weeks before the deadline."[113] Match Day in March was the fateful wedding, followed by a honeymoon period for the rest of the semester. Seniors relaxed and enjoyed themselves, and some held real weddings, as 85 percent of the senior class enjoyed a month of vacation in May.[114]

One often neglected aspect of medical students' lives was establishing a family, which could be a stabilizing as well as a destabilizing force. Medical school was stressful and busy enough on its own, yet many students married and had children while enrolled in medical school. Students had to find ways to juggle each of these priorities. For example, one medical student gave birth to a baby boy two weeks before the beginning of her sophomore year and was at the first day of class. Notwithstanding a busy schedule, most medical students clung to family life, seeing it not as a distraction but as a necessity. A 1991 graduate summed up the value of family life as follows.

> From the very first day of medical school, we were warned that doctors have the highest divorce rate of any profession in the country. The time, energy, and money required of medical school often forced family to take a reluctant back seat. Ironically though, it was precisely that time and energy requirement that made family life so important. Whether it was a parent, spouse, sibling, or child, the relationships with caring family members outside of the world of medicine made life much more tolerable. It seemed that the horrors of Microbiology or Pharmacology easily disappeared with the laughter of a newborn baby or the comradery of a caring sister.[115]

Conclusion

Medical education at Indiana University School of Medicine underwent dramatic changes from the mid-1970s to the mid-1990s not only because of implementation of the statewide education plan but also thanks to the impact of broad national trends. The administrators and faculty who trained these students marshalled existing resources and developed new ones in response. Through these two decades, Deans Beering and Daly oversaw an expansion in the size and complexity of the school, and in this sense the independence of the school (or at least the inability to control it) continued to grow despite the establishment of IUPUI. Even though the new campus only partially achieved the goal of integrating the medical school under a university administration close at hand rather than in Bloomington, the creation of IUPUI had a profound impact on IUSM. This ranged from the immediate functioning of faculty governance and numerous support services to the broader impact of the rapid establishment of a campus with multiple schools and tens of thousands of students.

The number of applicants grew, and the composition of entering classes changed even more, especially the proportion of women. In addition, the changing practice of medicine brought increased specialization and longer graduate training. Fortunately, there is a rich record of how students faced the daunting task of entering the healing profession. Despite these changes, the educational mission was hardly the only, and possibly not the main, endeavor of the school by the end of this period. As will be seen in the next chapter, from the budgeting standpoint at least, the research and clinical responsibilities of the IUSM grew and changed even more dramatically.

11

Tower of Babel or Paper Tiger: Research, Hospitals, and Clinical Practice at the Medical Center, 1975–1995

*F*rom its beginning, the IU School of Medicine was involved in more than the training of doctors. Because of the hospitals that quickly grew up around it and the research that was undertaken somewhat later, as early as 1930, leaders of the medical school were frequently using the term "medical center" to describe the complex of institutions and relationships that had been established west of the city and south of City Hospital.[1] Students at the medical school obviously benefitted from the many facets of the medical center, especially the opportunities for residents to receive clinical training in patient care, but from the 1970s to the 1990s, the clinical and research enterprises of the IU Medical Center (IUMC) became so large that their budgets far surpassed funds explicitly designated for the teaching mission.

The roots of the medical center concept can be traced back to the reforms advocated by the Flexner Report, which called for medical schools to be part of universities, to emphasize medical science, and to utilize teaching hospitals. Explicit in these reforms was defining and strengthening the teaching, research, and clinical service of medical centers. In response, a number of the top medical schools expanded their clinical resources through teaching hospitals and obtained research funds, especially from the Rockefeller Foundation. As a result, several US medical schools claimed to be the core of these integrated activities. In 1928, Columbia University Medical School and Presbyterian Hospital officially applied the name Columbia Presbyterian Medical Center to a new campus combining their research, teaching, and clinical facilities, and the concept was adopted by others, particularly after World War II.[2]

The priority claim of Columbia is questionable. At IUSM, the opportunity to be the core of a medical center arose just a few years after its establishment when the site for Long Hospital was chosen in 1911 next to City Hospital. In the next ten years an instructional building was added plus other hospitals thanks to the gifts of the friends of Riley and the Coleman family. In fact, the term "Indiana University Medical Center" was coined as early as 1919 by Dean Emerson at the dedication of the Medical Building, and it was used regularly in IU trustees minutes beginning after 1926 to refer to the school buildings and hospitals, which continued to expand in the 1930s with the addition of the dental school and Indiana Department of Health buildings. The trustees formally passed a resolution in April 1936 stating "that the official name of the Indianapolis Campus be 'Indiana University Medical Center.'"[3] After 1945, the new VA hospital, Larue Carter Memorial Hospital, and University Hospital continued the process, and at the same time the dramatic expansion of research began that added the final component of the IU Medical Center.

No one was more familiar with the complex multiple institutions of the IU Medical Center than Walter Daly who was educated and spent most his professional career there. As dean for a dozen years, he directed and promoted the medical center, but on two occasions, just before he left office and then several years after, Daly offered observations that more candidly reflect the difficulties involved in operations of the center. The first was made in his presidential address to the Central Society for Clinical Research that was published in the 1982 issue of its prestigious *Journal of Clinical and Laboratory Medicine*. At the time Daly was Chair of the Department of Medicine and it was just before he became dean. Focusing on the two elements added to medical instruction that were cornerstones of medical centers, he praised both the research and clinical care that were major scientific and economic forces which had raised the profile of IUSM locally and, to a certain degree, nationally. But he feared the two endeavors could work at cross purposes, because "research and general medicine have become contradictions."[4] He explained that academic medicine's culture had bifurcated into the language of general medicine (clinical care of patients) and the narrower focus of research. Students, he wrote, "have interested themselves in general medicine to a greater degree than their immediate predecessors," but in research the opposite was true. As he observed, "those who are attracted to research find their research experience in basic science laboratories and in the laboratories of subspecialists," which had become quite narrow and specific. The overall effect, Daly concluded, added to the sense of "a Tower of Babel."[5]

Reflecting back in an interview well after his retirement, Daly used another metaphor to describe the Medical Center, more from the perspective of administration but the result of the same difficulties stemming from such a large and fragmented enterprise. He called the medical center "a paper tiger." By this, he meant that it was little more than a renaming of the multiple responsibilities of the dean's office, which oversaw quite varied educational, clinical, and research activities. From his experience, Daly knew where the real power lay: within the various departments, centers, and hospitals.[6]

The novelty of the statewide teaching plan and the extensive work required to implement it have received a great deal of attention since it began at the end of the 1960s. On the other hand, these less visible changes in research and clinical practice may have been more significant, at least in the aggregate number of personnel added to the medical school and certainly as far as the budget was concerned. In 1971, the medical school reported $13 million in "sponsored research" for its accreditation review, and in 1983, externally funded award grants reached $17 million. A self-study LCME report a decade later, however, showed external grant income in 1993 of $72.8 million.[7] By 1995, more than one-third of the full-time faculty were wholly supported by grant funding, with most of the rest having at least part of their salaries paid from research projects. As will be seen later, the number of clinical faculty increased even faster, and income from hospital contracts and practice plans grew to dominate all other sources of funds for medical school activities.

Medical Research in Departments and Centers

This chapter cannot analyze all new research grants and growth of clinical activity at the IUSM, but it can illustrate the process by describing overall trends and their impact on a number of departments. Support for medical research in the United States saw its greatest increase in the period after the Second World War, with growth slowing by the 1980s and 1990s. The reverse was true in Indiana, where the main features of the expansion of research were only in place after the 1970s.[8] The key role was played by individual faculty members who were recruited nationally as well as graduates of the medical school who were retained and given increasing opportunities to conduct research. The careers of Deans Beering and Daly are examples of one (Beering) who was recruited to Indiana in midcareer as a medical researcher in the US military, and the other (Daly) who spent his career healing Hoosiers. External support was crucial to increased research at the medical school, but local funding was needed to make researchers competitive at the national level. This has been seen in earlier chapters describing the Riley Memorial Association support for pediatric research, and more significantly the new research centers and institutes established after the war including John Nurenburger's Institute for Psychiatric Research (1955), as well as the Krannert Heart Institute (1963), which helped John Hickam expand the research programs in the Department of Medicine, and the Regenstrief Institute (1967).[9]

The 1971 LCME accreditation study of research at the medical school shortly before Steven Beering became dean indicates the limits of this local support. The only units reporting over $300,000 in sponsored research were the departments of Medicine and Psychiatry. The rest of research was mostly by faculty in the medical science departments of Biochemistry, Neurology, Physiology, Pharmacology, and Medical Genetics, which was largely the result of new laboratories and recruiting after the opening of the new Medical Sciences Building in the late 1950s. Otherwise, the findings of the LCME report concluded, "emphasis on scholarly research activity is virtually absent in some departments."[10]

By the time of the next LCME visit in 1979, the committee reported, "Research activity has shown important increases since the last survey; it should be continued and encouraged." Of note was significant increase in sponsored research of Microbiology, Obstetrics and Gynecology, Radiology, and especially Pediatrics, where over $1 million in sponsored research was reported in the most recent academic year.[11] This success can be attributed to Beering and Daly following the precedent of Van Nuys and department chairs such as Hickam who supported research in a number of ways. First, they retained or brought back promising young local researchers, and they also recruited researchers established elsewhere to come to Indiana. In addition, they encouraged and took advantage of local philanthropy to support research as well as the hospital facilities they had long funded. The crucial role played by local philanthropy, especially to enable faculty to be competitive for large-scale national foundation and NIH grant funding, can be seen in the work of two of the most successful researchers at the medical school.

The first example of these nationally renowned researchers was Harvey Feigenbaum, a native of East Chicago, Indiana, who attended IU School of Medicine and then did his residency at Philadelphia General Hospital. He was recruited back to IUSM in 1962, where he joined other promising young faculty, including Suzanne Knoebel and David Hathaway at the research unit in Cardiology of the Krannert Institute, led by Charles Fisch. Feigenbaum, who is often referred to as the father of echocardiography in the United States, later recounted that he first became interested in the technique in 1963. Although there were precursors in Europe who tried to use ultrasound to view the heart, Feigenbaum had been working on catheterization techniques, and when he saw an advertisement from an ultrasound instrument manufacturer, he knew that it could not measure cardiac volume as advertised.[12] Through persistence and assembling people with the right expertise, he was able to perfect the equipment and demonstrate to his very skeptical colleagues the feasibility of cardiac ultrasound. In the process, he founded the American Society of Echocardiography and served as the first editor of its journal. He created a training program for cardiac sonographers and demonstrated the reliable diagnostic application of the technique. In addition to successfully obtaining grant money, Feigenbaum increased the national reputation of the unit and school. Among the junior scholars he mentored was Walter Daly during his early years in the Department of Medicine.[13]

The second example is Lawrence Einhorn, who attended Indiana University, went to medical school at Iowa, and returned to do his residency and join the faculty in oncology at IU School of Medicine in 1973. The following year, Einhorn, along with his collaborator John Donohue, began using platinum in combination chemotherapy to treat metastatic testis cancer (testicular cancer). Although results were discouraging at first, through careful monitoring of early detection, dosage, and length of treatment, the researchers achieved remarkable results that brought worldwide recognition to the IU Medical Center. When Einhorn did his first phase II study in 1974, the survival from this therapy was less than 10 percent for patients in their twenties and thirties. The new treatment he perfected was able to reverse the mortality of testicular cancer to a 95 percent cure rate. Of note, his research was initially supported by another local philanthropy, the Walther Oncology Center, the results from which were important for Einhorn to be successful in receiving steady funding from NIH.[14]

These two examples show that in addition to the genius of these two researchers, their success depended on substantial external support made possible by the enormous growth after 1945 of new government funding agencies such as NIH. As competition for large NIH grants increased, however, it was crucial to have results from pilot projects to support grant proposals. Young researchers were initially helped by new local philanthropic sources of medical research support that enabled them and other new researchers to get started. The local donors and medical research foundations

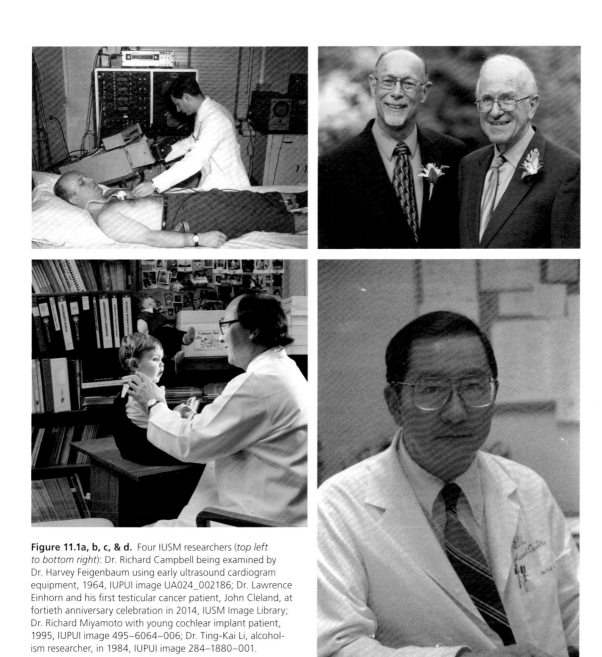

Figure 11.1a, b, c, & d. Four IUSM researchers (*top left to bottom right*): Dr. Richard Campbell being examined by Dr. Harvey Feigenbaum using early ultrasound cardiogram equipment, 1964, IUPUI image UA024_002186; Dr. Lawrence Einhorn and his first testicular cancer patient, John Cleland, at fortieth anniversary celebration in 2014, IUSM Image Library; Dr. Richard Miyamoto with young cochlear implant patient, 1995, IUPUI image 495–6064–006; Dr. Ting-Kai Li, alcoholism researcher, in 1984, IUPUI image 284–1880–001.

included those described in an earlier chapter: the Regenstrief Institute, the Showalter Trust, and the Walther Cancer Institute. These three organizations followed different paths toward maturation as they gained experience and knowledge working with their main grant recipient, the IU School of Medicine. In the case of Einhorn, the Walther funding dedicated to cancer research was a fortunate match of interests. Likewise, the Krannert Institute, which supported Feigenbaum, was for cardiology research.[15]

The Regenstrief Institute, as mentioned in an earlier chapter, had begun with a goal of improving health-care delivery, which was defined broadly enough to support Clem McDonald's research on medical records as well as clinical practice at the city hospital. In 1978, under new leadership, the institute was compelled by the IRS to stop its disbursement of funds in block grants to Indiana University and begin following the advice of a Scientific Advisory Committee (SAC) on the "medical and scientific merit" of potential projects. As a first step, the committee needed to decide on "new directions for both the Institute and the Foundation."[16] The committee was composed of Harvey Feigenbaum, Dean Beering, and Daly, who was chair of the Department of Medicine at the time. The SAC voted to focus on projects that would "improve the health delivery system" or would serve as "seed money" to fund early stage work with the promise to attract future external funding.[17] As Daly sought to build the research focus of the Department of Medicine, these funds served as a vital tool to help attract researchers, develop new projects, and respond quickly to new opportunities.[18] By 1988, the institute had three different research departments: management science research (the work of Clem McDonald described in an earlier chapter), computer science applications, and the department of medicine. Research sections in pediatric epidemiologic research, a vascular laboratory, and diagnostic radiological procedures were added later in the 1980s.[19]

The local foundation that eventually provided support for the broadest range of medical research at IUSM was the Showalter Trust. Previously, Showalter money (only half of which went to IUSM; the other half went to Purdue) was directed to supporting departments in the emerging areas of biochemistry, pharmacology, and rheumatology, rather than individual research projects. This changed gradually and quietly during the mid-1980s, with the encouragement of Daly to make funds available to help younger researchers. The Showalter Trust board was persuaded to shift its focus to providing seed money for pilot projects to obtain enough results to improve chances of obtaining larger external funding.[20]

Daly also tapped and increased internal sources of research support. Using the dean's funds, primarily from taxes on practice plan income (described below), he provided support to recruit new department chairs and key researchers, including funding for laboratory start-up and technicians. Other sources included project development funds from the university and IUPUI to promote collaboration across the campus and IU system. By the end of Daly's tenure, more than two hundred thousand additional square feet were under construction to house this research boom.[21]

Another example of Daly's commitment to research was the appointment in 1986 of a new associate dean of research, Ting-Kai Li, who was a dynamic young researcher in the area of alcoholism. Born in China, Li grew up around the globe as a son of Chinese diplomats. He took the fast track for a rising researcher with his MD from Harvard and residency at Peter Bent Brigham Hospital in Boston, where he was chief resident in 1965. After research at the Karolinska Institute in Stockholm, Daly recognized Li's talents and recruited him to IUSM in 1971. Li built up the Indiana Alcohol Research Center that became a nationally recognized program with long-term funding from the NIH's National Institute on Alcohol Abuse and Alcoholism. In addition to his own work, Li was a strong advocate for research support at the IUSM and across the IUPUI campus, including his strategy of "Research Investment Funds," which used indirect costs from existing grants to make awards to researchers for projects likely to generate additional indirect costs from external grants.[22]

Not every researcher could hope to achieve the success and have the impact of Feigenbaum and Einhorn, but thanks to judicious recruitment plus internal and local support for beginning research, by the 1990s the IUSM dramatically increased its external funding. As mentioned above, externally funded award grants rose from $17 million in 1983 to $72.8 million in 1993. Nonetheless, broadly speaking, IUSM researchers were late to the table nationally for grant funding; hence the 1994 LCME report found that research was "neither over nor under represented." It also noted, "Even though research programs have generally increased, there remains a serious unevenness in research productivity among various departments." Nonetheless, this represented substantial progress from two decades before, and the impact of research funding on staffing increases was substantial. By 1992, almost 44 percent of the basic science faculty and 32 percent of the clinical departmental funding were principal investigators on external grants.[23] Faculty now went through a more formal tenure process, with research (along with teaching and service) being one of the three areas for which standards had to be met. Prior to the 1980s, the tenure process was largely informal and under the purview of the dean. By the mid-1990s, faculty were required to show evidence of publications and "scholarly interest pursued independently of supervision or direction."[24]

The increase in research from the 1970s to the 1990s was reflected not only in tallies of external research funding but also in numerous noteworthy individual researchers as well as broader departmental programs and new research centers. The list of significant research is too long to cover adequately, but examples of individuals making extraordinary discoveries and achieving national and international recognition include Richard Myamoto in Otolaryngology and Pediatrics, Hal Broxmeyer in Immunology, and Darron Brown in Infectious Diseases.

Miyamoto applied cochlear implants to infants and received significant start-up funding from local organizations before securing long-term support from NIH. He also is an example of an IUSM medical school graduate (MD and residency in otolaryngology completed in 1975) who returned to become a faculty member at the IU Medical School after a fellowship at the University of Michigan under William House, where he participated in the first clinical trials of cochlear implants to assist hearing impaired infants. Among the local donors who supported his continued research at IUSM were the Psi Iota Xi Sorority, Indiana Lions Speech and Hearing, the Riley Memorial Association, and the DeVault family, which funded the DeVault Otologic Research Laboratory. The project required the work of surgeons as well as audiologists, including Mary Joe Osberger at IUSM. Based on the results of this research, and shortly before becoming chair of the department, Miyamoto successfully received funding from the National Institute on Deafness and Other Communication Disorders at NIH, which supported his research for the next twenty-five years.[25]

Hal Broxmeyer's work in cord blood treatment for leukemia was also dramatically successful and brought international recognition. He is an example of a successful researcher elsewhere (MD from NYU in 1973, and initial appointment at Cornell) who was recruited to IUSM in 1983. He received local support from the Walther Cancer Center, among other sources. The first successful umbilical cord blood transfusion was done in 1988, in collaboration with Rockefeller University and the Hôpital St. Louis in Paris.[26]

A final example is Darron Brown, who was recruited to the Infectious Diseases division at IUSM from the University of Rochester in 1989, where he received his MD ten years earlier. Brown helped discover the link between HPV and cervical cancer. Based on this research, he helped develop the technology underlying Gardasil and Gardasil 9, two of the three FDA-approved vaccines that have been used against infection by the human papillomavirus. According to the IU Simon Cancer Center, "He played a key role in the pre-clinical research into Gardasil, including demonstrating the effectiveness of a prototype vaccine, as well as the clinical testing of it."[27]

Of course, the departments already engaged in research before the 1970s also benefitted greatly from this added support from the school and local foundations. In the Department of Psychiatry and Institute for

Psychiatric Research, the 1970s brought new leadership and research priorities. Hugh Hendrie came to IU in 1975 as chair of the department and two years later he took over as the executive director of the Institute for Psychiatric Research. Gradually, as advances continued in psychiatry, the focus changed from basic research to clinically directed research. In 1986, John Nurnberger Jr. assumed the directorship of the institute his father created, and under his direction, the clinical thrust of the research program flourished thanks to almost $3 million in external support for research on bipolar illness, alcoholism, Alzheimer's disease, and anxiety disorders. The Larue D. Carter Hospital also received a National Institute of Mental Health Merit Program Award in 1990 to support the psychopharmacological research program of faculty member Joyce Small.[28]

The Department of Medicine continued to conduct the most research of any unit in the school, thanks to its size and the leadership of Hickam in the 1950s and 1960s. This trend continued thereafter, with grants and contracts growing from $6.5 million in 1982–83 to $24.8 million in 1992–93. When Daly became dean in 1983, August M. Watanabe became chairman of the Department of Medicine, and he helped support research in endocrinology and hematology. A separate Pharmacology Department was created in 1984, which recruited faculty and expanded research with the assistance of the Showalter Trust. Its first prominent recruit was D. Craig Brater in Clinical Pharmacology in 1984, at a time when only fifteen such programs existed in the United States. Biostatistics also became a separate division in 1988.[29] Other important new research in the department after the 1970s was in the rapidly growing field of transplant surgery. A Marrow Transplant Unit was established in 1984, followed by a cardiac transplantation program and then liver and kidney transplantation programs. Pediatric surgeon Jay Grosfeld, who started at Riley before becoming chair of the Department of Surgery in 1988, helped expand IU's leadership in transplants for both adults and children. John Brown, Peter Friend, and Mark Pescovitz were among the faculty recruited to expand the program at University Hospital.[30]

Two examples of departments in the period after the 1970s that developed new major research programs were Medical Genetics and Pediatrics. The work of Michael Conneally on isolating the gene for Huntington's Chorea and Joe Christian's twin studies were the result of their recruitment after Donald Merritt was brought to Indiana in 1961 from Washington to establish the new Department of Medical Genetics. Much like Hickam did when he joined the Department of Medicine a decade earlier, Merritt's department quickly became one of the most active research departments in the IUSM and joined the ranks of the top medical genetics departments in the country.[31]

Pediatrics had a long history of research and external support thanks to the Riley Hospital and the Riley Memorial Association, which had raised funds for it since the 1920s. When Morris Green became chairman in 1967, he and his successor, Richard Schreiner, deliberately built up research efforts to support and take advantage of the long-standing success in clinical care responsibilities of the department. This was mainly the work of a large number of individuals hired as part of an even more dramatic growth in clinical work (covered below), and their research gained higher visibility when Green began planning for a research center in 1986, shortly before his retirement. With donations from the Riley Memorial Association, the Herman B Wells Center for Pediatric Research opened in May 1990. As Green stated at the dedication, "We cannot have a great hospital for children unless we have a superior research unit and excellent clinical care." The first director, David A. Williams, was an IUSM graduate who was recruited back from Harvard and was also a Howard Hughes Medical Institute Investigator. He brought his hematology and oncology team to the Wells Center, which in turn helped it attract funds from the National Cancer Institute, leading to the 1994 opening of pediatric cancer center.[32]

As the Wells Center illustrates, the research center model, first pioneered at IUSM by the Krannert and Regenstrief Institutes, increasingly became the vehicle for research after the 1970s. Table 11.1, which is drawn from the 1994 LCME reports, illustrates this.

Besides its length, which reflects the growth of research, this list also demonstrates the frequent focus on disease or body part as the subject of research. This in turn reflects the long-term trend toward specialization in medicine during the twentieth century.[33] Another feature of the centers and institutes, although not shown in table 11.1, is the nature of their funding, which can be divided into three types: federal and other government funding, private funding, and philanthropy. These centers promoted collaborative research across departments and hospitals, though generally there was

Table 11.1. Institutes and Research Centers, IUSM, 1992–1993

Institute/Center	Budget ($ million)
Supported by local philanthropy	
Regenstrief Institute	2.9
Krannert Institute of Cardiology	0.5
Wells Research Center	1.0
Walther Oncology Center	1.0
NIH-supported centers	
General Clinical Research Center	
Alcohol Research Center	
Multipurpose Arthritis Center	
Indiana Alzheimer Disease Center	
Diabetes Research and Training Center	
Midwest Sexually Transmitted Disease Research Center	
Osteoporosis Research Center	
Other centers supported by private and government funds	
Bowen Research Center 1992	
Comprehensive Cancer Center	
Biomaterials & Biomechanics Center	
Institute for Psychiatric Research	

Source: LCME Self-Study, 1994, UA 073, In-U-Ar.

more focus on clinical than bench science, which reflects another broad trend in late-twentieth-century medical research. An example of an NIH-funded center was the Alcohol Research Center, established in 1986. The Wells Pediatric Center, which opened in 1988, was a hybrid of local, private funding and federal government grants; and the Walther Oncology Center was established in 1987, largely with private funding.[34]

Hospitals: "Blood and Guts," "The Mecca," "Vah Spa," and "The Riley"

The analysis of teaching and research at the medical school from the 1970s to the 1990s also requires examination of changes in hospital administration and clinical practice of the faculty. This period is especially important because it culminated in the plan at the end of Dean Daly's term for the consolidation with Methodist Hospital, which marked another major turning point in the school's history. Although referred to as a "medical center" beginning in the 1930s, in the eyes of most of the public, faculty, and students, the different hospitals had their own distinct cultures. For example, to the medical students, each facility had its unique style. Wishard was the "wild and wacky" hospital with patients in "all shapes and sizes," conditions, and lifestyles. But it was also the hospital with the sickest patients, the one where "blood & guts medicine" was taught.[35] University Hospital was known as "The Mecca" or "White Castle." It catered to patients with "strange diseases" and doctors who were interested in them.[36] Medical students also worked at the VA Hospital in Indianapolis, otherwise known as the "Spa," or the "Vah Spa." Students came to hate the way they had to fight the system in order to get the medical tests and procedures their patients needed. But they persevered because, as offended as they were with the bureaucracy of the VA system, these students cared enough to struggle through the red tape for their patients.[37]

Riley was a whole other ballgame for many medical students. One of them summed up what Riley stood for.

> Of all the places in the world, Riley will either make you believe in God or make you believe there is no God. Riley teaches you what heroism is, and courage, because those kids have it. They have it more and better than you would have had it if you were their age, or at least you feel that way. At Riley, though, you also get a glance at the void, because sickness and death for a kid doesn't seem to have any possible meaning and it makes you question sometimes. And Riley, more than anything, makes you work hard at being a healer, because you know you're not just saving a life, you're saving a life's worth of potential.[38]

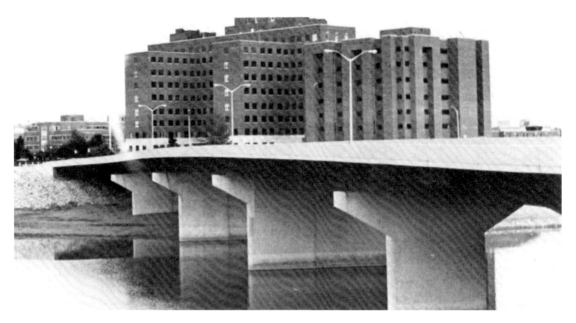

Figure 11.2. "'For a relaxing vacation, try the VA Spa.' The Indianapolis VA, 'flag hospital' of the Midwest, was full of frustration for the eager student who spent more time fighting with the system than fighting disease. Here we became acquainted with the 'gomers' and learned the rules of The house of God." *Caduceus* (1981): 29.

In contrast to the decentralization of medical education through the regional centers, the delivery of clinical care became more standardized and centrally controlled after the 1970s. Continuing the efforts started by their predecessors, Deans Beering and Daly worked to consolidate operation of the clinical facilities through management contracts with affiliated hospitals, sometimes rewriting contracts with old partners. The goal was to move closer to "one standard of care" across the medical center system. Daly especially used the concept of "medical center" to tie together the clinical care of the facilities at or near the medical school. According to a retrospective article by Stuart Kleit along with David and Daniel Handel, the key issue facing IUSM as well as other medical schools, in addition to finding the financial resources for meeting the educational mission of the school, was maintaining access to "a critical mass of clinical services adequate to meet the learning needs of their students, postgraduate trainees and researchers." The need for access to patients had long been met through partnerships with existing hospitals, but to IUSM officials, the changes in the health-care landscape suggested that a school the size of IUSM might require a system "well in excess of the [current] size needed to achieve the

Table 11.2. Hospitals in IU Medical Center, 1977

Hospital	Beds	Outpatient Visits
IU Hospitals: University, Long, and Riley	629	87,541
Wishard Memorial	567	203,817
Larue D. Carter Memorial	225	7,068
Veterans Administration	660	98,893
Total	2,081	397,249

Source: LCME Self-Study, 1979, UA 073, In-U-Ar.

missions." Beering and Daly worked hard with partner hospitals as well as an increasing number of ambulatory care facilities to achieve this goal.[39] Table 11.2 gives a picture of the various hospitals and their capacities in 1977.

Complicating these efforts of the IUSM and especially the hospital administration was the rapidly changing national picture of clinical care. IUSM trained two-thirds of the practicing physicians in Indiana, so any changes could have a major impact on how clinical care would be delivered in Indiana for decades to come. The creation of a robust academic medical center with six hospitals and numerous outpatients reflected the centripetal forces of modern health care, but it was also subject to the centrifugal forces of specialization and outpatient clinics. IUSM also was affected by the external pressures of suburbanization and new regional hospital systems, changing university climate, and increased regulation and governmental control. In the United States, an average hospital stay in 1975 was eleven days, but by 1995 it was three. At the same time, the long postwar hospital growth produced a surplus of hospital beds, particularly as an increasing number of procedures became outpatient. In fact, the number of hospital beds peaked in 1983.[40]

One of the key actors in creating a single standard of care within the medical center was Stuart Kleit, associate dean for Clinical Affairs. Kleit, who had been chief resident under John Hickam, was recruited back to IU in 1967 and rose to IUSM chief of Nephrology. Having worked closely with Daly in the Wishard agreements, Kleit was appointed in 1985 as associate dean for Clinical Affairs and interim director of Hospitals. This new position in the dean's office served the function of keeping the various players under the medical center umbrella.[41]

In addition to the change in hospital administration, the increased role of insurance and practice plans required more attention from the Dean's Office, beginning with improvement of care given at partner patient institutions. Of these, none was more important than the former city hospital, which in 1959 had been renamed Marion County General Hospital. Beginning in the late 1960s, the medical school and its faculty expanded their service to the hospital, culminating in a contract to direct medical services, a change that brought the clinical roles of IU doctors at Marion County General in line with the departmental duties of the medical school. Due to nearly constant crises that ensued, negotiations were needed to stabilize relationships with the hospital, which required an increase in the resources, provision of clinical experiences, and standardization of care. Beering took the dramatic step of committing IUSM to the administration of the hospital as both a strategic necessity and social justice priority. He asserted an unwillingness to settle for second-best care for the poor and underserved in the city of Indianapolis.[42]

The problems at Marion County General were multiple. It had a substantial low-income patient base, needing largely emergency and primary care. This was quite different from the IU hospitals, which provided referral or tertiary care. Reflecting the needs of the Marion County patients, Indiana had one of the highest infant mortality rates in the country, and Indianapolis was consistently ranked as one of the ten least healthy cities in the country.[43] Growing competition and declining infrastructure also meant that the hospital was losing some patients, such as in the critical area of obstetrical care, to other facilities that had begun to accept Medicaid. In addition, whereas IUSM doctors mostly staffed the county hospital, many did not have secure appointments in the medical school. In fact, IUSM did not have final control over hiring of the county hospital staff because the township trustees could fill positions not solely on the basis of merit or training but rather on local or political affiliation. Another problem was efficient use of equipment. Future dean Robert Holden, who was chief of the radiology service at the hospital, remembered there were often fifty to sixty people waiting for seven or nine rooms to get X-rays, hardly an optimal situation, while machines sat idle at University Hospital. Finally, Beering thought that only a handful of the top physicians at the hospital were dedicated to a successful partnership, and he hoped to use the key staff there to help build the new administration.[44]

One solution to the problem of efficiency that seemed "most logical" to Holden was to move medical service organization away from the internal hospital subservice model to a combined one for multiple hospitals.[45] The first attempt to organize such service across hospitals was gastroenterology, and although the plan was adopted for only a limited number of services, it was a precursor to what happened after the consolidation of hospitals that Holden oversaw after he became dean. The Department of Pathology, which had more experience coordinating referral laboratory facilities, was successful in combining operations at the county and university hospitals. Experienced physicians and other staff had "mixed reactions" to these changes that shook up the ways that things had been done. As an architect of the plan, Holden remained proud of the "stability of relationship" for the services that remained largely in place for two decades. With the new arrangement, he recalled, "the physician, patient, and relationship became supreme." Holden was above all convinced that the patient population at the county hospital was central to the education of medical students. In a period of increased specialization and rising costs, students benefitted from exposure to the full continuum of patients who would enter the door, including the impact of socioeconomics on health. He found that this environment helped teach students about empathy for homeless and recalcitrant patients, those not accepting of societal rules, and those with antisocial behaviors.[46]

In September 1975, the "consummation" of the management contract with Marion County coincided with the renaming of the facility as Wishard Memorial Hospital, whose namesake was William Niles Wishard, an early champion of the hospital.[47] No longer billed as a general hospital, Wishard and associated outpatient facilities focused on its extensive experience in treatment of complex trauma. Over the next few years, longtime Wishard workers as well as IUSM faculty adjusted to this new type of clinic-based service, with one standard of care. This process sent ripples across the medical center in such areas as the hiring, managing, and scheduling of nurses and other support staff; standardizing pay rates; and personnel policies. As examples of this change, Wishard received $250,000 in donations from community groups for an Adult Burn Unit. In addition, the medical school worked to address the critical nursing crisis at the hospital by recruiting one hundred new nurses, which led to more patient satisfaction and improved patient care. The new coordination of admissions increased University Hospital occupancy rates from 60 percent to 90 percent. In other metrics, the average length of stay was reduced to nine days, and collections increased by 25 percent within the first four years of implementation. From the perspective of the Wishard operators, the Health and Hospital Corporation of Marion County, these changes, plus the ability to liquidate debt, placed the hospital in a sound financial position.[48]

Besides Wishard, the other hospital that the medical school had a formal staffing agreement with was the Veterans Hospital. (Riley and University Hospitals were always run by the medical school.) The VA hospital, in the words of Daly, was like dealing with an "absent landlord." In the post–Vietnam War era, the provision of health care to veterans became a high-profile political issue. Congress changed VA health-care eligibility to provide free care for veterans with service-connected disabilities or low incomes, as well as other special groups of veterans and higher income, nonservice-disabled patients who could pay for part of their treatment. Late in the 1980s, the VA hospital began to dedicate resources to serving homeless and chronically mentally ill veterans. Although most actions were taken independently at the local level, nearly all administrative functions still needed to go through the VA system in Washington. Phillip Snodgrass was hired by Daly in 1973 to run the clinical services at the VA hospital, in part because it had a completely different patient base and payment system. National expansion in health care led to major building renovations that were completed in 1994, which allowed more room for outpatient, psychiatric services, and research space.[49]

During this time period from the mid-1970s to the mid-1990s, the University Hospital and Riley Hospital, run by directly by IUSM, also made significant additions to their facilities. In 1986, Riley Hospital opened a $56 million addition that included a Chronic Infant Care Unit (the Nurture Center) as well as modern patient units, expanded intensive care units, fourteen operating rooms, state-of-the-art imaging facilities, and, for the first time, a cafeteria. In addition, in 1991, the Herman B Wells Center for Pediatric Research opened with $5 million in funding from the RMA.[50] The main improvements to University Hospital included an outpatient center that opened in 1992, which included space for a later addition of clinical trial facilities.[51]

Departments and Clinical Practice

From the 1970s to the 1990s, the departments of the medical school, which were its organizational backbone for teaching and research as well as clinical practice, also changed their operations in response to larger changes in health care. Although they showed some common features, these responses varied quite a bit depending on the size, state of the art of practice, and historical culture of the department. A sample of some key departments—Medicine, Pathology, Pediatrics, and Psychiatry—will illustrate the different roles that departments played in following the agreements that the medical school made with hospitals and the development of their clinical practice plans.

The clinical operations of the Department of Medicine were the most important because it was by far the largest of the departments. Daly was chairman from 1970 until he became dean of the school in 1983, during

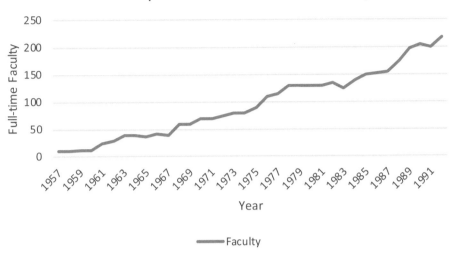

IUSM Department of Medicine Faculty

Figure 11.3. Number of Full-Time Faculty, IUSM Department of Medicine, 1958–1992, IUSM, Department of Medicine Annual Reports, 1957–1991, Department of Medicine History (1993).

which time the faculty grew from approximately seventy full-time faculty to 130, and the house staff and fellows from ninety-five to 140.[52]

As figure 11.3 shows, the number of full-time faculty in the department continued to grow to 217 by 1992, and it did not stop there. Part of the reason for the continued growth thereafter was the use of a newly established rank of clinical faculty appointment. At the urging of the medical school, in the early 1990s, Indiana University approved this nontenure track faculty rank to meet the growing need for physicians whose primary responsibilities were for clinical care and teaching but without research responsibility. The Department of Medicine made nine such appointments in the first year, and the number has grown considerably since then. For the whole IU School of Medicine, despite the increased number of tenure-line faculty, by 2012, the number of clinical rank faculty equaled them, and in 2016, the IUSM reported 742 clinical faculty compared to 605 tenure-line.[53]

The increase of clinical faculty (both tenure-line and the new clinical rank) to a large extent helped staff the newly developed practice plans, which were paid from new sources to reimburse clinical care through Medicare and Medicaid plus health insurance.[54] Ironically, as many observers pointed out at the time, this threatened a return to conditions at the beginning of the twentieth century, when students at the proprietary medical schools were taught by private practitioners on the side to supplement their income. In response, Flexner and other reformers called for full-time academic faculty to teach and do research. Earlier chapters have shown that the IU School of Medicine faced this major problem from its beginning and worked diligently over the years to create full-time positions in order to be less dependent on private practitioners who were part-time instructors. By 1970, however, Dean Irwin saw the establishment of practice plans, whereby department members formed a medical practice to offer clinical and diagnostic services to private patients, as a way to increase overall compensation. To be sure, private patients had been admitted to Long Hospital from the beginning, and part of the payment went to supplement physician faculty income, but the number of beds was limited. With the opening of University Hospital, however, the capacity to accommodate private patients increased dramatically, and it made practice plans not only possible but helpful in managing the billing and accounting. The first approvals came by the IU Board of Trustees in June 1971, and this quickly became a mainstay of the IUSM budget.

Individual departments, hospitals, and clinics had different arrangements so that a physician might be receiving revenue from various plans at the same time. According to Walter Daly, when he became chair after the sudden death of John Hickam, he found that Hickam had been working on a practice plan for the department, and it was relatively easy to implement.[55] In fact, in 1970, the department secretary, Nancy Baxter, began keeping track of private patients who were seen in the Clinical Building. She was not billing at this time, but she projected how much revenue could be created and how much should be retained by the department. This process was continued while awaiting state approval. Once obtained, the University Medical Diagnostic Associates was incorporated in 1971. Although this practice plan was set up outside of the Department of Medicine, it required an administrator as part of the operations of the department. The board members were primarily the heads of the sections in the department, and Daly recalled it was a "very substantial source of income."[56] According to department annual reports, the plan brought in $1.3 million of income in 1974, and it grew steadily to $4.9 million in 1984, reaching $14.8 million in 1991.[57]

In the Pathology department, the chair, Joshua Edwards, responded to growing income and services by creating in 1976 a not-for-profit corporation: University Anatomic Pathology Associates. Although Pathology had a long history of charging for services, even back to the alliance with the State Board of Health, the increase was significant. For example, in 1976, Pathology billed $457,609 for professional services, up 76 percent from the previous year. The nonprofit reporting requirements, as well as grants and increased clinical services, required more record keeping and administrative staff in the department chair's office.[58]

Dermatology is an example of a department that increased clinical services without establishing a practice plan. In 1963, it was made an independent department, and Victor Hackney was recruited from Stanford University to be the first chairman. The residency program and clinical service at the Marion County General Hospital and the clinical service at the IU hospitals were merged into the new department, and in the 1980s, other facilities were added. In 1976, Arthur Norins succeeded Hackney as chairman, and the number of faculty and dermatology residents continued to grow. The Hackney Laboratory for Investigative Dermatopathology was created in 1990 and developed a research program in molecular biology of the skin. When Norins stepped down in 1993, Evan Farmer was recruited from Johns Hopkins University to succeed him, in part because of his more general clinical focus, but also because of his research on dermatopathology, graft-versus-host disease, and clinical dermatology with emphasis on outcome studies.[59]

Another example of how department clinical practice worked was in the delivery of psychiatric services. Indiana had mental institutions long before a formal Department of Psychiatry was created in the 1930s. After 1945, more formal relations for residency training, and clinical rounds were established with the city hospital and the VA, but the establishment of Larue D. Carter Memorial Hospital, a new state mental institution built adjacent to the medical school, opened even more opportunities, especially after the creation of the Institute for Psychiatric Research in 1955.[60] More instructive of the era of the 1970s was a new management agreement in 1975 between Wishard Hospital and the IUSM Department of Psychiatry to develop the Midtown Community Mental Health Center. This community center, the first in the state of Indiana, was established in 1969 at Marion County General Hospital to provide a full range of psychiatric services. In 1975, IUSM faculty member Alan Schmetzer came to University Hospital and cofounded the Psychiatric Inpatient Service to work with Midtown, which quickly became a major teaching resource for the department's psychiatry residents and medical students.[61]

The national trend to close inpatient psychiatric wards in the early 1990s included Central State Hospital, where IUSM students had long trained. As a result, there was an increased need for more short-term inpatient services, and during this difficult transition, the work of Claire Assue illustrates how much the clinical activities of the Psychiatry Department and the mental hospitals were intertwined. Assue was superintendent of Larue D. Carter Memorial Hospital from 1981 to 1989, not only one of the first African American psychiatrist in the country to hold such a position but also serving at the helm of an institution during a time of tremendous change in the field of mental health. She received her MD from Howard University in 1954 and did an internship at Beth-El Hospital in Brooklyn. Following a short time at IUSM as a resident, she returned in 1958 to become a staff physician at Larue Carter and a clinical instructor in the Department of Psychiatry. She rose through the academic ranks, taking on administrative duties in patient services at Larue Carter Hospital, medical education for the Department of Psychiatry, and culminating as superintendent of the hospital in the 1980s. In these roles, she was a mentor to women coming through the program, and she helped recruit and train top students. Her mentorship and teaching were recognized nationally, and she was invited to become an examiner for the American Board of Psychiatry and Neurology.[62]

Once the various departmental practice plans were created, there was a long power struggle over control between the departments and the dean's office. This took on a degree of added urgency with changes in reporting requirements at the state and national level. After Daly became dean, he required all departments to transfer a front-end tax as a percentage of gross collections from practice (2–5 percent, he recalled, after some negotiation with all the departments). In addition, according to LCME reports, fellows were predominantly paid from the practice plans, with the remainder coming from hospital fees and grants.[63] On a schoolwide level, two major health-care entities were incorporated into the medical school in order to help support teaching and research: University Health Care in 1986, with a focus on primary care, and Indiana University Health Care Associates in 1987 for managed care patients. According to the new accounting, the clinical income increased but continued to comprise approximately one-quarter of the total school budget. It was not until the 1990s, however, that all the departmental practice plans were replaced by an overall IUMC system.[64]

A final example of a department with unusual clinical and hospital responsibilities, and one with probably the highest profile of all departments and hospitals in the medical center, was Pediatrics and Riley Hospital. After 1970, thanks to growth in both outpatient and inpatient visits, as well as increased support for neonatal care and research, both the hospital and especially the Department of Pediatrics grew significantly under two long-serving department chairs. Morris Green was named chairman of the Department of Pediatrics and the first physician-in-chief at Riley Hospital in 1967, and he served two decades in that role. Green was born in

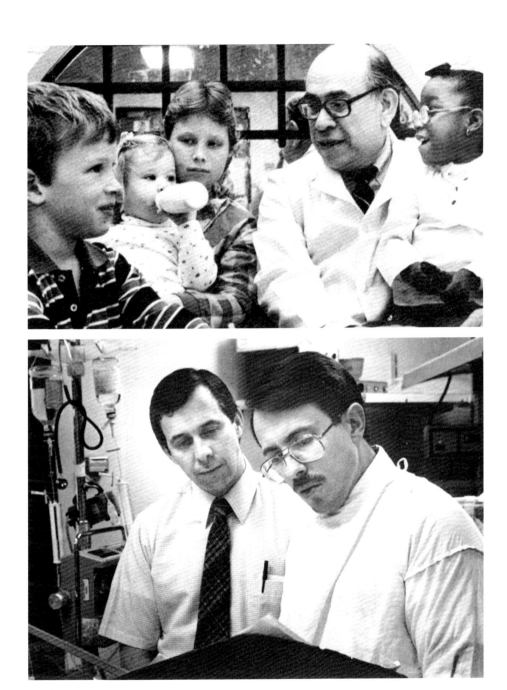

Figure 11.4a & b. Two chairs of Pediatrics: (*top*) Morris Green with children at Riley Hospital, March 1986, *Indiana Alumni Magazine* (March 1986): 28; (*bottom*) his successor as chair, Richard Schreiner, pictured with James Lemons (*left*) in the Newborn Intensive Care Unit, 1983, *Center Magazine* (1983).

Indianapolis, earned his AB degree from Indiana University in 1942, and earned his MD from IUSM in 1944. He completed a residency and served as an instructor at the University of Illinois College of Medicine. Green was appointed an assistant professor at Yale University in 1952, and in 1957, he was recruited back to IUSM by Lyman T. Meiks, chair of Pediatrics. As late as 1968, there were only four full-time faculty members in the Pediatrics Department.

The changes that occurred in the next twenty years through growth of services, increase in grant funding, and sustained recruitment are reflected by the number of faculty, which grew to forty-five physicians by the time of Green's retirement as chair in 1987. Likewise, the number of residents increased from four to fifty-four. Of course, this was also the result of broader changes in the field, including increased specialization. For example, a combined internal medicine and pediatric residency was instituted that eventually became the largest in the country. As mentioned above, in 1986, a Riley Hospital addition opened and included a Chronic Infant Care Unit, which served as a model for similar units in children's hospitals across the country. It also had modern patient units, expanded intensive care units, operating rooms, and state-of-the-art imaging facilities.[65]

Richard L. Schreiner followed Green in 1987 and served as chairman of the department and physician-in-chief until his retirement in 2009.[66] Schreiner is another example of a local native who left Indiana for college and medical school but then was recruited back to IUSM. He grew up in northern Indiana and attended St. Louis University (1963–67) and Washington University School of Medicine (1967–71). He completed his residency in pediatrics at St. Louis Children's Hospital, and after a fellowship in neonatology/perinatology at Riley Hospital and at the University of Colorado School of Medicine, Schreiner returned to join the faculty of the Indiana University School of Medicine in 1975. During his more than two decades as chair, the department grew from 45 to 250 faculty members. Key to this growth were twenty-two new endowed chairs, an increase in pediatric residents and fellows from fifty-four to 150, and growth of extramural NIH funding that raised the department's national ranking from sixtieth to seventeenth. The department faculty expanded clinical services in primary care throughout the Indianapolis area and in subspecialty services throughout the state.[67]

During the 1980s, Riley and the IU Medical Center gained national attention as the hospital that treated Ryan White one of the most highly publicized AIDS patients in the country. White was a thirteen-year-old from Kokomo, Indiana, who was diagnosed with AIDS following a contaminated blood transfusion for hemophilia at Riley in December 1984. Little was

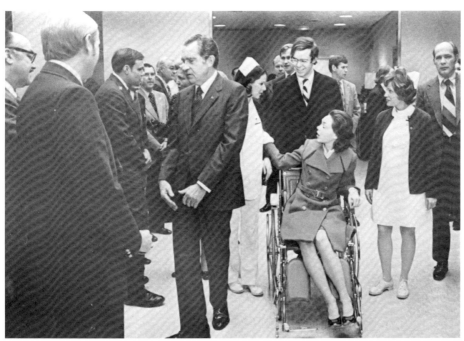

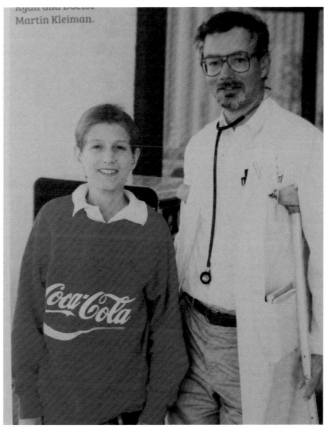

Figure 11.5a & b.
Famous patients and physicians: (*top*) Julie Nixon at University Hospital in 1974, IUPUI image 274–0274–01; (*right*) Ryan White with his doctor Marty Kleiman of the IUSM Pediatrics Department and Riley Hospital in 1986, photo by Jeanne White Ginder.

known about AIDS at the time, and Martin Kleiman, his physician and founder of the Section of Pediatric Infectious Disease at IUSM, predicted that Ryan only had a short time left to live. When his mother, Jeanne, tried to continue Ryan's life as normally as possible in the time he had remaining, his school tried to bar him from returning to class, and Ryan became the subject of a national debate about AIDS-related discrimination.[68]

At the IU Medical Center, media relations director Pam Perry recalled that University Hospital tried to protect the White family's privacy during Ryan's treatment and still provide information to the national media, which swarmed over the hospital during the five years Ryan struggled with the disease.[69] In the spring of 1990, when Kleiman and his team saw that White's struggle was nearing the end, the national media and celebrities such as Michael Jackson and Elton John descended on Indianapolis. Each day the physicians released information to the more than fifty reporters gathered in the University Hospital cafeteria, including one who tried to bypass security to reach Ryan's room. David Handel, director of University Hospital, established a kind of command post; IUPUI handled the additional security; and Perry informed the media, national political leaders such as First Lady Barbara Bush, and other celebrities who came to visit the dying boy, as well as the public bringing well wishes and sometimes dubious herbal remedies.[70] Ryan White died on April 8, 1990, one month before his high school graduation and only months before Congress passed the legislation bearing his name in August 1990, the Ryan White Comprehensive AIDS Resources Emergency (CARE) Act.

Other high-profile patients who brought national attention to the medical school include first daughter Julie Nixon Eisenhower, who was operated on for removal of an ovarian cyst in February 14, 1974.[71] She was in Indianapolis for an editorial board meeting of the *Saturday Evening Post* when she was hospitalized with bleeding. Attention was heightened because of the Watergate investigation going on at the time and Richard Nixon's visit to University Hospital for a few hours after the operation. Vice President Dan Quayle (who attended the Law School at IUPUI) was also a patient, as was Jerri Nielsen, who made national headlines in 1999 with her struggle to diagnose and treat her breast cancer at the isolated South Pole under the supervision of IUSM cancer specialist Kathy Miller.[72]

Toward the Joint Venture with Methodist Hospital

Walter Daly may have had second thoughts when he retrospectively called the IU Medical Center a paper tiger, but when he was dean, there was no stronger proponent of the institutions and relations that comprised the center and the purposes it served.[73] These included, above all, providing a common identity in order to receive and share credit for the scope and extent of medical activity that had been established with the medical school at its center. By the early 1990s, however, there were serious problems facing both the medical school and the idea of a medical center, some of which reflected national developments but others of which were local. The broader changes were in health-care finance, structure, and delivery as a result of rapidly increasing health-care costs, as well as the drive for health-care reform at the national and state levels. In addition, local hospitals were taking steps that threatened both the IU hospitals and those with whom the school had staffing agreements.

As a result, Daly began working behind the scenes, beginning in 1993, to examine the possible reconfiguration of the medical center. From a marketing perspective, he consolidated public relations for the medical school and medical center. In addition, he added several community and business leaders with diverse backgrounds to assist three trustees on a committee to advise on the rapidly changing health-care environment. Behind closed doors, key administrators from the dean's office and chairs of some of the biggest departments began discussions with Methodist Hospital of Indianapolis and Wishard Memorial Hospital about closer collaboration.[74]

A full examination of how the agreement of consolidation with Methodist Hospital was reached is beyond the scope of this chapter, but a published account by key participants provides an outline of some major steps.[75] According to coauthors Handel, Kleit, and Handel, the immediate reason the medical school began discussion about building new partnerships was the threat to the medical center's position as the tertiary care facility dependent on referrals from the rest of the state's hospitals. The statewide IUSM academic-clinical system began to be challenged when the major hospitals in Indiana that had also expanded in the postwar years began exploratory meetings about cooperating with each other to create their own statewide networks. For example, in October 1993, Community Hospital and St. Vincent Hospital in Indianapolis announced they had "teamed up" to coordinate care.[76] Although this particular plan was soon abandoned, variations on the expansion idea were pursued by other hospitals such as Methodist Hospital, where the top leadership struggled with whether or not to close the flagship downtown hospital complex. Its operations were threatened by high maintenance costs and the movement of much of the population it served to the suburbs. Officials announced a "beltway plan" with new medical plazas planned for the edges of the city, but when the Methodist board of directors also made the decision to continue to operate the downtown hospital, there was increased pressure to explore partnerships.[77]

Located less than two miles to the north of the IUSM campus, Methodist was the largest hospital in the state with 984 staffed hospital beds and numerous specialty and primary care facilities. Somewhat smaller, University Hospital and Riley together had 616 staffed beds, with more than half their patients coming from outside of the Indianapolis metropolitan area. The Handels and Kleit state that the discussions and debates were initially kept under wraps with little being shared with employees, physicians, many in leadership, or the public.[78]

Once the decision was made to begin discussions with Methodist, however, a small core planning committee was selected comprised of key staff, faculty, and an outside consulting firm that began drawing up plans for "system development." The committee included executives, board chairs, financial officers, and attorneys for the two organizations, plus the two chief medical officers, two Methodist physicians, and the chairs of IUSM Departments of Medicine, Pediatrics, and Surgery.[79] After examining a number of models, they soon decided against a typical merger where one party took over operations of the other. Instead, primarily because of the deep historical roots and name recognition of the hospitals, the committee decided on creating a new nonprofit organization, eventually named Clarian Health (and later changed to IU Health), which would develop and consolidate operations of the three hospitals: University, Riley, and Methodist. Clarian would be jointly owned and overseen by the IU trustees and the Methodist Health Group, which would have equal representation on a governing board. Although Daly showed "active involvement and strong support," he was not on the core committee. At both institutions, the physicians who normally ran general operations within the departments and facilities were "broadly" involved, but with only a few exceptions they were largely excluded from the process. Both institutions shared the same general missions and values, but it was agreed that IU would take the lead on medical education and Methodist on community services and clinics.[80]

In working on the educational mission, although the leaders of the consolidation praised the "open communication," those involved felt the process was interminable, and many faculty members felt left in the dark. Small committees worked on specific aspects of the project, such as human resources systems, but they were unaware of the broader details of the plan. Three leaders from each institution formed a new "Senior Executive Team" to coordinate the broad aspects of the consolidation. Highlighting the new operational complexity, executives at each hospital were responsible for the operations at the site as well as the assigned departments and services at all three hospitals. This model anticipated future growth if new hospitals were brought into the system, allowing some degree of local autonomy

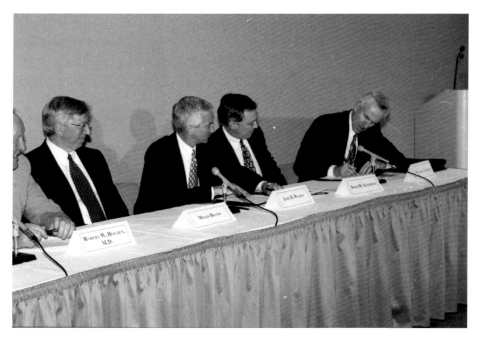

Figure 11.6. "IU, Methodist Announcement of Intent to Consolidate Hospitals," Methodist President William Loveday (*far right*) signs agreement as others look on (*to his right*): president of the Methodist Board of Directors David Goodrich, president of the IU Trustees John Walda, president of Indiana University Myles Brand, and IUSM dean Robert Holden. IUPUI image 596–6530–025.

and identity while conforming to being part of the larger system. Initially, the plan did not affect existing affiliation agreements with other hospitals, which was most critical for IUSM and its arrangements with Wishard, the VA, and Larue Carter.[81]

On March 9, 1995, after two years of negotiations, an agreement in principle was announced for the consolidation of the hospitals' operations.[82] Later, in the spring of 1995, more IUSM leaders were brought in to plan and develop the media relations strategies for the unveiling of the agreement to the many employees of the institutions and the public. Consultants supplied them with information about the demographics and experience of other medical centers. Another element was the extensive use of focus groups to determine public views of the agreement and Indianapolis health-care market.

The creation of the partnership still required quite a long list of approvals, including the IU trustees, the Methodist Group board, the Methodist Church Council, the state of Indiana, the IU faculty practice plans and IU Health Care, the Methodist, Riley, and IU Foundations. In addition, state and local medical accreditation was required, as well as federal oversight approval. The Methodist board approved the plan on April 25, 1996, and at the May 2, 1996, meeting of the IU Board of Trustees, the discussion and favorable vote on the agreement was broadcast from Bloomington to the Indianapolis campus.[83]

Among the most contentious problems in implementing the agreement was the need to accommodate the different practices and underlying cultures that had developed in the organization and practice of the clinical specialties in the various organizations, including Methodist Medical Group, M-Plan, Methodist outpatient centers, and the IU departmental faculty practice plans. Although this problem continued for years and was never fully resolved, in the following months, many different forums and information sessions were held with employees, faculties, vendors, and the public. Daly and members of the leadership team traveled the state to gain support for the agreement. In the speeches and publications, there was a strong focus on the advantages of the size of the $1.1 billion health-care system, touted as one of the largest in the country. In addition, a new shared compensation package was one of the first features to be consolidated.[84]

The leadership of Clarian included William Loveday, the CEO of Methodist Health Group who became CEO of Clarian.[85] In addition, John Walda, president of IU Board of Trustees, and David Goodrich, chair of the Methodist Health Group Board of Directors, served as cochairmen of the new board of Clarian Health. David J. Handel, director of hospitals at IU Medical Center, was named executive vice president of Operations of the new organization,[86] and Stuart Kleit, associate dean for Clinical Affairs and head of Graduate Medical Education at IUSM, was named executive vice president for Academic Affairs. The consolidation announced in the spring of 1995 was set to begin January 1, 1997. What was not released to the public and employees at that time was Walter Daly's decision to retire in November 1995.

Conclusion

Well after retirement, when Walter Daly was asked in an interview what he would most like to be remembered for, he quickly joked, "I just need to be forgotten." In fact, during the period from the mid-1970s to the mid-1990s, Daly participated in some important turning points as well as continuation of evolutionary changes in the history of the IU School of Medicine. The growth in medical research was part of a long-term national and widely publicized process that was not viewed as a sudden or dramatic change. Likewise, the implementation of the new statewide medical education plan, once decided, took place over two decades. The proposal to close some medical education centers in the early 1990s was surprising, but its defeat clearly demonstrated the strength of local political and economic interests in continuing the statewide program. Rather than consolidation, the reaction produced the opposite effect by energizing local interests to expand the scope of the regional centers that eventually led to offering all four years of medical school instruction at the eight sites outside of Indianapolis.

Daly mentioned in the same interview that as a junior faculty member in the late 1960s, he and others at the semiannual faculty meeting were simply asked to vote aye for the proposed statewide medical education plan.[87] His role in some key changes while dean, however, is more complex and is a subject worth further examination, although it is beyond the scope of this study. He appears to have had at least mixed feelings about the proposal in the early 1990s to consolidate some of the medical teaching centers, although he dutifully took the lead in presenting President Ehrlich's proposal. Likewise, he was not part of the inner circle that planned the Clarian Health agreement, although he similarly championed it for the short period he remained dean. His retirement in 1995 coincided with the implementation of the agreement, but it was also when he turned sixty-five, so it was not an early departure.

The creation of Clarian Health was an obvious and significant turning point in the medical school's history. Although the agreement that established Clarian attempted to preserve the tradition and names of the oldest institutions (Riley and Methodist), from the perspective of the history of the school of medicine, the merger meant that the dean ceased having main responsibility for running the school's hospitals, a feature of the institution dating back to the opening of Long Hospital in 1914. One result of the creation of Clarian Health was to put University and Riley Hospitals into a category more similar to the other hospitals that IUSM staffed: the VA, Wishard, and Larue Carter. The agreements with Riley and University were internal arrangements within IU, which was the co-owner, but a hospital administration separate from the dean's office now ran them. Two obvious but broad consequences included elimination of what had been a major responsibility of the dean—and often a bone of contention with the IU president that resulted in Dean Emerson's and Gatch's departure. But equally as obvious was a significant loss of control of a major source of income for the medical school: hospital fees and practice plans.

Robert Holden, the new dean given the task of implementing the Clarian Hospital agreement, looked back with mixed judgment about some of the broader results of the consolidation after two decades, and he noted,

"In a review of the consolidation approximately 20 years later, I think it can definitely be said that the clinical prowess of the system has been dramatically improved. The growth has allowed an accompanying improvement of facilities and enhanced outreach to the citizenry of the state. The patient population for training medical students and residents has as well been significantly improved."

Looking at the agreement from the longer perspective of his half century career in medicine, however, Holden warned,

> The above high-altitude overview gives some insight into the changes facing the School in its decision to enter into the agreement. It does not address the increased corporatization occurring throughout the nation in academic health centers. As a physician growing up through these changes 1960–2000's, I saw the emphasis on profit drive changes detrimental to a teaching and research faculty in medical schools. Our consolidation was very early in the national progression and while I believe it is successful, there are shortfalls which have not been addressed.[88]

These developments reflect broader influences on the school of medicine as it entered its second century.

12

Into the Second Century

The mid-1990s was a major turning point in the history of the Indiana University School of Medicine given the changes, both dramatic (hospital consolidations and statewide education) and gradual (research and clinical practice) that had taken place in the previous two decades. Rather than pause and consolidate, the school continued to change, and given its size, both the number and complexity of new developments were magnified. A few statistics will illustrate this.

When Robert Holden became the eighth dean of the IU School of Medicine in 1995, there were, according to a 1994 self-study for LCME accreditation, 902 full-time faculty in twenty-four departments. They taught 1,072 medical students on nine campus sites around Indiana plus 287 students in ten MS and PhD basic sciences programs.[1] This was in addition to training 694 residents and fellows in twenty-two specialties and subspecialties. Faculty conducted research that brought in over $72 million in external funding (1993), much of it done in research centers and institutes. The clinical departments of the school provided care for tens of thousands of patients that year in their practices ($138 million in revenue) while staffing four hospitals, including two very large general hospitals (the VA and Wishard) plus two specialty hospitals for children and psychiatric patients. The overall revenue of the school in fiscal year 1993 was over $295 million, more than a 280 percent increase in the revenue (adjusted for inflation) reported for fiscal year 1984.[2]

As this snapshot shows, the IUSM had become so large and complex by 1995 that its history in subsequent years is difficult to examine in great detail. This chapter therefore only outlines the main developments after 1995 in the areas of education, research, and clinical care. This serves as a framework within which to examine some of the more important changes

Table 12.1 Sources of Revenue, IUSM, Selected Years, 1984–2016

Source	FY 84	FY 93	FY 08	FY 16
Tuition and fees	4,660,806	12,381,032	41,174,669	60,000,000
% of Total	5.8	4.2	4.7	4.0
State and university	33,513,404	61,062,031	40,817,096	107,000,000
% of Total	41.7	20.1	4.6	7.1
Practice plan and services	2,026,848	107,519,546	372,658,230	545,000,000
% of Total	2.5	36.4	42.1	36.1
Affiliated hospitals and VA	8,444,496	28,186,260	122,834,070	458,000,000
% of Total	10	9.6	13.9	30.3
Grants and contracts	22,266,248	62,220,533	207,464,415	250,000,000
% of Total	27.7	21.1	23.5	16.5
Gifts and endowment	77,588	5,785,654	37,221,765	44,000,000
% of Total	0.1	2.0	4.2	2.9
Other (fees, labs)	9,375,758	17,912,482	62,447,471	48,000,000
% of Total	11.7	6.1	7.1	3.2
Total	80,365,148	295,067,538	884,617,716	1,512,000,000
Total (in 2016 dollars)	185,641,945	490,091,866	986,119,302	1,512,000,000

Note: Dollar amounts not adjusted for inflation except where noted.
Source: LCME Self-Study, 1984 to 2016, UA 073, InUI-Ar.

that have taken place since then. It also can help illustrate how the specific circumstances, some of which had persisted since the school's inception, combined with new demands and changes in the national health system to affect the school in the subsequent decades.

There have been three deans at IUSM since 1995. Robert Holden was the chair of Radiology when he became dean in 1995, but he served a relatively short term, only until 2000. He was succeeded by D. Craig Brater, a more traditional choice in that he had been chair of the Department of Medicine, like many of his predecessors. Brater served as dean until 2012, a term of service that was also more typical in length. The appointment of Jay Hess as his successor, a pathologist from the University of Michigan, was unusual in his medical specialization as well as in being an outside appointment, only the second time in the school's history.

By far the dominant feature in the history of the IU medical school since 1995 has been continued growth in all areas of activity: medical education, research, and clinical service. According to the self-study for the LCME accreditation in 2017, there were 2,085 full-time faculty (tenure line, clinical, and affiliate) in twenty-six departments teaching 1,350 students.[3] Graduate medical education had grown such that 235 residents were admitted in 2016, and research had grown to bring in $250 million in external funding in 2016, much of it in forty-one research centers and institutes. The two largest sources of revenue for the school were clinical practice ($545 million) and hospital affiliation ($458 million). Together, they represented two-thirds of the school's total revenue of $1.5 billion.

The main developments in the growth in operations during this time can be seen in the wealth of data that the medical school produced for accreditation and other reports. For example, table 12.1 lists sources of revenue for the IUSM for selected years as found in self-study reports for LCME accreditation. It shows growth in all activities but clearly not at the same rate.

Even though these are large aggregate figures, and there were significant changes in accounting during these three decades, especially for practice plans in the late 1980s, they offer useful snapshots that indicate broad changes. For example, according to LCME self-studies, the annual total revenue of the medical school (adjusted for inflation) increased 165 percent from 1983 to 1993 and tripled again from 1993 to 2016. The two specific categories that changed the most were the practice plans and hospital affiliations. As mentioned in the previous chapter, practice plans were a negligible part of reported income until Daly required that they appear in reports in fiscal 1989, and they immediately represented over 32 percent of income.[4] Thus, it inflated the overall revenue increase from FY 1984 to FY 1993. Excluding practice plan and hospital revenues, the medical school revenue increases were only 65 percent from FY 1984 to FY 1993. Once reported, however, practice plan income grew significantly in importance (to 43.5 percent in 2001[5]), but because there was even more rapid income growth from the new hospital arrangement, the practice plans declined to 36 percent of revenue in 2016. Affiliated hospital income was a stable contributor to medical school revenues throughout the 1980s and 1990s, at between 9 and 11.5 percent. Even after the Clarian agreement, hospital income rose slowly to 14 percent by 2008, but since then, it dramatically increased to over 30 percent of revenue by 2016.

The source of revenue that declined the most in importance during this time period was state and university contributions. Although steadily rising in dollar amount from $33 million in FY 1984 to $61 million in FY 1993 and $107 million in 2016, this represented only a 30 percent increase in constant dollars from 1984 to 1993, and 5 percent from 1993 to 2016. When compared to the rise in practice plan and hospital revenue, the percentage of revenue from state and university income therefore declined from almost 42 percent in 1984 to 20 percent in 1993 to only 4.6 percent in 2008, although there was a notable increase to 7 percent in 2016. Less dramatic but

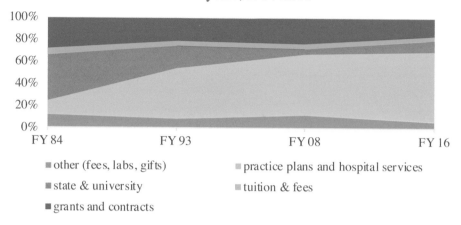

IUSM Revenue source as percentage of income,
selected years, 1984-2016

- other (fees, labs, gifts)
- state & university
- grants and contracts
- practice plans and hospital services
- tuition & fees

Figure 12.1. Revenue by Source as Percentage of Medical School Income. Source: figures from table 12.1.

noteworthy has been that external grants and contracts for research have been overshadowed in importance by practice plan and hospital income declining from 23.5 percent of all income in 2008 to 16.5 percent in 2016. In fact, adjusting for inflation, the dollar amount rose from $238.5 million to $250 million between 2008 and 2016. The steadiest share of income, although much lower as a percentage of the total, has been from tuition and fees. This was small comfort to students because these costs matched the 165 percent increase from 1983 to 1993 in overall revenue, and another 200 percent increase in the next twenty-three years (adjusted for inflation).

Figure 12.1 shows graphically these large increases in service income and a decline in state and local support, while the percentage provided from tuition income was surprisingly steady, matching the dramatic overall growth in income. It should be noted that this pattern largely followed national trends in medical school income, according to AAMC data.[6]

The broader underlying reason for the growth of all IU medical school activities was not simply the new medical discoveries and procedures that became available after the 1990s. It is true that such things as transplantation surgery and new imaging technology were widely adopted and costly, but there were other local influences that drove this growth, such as the cost of consolidation and expansion to compete with rival hospital systems in Indianapolis—St. Vincent, Community, and St. Francis—which challenged the supply of patients that the IU Medical Center had served for almost a century. From their beginning in the first part of the twentieth century, the

IU hospitals were established in response to state government demand for increased clinical care as well as for instruction of medical students and clinical research. The hospital merger and growth of practice plans were also responses to this new competition from other hospitals. A similar change took place in the other major demand on the medical school since its inception: the training of physicians.

Clarian Collaboration and Clinical Care

Even though there was expansion in all activities of the IU School of Medicine, after the agreement in 1995 between Riley and University Hospitals with Methodist Hospital, clinical practice and hospital administration grew the fastest. Clarian soon became a statewide hospital system, whereas the school maintained its agreements to staff the city, county, mental, and veterans hospitals, which also increased their services. The result was that growth and changes in clinical care overshadowed those in research and medical education. Despite the overall growth of activity, there were significant changes that varied in timing and impact.

When other hospitals became rivals to the medical center, this represented a major turning point in the history of the school and its hospitals. As this study has shown, for ninety years, the medical school was profoundly influenced by the hospitals it established for clinical care and instruction of students. From its start, in addition to training doctors, the new medical school was expected by the state legislature to increase the provision of medical care for citizens of the state. To this end, within fifteen years of its creation, the IU School of Medicine received funding to establish and run three new hospitals. Ever since, not only have the finances of the school been influenced by these and additional hospitals, but the careers of deans have also been determined as much by their ability to administer the school's hospitals as their expertise in patient care, medical research, or teaching. As mentioned in the previous chapter, the reason for the hospital consolidation in 1995 lay in local circumstances, which in turn were a reflection of broader national trends growing out of changes in the US health-care system during the last three decades of the twentieth century. Throughout the country, health-care institutions, including academic medical centers, increasingly promoted mergers at the local, regional, and national levels. Hospital consolidation frequently involved mergers with private hospitals after 1994.[7] In Indiana, the number of hospitals in local systems more than doubled from 2000 to 2008, rising from seventeen hospitals to thirty-seven.[8]

The man appointed dean in November 1995 who oversaw the IUSM hospital consolidation was radiologist Robert W. Holden. This continued the tradition of selecting internal candidates for dean, but it also reflected the growing importance of fields outside of the Department of Medicine, the home of most prior deans.[9] Medical specialization that had been driven a generation earlier by organ-specific disease pathways was now increasingly driven by technological innovations such as radiology and imaging that brought in insurance dollars. It was Holden's experience as a hospital administrator, having negotiated a recent agreement with Wishard Hospital, that helped him with the daunting task of building the Clarian alliance. The negotiations for the merger took two years, and the complicated process of implementation meant that clinical experiences were in flux for upper-level medical students and residents, as well as faculty and practitioners across the city.

Not surprisingly, the first step was to reduce administrative costs by eliminating duplication and consolidating operations such as finance, information systems, and human resources.[10] In addition a few new hospitals joined the system as provided for in the agreement. But "the most daunting task" according to the Handels and Kleit, who were part of the key leadership, was integrating clinical programs, which faced some obstacles. One was IU's tenure and promotion policies, which were crucial for faculty physicians, but there was even greater difficulty in what came to be called "cultural clashes." This meant physicians were not comfortable working in the consolidated setting, which turned out to depend on specialty. For example, those who were more successful, according to Handel et al., included heart disease, neurology, pathology, and radiology. There was also success in consolidating some features of medical education, such as combining all residencies and fellowships. More complicated but eventually also successful in monetary terms was the creation of a new, consolidated practice plan (IU Health Physicians) that allowed community physicians to be included. In FY 2012, the plan (whose name was shortened to IU Health) reported net patient revenue of $5.2 billion. The estimated combined equivalent for the merged systems in 1995 before consolidation was $862 million.[11]

The other hospitals in what had constituted the medical center also underwent significant change after the 1990s, including those not part of the new Clarian venture. For example, the VA Hospital expanded dramatically as a consequence of the Afghanistan and Iraq wars, beginning with a $25 million renovation in 2004 and the expansion of primary clinics in 2006.[12] Even more significant was the decision in 2009 by the Health and Hospital Corporation of Marion County to build a new Wishard Hospital in a location west of the IUPUI campus. Among other things, this required

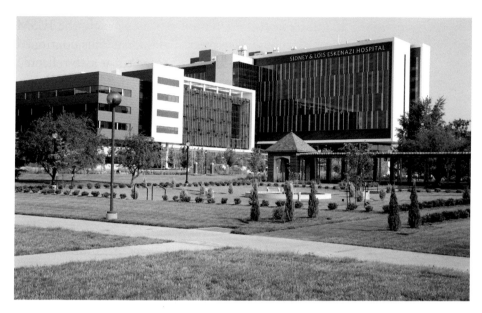

Figure 12.2. Eskenazi Health, new medical campus replacing old Wishard and City Hospitals, dedicated December 2013, Indiana University Health archives.

purchase of the site of Larue Carter Hospital, which relocated to a Veterans Hospital annex off campus. The new hospital also acquired and demolished the Union Building at the west end of the IUPUI campus and the abandoned State Health Department Building next to it. After a very successful bond issue, the new hospital was built, and following a major donation from Sidney and Lois Eskenazi, the name was changed to Eskenazi Health when it opened in 2013.[13] Most important for the medical school, and as mentioned earlier, the arrangements for staffing by the IUSM continued for both the VA and Eskenazi Health. Even though Riley Hospital was part of Clarian, it had its own funding resources (including a $40 million gift from the Simon family), which it used to build a $475 million, ten-story tower addition that began construction in 2006 and opened in phases beginning in 2010.[14]

Research

With the structure of the Clarian collaboration in place and the relationship fundamentally altered between hospitals and the medical school's clinical practice, D. Craig Brater was named dean in July 2000. Although this was a return to the practice of promoting the Chair of the Department of Medicine, Brater's appointment also suited his experience in expanding the research agenda of the school in the new era. Upon joining Indiana

University in 1986, he established the Division of Clinical Pharmacology within the Department of Medicine. Four years later, Brater became chairman of the Department of Medicine, the largest department at Indiana University and also the one most engaged in research.[15] Brater's support for research built upon the work of Ting-Kai Li and others described in the previous chapter, which in turn reflected a broader shift from organ-specific disease pathways to what was increasingly driven by molecular medicine as well as new technological imperatives.

Of necessity, the facilities on the campus expanded to accommodate the new research areas. In 1998, an addition to the VanNuys Medical Science Building was completed, and in September 2003, the Research II building was opened. This building included the Stark Neuroscience Research Center, established in 2000 thanks to a donation from Paul Stark and his wife. He was a Clinical Pharmacology faculty member who had been a leader of the clinical team at Eli Lilly and Company that developed Prozac. The center focused on applying advances in molecular, genetic, and imaging technologies to fundamental questions about brain function, dysfunction, and development.[16]

The hospital consolidation also led to reorganizing some existing research centers. For example, the Lilly Clinical Research Facility moved from Wishard to part of the new outpatient addition of University Hospital in 1998 despite concerns of some physicians that shifting from Wishard to University Hospital would hurt the quality of research.[17] Renovation to existing hospitals also facilitated the expansion of research. In 1999, the Roudebush VA Medical Center added additional space for IUSM faculty research, and the multimillion-dollar Riley Hospital Tower addition that opened in 2010, although primarily for clinical care, also housed significant pediatric research.

As key research projects grew, many were set up as research centers, often with external government and philanthropic support, as had been the case since the Krannert Center was created in the 1950s. That center and the Regenstrief Institute were primarily concerned with patient care, but after the 1980s, centers were established increasingly for laboratory bench research. For example, in 1997, both the IU Center for Aging Research and the National Center for Excellence in Women's Health opened, the latter with funding from the US Department of Health and Human Services. The following year, NIH funded the Mid-American Adolescent Sexually Transmitted Disease Cooperative Research Center to support research conducted not only by multiple departments at the medical school (biostatistics, pediatrics, and infectious diseases) but also partner universities (Northwestern, Louisiana State University, and the University of Iowa).[18] In

1999, the Core Center of Excellence in Molecular Hematology was funded by the National Institute of Diabetes and Kidney Diseases,[19] and the IUSM Division of Nephrology received significant NIH funding in 2003, leading to the establishment of the George M. O'Brien Research Center for Advanced Renal Microscopic Analysis.[20]

Several of these centers reflected the new emphasis on interdisciplinary medical research, which drew on faculty and resources from a number of departments and centers at the medical school. Indiana University also became increasingly involved with the application of scientific and medical research discoveries by establishing the Advanced Research and Technology Institute (ARTI) in 1996 to nurture research and economic development and to handle all IU-related intellectual property, trademarks, and business development.[21] As a result of these efforts, the medical school was able to establish significant research programs on the leading questions facing investigators as the school entered the twenty-first century, thanks to a combination of local and national funding. These included medical genetics, cancer, global health, translational research, and neuroscience.

One of the most dramatic new research initiatives was in the field of genetics and genomics, which was revolutionized by the discovery of the structure of DNA and the funding made available by the Human Genome Project of NIH. In the fall of 2000, the Lilly Endowment began discussions with the president of Indiana University about a grant in the field of biomedicine, a departure from the endowment's previous practice of avoiding support in health fields. Newly named Dean Brater of the School of Medicine suggested that funds go to support the rapidly growing field of genomics, and he and his new executive associate dean for Research Affairs, Ora Pescovitz,[22] appointed a steering committee of a dozen faculty to draft a proposal for the Indiana Genomics Initiative (INGEN) that was awarded a $105 million grant in December 2000, with another $50 million granted in 2003. This was the largest grant ever given by the Lilly Endowment and the largest received by the university. In addition to the unprecedented size, this grant was unusual in that it was not designated for a single research center; rather, the support went to six programs: genomics, bioinformatics, medical informatics, bioethics, education, and training. Nine service cores were also created to provide broad infrastructure support in such technical areas as genotyping, proteomics, imaging, and information technology.[23]

Another major area of research was cancer, and in the 1990s, researchers at the medical center took advantage of increased NIH funding from the National Cancer Institute (NCI) "Cancer Center Program," designed to provide combined support rather than funding multiple small, short-term projects at the same institution.[24] Individual researchers at IUSM such as

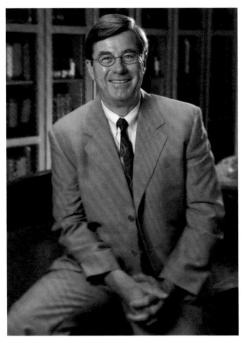
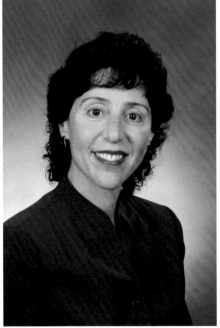

Lilly Endowment Inc. support to
Indiana's research infrastructure

INDIANA UNIVERSITY
SCHOOL OF MEDICINE

INCITE
2017
Collaborate and recruit talent to
build partnerships | $25 MILLION

PSI
2009
Recruited physician leaders to build
research programs | $60 MILLION

INGEN
2000
Built the foundation of cores, technologies
and talent to enable research | $155 MILLION

Figure 12.3a, b, & c. INGEN grant from Lilly Endowment, developed by IUSM dean Brater and associate dean for research Pescovitz, was largest gift in school's history. *Clockwise from top left*: D. Craig Brater (IUSM dean, 2000–2013), IUPUI Research and Creative Activity 28, no. 2 (spring 2006); Ora Pescovitz, IU Image Library; Lilly Endowment support to research infrastructure, 2000–17, "$25 million Lilly Endowment Grant to Help Grow Indiana's Life Science Sector," IUSM press release, July 12, 2017.

Lawrence Einhorn had been able to take advantage of NIH funding for cancer research, but the school did not apply to become a center until 1992, when a group led by Doris Merritt, who was then vice chancellor for Research at IUPUI, plus Victoria Champion from the School of Nursing and Steve Williams (who eventually became the director), submitted a proposal that was funded for a planning grant. This led to IU's designation as a clinical cancer center in 1999 with an initial grant of $6.3 million. At that time, there were only ten other clinical centers in the country, in addition to nine basic and forty comprehensive centers.[25] Funding has been renewed since then for this cross-department and cross-school center that involved faculty and resources from several schools, including Medicine, Nursing, Dentistry, Allied Health Sciences, Public Health, and schools of science at Purdue and IU-Bloomington.[26]

An important milestone in cancer research was marked with the opening of a new building on August 21, 2008, to house the renamed IU Simon Cancer Center. The new $150 million building received funding from numerous sources, including Indianapolis philanthropists Melvin and Bren Simon, who donated $25 million to the building project and $25 million to the research efforts at the center in memory of their son, Joshua Max Simon. This philanthropic gift followed a long history of charitable funding of hospitals at the medical school, which also included a $30 million gift in 2011 for the Eugene and Marilyn Glick Eye Institute.[27] The IU Simon Cancer Center marked an important departure because it was technically designated as an academic research center. Although patient care and some teaching were done, primarily in graduate medical education, the new addition marked the first hospital construction built without a primary focus on the teaching mission of the school.[28]

Another interdisciplinary center that benefitted from external funding was the IU Center for Global Health. Although the center was created in 2012, it housed the work that began over two decades earlier as a collaboration between IUSM and its partner medical school in Kenya.[29] There had been a few other overseas efforts involving medical school faculty besides the hospitals established in Europe during the two world wars. One exceptional postwar project was collaboration with the Jinnah Postgraduate Medical Center at the University of Karachi in Pakistan. Funded from 1957 to 1966 by a contract with the International Cooperation Administration (precursor to the US Agency for International Development), the program (originally known as the Basic Medical Sciences Institute) established a postgraduate master of science degree program, with the intent that graduates serve as faculty members at medical colleges throughout Pakistan.

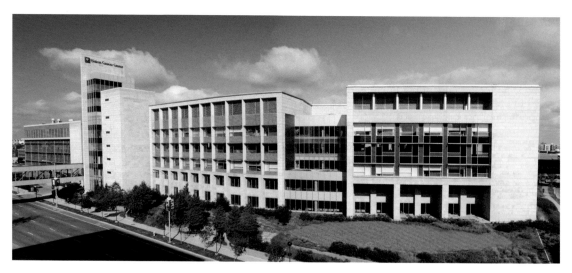

Figure 12.4. Indiana University Melvin and Bren Simon Cancer Center, a modern example of local philanthropy and NIH funding, IUSM Image Library.

Although it involved faculty from IUSM led by parasitologist William Hugh Headlee, the project was administered by the Office of the Dean of Research and Advanced Studies in Bloomington.[30]

The idea for the Kenya collaboration in the emerging field of global health was suggested by Bob Einterz (MD, 1981, from IUSM), who was hired after residency by the Department of Medicine in 1986 and immediately took a leave to work in Haiti. After his return, Einterz, along with Joe Mamlin (his division chief), and two other faculty members with experience in international health, Charles Kelley and Dave Van Reken, secured funding from the Moore Foundation in 1988 to visit sites in Nepal, Kenya, Ghana, and Liberia for potential collaboration with a medical school in a developing country to strengthen both medical schools and improve the health of the populations they served. The group selected as its partner Moi University in Western Kenya, where a new medical school was opened in 1990.

Activities began with a series of IUSM faculty members who made year-long visits, as well as visits from Kenyan medical faculty to Indiana, and regular rotations followed of medical students and residents between the two schools. The collaboration changed dramatically in the early 2000s in response to the AIDS epidemic that hit sub-Saharan Africa, including the Rift Valley in western Kenya. Eventually the program established a regional network of clinics under Kenya's Ministry of Health that were linked to

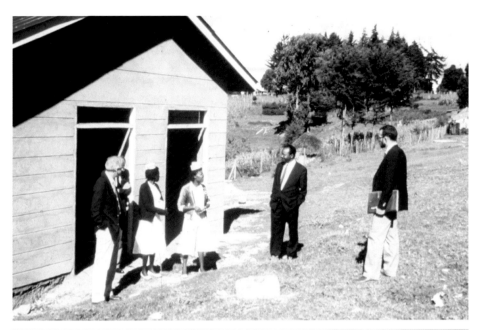

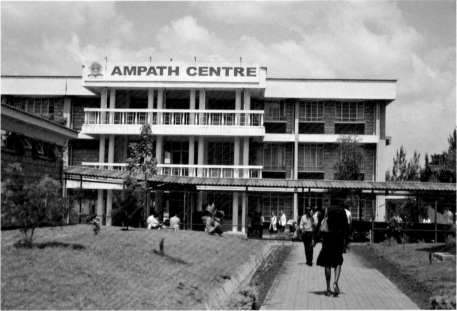

Figure 12.5a & b. IU-Kenya Program. (*top*) Bob Einterz and Joe Mamlin with local nurses and founding Dean Mengech of Moi University Medical School, during initial visit to Eldoret, Kenya in 1988, photo by Bob Einterz; (*bottom*) with funds secured by Indiana University, the AMPATH Centre was constructed in 2005 on the grounds of Moi Teaching and Referral Hospital to deliver clinical services for HIV infected individuals and house Moi University's research and training efforts to control the epidemic, photo by Bob Einterz.

expanded resources at the Kenyan medical school and its teaching hospital. In a dozen years, the number of HIV-positive patient enrollments exceeded two hundred thousand. The alliance among Moi Teaching and Referral Hospital, Moi University, and Indiana University also attracted several other North American medical schools as partners and became known as the Academic Model Providing Access to Healthcare (AMPATH). The program received additional funding from sources such as the Gates Foundation, the President's Emergency Plan for AIDS Relief (PEPFAR), and the US Agency for International Development (USAID). Although primarily focused on access to clinical care, the IU Center for Global Health became a significant research center in the field, and in 2014, it began offering a residency concentration in Global Health.[31]

Two other centers reflected the overlap of clinical practice and research, much like the cancer center. One was the Indiana Clinical and Translational Sciences Institute (CTSI), a statewide collaboration of Indiana University, Purdue University, and the University of Notre Dame, as well as public and private partnerships, whose goal was to "facilitate the translation of scientific discoveries in the lab into clinical trials and new patient treatments in Indiana and beyond." It was established in 2008 with a $25 million grant from the National Center for Advancing Translational Sciences (NCATS) of NIH, plus more than double that amount matched by the state, the universities, and other public and private partners. This research collaboration took advantage of NIH funding for a national network of 61 such centers. Another large-scale research endeavor taking part in a growing field was the Neuroscience Center that opened in 2013. It was the result of local investment by IU Health (which constructed the clinical building) and the IUSM (which financed the research building). It housed the Stark Neuroscience Center and was also a concrete example of the resources made possible by the hospital collaboration.

Because these centers were funded by grants, they were vulnerable to closure at the end of the grant period, or to being absorbed by other research centers. On the other hand, some centers grew to become departments. In the early 1980s, two biostatisticians joined the faculty of the Department of Medicine, and in 1984, they formed the Section of Biostatistics within the Regenstrief Institute for Health Care. The collaborative work soon extended beyond both the Department of Medicine and the School of Medicine. The section became an acknowledged division of the Department of Medicine in the late 1980s when the Center for Bioinformatics opened. In July 2011, it became a department within the newly established Fairbanks School of Public Health.[32]

Medical Education after 1995

After resisting efforts at consolidation in the early 1990s, the medical school's statewide system of medical education continued with few changes until 2006, when the decision was made to increase enrollment and add instruction of the third and fourth years at all centers. Unlike previous expansions that resulted from the state legislature calling for more physicians, according to Craig Brater, the impetus for this expansion came from an internal response to an AAMC statement on the physician workforce in 2006 that predicted physician shortages and called for an increase of 30 percent in medical school enrollment by 2015.[33] Even before the report was issued, other studies prompted Brater to ask his associate dean for education, Steve Leapman, to assemble a task force to study the situation in Indiana and issue a report. Members were drawn from the medical school faculty plus representatives from state agencies and associations. Their report of December 19, 2006, recommended that the medical school "boost its enrollment of medical students 30 percent to ensure an adequate supply of Indiana doctors in the coming two decades."[34]

The recommendation was to increase admissions gradually at the sites other than Indianapolis, because the eight other centers had the capacity to expand with relatively small additional cost as far as faculty or additional space. The plan was to add twelve students at a different center each year until by 2015, total enrollment would increase from 280 to 364 students. The centers would also add instruction for the third and fourth years by taking advantage of increased clinical instruction from physicians at hospitals in the communities around the state who were eager to expand their local medical centers.[35] The timing depended on funding, and when an appeal to the legislature for a $5 million budget increase was not successful, the implementation was slowed. Some funding came from Clarian/IU Health, but timing also depended on the retirement and hiring of new regional center directors. The South Bend campus added students in 2008, followed the next year by Northwest and Ft. Wayne. Then in 2010, Terre Haute expanded and implemented a program that had independently been planned with emphasis on rural medicine, and in 2012, the Bloomington and Lafayette programs expanded. Evansville and Muncie followed in the next two years, thus completing implementation of the program ahead of the 2015 deadline.[36]

Ironically, in 2013 Marian University in Indianapolis began teaching medical students at a new osteopathic medical school, directly contradicting the logic of the IU plan of statewide medical education.[37] Located just

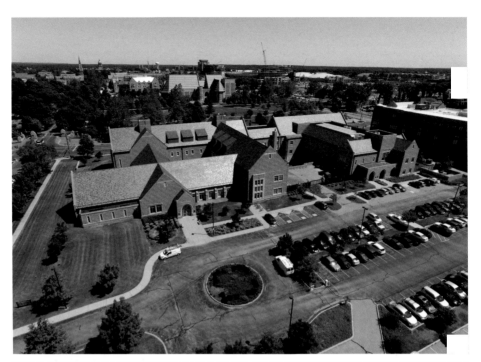

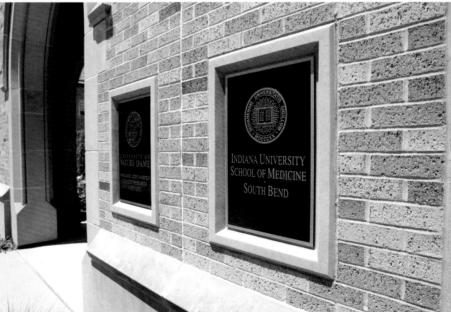

Figure 12.6a & b. IU South Bend medical center, operated in partnership with the University of Notre Dame and one of the statewide campuses of IUSM, IUSM Image Library.

Table 12.2 Some Features in Indiana Physician Workforce, AAMC 2015

	IN	Nat'l Avg	IN rank
No. of physicians (per 100,000)	222.6	265.5	38
Active female physicians	29.5%	33.3%	32
Medical students enrolled (public schools per 100,000)	21.4	17.5	21
Increase in medical student enrollment, 2004–2014	51.0%	33.4%	13
Medical students enrolled from in-state	71.8%	61.6%	19

Source: AAMC Facts & Figures 2016: Diversity in Medical Education, https://store.aamc.org/downloadable/download/sample/sample_id/210/

three miles from IUSM in downtown Indianapolis, this second medical school would not spread economic development or the training of physicians to another part of the state because of its location. It would also likely add to the number of graduating medical students leaving the state because it lacked adequate provisions for residencies in Indiana; it would not be part of a university with large laboratory resources in the sciences (although Marian University had a nursing school); and the school opened just as the IUSM completed its 30 percent increase in enrollment of entering students.

Statistics from the AAMC analysis of physician workforce in 2015 provide a larger context in which to view the impact of the expanded physician training at the IUSM and Marian University.

As table 12.2 shows, in 2014, Indiana had 222.6 physicians per 100,000 population, which ranked thirty-eighth in the country and lower than the national average of 265.5. The state ranked thirty-second in active female physicians, at 29.5 percent of all practitioners, slightly below the national average of 33.3 percent. On the other hand, the increased enrollment placed IUSM above the average of students enrolled per 100,000 inhabitants in public medical schools, 21.4 compared to 17.5. From 2004 to 2014, medical student enrollment in the state increased by over 50 percent, well above the national average increase of 33.4 percent. In keeping with tradition, Indiana was well above average in admitting students from in state (71.8 percent compared to 61.6 nationally), ranking it nineteenth in the country.[38]

There were some efforts to increase graduate medical education, with new residency and fellowship specialties made possible because of increased Medicare (and later Medicaid) funding and because of the expected need for more residency positions to accommodate the increase of MD graduates. This need had long been recognized as a problem. In fact, as shown in an earlier chapter, the statewide plan had originally been proposed to develop additional sites for graduate medical education.

Table 12.3. First-Year Residencies Filled in Indiana, 1967–1971, 2000–2016

Year	Total	Indpls IUSM	%	Other Indpls	%	Other IN	%	IUSM Grad	Resident/ Grad Ratio
				First-Year Residents in Indiana					
1967	117	66	56.4	29	24.8	22	18.8		
1968	139	78	56.1	31	22.3	30	21.6		
1969	126	57	45.2	34	27.0	35	27.8		
1970	145	57	39.3	44	30.3	44	28.3		
1971	180	93	51.7	43	23.9	44	24.4		
2000	319	191	60.0	61	19.1	67	21.0	264	1.21
2001	311	198	63.7	56	18.0	57	18.3	261	1.19
2002	305	183	60.0	63	20.7	59	19.3	273	1.12
2003	297	188	63.3	60	20.2	49	16.5	262	1.13
2004	308	203	65.9	57	18.5	48	15.6	258	1.19
2005	304	200	65.8	57	18.8	47	15.5	262	1.16
2006	309	200	64.7	61	19.7	48	15.5	258	1.20
2007	322	210	65.2	65	20.2	47	14.6	276	1.17
2008	327	208	63.6	67	20.5	52	15.9	260	1.26
2009	326	215	66.0	66	20.2	45	13.8	267	1.22
2010	318	203	63.8	65	20.4	50	15.7	264	1.20
2011	312	206	66.0	64	20.5	42	13.5	299	1.04
2012	360	229	63.6	74	20.6	57	15.8	291	1.24
2013	368	227	61.7	74	20.1	65	17.7	302	1.22
2014	377	235	62.3	78	20.7	64	17.0	298	1.27
2015	363	231	63.6	72	19.8	64	17.6	313	1.16
2016	373	235	63.0	76	20.4	62	16.6	319	1.17

Sources: IU Medical Center Annual Report, 1975–76; National Resident Matching Program, Report Archives, http://www.nrmp.org/report-archives/; AAMC enrollments, graduates data, https://www.aamc.org/data/facts/; IUSM, Scope, 2003–2006.

As table 12.3 shows, although the number of first-year residencies around the state increased following the statewide expansion, the predominance of positions in Indianapolis not only continued but increased and remained over 80 percent of the total.

Looking at graduate medical education from the national perspective, table 12.4 shows that the number of residents and fellows in Indiana was 21.4 per 100,000, well below the national average of 36.9, ranking Indiana thirty-ninth in the country.

Nor was the recent trend very encouraging. There was only a 9.1 percent increase in residency and fellow slots in Indiana from 2004 to 2014, compared to the national average increase of 14.4 percent, ranking the

Table 12.4. Residencies and Physician Practice, AAMC 2015

	IN	Nat'l Avg	IN rank
Number of residents and fellows (per 100,000)	21.4	36.9	39
Increase in residents and fellows, 2004–2014	9.1%	14.4%	44
Residents and fellows who had trained in-state	51.8%	38.7%	6
Practicing physicians who did residency/fellowship in-state	55.1%	47.2%	7

Source: AAMC, "2015 State Physician Workforce Data Book: Indiana Physician Workforce Profile," https://www.aamc.org/system/files/2019–08/indiana2015.pdf.

state forty-fourth. However, Indiana did a good job of retaining medical students, residents, and fellows who trained in the state. It ranked sixth in active physicians who received their MD in-state (51.8 percent versus 38.7 percent nationally) and seventh in practicing physicians who had been residents and fellows in the state (55.1 percent versus 47.2 percent).[39] Because Indiana lagged behind other states in increasing residency opportunities, this suggests that the focus of Indiana legislators and the IU Medical School on increasing medical school enrollment, to the exclusion of increasing in-state residencies) was successful as indicated by the high return rate of graduates to set up practice in the state.

As far as the organization and curriculum of the medical school, there were several changes after 1995, such as the addition of a new clinical department of Emergency Medicine in 1999, which had been preceded by a new residency program in 1997. But two changes involved significant reorganization of and an addition to the structure of the medical school in allied health and public health. As mentioned in earlier chapters, various health-related programs had grown up over the years since the Second World War on five different IU campuses, which were administered first in a Division and then a School of Allied Health Sciences. The administration and budget were separate but still technically under the IU School of Medicine, referred to as a "school within a school." The impetus for reorganization came first from Mark Sothman, who became Allied Health dean in 1997 and was concerned with the cost of laboratory and technology programs, which had limited numbers of students, because of equipment restrictions and the need for field experience placement demanded by accrediting agencies.[40]

In 2000, a study committee was created to recommend guidelines for determining which programs to continue and which might be transferred to other units. One new program in Health Information Administration was transferred to a new School of Informatics. Two programs in Health Science Education were discontinued when the School of Education declined to take

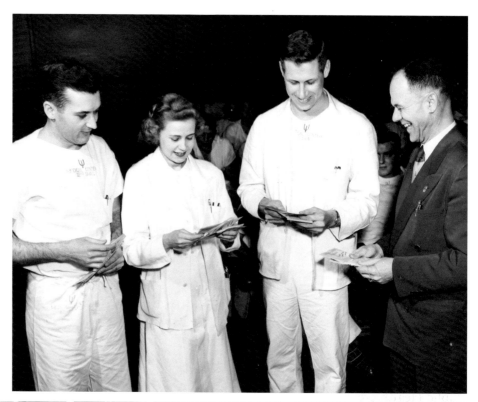

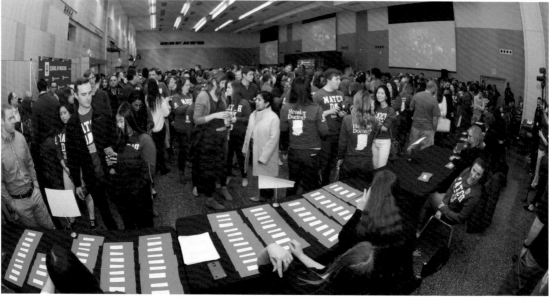

Figure 12.7a & b. Residents' match day, as well as the nature of IUSM students, has changed dramatically since the 1950s: (*top*) Residents match day, 1951, IUPUI image UA024_000361; (*bottom*) residents match day, 2019, IUSM Image Library.

them. The remaining programs were divided between the departments of the School of Medicine and the School of Allied Health which became a separate school in 2002 and was renamed Health and Rehabilitation Sciences in 2003. The latter included Occupational Therapy, Nutrition and Dietetics, Physical Therapy, and a recently added Therapeutic Outcomes Research degree program. The medical school retained the most popular programs closely associated with three departments. Pathology and Laboratory Medicine took over the BS in Cytotechnology, the BS in Clinical Laboratory Science, and the AS Certificate in Histotechnology. Emergency Medicine took over the AS in Paramedic Science; and Radiology took over the AS in Radiography, the BS in Medical Imaging, the BS in Nuclear Medicine, and the BS in Radiation Therapy.[41] In addition, the BS in respiratory therapy was taken over by Clarian/IU Health.

Public Health was the other new school created after the 1990s, after first being under the administration of the IUSM. As earlier chapters of this book have shown, the medical school's work in public health goes back even further, almost to its beginnings and the efforts of Dean Charles Emerson's Social Services Department. But the results can best be described as intermittent. The last initiative was a proposal in 1947 to establish a school of public health based around the medical school's Department of Public Health created in the 1930s, when the state Department of Health moved to the campus. That proposal was rejected by the IU trustees. The idea was not revived until over forty years later, although in the interim, the School of Public and Environmental Affairs (SPEA), with programs in Bloomington and Indianapolis, had filled the vacuum somewhat by developing a number of health-related programs in the 1980s, including public and environmental health as well as health administration.[42]

In 1993, Gerald Bepko, chancellor of IUPUI, secured the agreement of Dean Walter Daly to establish an ad hoc committee on a School of Public Health to explore "the creation of explicitly designated public health programs." He pointed out that because Indiana was surrounded by states with schools of public health, not only were people going elsewhere to obtain public health degrees, but there was also fear that "other universities . . . such as the University of Michigan or the University of Minnesota . . . will open programs in Indianapolis."[43] Committee members were drawn from several interested schools besides Medicine, including Nursing, Dentistry, Law, and SPEA, and the first meeting was held on February 3, 1994.

The initial strategy was to utilize existing resources in eight schools, including the Bloomington campus, with the first step to establish a graduate degree program. In 1997, a Department of Public Health was created in the

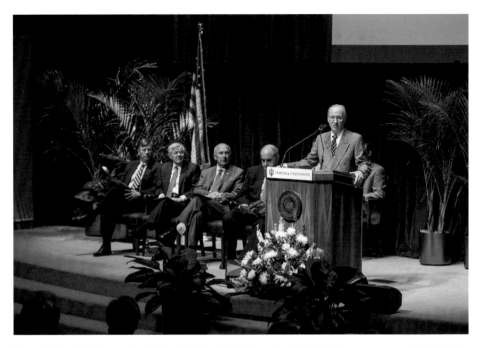

Figure 12.8. IUPUI Chancellor Charles R. Bantz (IUPUI chancellor, 2003–15) at announcement of Fairbanks Public Health School, September 27, 2012, with (*seated l. to r.*) IUSM dean D. Craig Brater, Fairbanks Foundation CEO Len Betley, IU trustee Phil Eskew, and IU president Michael McRobbie, photo by Chris Meyer/Indiana University.

School of Medicine, with Stephen Jay, a pulmonologist in the Department of Medicine, as chair. Later that year, a master's of public health (MPH) degree was approved. The first MPH students graduated in 2001, and the program was accredited the following year. Additional graduate degrees were added in subsequent years (e.g., a PhD in epidemiology in 2009), and health programs from SPEA were relocated so that in 2012, a separate School of Public Health was created, thanks also to a $20 million grant by the Fairbanks Foundation.[44] At the same time, the university announced that the School of Health, Physical Education and Recreation in Bloomington would be renamed the IU School of Public Health–Bloomington, with a "rural community focus." Thus was culminated almost a century of work in the field dating back to the efforts begun by Dean Charles Emerson.

In addition to these changes in public health and allied health sciences, plus the creation of an Emergency Medicine department, the IUSM responded to the impact of growing specialization by new efforts to attract students to primary care. Continuing throughout the school's history, IUSM struggled to find new ways to meet the primary care physician shortage, particularly in rural areas. The school found that despite the changes in the Indiana Plan, with an increased focus on statewide and primary care training and more graduates, more than one-fourth of Indiana's counties still had a shortage of primary care physicians. As a result, in 1997, a new program of rural health was announced involving Indiana State University and the IUSM site at Terre Haute. It differed from earlier programs by recruiting and supporting students from the undergraduate level through medical school and residency programs.[45]

The IUSM also expanded primary care training that continued development of the field of family medicine that had begun in the 1980s. One new program aimed at increasing provision of outpatient care beyond the partnerships with Wishard and the Regenstrief Clinics.[46] In July 1998, the Indiana University Methodist Family Practice Center allowed faculty to provide care and teaching experiences in family medicine without relying on outside providers. This program worked with the academic resources of the IUSM's Department of Family Medicine to restructure the Family Practice residency program and enhance training opportunities for residents and medical students in comprehensive care. As opposed to earlier internist or general medicine specialist, the family medicine perspective saw physicians as "involved with the patient's family and serving as the patient's advocate in all health-related matters," according to Deborah I. Allen, the Otis R. Bowen professor of family medicine and chair of the IU Department of Family Medicine.[47] These earlier and new programs led to nearly one quarter of the graduating class entering family practice residencies by the late 1990s, the tenth highest percentage in the nation.[48]

How did these changes affect the students who enrolled at the IUSM? The expansion of enrollment maintained the changed demographics that began in the 1980s. As figure 12.9 shows, in 2006, on the eve of the most recent expansion, the number of women graduates at the medical school had increased to half, 131 women out of a total of 261 graduates.

The percentage of students at IUSM indicating non-white ethnicity continued to grow with a record of over 30 percent of admissions in 2007, according to an AAMC report in 2007.[49] Most were Asian (20 percent), with black (5.4) and Hispanic (5.1) much lower. By 2015, black matriculants had doubled to 9.3 percent thanks to new diversity initiatives, additional financial support, and a conscious effort to recognize and publicize these gains.[50] Minority groups other than African American also increased, such that white admissions that year were less than 60 percent.[51] The school still drew nearly 90 percent of its student population from the Hoosier state but continued to gradually attract more out-of-state students each year.[52]

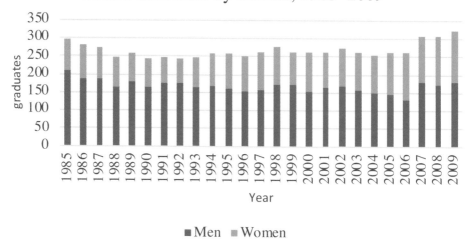

Figure 12.9. IUSM Graduates by Gender, 1985–2009, from Potter, "Learning Human Anatomy."

A final example of an experience that IUSM students shared with fellow students nationally was, unfortunately, the struggle with an increasing debt burden. Paying for medical school had always been a problem, but by the 1970s, it had grown to the point where in 1973–74, IUSM distributed scholarships to eight hundred fifty medical students. The largest, the IU Distinguished Scholarship ($4,000), was won by Linda Quinn, a student near the top of her graduating class who in total earned more than $6,000 in scholarships. Despite these awards, she anticipated owing more than $40,000 at graduation. By the 1990s, increased diversity and rising costs led to even greater need. IUSM records show that for the 1993–94 school year, of the 1,228 enrolled medical students, 685 requested financial aid, roughly evenly divided among students from each year. That year, 623 students actually received aid, with slightly more students in their junior and senior year receiving aid than freshman or sophomores. The average financial aid request was $2,483, although financial aid packages ranged from $500 to $6,100. This assistance targeted keeping talented Hoosier students in the state, because national recruiting was challenging. Recruiting a more diverse student body created more need for financial aid funds, but rather than simply distributing funds broadly, IUSM targeted large scholarships to attract top students while also working to increase the average award amounts. Daly made raising scholarship funds a priority by appealing to alumni and retiring faculty.[53]

Table 12.5. Cost of Tuition, IUSM 1984–2016

	1984–85	1993–94	2007–08	2016–17
In-state	3,600	8,170	25,140	34,019
Constant 2016 dollars	8,316	13,563	28,031	34,019
% increase 1984–85		63	237	309
Out-of-state	8,500	18,685	42,130	56,973
Constant 2016 dollars	19,635	31,017	46,974	56,973
% increase 1984–85		58	139	190
% increase overall IUSM revenue		164	431	714
% increase in US inflation		43	107	131

Source: LCME Self-Study, 1987, 1994, 2008, 2017, UA 073, InUI-Ar.

The obvious immediate cause of the problem was the increase in tuition that drove the average debt of students to more than $105,000 upon graduation by 2004. Table 12.5 shows that the rate of increase in in-state tuition increased at double or triple the rate of overall inflation in the US economy from 1984 to 2016.

Although this was not nearly as much as the overall revenues of the medical school, which increased at four to six times the national inflation average, it was small comfort to students. Among other things, this dramatic increase in cost for medical students continued the tradition of moonlighting in the attempt to make ends meet. Beyond the stress, the increased debt threatened the critical goals of increasing diversity and number of primary care physicians.[54]

One unexpected result of IUSM's regional campus system was to provide an incubator for curriculum innovation thanks to the smaller class sizes, which allowed for experimentation in medical education. On the Gary campus, for example, the pedagogy of problem-based learning was adopted, whereby students worked in small groups supervised by faculty facilitators.[55] An even more important pedagogical change in the instruction of all medical students after 1995 was the introduction of a competency-based curriculum in 1999. The roots of this change lay in the recognition that physician training occurred in a broader social context of growing awareness of medical mistakes and increasing distrust of physicians' authority.[56] Critics feared that medical schools had forgotten their "core mission" as a result of the expansion and emphasis on research and a corporate mentality.

In an effort to address these and other problems, the IUSM attempted what supporters termed a "second revolution."[57] Even before the hospital merger, the school began a thorough review of the curriculum. In 1992, faculty teams developed a curriculum called "The Indiana Initiative." It was based on Brown University's pioneering model of nine competencies, which moved away from the traditional subject-oriented curriculum to an integrated learning experience that emphasized not only basic clinical skills and medical diagnosis but also the social and community contexts of health care, moral reasoning and ethical judgment, and effective communication. Results elsewhere indicated that students judged to be deficient in certain competencies did not reflect this academically. This new system attempted to measure nonacademic components of the medical school experience, which some researchers called a "hidden" curriculum that continued even into residency.[58] Rather than being a replacement, the new curriculum was first implemented as an additional, parallel one at IUSM during the 1999–2000 academic years, with the first class to graduate under this system being the class of 2003.[59]

Although the university attempted to build support for the program, many faculty and students thought the new competencies were too subjective and difficult to assess. For example, students generally recognized the importance of the new curriculum goals, but some were concerned by the faculty's inconsistent knowledge of the competencies and a lack of sufficient communication about them. Some faculty members raised questions about how to document competency-related deficiencies and requirements of new routines and technologies. Other faculty challenged the potential underlying messages sent to students. Richard B. Gunderman, professor of radiology and pediatrics at IU School of Medicine, who had written widely on medical education, argued that "focusing on basic competencies can lead to the neglect of higher levels of educational excellence, such as expertise and mastery. By tending to promulgate a single set of standards for all programs, we may undercut educators' and learners' appreciation for innovation, style, and the love of surprises."[60] After a decade of implementation, IUSM researchers found that the curriculum was "well established and part of our institutional culture." To a certain extent, however, the critics were proved correct. Although most of the competency-related deficiencies were readily identifiable and correctable, deficiencies in professionalism and self-awareness were especially challenging.[61]

Conclusion

The period following the Clarian consolidation marked a new era for the IUSM in obvious ways, such as the administration of its own hospitals, as well as in some unanticipated ways, such as the consolidation of clinical services and employment of faculty. Its greatest impact was the result of the long-developing increased role of clinical practice in the responsibilities of the medical school faculty, which overshadowed even the dramatic rise in research during the previous decades. Despite these trends, the teaching mission of the school continued to adapt to the demand for more physicians who were trained in the changing technical and social skills needed to practice medicine in the twenty-first century. More will be said in the chapter that follows about broader changes after the mid-1990s, which includes, above all, that the size and complexity of the medical school and health care in the United States were beyond the predictability or control of a dean, university president, or state legislature. At the same time, the school strove to meet the challenge set forth by William Lowe Bryan in his January 22, 1903, presidential inaugural address, which called for "opening paths to those who care for human life."

13

The Case of IU Medical School

The history of the Indiana University School of Medicine has been part of the larger history of health care in the United State for more than a century. Like over one hundred other medical schools, IUSM grew dramatically in many ways since its beginning: the number of students it trained, the number of patients it cared for, and the research it conducted, all in response to the underlying scientific and social developments that have made health care almost 20 percent of the American economy. Given this larger context, it is therefore not surprising to find many similarities in the histories of medical schools. A number of these were deliberately self-imposed, because when IU's medical school was started at the beginning of the twentieth century, it joined other schools in the Association of American Medical Colleges, which had been formed to establish standards for medical education reform that resulted in similar admission requirements, as well as length and kind of instruction. In the 1950s, these standards became both more detailed and better enforced with the establishment of accreditation by the Liaison Committee for Medical Education, including regular site visits.

IU's medical school offers a case study of these broader, common changes, but like other schools, it also responded to these circumstances with its own local resources, individuals, and institutions that gave it a unique history and character. This book has shown the combination of broader influences and local differences in that history, beginning with the establishment of IUSM by multiple partners and continuing with the many developments that shaped the school's evolution. There are a number of themes that are helpful in understanding this complicated history and perhaps the future direction of the institution. First is that the school has roots that go back well into the nineteenth century. The university usually cites 1903 as the beginning of the medical school, when its new president,

William Lowe Bryan, called for the establishment of "a Medical Department with a two-year course of instruction." But it was not until 1908 that IU began offering a full four years of medical education when it took over the two largest medical schools in Indianapolis. The beginning of these private schools was the work of physicians returning to the city after the Civil War who saw the need, as John Bobbs put it, for "a medical school in Indiana . . . established on a scale and basis to compete in excellence, in eminence, in every appliance and means of instruction, with the very best schools of the age."

These proprietary schools grew and trained many of the physicians in the state but ultimately joined IU in order to keep pace with the rapid changes in medicine by the beginning of the twentieth century. In the process, and despite many efforts such as partnership with the City Hospital of Indianapolis that reinforced a working relationship with many of the physicians of the city, the medical education they offered fell short of the rising national standards for admissions and greater scientific and clinical training. Even though after 1908 the medical school's focus quickly became more statewide, and eventually national and international, its base remains to this day in an urban setting with close relationships to physicians and hospitals of its home city.

The consequences of the location of the medical school are important to understanding its history. To paraphrase a common saying, geography (along with demography) is destiny. Soon after 1908, the IUSM was the only medical school in a fairly populous state, located in the capital and biggest city. This gave the school the advantage of access to the largest concentration of both government and private resources for support, as well as patients in hospitals. The monopoly on medical education, however, also brought with it the burden of meeting expectations for training physicians. Indiana was not unique in this respect. Both Washington state and Colorado, among others, had similar responsibilities, but Indiana was perhaps most distinctive in how it increased the number of students to meet the demand for more doctors. By the time of the 2017 IUSM entering class of 353 students, the medical school of the University of Colorado admitted 183 students, the University of Washington admitted 270.[1] The means of achieving this growth in Indiana varied, from using facilities in Bloomington and Indianapolis to increasing and consolidating instruction at a larger medical campus in Indianapolis, and then the adoption of the statewide medical education system.

The medical school's response to its next most important obligation, clinical care, was also shaped to a great extent by local setting and resources. From its beginning, the school inherited a close relationship with the City Hospital, and it soon built three new hospitals and relocated its instructional building to a campus adjacent to its city partner. Both the IU facilities and adjacent hospitals grew in the last half of the twentieth century, and the medical school took increasing responsibility for staffing the adjacent institutions (City Hospital, a VA facility, and Larue Carter Hospital). This created a large medical center that the school and university proudly advertised as providing large and growing health-care resources to the state. One of the consequences, however, of the increased clinical responsibilities of the faculty at IU medical school was a threat by the end of the twentieth century to the Flexner reforms a hundred years before, which called for full-time research and teaching faculty. Patient care to instruct students was one thing, but as the school followed the national trend of relying more and more on clinical care for income, the clinical responsibilities of faculty competed with their time for teaching and research.

Another mixed result of the addition of hospitals to the medical school was that all the deans since Emerson found themselves extensively preoccupied by hospital administration. Emerson was an early and obvious casualty of the demands of balancing the needs of running large patient care facilities while integrating the newly acquired medical schools and upgrading medical instruction. Although subsequent deans avoided the dramatic showdown that befell Emerson, they all spent increasing time with legislators, architects and contractors, department chairs, and hospital staff, and their time for teaching and research dwindled. From this longer historical perspective, the creation of Clarian/IU Health from Riley, University, and Methodist Hospitals helped alleviate this problem, although at the expense of loss of control.

The establishment of the IU Medical Center would never have been possible without generous philanthropic support, another continuing theme in the history of the medical school. Initially focusing on hospital care, the tradition established by the Longs, the friends of Riley, and the Colemans (among others) continued and grew in the second half of the twentieth century and beyond. Although never sufficient to fully sustain these clinical care facilities, the philanthropic support was crucial in persuading the state government and national sources to fund the school. Moving into the last half of the twentieth century, philanthropy expanded to support medical research. Even more in need of "pump priming," research by the IUSM faculty relied on the resources of the Krannerts, Regenstrief, Showalter, and Walther to get them started on projects that eventually were competitive for national funding. To be fair, this was less in response to local demand and more the result of changing professional incentives and taking advantage of new external resources following the Second World War, especially from national foundations and NIH. The dramatic growth in obtaining external funding enabled the IU Medical Center to add major research contributions to its long established record of education and clinical care.

A great deal of attention in the history of medical schools has been paid to the role of deans. At IUSM, there have been only nine since Allison Maxwell's brief three-year tenure starting in 1908. Most have served from ten to fifteen years, which is longer than the national average (5.1 years between 1940 and 1992[2]), and many had similar background and training. For example, they usually had an Indiana connection of residence and/or training at the medical school; after Emerson (and until the current dean), the deans were promoted from within, and from the beginning all have been white males. Yet this history has certainly shown that deans had differences in style as well as administrative achievements. Charles Emerson's social conscience was obvious from his support of the Social Service Department. Willis Gatch was probably the best physician and surgeon, at least in the sense that he practiced the longest. Van Nuys was likely the best administrator, considering the times and circumstances when he worked and despite his lack of length and breadth of experience when he began. Glenn Irwin may have been the best liked, and Walter Daly was clearly the most historically conscious.

Looking at the deans from a broader perspective, despite the culture and tradition of centralized authority in medical schools, there were conflicting influences on the deans' power, especially after the mid-twentieth century. At IUSM, the dean's independence from university administration was reinforced by the location of the medical school fifty miles away from the main campus at Bloomington. In addition, the private medical schools that Indiana University took over brought with them a tradition of independence that continued because as a professional school, there were other authorities besides university administration to which the medical school answered for accreditation. But the dean's influence over the school itself was reduced as the sheer size of the operations of the school grew, especially after the Second World War, supported by greatly increased outside sources of revenue especially for research and clinical care. This added further to the number of those to whom the deans were responsible besides the IU administration. At the same time it increased the independence of the faculty, who were able to obtain their own funding from outside sources.

A final comment is warranted on the subject of missed opportunities. The two that seem most obvious are the delay in establishing sufficient and consistent support for public health, and the failure to consolidate medical instruction in one location. There is probably little disagreement that the medical school should have been earlier and more persistent in its commitment to public health. But there is less consensus whether the decisions concerning where to locate medical instruction were the optimal ones. It took fifty years to end the Bloomington and Indianapolis division, despite steady criticism from many sides. Equally important was the decision to not create a second medical school and instead to distribute medical instruction statewide. The latter question is likely to continue as a topic of discussion, because the recent creation of a second medical school in Indiana has ended IUSM's obligations tied to its monopoly of medical education in the state.

As mentioned at the opening of this study, there are many obvious ways of seeing the success of the IU School of Medicine. Missed opportunities notwithstanding, the main goal of this account has not been to make judgments but rather present an overall history of the school as a record to inform and help guide its future.

NOTES

1. The Indiana Way of Medical Education

1. Ludmerer, *Learning to Heal*, 3–4.
2. Ibid., 7–8.
3. Flexner, *Medical Education in the United States and Canada*, 221–22.
4. Liaison Committee on Medical Education (LCME), "Report: Indiana University School of Medicine," October 21–23, 1954, UA 073, Indiana University School of Medicine Records, 1848–2005, University Library Special Collections and Archives, University Library, Indiana University Purdue University Indianapolis (location of all subsequent LCME reports and studies).
5. Myers, *Medical Education*, 203.
6. Ibid.
7. LCME Report 1954; LCME Report, 1963.
8. Myers, *Medical Education*, vii–viii.
9. Woodburn, *History of Indiana University, 1820–1902*.
10. "The IU Physician" (Indiana University School of Medicine, 1978); Daly, "Indiana University Medical Center"; "A Brief History of the Indiana University School of Medicine."
11. Clark, *Indiana University*, 2: 65–100; 3: 381–438; Gray, *IUPUI*, 13–20.
12. Rothstein, *American Medical Schools*, 10.
13. It is noteworthy that for his multivolume history of Indiana University, Clark regretted not being able to include footnotes because "the text would run to such excessive length."

2. Learning and Practicing Medicine in the Nineteenth Century

1. Bobbs, "President's Address," 11–12.
2. Sulgrove, *History of Indianapolis and Marion County*, 281–82; Brayton, "Development of Medical Education in Indiana," 37.
3. Ludmerer, *Learning to Heal*, 14–15; Rothstein, *American Medical Schools*, 97.

4. In addition to Rothstein, *American Medical Schools*, 67–116, and Ludmerer, *Learning to Heal*, 9–28, see the other standard historian on this subject, Warner, *The Therapeutic Perspective*, and Warner, "The Maturation of American Medical Science."

5. Rothstein, *American Medical Schools*, 48, 57.

6. Rothstein, *American Medical Schools*, 24. For background, see Rosenberg, *The Care of Strangers*.

7. Cohen, *The Shaping of American Higher Education*, 58–61; Rothstein, *American Medical Schools*, 88, 94.

8. Sectarian physicians, along with associated organizations such as schools, societies, and journals, offered medical therapies not used by other sects or those offered by lay practitioners and people trained at sectarian medical schools. Allopathy was a system of medical practice that aimed to combat disease by use of remedies producing effects different from those produced by the target disease. "Is Medicine Attractive to Scholarly Men?" *JAMA* 41, no. 1 (August 1903): 317; "Indiana as a Factor in Medical Education: A Medical Department for the State University," *Indiana Medical Journal* (August 1903): 66; Ackerknecht, "Diseases in the Midwest"; Russo, "Pioneer Medicine in Indiana," 4–5; Starr, *The Social Transformation of American Medicine*, 7.

9. Anderson, *Internal Medicine Iowa*, 4–5; Pickard, *The Midwest Pioneer*, 35.

10. Rothstein, *American Medical Schools*, 15–29, 39–44.

11. Bobbs, "An Introductory Lecture," 13; Starr, *The Social Transformation of American Medicine*, 31, 37; Haber, *Quest for Authority*, 93.

12. Bobbs, "An Introductory Lecture," 11; Curran, *Introductory Lecture*, 16; Anderson, *Internal Medicine*, 4; Lears, *Fables of Abundance*, 41–43.

13. Myers, *Medical Education*, 14–17, 98–100; Smith, "'The Diploma Peddler,'" 26–47; Starr, *The Social Transformation of American Medicine*, 37, 58–59.

14. Stevens, "Synopsis of Early Laws," 21–22; Manhart, "The Indiana Central Medical College," 105–22.

15. Myers, *Medical Education*, 2–3; Zerfas, "Medical Education in Indiana," 139–48; Russo, "Pioneer Medicine in Indiana," 153–56. The chart was done by Howard R. Patton and first appeared in *Arbutus* 1935, p. 319. Some errors were analyzed by Rice, "One Hundred Years of Medicine in Indianapolis," 255–57.

16. Myers, *Medical Education*, 18–25; Brayton, "Development of Medical Education in Indiana," 16–19. For more, see documentaion for a recent historical marker for the medical school, accessed April 17, 2018, https://www.in.gov/history/markers/4403.htm.

17. Myers, *Medical Education*, 24–25; Brayton, "Development of Medical Education in Indiana," 18.

18. Rothstein, *American Medical Schools*, 71–72, 105–7; Ludmerer, *Learning to Heal*, 75–79; Warner, "The Fall and Rise of Professional Mystery," 310–41.

19. Kaufman, *American Medical Education*, 154–63; Rothstein, 144–49; Smiley, "History of the Association of American Medical Colleges 1876–1956," 512–25.

20. Sulgrove, *History of Indianapolis and Marion County*, 276.

21. Founders included Thomas B. Harvey, Robert N. Todd, George W. Mears, and William B. Fletcher. See *Proceedings of the Indiana Medical College*, April 29, 1869; May 1, 1869; May 6, 1869; May 15, 1869; May 17, 1869; June 3, 1869; June 30, 1869; July 20, 1869; August 3, 1869, UA 073, Indiana University School of Medicine Records, 1848–2005, University Library Special Collections and Archives, University Library, Indiana University Purdue University Indianapolis (hereafter referred to as InUI-AR). See also Daly, "The Origins of President Bryan's Medical School," 267.

22. *Proceedings of the Indiana Medical College*, July 20, 1869, UA 073, InUI-AR.

23. Badertscher, "A New Wishard Is on the Way," 348–49.

24. By the time the Bobbs Free Dispensary opened, William Fletcher, another prominent Indiana physician, founded the Indianapolis City Dispensary in 1870. Then in 1876, Indiana Medical College offered to operate it, but the city refused to give the college control because officials believed that the conditions for operation stipulated by Fletcher were too restrictive. *Proceedings of the Indiana Medical College*, January 1, 1872, UA 073, InUI-Ar; "Opening of the Indiana Medical College," 158–61; K. M. McDonell, "The Indianapolis City Hospital, 1833–1866," 1–2.

25. *Proceedings of the Indiana Medical College*, July 20, 1869, UA 073, InUI-Ar; Bobbs, "Address at the Opening of the Indiana Medical College," 15–17. In addition to Badertscher, there are many accounts of these institutions. See Dunn, *Greater Indianapolis*, 549–50; Rice, "History of the Medical Campus" 4: 91–93; Myers, *Medical Education*, 47; McDonell, "Care of the Sick Poor of Indianapolis to 1915," 2; Hale, Caring for the Community, 8–15.

26. Ludmerer, Learning to Heal, 102–122.

27. As quoted in Clark, *Indiana University* 2: 66; *Indiana University Annual Report* (hereafter referred to as *IU AR*), *1870–1876*, 37; Myers, *Medical Education*, 48; Brayton, "Development of Medical Education in Indiana," 38–39.

28. *IU AR*, *1870–1876*, 37.

29. *IU AR*, *1870–1876*; *Proceedings of the Indiana Medical College*, July 3, 1871, UA 073, InUI-Ar.

30. *IU AR*, *1874–1875*, 27.

31. *IU AR*, *1870–1871*, 37.

32. *Proceedings of the Indiana Medical College*, April 25, 1873; April 10, 1874; May 26, 1874; September 4, 1874; January 22, 1875; June 25, 1875; May 19, 1876; UA 073, InUI-Ar. In his article, Daly incorrectly states that the Indiana Medical College was affiliated only with Indiana University during the 1875–1876 academic school year. Daly, "The Origins of President Bryan's Medical School," 268.

33. Lemuel Moss, "Professional Schools," *IU AR*, *1876–1877*, 44–45.

34. Woodburn, *History of Indiana University*, 280–81; Harling, *Indiana University*, 169, 176–77.

35. *IU AR 1870–1876*; *Proceedings of the Indiana Medical College*, February 13, 1871; February 24, 1871; UA 073, InUI-Ar; "Opening of the Indiana Medical Colleges," 149; Starr, *The Social Transformation of American Medicine*, 4–5; Ludmerer, *Learning to Heal*, 47; Haber, *The Quest for Authority and Honor in the American Professions*, xii–xiii.

36. Kemper, *A Medical History of Indiana*, 165–67.

37. Kirk, "The State Board of Medical Registration," 51–53. See also in Russo, Charles N. Combs, "History of the Indiana State Medical Association," 7–29; and Albert Stump, "Regulation of the Practice of Medicine in Indiana since 1897," 53–59.

38. For background, see Haller, *A Profile in Alternative Medicine*; Haller, *The History of American Homeopathy*.

39. *Proceedings of the Indiana Medical College*, September 25, 1870, October 4, 1870, UA 073, InUI-Ar; Starr, *The Social Transformation of American Medicine*, 96–98.

40. Medical College of Indiana, "The Medical College of Indiana Catalogue . . . , Announcement," UA 073, InUI-Ar.

41. *Proceedings of the Indiana Medical College*, September 24, 1875; October 8, 1875; May 4, 1876; October 22, 1877; September 13, 1877; September 18, 1877; February 12, 1878, UA 073, InUI-Ar; Brayton, "History of the Indiana Medical College," 5.

42. *Proceedings of the Indiana Medical College*, August 7, 1876; August 14, 1876; September 5, 1876; March 30, 1878, UA 073, InUI-Ar; Manhart, "The Indiana Central Medical College," 9; Daly, "The Origins of President Bryan's Medical School," 269.

43. *Proceedings of the Indiana Medical College*, May 2, 1878; May 24, 1878; June 12, 1878; June 27, 1878; July 18, 1878, UA 073, InUI-Ar; Brayton, "The Development of Medical Education in Indiana," 37. Daly,"The Origins of President Bryan's Medical School," 268, incorrectly stated that the Indiana Medical College and the College of Physicians and Surgeons merged to become the Medical College of Indiana in 1876 and did not mention any affiliation with Butler University.

44. Brayton, "Development of Medical Education in Indiana," 39–40; MacDougall, "Joseph Eastman, M.D.," 28; Earp, "Joseph Eastman," 207.

45. "First Annual Announcement of the Central College of Physicians and Surgeons"; John F. Barnhill, "An Epoch of Medical Education," 54.

46. The Ryan Building was a flatiron building at the northwest corner of Indiana Avenue and Tennessee Street (later renamed Capitol Avenue). The new site was another flatiron building at the intersection of New York, Delaware, and Massachusetts streets. On the Block Building, see MacDougall, "Joseph Eastman, M.D.," 27.

47. Potter, "Microscopic Laboratories," 7–8; *Indianapolis City Directory, 1882–1889*; Brayton, "History of the Indiana Medical College," 5–6.

48. Barnhill, "An Epoch of Medical Education," 55; Brayton, "History of the Indiana Medical College," 5–6; Haber, *The Quest for Authority and Honor in the American Professions*, 321.

49. J. W. Marsee, a well-known surgeon who later became dean of the school, and Alembert W. Brayton, editor of the *Indiana Medical Journal*, finally convinced the college to purchase one dozen microscopes for use in the lab. Potter, "Microscopic Laboratories," 7–8. Medical College of Indiana, Faculty Minutes, September 1889, October 4, 1889, UA 073, InUI-Ar. Potter quickly rose to the rank of professor at MCI in 1892 and joined Brayton as an editor of *IMJ*. He

remained on the faculty at MCI until it was taken over by the new Indiana University School of Medicine, and he remained there until his untimely death in 1915. See Wynne, "Dr. Theodore Potter," 192–93; Bodenhamer, Barrows, and Vanderstel, *The Encyclopedia of Indianapolis*, 1130; Ludmerer, *Learning to Heal*, 129–30.

50. Ludmerer, *Learning to Heal*, 74; Barnhill, "An Epoch of Medical Education," 55; Sowder, "Address," 242–43.

51. Medical College of Indiana, Faculty Minutes, May 23, 1890; June 16, 1890, UA 073, InUI-Ar.

52. "Smoldering Ruins," *Indianapolis News*, November 3, 1894; "A Disastrous Fire," *Indianapolis Journal*, November 3, 1894; "Fire Destroys Gas Company Building—Indiana Medical College and Scottish Rite," *Indianapolis Sentinel*, November 3, 1894. Medical students even participated in dissection while under the influence of alcohol. In 1898, the *Indianapolis Sentinel* reported that a medical student was so drunk that he fell into the vats of brine used to store cadavers. This same student was reportedly drunk during his entire medical school experience ("Into a Pickling Vat," *Indianapolis Sentinel*, November 22, 1898). Whether or not any of this was true, the article is representative of typical attitudes the general public held about the irresponsible behavior of medical students; Bonner, *To the Ends of the Earth*, 215–16; Ludmerer, *Learning to Heal*, 91.

53. The Lomax Building was the first building dedicated to medical education since the LaPorte University Medical School closed in the 1850s. Theodore Potter, "A Brief History," 11; "Smoldering Ruins," *Indianapolis News*; "A Disastrous Fire," *Indianapolis Journal*; "Fire Destroys Gas Company Building," *Indianapolis Sentinel*; Myers, *Medical Education*, 59–60.

54. In fact, as will be seen in a later chapter, the successors to all these institutions except Butler became part of IUPUI. See Gray, *IUPUI*.

55. Joseph Eastman, Samuel E. Earp, and Allison Maxwell to Joseph Swain, Folder 5, Box 1, Collection C126, Indiana University Archives, Bloomington (hereafter cited as C126 InU-Ar); "The Medical College of Indiana of the University of Indianapolis" (1899–1900), 89–91; "Indiana as a Factor in Medical Education," 68.

56. Daly, "Essay on Medical Education."

57. Barnhill, "An Epoch of Medical Education," 56–57; Sowder, "Address, The Central College of Physicians and Surgeons," 243. In 1893, Johns Hopkins opened with a four-year curriculum, and other leading schools made four years of study compulsory. By the early 1900s, most medical schools had a four-year curriculum, and those failing to do so did not survive long after the Flexner Report was published in 1910. Ludmerer, *Learning to Heal*, 74.

58. James W. Fesler to Joseph Swain, June 15, 1901, Folder 5, Box 1, C126, InU-Ar; Van Allen, *Keeping the Dream,* 95; Fesler to Swain, June 15, 1901; Albert Rabb, [Sr.] to Swain, June 13, 1901, W. E. Henry to Swain, June 14, 1901, W. S. Blatchley to Swain, Folder 5, Box 1, C126, InU-Ar; Clark, *Indiana University* 2: 33–36; "W. E. Henry Dies in West," *Indianapolis Star*, March 21, 1936.

59. Eastman's sons were Thomas B. and Joseph Rilus Eastman, who had also become physicians. Fesler to Swain, June 15, 1901; Cottman, *Centennnial*

History of Indiana, 7; Bodenhamer, Barrows, and Vanderstel, *The Encyclopedia of Indianapolis*, 523.

60. Board of Trustees Minutes, Central College of Physicians and Surgeons, January 2, 1902; January 14, 1902; March 3, 1902; March 24, 1902. See also Medical Colleges—Central College of Physicians and Surgeons, Reference Files, Indiana University Archives, Bloomington; Rice, *The Hoosier Health Officer*, 38.

61."Twenty-Five Indictments in Grave-Robbing Cases Returned by Grand Jury," *Indianapolis Sentinel*, October 26, 1902; "New Names in Ghoul Cases," *Indianapolis Sentinel*, October 28, 1902; Inghram,"Formal Opening of the New Home," 395.

62. Examples of the large amount of scholarship on this are Sappol, *"A Traffic of Dead Bodies"*; Warner and Rizzolo, "Anatomical Instruction," 403–14.

63. Medical College of Indiana, Faculty Minutes, January 5, 1883, UA 073, InUI-Ar. For a summary of the early anatomy laws enacted in Indiana, see Myers, *Medical Education*, 92–95; Rothstein, *American Medical Schools*, 90; Warner, *Against the Spirit of* System, 207–8.

64. *Proceedings of the Indiana Medical College*, May 25, 1872; April 7, 1876; July 5, 1877, UA 073, InUI-Ar; Medical College of Indiana, Faculty Minutes, August 2, 1878, UA 073, InUI-Ar; "Twenty-Five Indictments in Grave-Robbing Cases Returned by Grand Jury," *Indianapolis Sentinel*; "Arrest of Dr. F. M. Wright," *Indianapolis Sentinel*, December 31, 1902; "Detectives on Trail of Two More Well-Organized Gangs of Grave Robbers," *Indianapolis Sentinel*, October 2, 1902; "May Free the Ghouls," *Indianapolis Sentinel*, February 27, 1903; "State Anatomical Board," *Indianapolis Sentinel*, March 9, 1903. For a summary regarding the details of this law, see Myers, *Medical Education*, 95–97; interview with Goethe Link, May 20, 1977, 32, Center for the Study of History and Memory, Indiana University, Bloomington.

65. Ludmerer, *Learning to Heal*, 87.

66. "The Medical College of Indiana, Department of Medicine of the University of Indianapolis" (1900–1901), 2; "Central College of Physicians and Surgeons"; "The Natural Method of Teaching Medicine: Methods of the Indiana Medical College and of Johns Hopkins Medical School," *Indiana Medical Journal* (Jul 1901–Jun 1902): 185.

67. A. W. Brayton to Bryan, June 1903, Box 1, C126, InU-Ar; "Medical Activity in the State Universities," 1726; Barnhill, "An Epoch of Medical Education," 55.

68. Bobbs, "President's Address," 11.

3. Making Medicine Modern, 1900–1912

1. Rothstein, *American Medical Schools*, 142–43, 150; Ludmerer, *Learning to Heal*, 95–101, 108–13.

2. Brayton, "Development of Medical Education in Indiana," 73–130; Myers, *Medical Education*, 121–54; Clark, *Indiana University*, 2: 65–93; and Daly, "The Origins of President Bryan's Medical School," 265–84.

3. In 1902, Bryan reported to the board that there were 748 students enrolled and that only 85 of them were registered in the School of Law, then IU's only professional school. Purdue's enrollment that year was 1,006. Clark, *Indiana University* 1: 218–20, 223–24, 234–35; Woodburn, *History of Indiana University*, 375, 385–88; Stypa, "Purdue Girl."

4. William Bryan, President's Reports to the Indiana University Board of Trustees, November 6, 1902, March 2, 1903, Presidents' Reports to the Indiana University Board of Trustees, Collection C654, Indiana University Archives, Bloomington (hereafter cited at C654, InU-Ar); Clark, *Indiana University* 2: 7; Myers, *Medical Education*, 22, 123; Bryan, Inaugural Address, January 21, 1903, President William Lowe Bryan speeches, Collection C71, Indiana University Archives, Bloomington (hereafter cited as C71, InU-Ar).

5. Before becoming president of IU, Bryan also studied in Paris and Würzburg. Woodburn, *History of Indiana University*, 399; Clark, *Indiana University* 2: 7; Ward W. Moore, "History of the School of Medicine in Bloomington," 2, paper delivered to the John Shaw Billings Society, Indiana University School of Medicine, November 12, 1990. Mall taught at Clark University from 1889 to 1892. Harvey, *Adventures in Medical Research*, 100–101.

6. Clark, *Indiana University*, 1: 223–24, 234–35; Bannister, *Indiana University*, 177–78; Moore, "History of the School of Medicine in Bloomington," 1–2. Jordan's interest in biology led him to become a champion of eugenics at Stanford. For more on Jordan and the eugenics movement, see Lombardo, ed., *A Century of Eugenics in America*, 16.

7. Clark, *Indiana University* 2: 12; Myers, *Medical Education*, 20; Bryan, "Indiana University and Medical Education," March 1, 1906, Folder 23, Box 1, Collection C126, Indiana University Archives, Bloomington (hereafter cited as C126, InU-Ar); "Restrictions on Medical Education in Indianapolis," 212.

8. Topping, *A Century and Beyond*, 155; Daly, "The Origins of President Bryan's Medical School," 273–75.

9. Bryan, President's Reports, March 27, 1903, Box 2, C654, InU-Ar; Minutes; Indiana University Board of Trustees, March 27, 1903, Box 2, C218, (hereafter cited as C654, InU-Ar); Myers, *Medical Education*, 122–23; Moore, "History of the School of Medicine in Bloomington."

10. Russo, *One Hundred Years of Indiana Medicine*; Myers, *Medical Education*, 64.

11. Russo, "Pioneer Medicine in Indiana," 8; Myers, *Medical Education*, 64; Fesler to Bryan, March 6, 1903, Folder 6, Box 1, C126, InU-Ar; Bryan, President's Reports, March 28, 1904, Box 2, C654, InU-Ar.

12. Bryan to A. W. Brayton [1903, never sent], Folder 5, Box 1; Bryan, President's Reports, March 28, 1904, Box 2, C654; Bryan to William T. Gott, January 27, 1904, Folder 6, Box 1; Fesler to Bryan, July 28, 1903, Folder 5, Box 1; Henry Jameson to Bryan, July 31, 1903, Folder 15, Box 1, C126, InU-Ar; Bryan to Myers, August 5, 1903, Box 90, Indiana University President's Office correspondence, Collection C270, Indiana University Archives, Bloomington (hereafter cited as C270, InU-Ar); Bryan, President's Reports, November 6, 1903, Box 2, C654, InU-Ar.

13. Moore, "History of the School of Medicine in Bloomington," 2; Bryan, President's Reports, March 27, 1903, Box 2, C654, InU-Ar; Bryan to Myers, June 29, 1903, Myers to Bryan, July 2, 1903, Box 90, C270, InU-Ar; Myers, *Medical Education*, 123, 125.

14. "New College," *Indiana University Daily Student (IDS)*, September 12, 1903; Moore, "History of the School of Medicine in Bloomington"; Myers, *Medical Education*, 126–27; Myers to Pohlman, August 2, 1904, Box 98, C270, InU-Ar.

15. Moore, "History of the School of Medicine in Bloomington," 2; Myers, *Medical Education,* 127; Clark, *Indiana University* 2: 12–13, 32. Science Hall was dedicated on January 21, 1903, and was later named after Ernest H. Lindley (Clark, *Indiana University* 2: 12).

16. The State Board of Medical Registration and Examination governed IU's right to cadavers. "New College"; Bryan to Myers, August 5, 1903; Myers to Bryan, July 7, 1903, Box 90. Bryan to Myers, August 15, 1903; Myers to Bryan, August 18, 1903; Myers to Bryan, September 9, 1903, Box 90, C270, InU-Ar. Bryan, "President's Reports," November 6, 1903, Box 2, C654, InU-Ar. Fesler to Bryan, November 16, 1903, Box 44, C270, InU-Ar; Myers, *Medical Education,* 100–102, 127. Rice, *One Hundred Years of Medicine*, 44.

17. Daly offers a slightly different account; see Daly, "The Origins of President Bryan's Medical School," 273. Bryan, "The situation with regard to the medical school of IU. . .," January 1904, Fesler to Bryan, November 21, 1904, Folder 55, Box 1, C126, InU-Ar. Myers, *Medical Education*, 102–3, 131–32. Fesler to Bryan, February 9, 1904; Fesler to Bryan, November 22, 1904, Folder 6, Box 1, C126, InU-Ar. Indiana University Board of Trustees Minutes, January 6, 1904; March 29, 1904; November 22, 1904, Indiana University Board of Trustees Minutes, http://webapp1.dlib.indiana.edu/iubot/welcome.do;jsession id=8D63E4C2F845A8E9EA76D3C653FAC896 (hereafter cited as IU BOT). Barnhill to Bryan, IU Board of Trustees, November 22, 1904, Box 10, C270, InU-Ar. Bryan, President's Reports, June 15, 1905, Box 2, C654, InU-Ar. "New Turn in Medical School Controversy," *Indianapolis News*, February 23, 1906.

18. Bryan, Presidents Reports, April 3, 1905, Box 2, C654, InU-Ar; AAMC, "Minutes of the Fifteenth Annual Meeting, 44.

19. For some contemporary documents on the negotiations that began in May 1905 when the officers of the MCI submitted a proposal for union with Purdue and the reactions, see Bryan, Presidents Reports, June 15, 1905, Box 2, C654, InU-Ar; Charles Major to Stone, August 23, 1905; Stone to George Kahlo, September 11, 1905, Series 1, UA 0049, Purdue University Archives and Special Collections (hereafter cited as PU-Ar); "To Become Part of Purdue University," *Indianapolis News*, August 31, 1905; Henry Jameson, George J. Cook to— (form letter), September 8, 1905, Folder 20, Box 1, C126, InU-Ar; Stone, "The New School of Medicine," 9; "Purdue Gets School, Medical College Formally Transferred to University," *Lafayette Courier*, September 1, 1906; "Medical Schools to Fight to a Finish," *Indianapolis Star*, November 30, 1906. For secondary accounts, which are limited, see Phillips, *Indiana in Transition*, 97–99; *A Biographical Directory of the Indiana General Assembly* (Indianapolis: Select Committee on the Centennial History of the Indiana General

Assembly, 1980) 1: 163; Topping, *A Century and Beyond*, 159–61; Robert Kriebel, "Focus on History, Purdue, IU Clashed on Med School," *Lafayette Journal and Courier*, January 19, 1997.

20. According to the terms of the agreement, the Central College would turn over to Purdue its equipment, students, alumni, and that part of the tuition fund left after the school's current operating expenses up to that point in the current term were paid. However, Purdue did not accept Central College's debt, and significantly, the school's building on North Senate Avenue remained the property of the medical college corporation. The Central College Board of Trustees immediately appointed a committee to arrange for the sale of the building to cover the institution's outstanding mortgage. Board of Trustee Minutes, Central College of Physicians and Surgeons, September 25, 1905, Medical Colleges—Central College of Physicians and Surgeons, Reference files, Indiana University Archives, Bloomington (hereafter cited as Reference files, InU-Ar); "Medical Colleges Are Consolidated," *Indianapolis Star*, September 26, 1905; "Medical Colleges Are Consolidated," *Indianapolis Sentinel*, September 26, 1905; Stone to Kahlo, September 11, 1905, Stone Papers, UA 073, Indiana University School of Medicine Records, 1848–2005, University Library Special Collections and Archives, University Library, Indiana University Purdue University Indianapolis (hereafter cited as InUI-Ar); "Pertinent Facts Concerning the Union of Medical Colleges in Indiana," *The Central States Medical Monitor* 9 (February 15, 1906): 493–94; "College May Join State University," *Indianapolis Star*, September 25, 1905; "George D. Kahlo, Obituary"; Scherrer, "A True Statement of Facts," 63; Board of Trustee Minutes, Central College of Physicians and Surgeons, September 25, 1905; "Combined with Purdue," *IDS*, September 27, 1905.

21. "President Stone Stops Dissention," *Lafayette Courier*, September 28, 1905; Muller, "The Indiana University School of Medicine," 9; Topping, *A Century and Beyond*, 150–51.

22. Christian B. Stemen to Stone, Stone to Stemen, September 25, 1905; Stone to Stemen, September 29, 1905; Wishard to Stone, October 4, 1905; October 4, 1905; W. O. Goss to Stone, October 3, 1905, Stone Papers, UA 073, InUI-Ar. "Purdue Adopts Medical College," *Fort Wayne News*, October 5, 1905; "Merger of Medical Colleges Completed," *Indianapolis News*, October 9, 1905.

23. William Lowe Bryan, President's Reports to the Indiana University Board of Trustees, October 5, 1905, Box 2, C654, InU-Ar.

24. Stone, "The New School of Medicine," 9–10; "Purdue Adopts Medical College," "Indiana May Have War with Purdue, Growing Resentment at Bloomington over Alleged Encroachments of Rivals," *Indianapolis Star*, January 9, 1906; "Indiana's Threat," *Lafayette Courier*, January 10, 1906; "Glaringly Yellow," ed., *IDS*, January 17, 1906; "Great Fight Ahead," ed., *Indianapolis News*, February 23, 1906; Stone to Bryan, October 20, 1906, Folder 30, Box 1, C126, InU-Ar.

25. Myers, *Medical Education*, 138; Myers, "Report of the Medical Department," IU BOT Minutes, October 30, 1906; "The State and Medical Education," ed., *Indianapolis News*, January 27, 1906.

26. Bryan, memo for the record, October 31, 1905, Folder 7, Box 1, C126, InU-Ar.

27. Bryan, President's Reports, January 4, 1906.

28. "The College Prospects," 19; Myers, *Medical Education*, 138; Bryan, "Indiana University and Medical Education"; "Hold Indiana University Is Acting within Law," *Indianapolis Star*, April 29, 1906.

29. "New Turn in Medical School Controversy," *Indianapolis News*, February 23, 1906; Bryan to B. F. Shively, January 31, 1906, Box 111, C270, InU-Ar; Myers, *Medical Education*, 139; "Instructions for the New Medical School," *Indianapolis Star*, March 29, 1906. Members of the Committee for the Sale of the Property of the Central College of Physicians and Surgeons included Charles R. Sowder, who later joined a lawsuit against Purdue with Simon P. Scherer, and Barnhill, who by this time was sympathetic to IU. On Maxwell, see "Memorial to Dr. Allison Maxwell," 173–75.

30. As summarized and quoted in length in Brayton, "Development of Medical Education in Indiana," 86–89.

31. Ibid.

32. "Resigns Position in Purdue Medical School," *Indianapolis News*, January 31, 1906.

33. Fesler to Bryan, January 31, 1906; Bryan to Shively, January 31, 1906, Box 44, C270, InU-Ar. Myers, *Medical Education*, 139; "Resigns Position in Purdue Medical School"; "Buy Medical School Building," *IDS*, January 31, 1906.

34. Jameson drafted the report and forwarded it to Stone for his revisions, and then Jameson, Kahlo, and Stemen signed it as the deans of the private medical schools that formed the Indiana Medical College in October 1905. American Medical Association (AMA) to Jameson, February 26, 1906; Jameson to Stone, February 3, 1906; Jameson to Stone, February 5, 1906; Jameson to Stone, February 21, 1906, Medicine; Stone to Stemen, Stone Papers, UA 073, InUI-Ar. Jameson, Kahlo, Stemen to Dear Sir, February 1906, Folder 20, Box 1, C126, InU-Ar. Bryan, memo for the record, October 31, 1905; Jameson, Kahlo, Stemen to Dear Sir; "Set Forth Reasons for the Consolidation," *Indianapolis News*, February 24, 1906; "Relation of the Indiana Medical College to the State University," *IMJ* 24 (February 1906): 347–48.

35. Jameson to Stone, March 26, 1906; Stone to Jameson, March 27, 1906, Stone Papers, UA 073, InUI-Ar. "Obstacle for New Medical School," *Indianapolis Star*, March 25, 1906.

36. For the role of the AAMC in the Flexner Report described below, see Ludmerer, *Learning to Heal*, 169.

37. "Medical Case Argument," *Indianapolis News*, April 14, 1906; "McMaster Decides Against Purdue," *IDS*, May 23, 1906; Clark, *Indiana University* 2: 74. Ultimately, on December 19, 1908, the plaintiffs dismissed the case (Docket No. 70880-1, Archives of the Marion County Superior Court, Indianapolis, Indiana). "Medical College Dispute," ed., *Lafayette Courier*; "New Hospital Plan," *Indianapolis Star*, April 14, 1906; "Step toward New Medical College," *Indianapolis Star*, April 7, 1906; "Medical College Names Its Faculty," *Indianapolis Star*, April 28, 1906; "New School of Medicine," *Indianapolis News*, May 23, 1906.

38. Barnhill, "An Epoch of Medical Education," 60.

39. "Spurn Indiana Medical College's Overtures," *Indianapolis News*, April 5, 1906; "Obstacle for New Medical School"; "Buy Building for a Medical College," *Indianapolis Star*, March 15, 1906; Kahlo et al., Jameson to Stone, March 28, 1906, Stone Papers, UA 073; "Letter to the President and Board of Trustees of the Central College of Physicians and Surgeons," March 19, 1906, "Dr. J. F. Barnhill No Longer with School," Medical Colleges—Central College of Physicians and Surgeons, Reference files, InU-Ar.

40. "Step toward New Medical College," *Indianapolis Star*, April 7, 1906; "Medical College Names Its Faculty," *Indianapolis Star*, April 28, 1906; "New School of Medicine," *Indianapolis News*, May 23, 1906.

41. Myers, "Report of the Medical Department," October 30, 1906, C270, InU-Ar; Myers, *Medical Education*, 141; "To Confer Degrees in Medicine at I.U.," *Indianapolis Star*, July 21, 1906; "First Bulletin Out," *Indianapolis Star*, August 3, 1906.

42. Not only did IMC control the City Hospital, but it also influenced other private hospitals and public institutions, including St. Vincent Hospital, Door of Hope Maternity Hospital, and Eleanor Hospital for Children. Bryan to Maxwell, May 21, 1906, Box 82, C270, InU-Ar; "Purdue Graduates 122 Young Medics," *Indianapolis News*, May 15, 1906; Myers to Bryan, August 1, 1906, Box 90, C270, InU-Ar; Barnhill, "An Epoch. . .," 60; Jameson to Stone, March 26, 1906, Stone Papers, UA 073, InUI-Ar; Indiana Medical College, "The School of Medicine of Purdue University," *First Annual Catalogue and Announcement, 1906–1907*, UA 073, InUI-Ar; "Summer Medical Courses," *Indianapolis News*, May 2, 1906.

43. Scherer to Bryan, June 25, 1906; Bryan to Maxwell, June 28, 1906, Box 82, C270, InU-Ar. Ludmerer, *Learning to Heal*, 157.

44. Barnhill, "An Epoch. . .," 60; Bryan to Maxwell, June 28, 1906; "Hospital Feature of New Medical College," *Indianapolis News*, July 18, 1906; Myers to Bryan, December 15, 1909, Box 90, C270, InU-Ar; Myers, *Medical Education*, 140; "New College Prospers," *IDS*, October 11, 1906.

45. Barnhill, "An Epoch. . .," 60; Scherer, "A True Statement. . .," 64; "New Hospital to Open," *Indianapolis Star*, September 13, 1906; "New Hospital Opens," *Indianapolis Star*, September 14, 1906; "Formal Opening of New State College Hospital," *Indianapolis News*, September 14, 1906; Clark, *Indiana University* 2: 74; "New College Prospers," *IDS*, October 11, 1906; Bodenhamer, Barrows, and Vanderstel, *The Encyclopedia of Indianapolis*, 592–93.

46. "Physicians Favor Only One Big Medical School," *Indianapolis News*, March 1, 1906; "Denounce Effort to Split School," *Indianapolis Star*, March 1, 1906; "Medical School Wrangle," *Indianapolis News*, May 2, 1906; Shively to Bryan, April 19, 1906, Box 111, C270, InU-Ar; Stone, Address at Banquet of Grad Med Class, May 10, 1906, Box 1, UA 073, Winthrop E. Stone Papers, InUI-Ar; Bryan to Fesler, July 12, 1906, Box 44, C270, InU-Ar.

47. Because the Purdue trustees had formally entered the union with the MCI with Hanly's approval, it was generally known that Indiana's governor opposed Indiana University in the medical school controversy. Sources in the extensive archival record include Stone to James Frank Hanly, November 17,

1906; Jameson to Stone, November 23, 1906; Stone to Hanly, January 2, 1907; Hanly's Secretary to Stone, November 3, 1906, Letter book, no. 45; Hanly to Stone, February 18, 1907, Letter book, no. 47; Hanly to A. W. Brayton, April 16, 1906, Hanly Papers, UA 073, InUI-Ar.

48. Representative examples of the great interest include Bryan to Stone, October 24, 1906; Stone to Bryan, October 31, 1906, Box 119, C270, InU-Ar. Bryan to Shively, November 3, 1906, Box 111, C270, InU-Ar. John N. Hurty to Stone, May 11, 1906; Stone to George Ade, December 29, 1906, UA 073, InUI-Ar. Myers to Bryan, August 1, 1906, Box 90, C270, InU-Ar. Jameson to Barnhill, May 8, 1906, Folder 8, Box 1, C126, InU-Ar. Sidney K. Ganiard to Woodburn, October 6, 1906, Folder 8, Box 1, C126, InU-Ar; Stone to Hanly, November 17, 1906.
For examples of press coverage, see "The Other Side," *Bloomington Telephone*, February 5, 1907; Barnhill, "An Epoch. . .," 61; "Medical Schools to Fight to a Finish," *Indianapolis Star*, November 30, 1906; "Indiana Will Win," *Bloomington Telephone*, January 25, 1907.

49. Stone to A. W. Brayton, April 16, 1906; Bryan to Stone, October 24, 1906; Bryan to Stone, October 24, 1906; Stone to Bryan, October 31, 1906; Stone to George Ade, December 29, 1906, Stone Papers, UA 073, InU-Ar. Bryan to Shively, November 3, 1906, Box 111, C270, InU-Ar.

50. "Fight for Purdue," *Lafayette Courier*, October 18, 1906. Ade to Stone, December 27, 1906; Major to Stone, October 16, 1906, Stone Papers, UA 073, InUI-Ar.

51. Oscar E. Bland, an attorney from Linton, Indiana, who represented Greene, Monroe, and Owen counties in the Senate, authored a competing bill to permit Indiana University's operation of a medical school in Marion County. Will R. Wood, Joint Resolution, January 1907, Folder 16, Box 1, C126, InU-Ar; "Bill Introduced Today," *IDS*, January 15, 1907; "Medical School Fight Now Begun," *IDS*, January 16, 1907; "Medical School Fight Opens," *Indianapolis Star*, January 17, 1907; "Facts for Lawmakers," *Bloomington Telephone*, January 18, 1907; "Fight Will Be Bitter," *Lafayette Courier*, October 26, 1906; Moore, "History of the School of Medicine in Bloomington," 7; *A Biographical Directory of the Indiana General Assembly* 2: 41, 123, 451; Clark, *Indiana University* 2: 80.

52. "Senate Thronged for Medical Fight," *Indianapolis Star*, January 23, 1907; "Indiana Will Win," *Bloomington Telephone*, January 25, 1907; Barnhill, "An Epoch. . .," 61; "To the Front," *Bloomington Telephone*, January 29, 1907; "The Medical Situation," *Purdue Exponent*, January 24, 1907; "Both Sides Are Heard," *IDS*, January 23, 1907; "Indiana Will Win"; "Medical Bill Reported," *IDS*, January 18, 1907; "School Fight on the Floor," *Indianapolis Star*, January 18, 1907; Myers, *Medical Education*, 164; Clark, *Indiana University* 2: 81–83.

53. Bryan, "Senate Testimony, January 22, 1907," C270, InU-Ar. Purdue's president also explained that nothing in the Morrill Act of 1862, the act of Congress under which Purdue was founded prevented the school from establishing a school of medicine. "From the very nature of its plans and its courses it is logical that Purdue should teach medicine," he added. "Senate Thronged for

Medical Fight"; "The Medical Situation," *Purdue Exponent*, January 24, 1907; "Both Sides Are Heard," *IDS*, January 23, 1907.

54. Each school asked for over $300,000 for the next biennium. However, the 1907 legislature awarded Purdue only $100,000; and Indiana University received $99,475. "Compromise Talked"; "Dr. B. D. Myers on Medical Fight," *IDS*, February 6, 1907; "Indiana Suffers," *Bloomington Telephone*, February 12, 1907; "State Must Hold Down Its Expenses," *Indianapolis Star*, February 12, 1907; "A Great University," *Indianapolis News*, March 1, 1907; "Indiana Medical Bill Fails Again," *IMJ* 25 (March 1907): 360; "Indiana Medical College," *IMJ* 25 (April, 1907): 393; Clark, *Indiana University* 2: 87.

55. "Medical College Fight Breaks Out in Senate," *Indianapolis News*, March 6, 1907; "Before the Senate," *Bloomington Telephone*, March 8, 1907; "Indiana University Medical School Bill Fails Again," *IMJ* 25 (March, 1907): 359–60; Clark, *Indiana University* 2: 87; "No Medical School to Be Authorized," *Indianapolis Star*, January 30, 1907; "Outlook Not Black," *Bloomington Telephone*, February 1, 1907; "Compromise Talked," *Bloomington Telephone*, February 1, 1907; "House Treats Purdue the Same as Indiana"; "Purdue Bill Killed Today," *IDS*, February 1, 1907; Clark, *Indiana University* 2: 85

56. Editorial, "The Medical Student," *The Medical Student* 5 (April 1907): 20; Harris to Stone, February 27, 1908, Stone Papers, UA 073, InUI-Ar; "Maybe One School, Project to Unite All State Institutions," *Lafayette Courier*, December 30, 1906; Clark, *Indiana University* 2: 86.

57. "Strong State School of Medicine Probable," *Indianapolis News*, March 12, 1907; "The Medical Situation," 18.

58. Stone, Address at Banquet of Grad Med Class, 10 May 1906; Stone, Remarks, Graduates of Medical School, May 1, 1907, Box 1, Winthrop E. Stone Papers, InPU-Ar; Stone to All Trustees, April 16, 1907, Stone Papers, UA 073, InU-Ar. For examples of trustee reactions, see Joseph D. Oliver to Stone, April 18, 1907; Harris to Stone, April 24, 1907, Medicine, School of, 1905–1907, InPU-Ar. "Indiana Medic Notes," *Purdue Exponent*, March 17, 1907; Stone, "The Evolution of Medical Education in Indiana," *IMJ* 25 (June 1907): 471.

59. Association of American Medical Colleges, "Minutes of the Fifteenth Annual Meeting, May 6, 1907" (Chicago: AMA, 1907), 22.

60. In the summer of 1907, Bryan, Myers, Barnhill, Sowder, and Frank F. Hutchins each contributed five hundred dollars to help pay off State College's debts, which were in excess of $2,000. Myers to Bryan, June 13, 1907, Box 90, C270, InU-Ar; Myers, *Medical Education*, 146. In August 1907, "charitably disposed persons" contributed or pledged nearly $4,000 to cover the State College Hospital operating deficit. Myers to Bryan, August 1, 1907, Box 90, C270, InU-Ar.

61. Myers, *Medical Education*, 147. On problems at both institutions, see Jameson to Stone, September 16, 1907, Stone Papers, UA 073, InU-Ar; *Bulletin of the Purdue School of Medicine, 1907–1908*, 2; "Indiana University to Continue Its Fight," *Indianapolis News*, May 18, 1907; Bryan, "Medical School Commencement," May 18, 1907, Bryan Speeches, Box 1, C71, InU-Ar; "Graduation Exercises of the State College of Physicians and Surgeons," 242–44; "Indiana University School of Medicine," 297; Bryan to Fesler, October 7, 1907,

Box 44, C270, InU-Ar; Myers, *Medical Education*, 145–46; Jameson to Stone, September 16, 1907, Stone Papers, UA 073, InU-Ar; IU BOT Minutes, August 18, 1907; November 6, 1907.

62. Wishard related his account of early discussions leading to the 1908 compromise agreement thirty years later, in 1938. He mistakenly identified the date of these discussions. "Statement of Dr. William N. Wishard relative conditions agreed upon when Purdue Medical School was transferred to Indiana University in 1908. To the Special Committee of the Indiana State Medical Association, Dr. F. S. Crockett, Chairman" [enclosure]; Wishard to Bryan, October 6, 1938, Medicine, School of—Survey 1910, C270, InU-Ar. From the dates of Edwards's letters, these discussions occurred during October and November 1907 rather than March or April 1908. John H. Edwards to Bryan, October 18, 1907; Edwards to Bryan, November 4, 1907, [enclosure] to Edwards, November 2, 1907, C270, InU-Ar. In notes Stone made about the events leading up to the resolution of the medical school controversy, he also identified Wishard as the individual who held preliminary discussions with Edwards about the possibility of a compromise between Purdue and IU prior to December 16, 1907. Stone, "Notes on events leading to resolution of the medical school controversy [1908], School of Medicine, 1905–1907," Stone Papers, UA 073,

63. Myers, *Medical Education*, 148. Bryan, President's Reports, November 5, 1907; April 3, 1908, Box 3, C654, InU-Ar. Bryan to Stone, December 16, 1907; Stone to Harris, January 8, 1908; Bryan to Stone, February 4, 1908; Harris to Stone, February 15, 1908, Stone Papers, UA 073, InU-Ar. Stone to Bryan, December 19, 1907, Folder 30, Box 1, C126, InU-Ar. Bryan to Shea, Rose, Shively, January 7, 1908, Bryan Letter Press Books, InU-Ar; Bryan, President's Reports, April 3, 1908, Box 3, C654, InU-Ar.

64. Harris to Stone, February 27, 1908; Stone to Bryan, February 28, 1908, Folder 30, Box 1, C126, InU-Ar. Harris to Stone, March 26, 1908; Harris to Stone, March 27, 1908; Stone to Harris, March 30, 1908, Stone Papers, UA 073, InUI-Ar Stone to Bryan, March 27, 1908, Folder 30, Box 1, C126, InU-Ar. "State Medical College Fight May End Soon," *Indianapolis News*, March 24, 1908.

65. Minutes, Indiana University Board of Trustees, April 3, 1908, Box 2, C218, Trustees Minutes, InU-Ar; IU BOT Minutes, April 4, 1908; To the Special Committee of the Indiana State Medical Association, Dr. F. S. Crockett, Chairman [enclosure]; Minutes of the Faculty of the Indiana Medical College, April 8; Clark, *Indiana University* 2: 92.

66. "Medical Colleges Joined Under IU," *Indianapolis Star*, April 6, 1908; "Medic Controversy Settled," *Purdue Exponent*, April 7, 1908; "Medical Consolidation," *IDS*, April 10, 1908. Stone to Harris, April 6, 1908; Stone to Beem, April 8, 1908, Stone Papers, UA 073, InUI-Ar.

67. Bryan, President's Reports, October 5, 1905; Bryan to Charles P. Emerson, January 12, 1912, C270, InU-Ar.

68. Wells, *Being Lucky*, 111; Clark, *Indiana University* 2: 65.

69. Major to Stone, April 6, 1908; Joseph D. Oliver to Stone, April 7, 1908; L. Ert Slack to Stone, April 6, 1908; Harris to Stone, April 7, 1908; David E. Beem to Stone, April 7, 1908, Stone Papers, UA 073, InUI-Ar. "President Stone

Honored," *Lafayette Journal*, June 27, 1908; "Present Watch to Stone," *Indianapolis News*, June 27, 1908.

70. The committee included Miles F. Porter, James H. Ford, Frank B. Wynn, John F. Barnhill, Edmund D. Clark, Alois B. Graham, Frank F. Hutchins, and Burton D. Myers. Bryan to Jameson, April 23, 1908, Box 67, C270, InU-Ar; Bryan to John F. Barnhill, Edmund D. Clark, Frank B. Wynn, Miles F. Porter, April 23, 1908, InU-Ar, Bryan to Fesler, Shea, et al., May 6, 1908, Bryan Letter Books, InU-Ar; Myers, *Medical Education*, 150; Myers's Copy of the Minutes of the Committee on Medical Organization, May 8, 1908, Reference files, InU-Ar.

71. Bryan to Jameson, May 17, 1908, Bryan Files, UA 073, InUI-Ar; E. F. Hodges to Bryan, June 17, 1908, Folder 56, Box 1, C126, InU-Ar; Report of the Indiana University School of Medicine, June 9, 1916, Box 6, C654, InU-Ar.

72. Bryan to Fesler, Hill, et al., May 6, 1908; Barnhill to Bryan, June 18, 1908, Folder 56, Box 1, C126, InU-Ar. Myers, *Medical Education*, 150.

73. As for Myers, he was officially appointed the secretary of the school for Bloomington. Maxwell was unable to dedicate much of his time to the school, so Wishard and Wynn performed important roles, first as members of the Advisory Committee and then as members of the Executive Committee. Because he had played such an important part in ending the medical school controversy with Purdue, Bryan especially wanted Wishard's "counsel and friendship." These discussions are found in extensive archival records. See, for example, Bryan correspondence with Fesler, Barnhill, Jameson, Maxwell, Myers, *inter alia* from May to July 1908 in Bryan Letter Books, Bryan Files; C270, InU-Ar. See also Myers, *Medical Education*, 150.

74. *Indiana University Bulletin*, July 1908, 4, 56–70; Myers to Bryan and the Indiana University Board of Trustees, March 23, 1909, Bryan Files, Box 90, C270, InU-Ar.

75. William P. Best, Orlando S. Coffin to Bryan, July 3, 1908; A. Duthie, N. D. Woodard, E. M. Haggard to Bryan, July 4, 1908, Bryan Files, InU-Ar. Bryan, President's Reports, November 9, 1909, Box 3, C654, InU-Ar.

76. To the Faculty of the Indiana University School of Medicine, August 11, 1908, Bryan Files, Box 43; Myers to Bryan, August 28, 1908, Bryan Files, Box 90, C270, InU-Ar; Maxwell to Bryan, August 28, 1908, Box 82, C270, InU-Ar; D. W. Weaver, O. S. Runnels to Bryan, September 26, 1908, Bryan Files, InU-Ar; IU BOT Minutes, December 31, 1908. Bryan to Wishard, October 3, 1908; Bryan to Woodard, H. C. Martindale, N. E. Harold, April 14, 1911; Bryan to Woodard, H. C. Martindale, N. E. Harold, April 26, 1911, Bryan Files, InU-Ar. Myers, *Medical Education*, 78, 81, 156.
On unorthodox medical sects, see Rogers, *An Alternative Path*, 87–90; Starr, *The Social Transformation of American Medicine*, 107–8.

77. Myers, *Medical Education*, 78.

78. Bryan, President's Reports, March 25, 1909, Box 3, C654, InU-Ar.

79. Sowder to Bryan, November 10, 1908; Barnhill to Bryan, November 10, 1908, Bryan Files, InU-Ar. IU BOT Minutes, November 9, 1908; December 8, 31, 1908; June 24, 1909.

80. As quoted in Myers, *Medical Education*, 159.

81. Wishard to Bryan, March 16, 1909, Bryan Files, Box 134, C270, InU-Ar; Myers, *Medical Education*, 159; Ludmerer, *Learning to Heal*, 184. Despite the immediate difficulties it would impose, Wishard later understood the need to raise admissions standards so that IU's requirements were consistent with those of professional schools at other universities. See Wishard to Bryan, April 13, 1909, Bryan Files, Box 134, C270, InU-Ar.

82. Myers to Bryan, October 5, 1915, box 188, Indiana University President's Office correspondence, 1913–37, Collection C286, Indiana University Archives, Bloomington (hereafter cited as C286, InU-Ar).

83. Myers, *Medical Education*, 158–61.

84. Minutes, Indiana University Board of Trustees, Box 2, C218, Trustees Minutes, InU-Ar; Maxwell to Bryan, July 5, 1909, Bryan Files, Box 82; Myers to Bryan, December 15, 1909, Bryan Files, Box 90, C270, InU-Ar. Myers to Bryan, November 5, 1909, Myers to Bryan, November 16, 1909, Bryan Files, Box 90, C270, InU-Ar.

85. Brown, *Rockefeller Medicine Men*, 145, 153–54; Ludmerer, *Learning to Heal*, 182; Ludmerer, *Time to Heal*, 5, 7.

86. The other medical schools established according to modern principles included Oklahoma (organized in 1898), West Virginia (1902), Wake Forest (1902), Mississippi (1903), Fordham (1905), Utah (1906), and Wisconsin (1907). Ludmerer, *Learning to Heal*, 81.

87. Flexner, *Medical Education*, 220.

88. Henry S. Pritchett to Bryan, December 8, 1909; Flexner to Bryan, February 28, 1910, President's Reports, June 10, 1910, Box 99, C270, InU-Ar. Flexner, *Medical Education*, 220; Bryan to Ernest O. Holland, May 14, 1910, Box 60; Bryan to Pritchett, December 2, 1910, Box 99; Myers to Bryan, IU Board of Trustees, March 23, 1908, Box 90. President's Reports, March 25, 1909; June 17, 1910, Box 3. Pritchett to Bryan, April 20, 1909; Flexner to Bryan, February 28, 1910, Box 99, C270, InU-Ar.

89. In Ludmerer, *Learning to Heal, 185,* the author asserted that Indiana University was one among a group of schools that objected to Flexner's findings. However, when IU professor Ernest O. Holland revealed Flexner's concerns about the medical school to Bryan, the president replied that his impression was the "reverse." Instead, Bryan believed that the report reflected favorably on Indiana University and, at the same time, acknowledged the correctness of its criticisms. Holland to Bryan, May 10, 1910; Bryan to Holland, May 10, 1910, Box 60, C270, InU-Ar. Bryan, President's Reports, June 17, 1910, Bryan Files, InU-Ar.

89. Minutes, IU BOT, March 8, 1910.

90. Ibid. For these exchanges, see Pritchett to Bryan, December 9, 1909; Bryan to Pritchett, December 18, 1909, enclosure: "Indiana University School of Medicine"; Bryan to Pritchett, February 18, 1910; Bryan to Pritchett, February 24, 1910; Flexner to Bryan, February 28, 1910; Pritchett to Bryan, January 4, 1910, Box 99, C270, InU-Ar.

91. President's Reports, March 7, 1910, Box 3, C654, InU-Ar; IU BOT Minutes, March 8, 1910. Holland to Bryan, May 9, 1910; Bryan to Holland, May 14, 1910, Bryan Files, InU-Ar.

92. IU BOT Minutes, March 8, 1910.

93. Myers to Bryan, November 5, 1909, Box 90, C270, InU-Ar.

94. Myers to Bryan, November 5, 1909; Myers to Bryan, March 23, 1909; Myers to Bryan, [June 1909?], Bryan Files, Box 90, C270, InU-Ar. Bryan, President's Reports, November 8, 1909, Box 3, C654, InU-Ar.

95. Myers to Bryan, IU Board of Trustees, March 7, 1910, Box 90, C270, InU-Ar; Bryan, President's Reports, June 10, 1910. For the IU Board of Trustees' resolution regarding its policy against fee-splitting among IU School of Medicine faculty, see Minutes, IU Board of Trustees Minutes, March 9, 1910, Box 2, C218, Trustees Minutes, InU-Ar.

96. Minutes, Indiana University Board of Trustees, June 20, 1910; June 22, 1910, Box 3, C218, Trustees Minutes, InU-Ar.

97. Bryan to [IU School of Medicine] Faculty, August 13, 1910, Folder 20, Box 1, C126, InU-Ar; Myers to Bryan, IU Board of Trustees, March 7, 1910, InU-Ar; *Bulletin, Indiana University School of Medicine, 1908–1909*, 258–59; Bryan, President's Reports, June 10, 1910.

98. Porter to Bryan, August 20, 1910, Folder 34, Box 1, C126, InU-Ar; K. K. Wheelock to Bryan, August 29, 1910, Folder 34, Box 1, InU-Ar; Amelia R. Keller to Bryan, August 19, 1910, Folder 34, Box 1, C126, InU-Ar; Moses Thorner to Bryan, August 31, 1910, Folder 34, Box1, C126, InU-Ar; Maxwell to Bryan, October 14, 1910, Bryan Files, Box 82, C270, InU-Ar. Folder 34 in Box 1 of collection C126 at University Archives Bloomington (InU-Ar) contains more letters too numerous to cite written in response to Bryan's circular to the faculty dated August 13, 1910.

99. Keller to Bryan, August 19, 1910; *Bulletin, Indiana University School of Medicine, 1908–1909*, 258–59.

100. Correspondence and Reports, 1915–22, Division of Infant and Child Hygiene, Indiana State Board of Health, R6744, In-Ar; Emerson to Bryan, December 18, 1930, Bryan Files, InU-Ar; Ritchie, "Obituary: Dr. Ada Estelle Schweitzer."

101. Ludmerer, *Learning to Heal*, 99. For the case of IUSM, see subsequent chapters and the overview by Potter, "Learning Human Anatomy."

102. Minutes, IU Board of Trustees, December 8, 1908; December 31, 1908, Box 2, C218, Trustees Minutes, InU-Ar. Myers, "Black Graduates of Indiana University School of Medicine, 1908–1989," Historical Collections, University Library Medical Library, Indiana University Purdue University Indianapolis (hereafter cited as InU-M). Interview with Rawls, December 13, 2001, 1, 9, Center for the Study of History and Memory (InU-CSHM); IU School of Medicine Graduating Class Composite Photographs, History of Medicine Collections, InU-M; Wells to Glenora English McFadden, August 22, 1945, Box 83, Indiana University President's Office records, Collection C213, Indiana University Archives, Bloomington (hereafter cited as C213, InU-Ar). According to George H. Rawls, *History of the Black Physician in Indianapolis 1870 to 1980*, 4, Clarence Lucas Jr. and Carolyn Lucas Dickson, two children of Clarence Lucas Sr., also earned medical degrees.

103. From 1923 to 1932 there were three to six Jewish medical graduates at IUSM, and there were ten graduates in 1933. Thos. A. Cookson, Registrar to J.

B. H. Martin, IUSM Administrator, March 6, 1934, William Lowe Bryan papers, Collection C69, Indiana University Archives, Bloomington; Wells to John W. Van Nuys, December 1, 1941, C213, InU-Ar.

104. Lotys Benning Stewart, "They Achieve," *Indianapolis Star*, October 1, 1944; Bonsett, "Medical Museum Notes," 425.

105. Bryan to Allison Maxwell, June 16, 1911, Bryan Letter Books, InU-Ar; Allison Maxwell to Bryan, June 19, 1911, Bryan Files, InU-Ar.

106. Like officials of other schools across the country in the years following the release of *Medical Education in the United States and Canada*, Bryan conferred with Flexner and Pritchett and several other leaders in medical education before launching IU's search for a medical school dean in spring 1911. The other physicians considered for the IU School of Medicine deanship show how serious Bryan was in conducting a national search: Channing Frothingham, who taught at Harvard University Medical School; Wilder Tileston, an assistant professor of medicine at Yale; Rufus I. Cole, who became the first director of the hospital for the Rockefeller Institute for Medical Research; Thomas R. Boggs, who was a member of the medical faculty at Johns Hopkins; and Nellis Taylor, who belonged to the College of Physicians and Surgeons faculty at Columbia. For background, see Muller, "The Indiana University School of Medicine," 19; Clark, *Indiana University* 2: 96; Ludmerer, *Learning to Heal*, 188.

107. On Emerson, see Glenn W. Irwin, Jr., "Charles P. Emerson, M.D., Dean of the Indiana University School of Medicine, 1911–1932," paper delivered to the John Shaw Billings Society, Indiana University School of Medicine, January 14, 1990; Muller, "The Indiana University School of Medicine," 19; Myers, *Medical Education*, 163; Clark, *Indiana University* 2: 96. Myers to Bryan and the IU Board of Trustees, March 7, 1910; Bryan to Emerson, June 3, 1911, Bryan Files, Box 42, C270, InU-Ar. Bryan, President's Reports, June 16, 1911, Box 4, C654, InU-Ar. Flexner to Bryan, June 24, 1911; Bryan to Pritchett, July 4, 1911, Box 99, C270, InU-Ar. Bryan to Wishard, June 15, 1911, Box 134, C270, InU-Ar. On so-called social medicine, see "Department of Social Service Is Explained," *Indianapolis News*, October 24, 1911; Piepho, "The History of the Social Service Department," 5–7; Rogers, *Seventy Years of Social Work*, 13; Rosenberg, *The Care of Strangers*, 313; Bodenhamer, Barrows, and Vanderstel, *The Encyclopedia of Indianapolis*, 541–42.

108. Myers to Bryan, IU Board of Trustees, March 10, 1910; Bryan to Wishard, June 15, 1915, Bryan Files, InU-Ar.

109. Bryan to Wishard, June 15, 1915; Bryan to William H. Welch, June 15, 1915; Bryan to Flexner, July 4, 1915; William Welch to Bryan, June 9, 1911; Bryan to Fesler, Shively, Shea, et al., July 7, 1911, Bryan Letter Books. Bryan to Edna Henry, July 4, 1911, Box 58; Bryan to Wishard, July 4, 1911, Box 134, C270, InU-Ar; Bryan to Pritchett, Bryan Files, Box 99; Lewellys F. Barker to Bryan, July 20, 1911, Box 10, C270, InU-Ar; IU BOT Minutes, July 3, 1911; Myers, *Medical Education*, 163–66.

4. Charles Emerson and the Creation of the Medical Center, 1912–1932

1. Emerson to Bryan, May 8, 1923, Box 87, Indiana University President's Office correspondence, Collection C286, Indiana University Archives, Bloomington (hereafter cited as C286, InU-Ar).

2. In addition to Ludmerer, *Time to Heal*, and Paul Starr, *The Social Transformation of American Medicine*, other examples of scholarship on hospitals include Stevens, *In Sickness and in Wealth*, and Charles Rosenberg, *The Care of Strangers*.

3. Myers lamented, "I have thought so much and talked so much of a hospital of our own, that I cannot resist the temptation to express my willingness and wish to work actively in the realization of the things for which for the past five years I have urged as essential." Myers to Bryan and the IU Board of Trustees [1910], Box 126, C270, InU-Ar.

4. Bryan to Pritchett, February 24, 1910, C270, InU-Ar; "$200,000 as a Gift for a New Hospital," *Indianapolis News*, January 26, 1911. By raising the consciousness of the American public about the plight of medical education, an editorial in the *Journal of the American Medical Association* hoped that Flexner's survey would "call the attention of men of wealth to the need of endowment for medical education." "Carnegie Foundation Report," 1949. For background, see Ludmerer, *Time to Heal*, 5; Ludmerer, *Learning to Heal*, 220–29.

5. Born in New Maysville, Indiana, in 1843, Robert W. Long was the son of William Long, a pioneer physician. After attending Franklin College, he enlisted in the Indiana Seventy-Eighth Infantry shortly after the opening of the Civil War. When his term of duty had expired, he began the study of medicine in his father's office. He took one term of lectures at the Rush Medical College but graduated from Jefferson Medical College in Philadelphia in 1869. In 1875, he moved to Irvington, which was then a separate town on the outskirts of Indianapolis, and began a lucrative practice. In 1890, Long moved his office into the capital city, where he spent much of his time investing in real estate. For many years, he served as a member of the Central College of Physicians and Surgeons Board of Trustees. Although Barnhill was Long's partner for only two years, the men remained fast friends. Some descriptions of how Long came to donate money for a hospital to the university appear to have been embellished and romanticized to a certain extent and contain some factual inaccuracies. Among contemporary accounts are Henry, "Dedication of the Robert W. Long Hospital," 407; "Dr. Robert W. Long Dies at His Home," *Indianapolis News*, June 18, 1915; Earp, "Death of Robert W. Long," 314–18.

6. Robert W. and Clara J. Long to the Trustees of Indiana University, January 24, 1911, Folder 9, Box 75, Thomas R. Marshall Papers, Indiana Memory Digital Collections, Indiana State Library; Rice, "History of the Medical Campus, Chapter VI: Indiana University Chooses a Medical Campus," 139; Myers, *History of Medical Education*, 167; Glenn W. Irwin Jr. et al., *A Brief History of the Indiana University School of Medicine*, 8, unprocessed papers, Indiana University School of Medicine Records, 1848–2005, University Library Special Collections and Archives, University Library, Indiana University Purdue University Indianapolis (hereafter cited as UA 073, InUI-Ar).

7. Robert W. and Clara J. Long to the Trustees of Indiana University; "$200,000 as a Gift for a New Hospital"; Marshall to Sixty-Seventh General Assembly, January 26, 1911, Folder 9, Box 75, Marshall Papers.

8. Bryan to Pritchett, December 2, 1910, C270, InUI-Ar; Marshall, Speech to University Presidents, October 14, 1909, folder 4, box 74, Marshall Papers; "Military Park Chosen as Site for Hospital," *Indianapolis News*, February 2, 1911; Earp, "Death of Robert W. Long," 317; Robert W. and Clara J. Long to the Trustees of Indiana University; Rice, "History of the Medical Campus, Chapter VI," 139; Myers, *Medical Education*, 167; Irwin Jr. et al., *A Brief History of the Indiana University School of Medicine*, 8; "Dr. Robert W. Long Dies at His Home."
The Long gift was even larger than that of John Purdue nearly one-half century earlier, when Purdue pledged $150,000 to establish a university in Tippecanoe County. (Inflation was negligible or likely negative.) Topping, *A Century and Beyond*, 55.

9. Indiana Centennial Celebration Committee, *Suggestive Plans*, 86. Founded with the city in 1820, Military Park was bounded by West, New York, and Blackford Streets and the Central Canal. The militia used the park as a training ground, and later it was used as Civil War Camp Sullivan. Following the war, the grounds were improved with a fountain, pool, and shelter. In 1909, George E. Kessler, the internationally known landscape architect and urban planner, first conceived the idea of building a state government complex west of the Statehouse. Proponents defended their plan by stating that the hospital would occupy only one-fourth of the park. "Dr. Henry Jameson to Succeed Merritt," *Indianapolis Star*, September 15, 1906; "Military Park Chosen as Site for Hospital."

10. For more detail on the dispute, see Jones, "The Greatest Outrage."

11. Long to Bryan, April 12, 1911, Box 78, C270, InU-Ar; President's Reports, June 16, 1911, Box 4, C654, InU-Ar; George W. Curtis to Bryan, June 25, 1911, Box 35, C270, InU-Ar; Bryan, Minutes, IU Board of Trustees, July 3, 1911, Box 3, C218, InU-Ar; *Indiana Biographical Series* 2:94–95, Indiana Division, Indiana State Library; Bodenhamer, Barrows, and Vanderstel, *The Encyclopedia of Indianapolis*, 895–96.

12. The original tract of land proposed by the city was bounded by Caldwell and Porter Streets between Walnut Street and Fall Creek ("Proposed Grouping of 3 Medical Units"). Porter and Caldwell Streets no longer exist, but this site was situated approximately where James Whitcomb Riley Hospital for Children is located on the IU Medical Center campus. Rice, "History of the Medical Campus, II," 36; Bryan to State Senators, June 24, 1911, C270, InU-Ar; Bryan to Long, July 1, 1911, Box 78, C270, InU-Ar; Ludmerer, *Time to Heal*, 21; "News, Notes, and Comments," 90.

13. "The Hospital Site Again," *Indianapolis Star*, December 13, 1911; "Long Site Provided by Committee," *Indianapolis Star*, January 5, 1912.

14. Opening Dedication Program, Robert Long Collection, Historical Collections, Ruth Lily Medical Library, Indiana University Purdue University Indianapolis (hereafter cited as InU-M).

15. The main building was seventy-five feet by forty-five feet, with a central corridor extension of forty feet by twenty-six feet, and two wings seventy-six by thirty-six feet. It was originally heated by steam heat and forced ventilation. The upper roof decks were enclosed to form a tuberculosis ward. Henry, "Dedication of the Robert W. Long Hospital," Long Collection, InU-M.

16. Rice, "History of the Medical Campus, Chapter VI," 140; Myers, *Medical Education*, 168. This new site was bounded by Hiawatha Street to the east and Porter and Elwood Streets to the west and southwest. At this time, West Michigan Street to the south was paved in brick. See "Long Site Provided by Committee."

17. Having confronted the challenges of site and budget, the weather dealt the completion of Long Hospital another setback. Beginning on Easter Sunday, March 23, 1913, heavy rains in Indianapolis caused the waters of Fall Creek and White River to flood, and the almost completed Long Hospital was on precariously low ground. Compared to the damage throughout Indiana and the entire Midwest, the impact of the "Great Flood" on Long Hospital was minimal, but it further delayed the opening as the facilities in the basement were renovated, costing the university another three thousand dollars. Rice, "History of the Medical Campus, VI," 140–41; Emerson to Meyers, March 31, 1913, Box 42, C270, InU-Ar; Gray, *IUPUI*, 16–18; Germano, "A View of the Valley."

18. Henry, "Dedication of the Robert W. Long Hospital," 394;

19. "Dr. Long Presents Hospital to the State," *Indianapolis News*, June 15, 1914. Long died almost exactly a year later.

20. Ibid. On Flexner and American medical education, see the previous chapter. Since the late nineteenth century, medical schools were no longer commercial enterprises but rather university based. In the West and the South, with a few exceptions, the states controlled medical education. Brown, *Rockefeller Medicine Men*, 177; Fosdick, *Adventure in Giving*, 166; Ludmerer, *Time to Heal*, 4.

21. With a model teaching hospital, the School of Medicine seemed more qualified to receive such an endowment than ever before, and Pritchett even went so far as to suggest that IU officials should indicate the terms for such a gift. The foundation president informed Bryan that the Carnegie Foundation had decided to endow the Vanderbilt University School of Medicine with one million dollars first because medical education in the South was so weak. Bryan to Pritchett, March 18, 1913, Box 213, C286, InU-Ar; Bryan, President's Reports, June 13, 1913, Box 4, C654, InU-Ar. Bryan to Pritchett, December 10, 1910; Bryan to Pritchett, March 18, 1913; Bryan, President's Reports, June 13, 1913, InU-Ar. Ludmerer, *Learning to Heal*, 193–94; Jacobson, *Making Medical Doctors*; Brown, *Rockefeller Medicine Men*, 165, 176–77. The Rockefeller General Education Board also determined that creating a model institution for the South was a first priority and gave an additional four million dollars to the Nashville, Tennessee, school. See Ludmerer, Learning to Heal, 193–94.

22. Bryan to Pritchett, March 18, 1913; S. D. Miller to Elihu Root, May 27, 1918, C286, InU-Ar; Flexner to Emerson, November 28, 1921, UA 073, InUI-Ar; Bryan to Emerson, April 26, 1922, Box 87, C286, InU-Ar; Emerson to Bryan, November 8, 1922, "Indiana University School of Medicine: Historical,"

Box 87, C286, InU-Ar; Fosdick, Adventure in Giving, 168; Brown, Rockefeller Medicine Men, 176–87; Ludmerer, Time to Heal, 193.

23. That realization also limited Emerson's plans. Pritchett to Bryan, January 10, 1910, C270, InU-Ar. Bryan to Emerson, November 10, 1914, Box 86, C286 InU-Ar. Emerson to Bryan, October 23, 1923, Box 87, C286, InU-Ar. Emerson to Bryan, November 4, 1922, "Indiana University School of Medicine: Historical"; Bryan to Pritchett, March 18, 1913; J. J. Pettyjohn to James P. Goodrich, September 25, 1920, Documents and Reports: Indiana University, Box 156, James P. Goodrich Papers, Indiana Archives and Records Administration (hereafter cited as In-Ar). Brown, Rockefeller Medicine Men, 155; Ludmerer, Learning to Heal, 192.

24. *Indiana Statutes relating to Township Trustees: Concerning Their Duties, Powers and Prohibitions* (Indianapolis: Wm. B. Burford, 1915), 53.

25. Indiana University Catalog (Bloomington: Indiana University, 1915); Flowers, *A Legacy of Leadership*; Rock, "A History of the Indiana University Training School for Nurses."

26. After she left Indiana, Fitzgerald spent fifteen years establishing nursing programs in several different countries, including in Eastern Europe after the First World War and in Asia while working for the International Health Board of the Rockefeller Foundation. In 1930, she returned to work in New York. Her papers are at the Johns Hopkins Medical Archives.

27. Marriner-Tomey, *Nursing at Indiana University*, 9–10; Rock, "A History of the Indiana University Training School for Nurses," 55–57; Number of Graduates, 1917–1928, Box 1, School of Nursing Records, UA 025, InUI-Ar.

28. The nursing program remained under the administration of the medical school until it became its own school in 1965. Rock, "A History of the Indiana University Training School for Nurses; Flowers, A Legacy of Leadership."

29. Bryan, President's Reports, June 16, 1911; Emerson, Report to the President and Members of the Board of Trustees, November 1, 1911, President's Reports, C270, InU-Ar.

30. Emerson, Dean's Report, Bryan, President's Reports, June 4, 1912, C270, InU-Ar.

31. Willis D. Gatch to Emerson, n.d., Folder 67, Box 1, Collection C126, Indiana University Archives, Bloomington (hereafter cited as C126, InU-Ar); Gatch to Bryan, January 1, 1949, Box 2, C69, InU-Ar; Henry Mills Hurd to Emerson, July 31, 1911, Folder 67, Box 1, C126, InU-Ar; William H. Welch to Bryan, September 11, 1911, C270, InU-Ar; Bodenhamer, Barrows, and Vanderstel, *The Encyclopedia of Indianapolis*, 609–10; Battersby, *Dr. Gatch as I Knew Him*, 37. Battersby's account contains some factual errors. For example, Gatch graduated from IU in 1901 rather than in 1903. He attended IU during Joseph Swain's administration rather than David Starr Jordan's. Nevertheless, this booklet is important because it reveals much about Gatch's character.

32. Gatch to Emerson, n.d., Folder 67, Box 1, C126, InU-Ar; Hurd to Emerson, July 31, 1911; William H. Welch to Bryan, September 11, 1911; Ludmerer, *Time to Heal*, 94; Bodenhamer, Barrows, and Vanderstel, *The Encyclopedia of Indianapolis*, 609. Washington University's medical school had followed a similar path to that of IU, having taken over two proprietary schools at the

turn of the twentieth century. It was likewise responding to similar criticism from the Flexner report at the time Gatch was hired, but unlike IU, Washington University was successful in obtaining an endowment of $750,000 from the Rockefeller General Education Board in 1914. See "Origins and History of the Washington University School of Medicine," accessed August 16, 2017, http://beckerexhibits.wustl.edu/wusm-hist/index.htm; and Schneider, "The Men Who Followed Flexner: Richard Pearce, Alan Gregg, and the Rockefeller Foundation Medical Divisions, 1919–1951," in *Rockefeller Philanthropy and Modern Biomedicine*, 9.

33. Bryan to Emerson, September 18, 1911, Bryan Letter Books, Box 147, C270, InU-Ar. William H. Welch to Bryan, September 11, 1911; Minutes, IU Board of Trustees, November 3, 1911, Box 3, C218, InU-Ar. Emerson, Report to the President and Members of the Board of Trustees, November 1, 1911; Gatch to Emerson, September 23, 1911, Folder 68, Box 1, C126, InU-Ar.

34. George S. Bond to Emerson, April 8, 1914, Box 86; Emerson to Bryan, April 13, 1914, Box 86; Bond to Emerson, May 22, 1914, Box 87; Emerson to Bryan, June 11, 1914, Box 87; Emerson to Bryan, June 5, 1916, Box 86, C286, InU-Ar; Edwin N. Kime to Elvis Stahr, June 6, 1966, enclosure: Memorial Volume, Golden Anniversary Reunion, Class of 1916, IU School of Medicine, 14–17, Box 111, InU-Ar; Harvey, *Adventures in Medical Research*, 19; Indiana University, The Indiana University Catalogue (Bloomington: Indiana University, 1931), 340.

35. Indiana University Catalog, 297. For national comparisons, see Ludmerer, Time to Heal, 24.

36. Emerson to Bryan, September 30, 1914, Box 87, C286, InU-Ar.

37. In 1912, this group succeeded the Executive Committee as the faculty's governing body and did the work formerly done by the old Advisory, Educational, and Curriculum Committees. Barnhill, Gatch, Myers, Oliver, Wynn, and Wishard were among its members. Indiana University Catalog.

38. "Dr. John H. Oliver," Wishard Scrapbook (Indianapolis Medical Society, 1940), 36, The Program of Digital Scholarship at IUPUI University Library.

39. According to the Indiana University *News Gazette* (July 1915), paying patients were charged fifteen dollars per week and up to twenty-five dollars per week for private rooms, with fees for special services such as an operating fee of five dollars. Paying patients continued under their family doctor or a member of faculty. Bodenhamer, Barrows, and Vanderstel, *The Encyclopedia of Indianapolis*, 1065; Bryan, President's Reports, June 4, 1912, C270, InU-Ar; Emerson to Bryan, July 22, 1914, Box 87, C286, InU-Ar; Wishard to Emerson, July 29, 1914, Folder 3, Box 2, UA 073, InUI-Ar; Emerson to Bryan, August 1, 1914, Box 87; Emerson to Bryan, October 29, 1914, Box 86, C286, InU-Ar; "Robert W. Long Hospital," [1914], Folder 19, Box 2, UA 073, InUI-Ar; Bulson to Emerson, December 20, 1922, Box 86, C286, InU-Ar; Myers, *Medical Education*, 170.

40. Emerson, "Indiana University School of Medicine," 40.

41. Bryan to Emerson, October 15, 1914, Box 86, C286, InU-Ar.

42. See Emerson, "Medical Social Services of the Future," 333–42. The Indiana University School of Social Work in fact claims the Medical Service

Department as its founding organization. See Rogers, *Seventy Years of Social Work Education*.

43. Beecher and Altschule, *Medicine at Harvard*, 156–57.

44. Minutes, IU Board of Trustees, July 3, 1911, InU-Ar; Bryan to Fesler, Shively, Shea, et al., July 7, 1911, Bryan Letter Books, Box 146, C270, InU-Ar; Myers to Bryan, February 18, 1909, Box 90, C270; Emerson to Bryan, March 10, 1921, Box 87; Emerson to Bryan, June 27, 1931, Box 87, C286, InU-Ar; Bryan to Edna Henry, July 4, 1911, Box 58, C270, InU-Ar; Myers, *Medical Education*, 163–66; Piepho, "The History of the Social Service Department," 4–5; Rosenberg, *The Care of Strangers*, 313.

45. Piepho and Rogers state that Ulysses G. Weatherly first discussed the need for establishing a social service department at the IU School of Medicine as a laboratory for the Department of Economics and Social Work "at the same time that plans were underway for" Long Hospital in 1911. However, in February 1909, Burton D. Myers was already formulating a plan for a social service department in connection with the IU School of Medicine. Myers to Bryan, February 9, 1909, Box 90, C270, InU-Ar, February 18, 1901, Box 31, C174, InU-Ar; Bryan to Emerson, June 10, 1912, Box 86, C286, InU-Ar; Myers, *Medical Education*, 163–66; Rogers, *A Digest of Laws*, 3–26. Clark, *Indiana University* 2:301, has high praise for Weatherly, who joined the Indiana University faculty in 1895 and remained until his retirement in 1935, having served as president of the American Sociological Association in 1923. Henry received her undergraduate degree from Indiana University in 1897, and she later completed her master's and doctoral degrees at the same institution. Before her appointment at IU, she had been instrumental in organizing the Associated Charities in Anderson and had worked with the Indianapolis Public Schools. Her work in the IU Social Services Department began in September 1911. Indiana University Board of Trustees Minutes, June 17, 1911, Indiana University Board of Trustees Minutes, http://webapp1.dlib.indiana.edu/iubot /welcome.do;jsessionid=8D63E4C2F845A8E9EA76D3C653FAC896 (hereafter cited as IU BOT); Henry to Bryan, June 18, 1911, Box 58, C270, InU-Ar; Myers, *Medical Education*, 164; Rogers, *A Digest of Laws*, 13, 15; John A. Offord, "The Boon of Health," *The New York Observer*, January 18, 1912; Bodenhamer, Barrows, and Vanderstel, *The Encyclopedia of Indianapolis*, 506–7.

46. Piepho, "The History of the Social Service Department," 16–29; 34–35.

47. This was not uncommon. On the general relationship between eugenics and public health, see Brandt and Gardner, "Antagonism and accommodation," 707–15. As stated above, the IU School of Social Work dates its founding from Emerson's Social Service Department. See Rogers, *Seventy Years of Social Work Education*, 3. In his book *Racial Hygiene*, Rice listed himself as "Chairman, Indiana Eugenics Committee."

48. Piepho, "The History of the Social Service Department," 40–48. See also Bush et al., "Indiana University School of Social Work," 83–100.

49. Piepho, "The History of the Social Service Department," 31.

50. Bobbs Dispensary and City Dispensary merged into the City Dispensary in 1909, and IUSM took over the operations as a part of their clinical facilities. Edna Henry, Report of the Social Services Department, May 31, 1913, Bryan,

President's Reports, InU-Ar; Bryan to Fesler, July 14, 1914, Box 94, C286, InU-Ar; Piepho, "The History of the Social Service Department," 29–30, 34–36.

51. Bryan to Emerson, October 15, 1914, Box 86, C286, InU-Ar.

52. Ibid.

53. Bryan to Fesler, July 14, 1914, Box 94, C286, InU-Ar; Emerson to Bryan, December 29, 1914, Box 87, C286, InU-Ar; Reiser, *Technological Medicine*, 14–30; Rothman, *Beginnings Count*; Piepho, "The History of the Social Service Department," 23.

54. Piepho, "The History of the Social Service Department," 5–7; Emerson to Bryan, October 15, 1914; Emerson to Bryan, February 28, 1920; Bryan to S. E. Smith, May 26, 1924, Box 243, C286, InU-Ar.

55. Moreover, Bryan's estimates only included the operation of two floors of the hospital. With the opening of the third floor, the university president was sure that the absolute deficit would be greater, although it would lower the per capita cost. "There are many things which might be said about this," Bryan said, "but the important one is that we can not meet the proposed deficit, and, therefore, must not incur it." Emerson to Bryan, October 15, 1914, InU-Ar. Bryan to Emerson, November 25, 1914, InU-Ar. Emerson to Bryan, November 30, 1914; Bryan to Emerson, December 1, 1914, Box 87, C286, InU-Ar. Minutes, IU BOT, December 1, 1914, InU-Ar. Flowers, A Legacy of Leadership.

56. Minutes, IU BOT December 2, 1914; Rice, "History of the Medical Campus, Chapter VIII: The School of Nursing," 187. Emerson to Bryan, December 29, 1914; Emerson to Bryan, March 1, 1915, Box 87, C286, InU-Ar.

57. Emerson, Report to the IU Board of Trustees, June 9, 1916, Box 6, C654, InU-Ar.

58. Ibid. See also Emerson to Bryan, February 18, 1914, Box 87, C286, InU-Ar; Minutes, IU Board of Trustees, November 3, 1911; June 15, 1912, Box 3, C218, InU-Ar; Emerson to Bryan, February 18, 1914, InU-Ar; Emerson to Bryan, April 14, 1916, Box 87, C286, InU-Ar.

59. Emerson to Bryan, February 18, 1914; Emerson to Bryan, September 15, 1914, Box 87, C286, InU-Ar.

60. Emerson to Bryan, February 18, 1914; Emerson to Bryan, September 15, 1914. Eastman (1869–1919) was a professor of obstetrics and trained at the Central College of Physicians and Surgeons, as well as in Europe. For a more favorable view of Eastman, see, Dunn, 663; *Indianapolis Medical Journal* 20 (1919): 659.

61. Wynn to Emerson, November 1, 1915, Folder 9, Box 2, UA 073, InUI-Ar; "Dispensary Situation at Indianapolis," 69; Bodenhamer, Barrows, and Vanderstel, *The Encyclopedia of Indianapolis*, 507.

62. Kathi Badertscher, "A New Wishard Is on the Way," 345–82. Burdsal (1839–1912) developed a paint manufacture business in Indianapolis in 1877 and incorporated it in 1892. This donation and the hospital made news across the country. Dowling, *City Hospitals*, 78, 93; Vogel, *The Invention of the Modern Hospital*, 66–67; Catlin-Leguto, *The Art of Healing*, 2; Hale, *Caring for the Community*, 53–56; Rice, "History of the Medical Campus, Chapter X," 235–39; Cleland, "The Mural Decorations of the City Hospital," 395–99.

63. "Dispensary Situation at Indianapolis."

64. Emerson, Report to the IU Board of Trustees, IU BOT Minutes, June 9, 1916.

65. IU School of Medicine Educational Committee to the IU Board of Trustees, June 30, 1916, Folder 17, Box 1, E127, InU-Ar. The coincidence was such that some of the old enemies of the school suggested that the fire "was not entirely accidental," but rather was started to force the state legislature to fund construction of a new educational building. City officials ruled out arson.

66. Rice, "History of the Medical Campus, Chapter V," 119; Myers, *Medical Education*, 170. For documentation on this complex story, see Emerson, Statement regarding Medical School Building Fire, December 1916, C286, InU-Ar; Financial Committee Minutes, IU School of Medicine, January 5, 1917, Box 16, A85-3, InUI-Ar; "Indiana University, Its Resources and Needs," Documents and Reports, Indiana University, 1917–1921, Box 156, James P. Goodrich Papers, In-Ar.
The story elicited extensive newspaper accounts. "Medical School Fire," 33; "Fire Fails to Stop Medical Class Work," *Indianapolis Star*, December 5, 1916; "Fire at School of Medicine; Loss Big," *Indianapolis News*, December 7, 1916; "Considers Repairs, but Expects to Ask Legislature for New Structure," *Indianapolis Star*, December 22, 1916.
The Indiana Dental College was a private proprietary school that became the Indiana University School of Dentistry in 1925. See subsequent chapter and Rice, "History of the Medical School Campus, Chapter IX: The Dental College," 216.

67. The governor did not help matters by favoring only a plan to fund the new building with budget cuts from the Indiana State Normal School and Purdue. The legislature also argued about the role of the educational levy and the general fund in funding higher education. "Indiana University, Its Resources and Needs," 214; Fesler to Bryan, January 29, 1917, Box 94, C286, InU-Ar; Myers, *Medical Education*, 171.

68. Fesler to Bryan, March 7, 1917, Box 94; Bryan to S. E. Smith, March 9, 1917, Box 242; Bryan to S. E. Smith, March 11, 1917, Box 242; Bryan to Fesler, April 4, 1917 (board letter), Box 94, C286, InU-Ar.

69. Connor McBride, "Base Hospital 32: Lilly Base Hospital," accessed August 17, 2017, http://www.worldwar1centennial.org/index.php/indiana-in-wwi-stories/2434-base-hospital-32.html, which relies heavily on Hitz, *A History of Base Hospital* 32. See also Inlow, "The Indiana Physician in World War I," 92–105. The records of the hospital, including a summary history, are in InUI-Ar archives, MSS 015. For background, see Lynch, *The Medical Department of the United States Army in the World War 1*: 92–105. The first six Red Cross hospitals were organized by 1916 and included Harvard, Lakeview (Cleveland), and Bellevue Hospital in New York.

70. Bernard D. Karpinos and Albert J. Glass, "Disqualifications and Discharges for Neuropsychiatric Reasons, World War I and World War II," accessed May 24, 2018, http://history.amedd.army.mil/booksdocs/wwii/NeuropsychiatryinWWIIVolI/appendixa.htm.

71. Walter J. Daly, "Essay on Medical Education: Historical Perspective," October 6, 2010, 6, unprocessed papers, UA 073, InUI-Ar; Phillips, *Indiana in*

Transition, 126–27, 611–12; "Indiana University, Its Resources and Needs," Documents and Reports, Indiana University, 1917–21. For a list of the faculty members who participated in World War I, see Myers, *Medical Education*, 172. For the role of World War I in changing medical education, see Bonner, *Becoming a Physician*, 306–12; Rothstein, *American Medical Schools*, 155–56.

72. "IU Medics to Get New Home Soon"; Minutes, IU Board of Trustees, June 9, 1917, Box 4, C218, InU-Ar; Emerson to Bryan, September 29, 1917, Box 87; Emerson to Bryan, [Fall 1918], Box 87, C286, InU-Ar; Myers, *Medical Education*, 172; Bryan to Goodrich, April 28, 1917, Documents and Reports: Indiana University, Box 156, James P. Goodrich Papers, In-Ar; "Indiana University, Its Resources and Needs," Documents and Reports, Indiana University, 1917–1921. Bryan to Fesler, April 27, 1917; Bryan to Fesler, April 10, 1917, Box 94. Smith to Bryan, April 13, 1917, Box 94; Fesler to Bryan, April 17, 1917, Box 94, C286, InU-Ar.

73. Goodrich to Bryan, March 5, 1918, Folder 4, Box 137, James P. Goodrich Papers, In-Ar.

74. Goodrich to Bryan, March 7, 1918, C286, InU-Ar. Minutes, IU Board of Trustees, March 8, 1918; April 17, 1918; June 6, 1918; Box 4, C218, InU-Ar. Myers, *Medical Education*, 173; Rice, "History of the Medical Campus, Chapter V," 120.

75. Medical School Ground Broken," *Indianapolis Star*, June 18, 1918; Myers, *Medical Education*, 173–74.

76. Ibid.

77. "Indiana University School of Medicine, in Its New Home, Joins in the Great Work of the R. W. Long Hospital," *Indianapolis Star*, November 2, 1919; Myers, *Medical Education*, 174–75; Rice, "History of the Medical Campus, Chapter V: The Medical School Building," 120.

78. Bryan to Gatch, January 31, 1936; April 20, 1936, Indiana University President's Office correspondence, Collection C286, Indiana University Archives, Bloomington (Indiana University President's Office correspondence, 1913–1937).

79. Ibid.

80. Architect's Blueprints, Physical Plant, Box 2, UA 059, InUI-Ar; "Three Buildings Costing $1,000,000 Will Be Built at the Indiana University Medical Center This Year," *Indianapolis Star*, June 19, 1927; *Indianapolis Sunday Star*, July 23, 1934: Clipping File, Indiana State Library, Indianapolis.

81. "Emerson Hall Remodeling, 1961–1964," UA 073, InUI-Ar.

82. Smith was superintendent of the Northern Indiana Hospital for the Insane in Logansport from 1888 to 1891, when he moved to the Indiana State Hospital in Richmond. While at Richmond from 1891 to 1923, he greatly expanded the facility to forty-four buildings on nearly one thousand acres of land. He led the Indiana Board of Charities in 1910 and the American Medico-Physiological Association. For history of the Provost Office, C173, InU-Ar. No successor was named when Smith died in 1928.

83. Myers to Bryan, October 2, 1925, Box 188, C286, InU-Ar; Emerson to the IU Board of Trustees, November 1, 1927, Box 87, C286, InU-Ar; "Concerning Faculty Salaries," 40; Emerson to S. E. Smith, June 1, 1927, C 173InU-Ar.

84. Van Allen et al., *Keeping the Dream*, 9–11.

85. "Big Hospital to Be Memorial to Riley," *Indianapolis News*, August 21, 1917; Van Allen et al., *Keeping the Dream*, 13–14; Van Allen, *James Whitcomb Riley*, 270–71.

86. Osgood, "Education in the Name of 'Improvement,'" 272–99; Preston and Haines, *Fatal Years*, 52–53; Meckel, *Save the Babies*, 124; Katz, *In the Shadow of the Poorhouse*, 113–15; Madison, *The Indiana Way*, 171; Van Allen et al., *Keeping the Dream*, 7.

87. Osgood, "The Menace of the Feebleminded," 258; Indiana Committee on Mental Defectives, 8. The committee issued two earlier reports in 1916 and 1919. See also "Big Hospital to Be Memorial to Riley."

88. Koch, "Not a 'Sentimental Charity,'" 69–70.

89. Halpern, *American Pediatrics*, 56–60; Kohler, *Partners in Science*, 41–43; Stern, "Making Better Babies," 742–52.

90. "Big Hospital to Be Riley Memorial"; AR IUSM, June 9, 1916; Emerson to Bryan, September 29, 1917, Box 87, C286, InU-Ar; Emerson to Bryan [Fall 1918]; Emerson, Report of the IU School of Medicine, October 15, 1917, President's Reports, Box 7, C654, InU-Ar; Emerson to Bryan, September 13, 1919, Box 87, C286, InU-Ar; Emerson, Report of the IU School of Medicine, October 27, 1919, President's Reports, Box 8, C654, InU-Ar; Emerson to Bryan, March 5, 1920, Box 87, C286, InU-Ar.

91. "Child Hospital Given Support," *Indianapolis Star*, August 26, 1917; "Indiana University, Its Resources and Needs"; L. C. Huesmann to Goodrich, October 23, 1918; Minutes, Organizational Meetings, Riley Memorial Association Papers, Riley Memorial Hospital, Indianapolis, Indiana (hereafter cited as RMA); "Committee to Confer Today with M'Cray," *Indianapolis Star*, January 29, 1921.

92. Emerson approached the Child Welfare Association's president, Albion Fellows Bacon, for her help. In 1913, during his first year in Indianapolis, he had become acquainted with Bacon when he supported passage of Indiana's first statewide housing law, for which she largely had been responsible. Edmondson, "The Indiana Child Welfare Association."

93. Minutes, Organizational Meetings, January 21, 1921; February 1, 1921, RMA. "Committee to Confer Today with M'Cray"; "Riley Admirers Dedicate Poet's Home on Lockerbie Street as Public Shrine and Pledge Aid to Memorial Hospital," *Indianapolis Star*, April 14, 1922; Van Allen et al., *Keeping the Dream*, 14.

94. "Hits at Tax Levy for State's Universities"; "Riley Hospital Bill Is Passed," *Indianapolis Star*, March 2, 1921.

95. Minutes, Organizational Meetings, March 9, 1921, RMA; Report of F. E. Schortemeier, Secretary, James Whitcomb Riley Association for the year 1921, January 11, 1922; Bryan to Dr. and Mrs. S. E. Smith, February 24, 1921, Box 243, C286, InU-Ar. Minutes, Organizational Meetings, March 9, 1921, RMA.

96. Van Allen et al., *Keeping the Dream*, 12. Smith, Bryan, and Fesler were selected to represent the IU Board of Trustees on this joint committee with the Riley Memorial Association along with Benjamin F. Long, George A. Ball, and Ira Batman. As president of the university, Bryan was elected the committee's chairman. Hugh McK. Landon, William C. Bobbs, Louis C. Huesmann,

Carleton B. McCullough, and Lafayette Page were designated as representatives of the Riley Memorial Association, which officially incorporated on April 9, 1921. Minutes, Organizational Meetings, March 9, 1921, RMA; Bryan to S. E. Smith, March 23, 1921, Box 243, C286, InU-Ar; Minutes, IU Board of Trustees, March 28, 1921, Box 5, C218, InU-Ar; Bryan to S. E. Smith, March 29, 1921, Box 243, C286, InU-Ar; Articles of Incorporation, April 9, 1921, RMA.

97. The committee "spent several weeks calling on physicians, nurses, and hospital business officials, for advice . . . and personally investigated children's hospitals in Chicago, Iowa City, Boston, New York, Philadelphia, Baltimore, Washington, Detroit, and St. Louis." Minutes, Organizational Meetings, March 9, 1921, RMA

98. Questions arose about the legality of acquiring portions of this property through condemnation proceedings. Finally, the city promised "to carry through a measure for . . . building . . . a park" covering approximately one hundred twenty-five acres from the hospital site to the White River, which would have the IU School of Medicine complex as its centerpiece. Report of F. E. Schortemeier, January 11, 1922. Minutes, Joint Executive Committee, April 6, 1921; April 22, 1921; April 27, 1921; May 4, 1921; June 22, 1921; July 6, 1921; July 13, 1921; August 10, 1921; September 1, 1921; October 12, 1921, RMA. Schortemeier to Bryan, May 12, 1921; Schortemeier to Bryan, May 19, 1921, C286, InU-Ar; "First Frame House Here, Built by Riley Ancestor, Stands on Riley Hospital Site," *Indianapolis Star*, September 18, 1921; "How the James Whitcomb Riley Hospital Will Look When Completed," *Indianapolis News*, July 8, 1922; "Governor and Mayor Break Ground for the First Unit of Riley Memorial," July 12, 1922; Van Allen et al., *Keeping the Dream*, 15–16.

99. Buildings and Building Improvements, [1920], C286, InU-Ar; Schortemeier to Bryan, May 12, 1921; "Riley Admirers Dedicate Poet's Home"; Anderson, 40.

100. Daggett designed the hospital to be built in stages with the first part of the hospital to include offices, public wards, private rooms, operating rooms, and nurse and intern quarters, to be followed by the orthopedic convalescent clinic and pediatric medical wards. A third addition was designed to house the surgical department, operating pavilions, and an infant ward. Van Allen et al., *Keeping the Dream*, 16.

101. Minutes, Joint Executive Committee, June 1, 1921, RMA; "How the James Whitcomb Riley Hospital Will Look When Completed"; Report of F. E. Schortemeier, January 11, 1922; Minutes, Joint Executive Committee; "How the James Whitcomb Riley Hospital Will Look When Completed"; "Riley Admirers Dedicate Poet's Home"; "Governor and Mayor Break Ground"; "Name Riley 'Gym' for Ball Family," *Indianapolis Star*, September 20, 1922; "140 Members of Rotary Club Volunteer Aid in Drive for Riley Memorial Fund," *Indianapolis Star*, September 20, 1922; "Subscribe $81,375 to Riley Hospital," *Indianapolis Star*, February 21, 1923; Van Allen et al., *Keeping the Dream*, 16.

102. "Riley Hospital Is Birthday Tribute," *Indianapolis News,* October 7, 1924; "A Perfect Memorial," *New York Times*, October 10, 1924; Van Allen et al., *Keeping the Dream*, 16.

103. *Acts of Indiana General Assembly*, 1921, chap. 266, 834; Minutes, Joint Executive Committee, March 1, 1922, RMA; Morris Green, "The History of the James Whitcomb Riley Hospital," unpublished paper, n.d., RMA; "Some Odds and Ends," *Indianapolis Star*, June 4, 1921.

104. Emerson to Bryan, May 24, 1922, Box 87, C286, InU-Ar; "Editorial Notes," *Journal of the Indiana State Medical Association* 15 (March 1922): 101, 329; Myers to Bryan, October 30, 1922, Box 188, C286, InU-Ar; Starr, *The Social Transformation of American Medicine*, 253.

105. "Riley Hospital Is Birthday Tribute," *Indianapolis News*, October 7, 1924; "A Perfect Memorial," *New York Times*, October 10, 1924; Van Allen et al., *Keeping the Dream*, 16.

106. James Whitcomb Riley Hospital for Children, Movement of Patients, November 1, 1924 to August 31, 1925; *Indiana University Hospitals Bulletin, Riley Hospital Service Committees* 3 (April 3, 1928).

107. Van Allen et al., *Keeping the Dream*, 17; Emerson to Oliver, August 22, 1924, Folder 33, Box 3, UA 073, InUI-Ar; Minutes, IU Board of Trustees, September 23, 1924; Oliver to Emerson, September 23, 1924, Box 2, UA 073, InUI-Ar.

108. Gatch to Bryan, October 7, 1931, Box 104, C286, InU-Ar.

109. Schedules, Courses, and Clinics, 1921–22, Folders 19, 22, Box 3, UA 073, InUI-Ar; Schedules, Courses, and Clinics, 1922–23, Folders 20, 21, 23, 24, 25, Box 3, E126, InU-Ar; Olga Bonke Booher, interview by Chad Berry, August 18, 1992, Indiana Medicine 1993, Indiana University Center for the Study of History and Memory, Bloomington; Emerson to Bryan, November 21, 1923, Box 87, C286, InU-Ar; Ludmerer, *Time to Heal*, 66; Thompson, "This Important Trust."

110. Emerson to Bryan, July 21, 1920, Box 87, C286, InU-Ar. For more on the rise of obstetrics and the problem of unwed mothers, see Maternal Health League of Indiana; Kunzel, *Fallen Women, Problem Girls*; Thompson, "This Important Trust"; Apple, *Perfect Motherhood*; Lovett, *Conceiving the Future*.

111. William H. Coleman to the IU Board of Trustees, December 16, 1924, C286, InU-Ar; S. E. Smith to George A. Ball, December 30, 1924, Box 1, C173, InU-Ar; Minutes, IU Board of Trustees, January 30, 1925, Box 6, C218, InU-Ar; Thompson, *"This Important Trust,"* 73. The Coleman family also funded the Suemma Coleman Home for Unwed Mothers, which provided adoption and services for young women until it closed its doors in 1975.

112. S. E. Smith to Edward L. Jackson, June 15, 1925, Box 243, C286, InU-Ar; "Indiana University and the Legislature," 175–77; "Help Others Help Themselves," *Richmond Palladium*, January 10, 1925.

113. Minutes, IU Board of Trustees, January 26, 1926; June 7, 1926, Box 6, C218, InU-Ar. "Coleman Hospital, 1927–1967," 13–18. For more on Jackson (1873–1954), who was a member of the Indiana branch of the Ku Klux Klan and became involved in several political scandals, but was not convicted, see Gugin and St. Clair, *The Governors of Indiana*; Moore, *Citizen Klansmen*.

114. Jackson to S. E. Smith, June 23, 1925, Box 243, C286, InU-Ar. Minutes, IU Board of Trustees, January 26, 1926; June 7, 1926, Box 6, C218, InU-Ar. S. E. Smith to Bryan, September 23, 1927, Box 243, C286, InU-Ar; "William

H. Coleman Hospital, IU Medical Unit, Dedicated," *Indianapolis Star*, October 21, 1927; "Dedication of the William H. Coleman Hospital for Women," 42; Thompson, 75.

115. Dishman, "Coleman Hall," 622–23; "Coleman Hospital, 1927–1967," 13–18; Steven C. Beering to Irwin, April 16, 1979, Capital Improvements/Coleman Hall, Box 1, A2000/01–004, InIP-Ar; Herman W. Blomberg to Raymond Casati, April 20, 1979, Capital Improvements/Coleman Hall, Box 1, A2000/01–004, InIP-Ar. The Division of Allied Health became the School of Allied Health Science in April 1991 (Minutes, IU Board of Trustees, April 6, 1991, Box 50, C218, InU-Ar).

5. New Medical Education, 1912–1932

1. Pinel, *The Clinical Training of Doctors*, 77–79, 85–93.

2. Emerson, "Report on the Condition of the Indiana University School of Medicine," December 1914, Emerson to Bryan, May 29, 1915, Indiana University President's Office correspondence, Collection C286, Indiana University Archives, Bloomington, (hereafter cited as C286, InU-Ar).

3. Walter Daly, "Essay on Medical Education: Historical Perspective," October 6, 2010, 10–11, unprocessed papers, Indiana University School of Medicine Records, 1848–2005, University Library Special Collections and Archives, University Library, Indiana University Purdue University Indianapolis (hereafter cited as UA 073, InUI-Ar).

4. William D. Day, interview by Chad Berry, July 20, 1993, Indiana Medicine, 1993, Indiana University Center for the Study of History and Memory (hereafter cited as CSHM); Edith Schuman, interview by Steven Stowe, May 25, 1993, Indiana Medicine, 1993, CSHM; Durward W. Paris, interview by Patrick Ettinger, June 17, 1994, Indiana Medicine 1993 CSHM.

5. Daly, "Essay on Medical Education," 10–11.

6. Margaret M. Newhouse, interview by Patrick Ettinger, August 3, 1994, Indiana Medicine, 1993, CSHM; Frank Ramsey, interview by Patrick Ettinger, February 5, 1993, Indiana Medicine, 1993, CSHM; Daly, "Essay on Medical Education," 10–11.

7. Ludmerer, *Let Me Heal*, 4. See, for example, Steinecke, and Terrell, "Progress for Whose Future?" 236–45.

8. Daly, "Essay on Medical Education," 4; Burton D. Myers, *History of Medical Education in Indiana* (Bloomington: Indiana University Press, 1956), 136; Bryan to Pritchett, March 18, 1913, C286, InU-Ar; "Dr. Long Presents Hospital to the State."

9. Based on Daly's review of Myers's correspondence housed in the UA 073, InUI-Ar. Daly, "Essay on Medical Education," 7.

10. Ibid., 9. The most extensive study of black physicians in Indianapolis at this time is by Erickson, "African-American Hospitals."

11. Three transferred to the University of Pennsylvania, and three transferred to Rush Medical College. Two transferred to Cincinnati, and one each went to Columbia, Western Reserve, the University of California, and Stanford. Daly, "Essay on Medical Education," 7.

12. Ibid.

13. Hurty held various titles at IUSM, including professor of bacteriology, and at Purdue in pharmacy. See Bennett and Feldman, "'The Most Useful Citizen of Indiana,'" 34–43; Paris interview; George W. Macy, interview by Patrick Ettinger, June 8, 1994, Indiana Medicine, 1993, CSHM; Schuman interview; Day interview; Hugh K. Thatcher, interview by Chad Berry, March 3, 1994, Indiana Medicine, 1993, CSHM; Daly, "Essay on Medical Education," 11.

14. "Dr. Thurman Rice, 1888–1952," 271.

15. Daly, "Essay on Medical Education," 10; Arthur B. Richter, interview by Chad Berry, September 7, 1992, Indiana Medicine, 1993, CSHM. J. D. Hayden, To Whom It May Concern at IUMC, October 29, 1924; Robert E. Neff to Mr. Rowlands, November 15, 1924, Box 14, UA 073, InUI-Ar.

16. Schuman interview; Daly, "Essay on Medical Education," 9.

17. "Student Training Corps 1917–1918," and "Summary of Information for Statistical Purposes," Box 8, UA 073, InUI-Ar; Schuman interview; "Dr. Thurman Rice, 1888–1952."

18. Frank P. Albertson, interview by Patrick Ettinger, October 28, 1993, Indiana Medicine, 1993, CSHM; Schuman interview.

19. Mary Keller Ade, interview by Chad Berry, March 18, 1993, Indiana Medicine, 1993, CSHM; Newhouse interview.

20. Naomi Dalton, interview by Steven Stowe, March 25, 1993, Indiana Medicine, 1993, CSHM; Schuman interview; Ade interview; Newhouse interview; Ramsey interview.

21. The terms were still fluid until the formation of the national placement system in 1952, which helped to create a unified system. See Stevens, "Graduate Medical Education," 1–18; Etheridge, "Graduate Medical Education: Then and Now," 166–67; Lister, "The History of Postgraduate Medicine Education," 728–31; and Cohen, *House Officer*.

22. Ludmerer, *Let Me Heal*.

23. In general, school records were kept only for those who stayed in Indiana for hospital appointments. See "Resident Student," UA 073 InUI-Ar.

24. Specialists of this earlier era typically were "informally credentialed" by their experience and the recognition of their fellow physicians and communities. Most specialty boards were not organized until the late 1930s, by which time the 1914–15 graduates were well established in practice, whether general or specialty. See Daly, "Essay on Medical Education," 11–12, 18.

25. Piepho, "History of the Social Service Department," 5–7; Emerson to Bryan, October 15, 1914, Box 243, C286, InU-Ar.

26. Piepho, "History of the Social Service Department," 35–36.

27. Emerson to Bryan, September 20, 1913; Emerson to Bryan, November 9, 1922; Myers to Fesler, November 12, 1931, C286, InU-Ar.

28. IU BOT Minutes, June 25, 1925; *Indiana University Alumni Quarterly* 12 (October 1925): 497.

29. Initial gifts to the Huesmann Foundation totaled approximately $60,000, which allowed for the establishment of a research fellowship of $2,500 a year in the Department of Pediatrics. Emerson to the IU Board of Trustees, November 15, 1927; Landon to Bryan, November 6, 1926; Bryan to Emerson, January 9,

1929; Emerson to Bryan, June 24, 1931, C286, InU-Ar. See also Van Allen et al., *Keeping the Dream*, 20.

30. Bryan, [untitled], Notes and Memoirs, William Lowe Bryan papers, Collection C69, Indiana University Archives, Bloomington (hereafter cited as C69, InU-Ar). In 1969, Bryan's executive secretary, Ruth McNutt, who had been secretary to Indiana Governor Samuel M. Ralston between 1913 and 1917 and came to work for Bryan from 1917 until his retirement, recalled that Charlotte suffered from mental problems and that Bryan felt that he could not leave her alone for long periods of time. See Ruth J. McNutt, interview by Thomas D. Clark, May 27, 1969, History: Indiana University 1968–81, CSHM.

31. Bryan, Notes and Memoirs. Longtime IU trustee John S. Hastings claimed that Emerson and Bryan never spoke to one another again in person after this incident. See John S. Hastings, interview by Thomas Clark, November 19, 1970, History: Indiana University 1968–81, CSHM. Although this is very unlikely, because Emerson remained active as dean for another decade, Ruth McNutt claimed that she did not know Emerson. See McNutt interview.

32. Battersby, *Dr. Gatch as I Knew Him*.

33. Emerson to IU Board of Trustees, November 15, 1927; Bryan to Emerson, December 8, 1927; Emerson to Bryan, February 17, 1928, C286, InU-Ar.

34. Bryan to Emerson, December 8, 1927; Bryan to Fesler, December 8, 1927; Fesler to Bryan, December 9, 1927, C286, InU-Ar.

35. Emerson to Bryan, December 14, 1927, C286, InU-Ar.

36. Emerson to Smith, January 18, 1928; January 31, 1928; Smith to Emerson, February 3, 1928, C286, InU-Ar.

37. Emerson to Bryan, February 17, 1928.

38. Bryan to Gatch, February 18, 1928, C286, InU-Ar; Olga Bonke-Booher interview, November 1, 2000, unprocessed papers, UA 073, InUI-Ar.

39. Fesler to Bryan, December 9, 1927; S. E. Smith to Emerson, February 20, 1928, C286, InU-Ar.

40. Piepho, "History of the Social Service Department," 105–7.

41. Ibid.

42. Emerson to Bryan, June 13, 1928, C286, InU-Ar.

43. Myers to Bryan, May 13, 1930; Bryan to Emerson, June 12, 1930, C286, InU-Ar.

44. IU School of Medicine Finance Committee, June 17, 1930, Box 16, A85–3, InUI-Ar; Thompson to Emerson, September 2, 1930, Janet Thorton, "Recommendations to the Development of a Social Service Department in the Indiana University Hospitals, May 29, 1931," C286, InU-Ar; Piepho, "History of the Social Service Department," 104–7.

45. Starr, *The Social Transformation of American Medicine*, 180–97.

46. Fesler to Bryan, June 18, 1930; Fesler to Bryan, July 11, 1930, C286, InU-Ar. Gatch's complaints were likely influenced by the way Emerson handled his appointment as chair of Surgery. But they may also reflect the persistent misogynistic bias in medicine. Whereas these examples of overstaffing were all female employees, in other settings Gatch complained that the hospitals were understaffed when referring to the male doctors.

47. Emerson to Bryan, March 6, 1931, C286, InU-Ar.

48. The position was referred to as a "commissioner of the Committee of Evaluation Movement in Asia," most likely as part of efforts to certify Western-trained physicians in China. Emerson to Bryan, March 6, 1931, C286, InU-Ar; Xu, *Chinese Professionals and the Republican State.*

49. IU BOT Minutes, July 23, 1931; June 11, 1932; Emerson to Bryan, February 2, 1931; Bryan to Emerson, February 5, 1931; Emerson to Bryan, February 14, 1931; Bryan to Emerson, February 23, 1931; Bryan to Emerson, June 16, 1931, C286, InU-Ar. *Indiana University Alumni Quarterly* 18 (July 1931): 378.

50. IU BOT Minutes June 10–13, 1932–33; "Indiana University News Notes," 468.

51. On entering class sizes, see chapter 9, table 9.2. In 1932, IUSM admitted 123 students, whereas Wisconsin, Minnesota, and Michigan admitted between 120 and 131 each. Illinois was the largest (178). Harvard admitted 125, and the University of Pennsylvania admitted 131 students that year.

52. Illinois and Colorado largely followed a similar path, with medical centers developed in the largest cities of their states, away from the state universities. This was not the case with Iowa, but along with Colorado it had the advantage of receiving support from the Rockefeller Foundation for medical school expansion. Iowa received $2.2 million in 1922 for construction of its university hospital, and in 1925, the RF gave $700,000 to the University of Colorado to help it move its medical school from Boulder to Denver. Brown, *Rockefeller Medicine Men,* 183.

53. Piepho, "History of the Social Service Department," 104.

54. Scholars such as Martin Pernick, "Eugenics and Public Health in American History," have shown the similarities of many features of public health and eugenics. In addition to Stern, "We Cannot Make a Silk Purse," 3–38, examples of recent research on eugenics in Indiana are Carlson, "The Hoosier Connection," 11–25, and Lantzer, "The Indiana Way of Eugenics," 26–42.

55. It was a slow and complicated process everywhere. Hopkins created the first public health school in 1916, followed quickly by Harvard (both with significant Rockefeller funding), but by 1936 there were only ten schools in the United States. The others were Columbia University, University of Michigan, University of California at Berkeley, Massachusetts Institute of Technology, University of Minnesota, University of Pennsylvania, Wayne State University, and Yale University. Michigan's first degrees in public health were offered in the Medical School in 1915. However, in 1920 a separate graduate School of Hygiene was created, which became a School of Public Health only in 1941. See Rosenstock et al., "Public Health Education in the United States," 39–65; Fee, "Who Will Keep the Public Healthy?"

56. Of note, the school was established with the support of a local philanthropy, the Fairbanks Foundation. But in another twist and a sign that the Bloomington-Indianapolis split continued to be a potential problem, a second School of Public Health was established at the same time in Bloomington. See chapter 10.

6. Leadership Change and the Great Depression, 1932–1941

1. Fesler to Myers, January 11, 1934, William Lowe Bryan papers, Collection C69, Indiana University Archives, Bloomington (hereafter cited as C69, InU-Ar).

2. Clark, *Indiana University*, vol. 2; Woodburn et al., *History of Indiana University*, vol. 2.

3. Weisz, *Divide and Conquer*, 127–46; Stevens, *American Medicine*.

4. "IU Medical Center Wins Recognition at Dedication of $600,000 Clinical Unit," *Indianapolis Star*, May 15, 1938; Wells, "Remarks at the Dedication of the School of Medicine Building," November 21, 1937, Indiana University President Herman B Wells speeches, Collection C137, Indiana University Archives, Bloomington (hereafter cited as C137, InU-Ar).

5. The history of the School of Dentistry is outside the scope of this book, but it has a rich parallel history. See Rice, "History of the Medical Campus, Chapter IX: The Indiana Dental College," 211–16; Carr, "History of the Indiana Dental College"; "School of Dentistry, 1957" and "History up to 1974," Box 12, Indiana University School of Dentistry Records, 1934–2003, University Library Special Collections and Archives, Indiana University Purdue University Indianapolis.

6. Bryan to Gatch, February 18, 1928, Indiana University President's Office correspondence, Collection C286, Indiana University Archives, Bloomington (hereafter cited as C286, InU-Ar); Booher interview; Clark, *Indiana University* 2: 96–97; Lois Ann Piepho, "The History of the Social Service Department," 104.

7. The survey was conducted by Robert E. Neff, a former IU hospital administrator. Neff graduated from IU in 1911, became the auditor for Long Hospital in 1920, and eventually was the first professional administrator at Methodist Hospital in Indianapolis in 1945. "Suggestions for Administrative Improvements in the Indiana University Hospitals," August 22, 1930; Neff to Bryan and the IU Board of Trustees, May 4, 1931; Bryan to E. T. Thompson, July 14, 1931; [Gatch], "Proposed Changes in the Organization and Administration of the Medical School," [September 5, 1931], C286, InU-Ar. "Indiana University, School of Medicine Records of the Registrar, 1915–1956, Collection #127." As mentioned in chapter 3, the Bloomington Department of Economics and Sociology continued to operate programs like those of the Social Service Department in Indianapolis that eventually became the School of Social Work after the Second World War.

8. Battersby, *Dr. Gatch as I Knew Him*, 2.

9. Edmund L. Van Buskirk, interview by Patrick Ettinger, June 30, 1993, interview 93-015, transcript, 4, 13, CSHM.

10. Donald E. Bowman, "The Dean's Intuition," November 1985, Box 1, Dept. of Biochemistry Records, UA-63, University Library Special Collections and Archives, University Library, Indiana University Purdue University Indianapolis; Battersby, *Dr. Gatch as I Knew Him*; George T. Lukemeyer, interview by Elizabeth J Van Allen, December 19, 2000, UA 071 Oral History, InUI-Ar.

11. [Gatch], "Report on the Administration of the Medical School and University Hospitals," (1931 Report on Administration of IUSM) November 1931, Indiana University School of Medicine Records, 1848–2005, University Library Special Collections and Archives, University Library, Indiana University Purdue University Indianapolis (hereafter cited as UA 073, InUI-Ar).

12. Battersby, *Dr. Gatch as I Knew Him*; Ludmerer, *Time to Heal*, 79, 88; Stevens, *American Medicine and the Public Interest*; Weisz, *Divide and Conquer*; Kenneth M. Ludmerer, *Let Me Heal*, 87–94.

13. *Indiana Senate Journal* (1923): 6; Martin, *Indiana*, ch. 14; Madison, *Hoosiers,* 289–95; Kotlowski, *Paul V. McNutt and the Age of FDR*, 100–27.

14. Martin, *Indiana*, 253–54; Blake, *Paul V. McNutt*. The Democrats won ninety-one of one hundred House seats and forty-three of fifty Senate seats.

15. Paul V. McNutt, "Inaugural Address of Governor Paul V. McNutt of Indiana," delivered in Indianapolis, January 9, 1933. At his inauguration, Governor McNutt articulated the challenges the state faced but also his intention "to prove that government may be a great instrument of human progress." When McNutt took office, he reduced a bureaucracy of over "one hundred distinct and largely independent departments and agencies" into eight departments.

16. "An Intensive Post-Graduate Course," xv; "Reorganization of the State Board of Health," 209; Rice, "History of the Medical Campus, Chapter X," 236; Clyde G. Culbertson, interview by Steven Stowe, April 29, 1992, Indiana Medicine, 1993, CSHM; Hull, "History of the Department of Pathology," 2–4. For the broader context, see Madison, *Indiana Through Tradition and Change,* 217–19; Linda Gordon, *Pitied but Not Entitled*, 200–1.
Although the reorganization enabled greater government intervention in many facets of Indiana life, it was far from uniformly progressive.   For example, in the decades leading up to this reform, doctors had criticized the State Board of Health's activities, especially in its Division of Infant and Child Hygiene, which they claimed put the state in competition with private practitioners. At the federal level, this same impulse led the AMA to persuade Congress to discontinue the Sheppard-Towner Act. The *Journal of the Indiana State Medical Association* declared that the new setup was designed "to correct . . . abuses, improve the quality of the proper services of the State Board of Health, and to effect a saving of probably $75,000."

17. Bryan to Gatch, December 1, 1934, C286, InU-Ar; Clark, *Indiana University* 2: 254–64. "The Living New Deal," referenced June 9, 2016, https://living newdeal.org/map. The Public Works Administration was created in 1933 as part of the National Industrial Recovery Act to pay for large-scale projects proposed by states and other governmental entities. For national comparisons of the program, see Smith, *Building New Deal Liberalism*.

18. Smith, *Building New Deal Liberalism*. For the situation across the state, see Topping, *A Century and Beyond*, 254–60.

19. The definitive work on Wells is by Capshew, *Herman B Wells*. Bryan had clearly felt the time to leave the presidency was at hand for several years. Nonetheless, he found it hard to relinquish control in the tumult of the 1930s. His decision was made easier by the legislature's passage of a law that established

a pension system for Indiana University. See also, Clark, *Indiana University* 2: 363–66, 384–87, 400–1.

20. The first indication of the findings of the self-study was in remarks at the dedication of the new medical building in Bloomington. See Wells, "Remarks at the Dedication of the School of Medicine Building" [20 Nov. 1937], Box 1, C137, InU-Ar. In Wells's files, this speech is misdated November 21, 1937. In his book, *The History of Medical Education in Indiana* (p. 189) Myers listed November 29, 1937, as the dedication date. Both of these dates are incorrect. According to the *Indianapolis News* and the *Indiana Alumni Quarterly*, the building was dedicated on November 20, 1937 ("Dedication Rite Tomorrow for IU Unit"; "Dedication of the Medical School Building").

21. Weiskotten et al., *Medical Education in the United States*, 5; Rothstein, *American Medical Schools*, 142–43.

22. Although enrollment figures increased, during the 1930s, on-time completion and drop-out rates increased, partially due to the economic conditions, with many students moonlighting or dropping out to pay for classes.

23. Weiskotten, *Medical Education in the United States*, 5–6.

24. Gatch to Bryan, December 4, 1934, C286, InU-Ar; Myers to Gatch, March 19, 1935, C69, InU-Ar; Myers to Bryan, IU Board of Trustees, April 2, 1935. The overcrowding was no secret. See, for example, "Owen Hall Crowded; Medics Turned Away," *IDS*, September 22, 1928.

25. William D. Cutter to Bryan, March 5, 1935; "Divided Medical School Is Rapped," *Indianapolis News*, October 5, 1937; Cutter to Gatch, July 28, 1937, Box 377–79; Confidential Report on the Council on Medical Education and Hospitals to the Schools of Medicine of the United States and Canada, Evaluation, Indiana University School of Medicine, 1937, Box 377–79, Indiana University President's Office records, Collection C213, Indiana University Archives, Bloomington (hereafter cited as C213, InU-Ar); Gatch to Wells, October 1, 1938, UA 073, InUI-Ar; Ludmerer, *Time to Heal*, 62–63.

26. Weiskotten, *Medical Education in the United States*, 32.

27. Ibid., 31–32.

28. "Divided Medical School Is Rapped."

29. Ibid. See also "Split-Course Medical School at I. U. Scored by Doctor, Defended by Dean," *Indianapolis Star*, October 6, 1937.

30. Gatch to Franklin Crockett, September 23, 1938, Box 377–79, C213, InU-Ar; "Medical School Merger Studied," *Indianapolis News*, October 5, 1938.

31. On the occasion of the new PWA Medical Building in Bloomington that opened in 1937, IU historian Clark said that by constructing a "pretentious" building for the departments of anatomy and physiology on the university's main campus, it looked "as though the intent [was] to retain indefinitely the first year of medical training at Bloomington." See "Divided Medical School Is Rapped." For background, see Clark, *Indiana University* 2: 254–64.

32. Medical School Problem [July 2, 1940]; IU BOT Minutes, June 3, 1940; Gatch to Wells, June 11, 1940, Box 377–79, C213, InU-Ar.

33. Myers to Bryan, May 21, 1935; Bryan to Wildermuth, May 20, 1935; Gatch, Report to the IU Board of Trustees, June 14, 1935, Gatch to Bryan, May 24, 1935; IU BOT Minutes, June 14, 1935.

34. Ludmerer, *Time to Heal*, 62.

35. Daly, "Essay on Medical Education: Historical Perspective," 7, unprocessed papers, UA 073, InUI-Ar.

36. Gatch to Bryan, May 24, 1935; Gatch, Report to the IU Board of Trustee, June 14, 1935, C69, InU-Ar.

37. See next chapter, table 8.1.

38. Myers to Wells, June 12, 1940, Box 377–79, C213, InU-Ar; Minutes, Executive Committee of the IU Medical Center, July 25, 1940, UA 073, InUI-Ar; "Procedures for the Admission of Medical Students," July 12, 1940, UA 073, InUI-Ar. The aptitude test was begun in 1926 as the Scholastic Aptitude Test for Medical Students and was later renamed Medical College Admission Test.

39. Minutes, Executive Committee of the IU Medical Center, July 25, 1940, UA 073, InUI-Ar; "Procedures for the Admission of Medical Students," July 12, 1940, UA 073, InUI-Ar; Battersby, *Dr. Gatch as I Knew Him*, 1.

40. Requirements adopted by the Medical Council of the IU School of Medicine, for the direction of the Committee on Admissions, June 1, 1935, Reference files, Indiana University Archives, Bloomington (hereafter cited as Reference Files, InU-Ar); "At the Medical Center," *Indiana University Alumni Quarterly* 23 (Summer 1936): 318–19.

41. See, for example, Steinecke and Terrell, "Progress for Whose Future," 236–45.

42. Herbert O. Chattin, interview by Patrick Ettinger, October 3, 1994, Indiana Medicine, 1993 (CSHM), 14, 16.

43. Byron Kilgore, interview by Patrick Ettinger, March 17, 1994, Indiana Medicine, 1993 (CSHM), 10, 13.

44. Norma Erickson, "African-American Hospitals and Health Care," 97; Rawls, *The History of Black Physicians in Indianapolis*; Badertscher, "A New Wishard Is on the Way," 366, 369.

45. Bryan to Gatch, October 5, 1933, C286, InU-Ar; Bryan Report to Board of Trustees, October 14, 1933.

46. Bailey to McNutt, September 11, 1933, Box 191, C286, InU-Ar.

47. Dalton interview.

48. William M. Sholty, interview by Patrick Ettinger, June 30, 1993, Indiana Medicine, 1993, CSHM, 5–6, 10.

49. Otis Bowen, interview by Philip Scarpino, January 23, 2007, Randall L. Tobias Center for Leadership Excellence, IUPUI, Indianapolis, IN. For additional information on his time at IU, see Bowen and Du Bois, *Doc: Memories from a Life in Public Service*, 21–38.

50. Bowen interview.

51. George L. Compton, interview by Patrick Ettinger, June 23, 1994, Indiana Medicine, 1993, CSHM.

52. Charles Fisch, interview by Chad Berry, 2 September 1992, Indiana Medicine, 1993, CSHM.

53. Bowen interview.

54. Fisch interview.

55. Victor J. Vollrath, interview by Patrick Ettinger, November 9, 1994, Indiana Medicine, 1993, CSMH.

56. Compton interview.

57. Compton interview.

58. Fesler to Bryan, March 1, 1933; Gatch to Bryan, January 24, 1934, C286, InU-Ar.

59. Gatch to Bryan, August 18, 1932; Fesler to Bryan, March 1, 1933; Gatch to Bryan, January 24, 1934, C286, InU-Ar. J. B. H. Martin to IU Medical Center employees, May 5, 1933; J. W. Carr to Gatch, August 7, 1934, C69, InU-Ar.

60. Chattin interview.

61. Dalton interview.

62. Brice E. Fitzgerald, interview by Patrick Ettinger, February 24, 1994, Indiana Medicine, 1993, CSHM.

63. Fitzgerald interview.

64. L. B. Miller, interview by Chad Berry, October 16, 1993, Indiana Medicine, 1993, CSHM.

65. Rock, "A History of the Indiana University Training School for Nurses," 33–34.

66. "Early History of IU School of Nursing by Nellie Brown, 1951" and "Correspondence Ethel P. Clarke, 1920–1929," Box 1, UA 025, Indiana University School of Nursing Records, 1914–2002, University Library Special Collections and Archives, University Library, Indiana University Purdue University Indianapolis.

67. "Early History of IU School of Nursing by Nellie Brown, 1951"; Myers to Bryan, Emerson, Gatch, Turner, June 25, 1930, Bryan to Fesler, August 29, 1930, Emerson to Bryan, September 10, 1930, Emerson to Bryan, December 14, 1930, C286, InU-Ar.

68. 1931 Report on Administration of IUSM.

69. Bryan to Ora L. Wildermuth, October 1, 1931; Neff to Bryan and the IU Board of Trustees, May 4, 1931, C286, InU-Ar. 1931 Report on Administration of IUSM.

70. Neff to Bryan and the IU Board of Trustees, May 4, 1931; 1931 Report on Administration of IUSM.

71. See later, and for example, Gatch to Wells, September 2, 1943, UA 073, InUI-Ar.

72. Rock, "A History of the Indiana University Training School for Nurses," 63.

73. Ibid., 61.

74. Gatch to Wells, January 6, 1939, UA 073, InUI-Ar; Wells to Gatch, January 10, 1939, Box 377–79; Culbertson to Wells, January 20, 1939, Box 377–79; Lute Troutt to Wells, September 18, 1939, Box 377–79. [Gatch], Report to the Board of Trustees, for the year 1936–1937, June 10, 1937; [Gatch], Report to the IU Board of Trustees for the Fiscal Year Ending, July 1, 1940, Box 377–79, C213, InU-Ar. Martin, "The Medical Center of the University of Indiana"; Emerson to Thomas A. Cookson, November 1, 1926, C286, InU-Ar.

75. Kahmann was the first occupational therapist elected president of the American Occupational Therapy Association. During World War II, she was called to Washington, DC, to serve as chief of the Occupational Therapy Section in the US Surgeon General's office. See "Therapist is Pioneer," *Indianapolis Times*, October 20, 1957; "Physical, Occupational Therapist to Retire from

Riley Hospital," *Fort Wayne Journal-Gazette*, August 11, 1975; Anderson, *The Uneasy Equilibrium*, 72; Annual Report of the James Whitcomb Riley Hospital for Children, Fiscal Year 1930–1931, Riley Memorial Association Papers, Riley Memorial Hospital, Indianapolis, Indiana (hereafter cited as RMA).

76. Ludmerer, *Time to Heal*, 79, 83–89.

77. Gatch, Report to the IU Board of Trustees, June 14, 1935; Gatch to P. W. Bailey, October 31, 1938, UA 073, InUI-Ar. Gatch to Wells, September 14, 1938; Report of the Self-Survey Committee of the Medical Center, January 9, 1939; [Gatch], [Address on changes in medical education], UA 073, InUI-Ar. *Indiana University Medical Center Quarterly* 1, no. 1 (1939): 23.

78. Badertscher, "A New Wishard Is on the Way," 366, 369; Rawls, *History of the Black Physician in Indianapolis*.

79. 1931 Report on Administration of IUSM; Culbertson interview.

80. "The Work of the Indiana University Medical Center," S. E. Smith to Bryan, February 3, 1919; Myers to Bryan, March 14, 1932; Fesler to Bryan, April 13, 1931; J. B. H. Martin to Bryan, December 24, 1932; Gatch to Bryan, August 7 1933, C286, InU-Ar. Gatch to Bryan, April 21, 1937; F. Katherine Bailey to Paul V. McNutt, September 11, 1933, Reference Files, InU-Ar. On Neff, see note 7, above.

81. Hale and Wilson, *Through the Years*, 38. According to [Gatch], "Report on the Administration of the Medical School and University Hospitals," the dean split the duties in the department among its most capable men. He appointed J. O. Ritchey, who later become head of the department, chief of medical service at Long Hospital. Leon G. Zerfas, who headed the Lilly Clinic, which Eli Lilly and Company established at City Hospital in 1926, became chief of medical education. In addition, he assigned George Bond the didactic portion of the internal medicine curriculum. Cecil L. Rudesill took charge of the department's laboratory work, John A. MacDonald took responsibility for postgraduate education, and M. Joseph Barry supervised work in the dispensary.

82. As he did in other fields, Gatch retained a local practitioner, Lacy Shuler, as chairman of the division and appointed George J. Garceau to be Riley Hospital's orthopedic surgeon with responsibility for complete care of all orthopedic patients. Hale and Wilson, *Through the Years*, 38.

83. [Gatch], "Report on the Administration of the Medical School and University Hospitals"; Gatch to Bryan, April 2, 1932; E. T. Thompson, IUSM Annual Report, 1931–1932, C286, InU-Ar. Holden and Klatte, "History of the Indiana University School of Medicine's Department of Radiology," Center and Departmental Histories, UA 073 InUI-Ar. Although the Department of Radiology's brief history prepared for the ninetieth anniversary of the IU School of Medicine stated that Wright's full-time appointment was in 1928, Bryan's correspondence revealed that he was not recommended for this until August 1931. Bryan to Emerson, August 4, 1931, C286, InU-Ar; Hale and Wilson, *Through the Years*, 25–30.

84. *IUMC Quarterly*, 1932, UA 073, InUI-Ar; *Quarterly Bulletin Indiana University Medical Center* (hereafter cited as QB) 4, no. 1 (1943): 24; Hale and Wilson, *Through the Years*, 24.

85. Neff to Bryan and the IU Board of Trustees, May 4, 1931; 1931 Report on Administration of IUSM; Bryan to E. T. Thompson, July 30, 1931, C286, InU-Ar. Piepho, "The History of the Social Service Department," 107.

86. 1931 Report on Administration of IUSM; Myers to Gatch, August 3, 1931.

87. The 17.6 percent cut was less than the overall decline nationally in state support for higher education, which was 32.7 percent from 1931 to 1933. See Snyder, ed., *120 Years of American Education*, 89. The problem was declining revenue, which New Deal Indiana Governor McNutt (as well as others around the country) sought to remedy by a sales and income tax. Government expenditures actually remained stable, so cuts in higher education were prompted by shifts to cover increased spending on things such as poor relief. See Kotlowski, *Paul V. McNutt and the Age of FDR*, 127–55; Snell, "State Finance in the Great Depression."

88. Neff to Bryan and the IU Board of Trustees, May 4, 1931; Gatch to Bryan, April 21, 1937; Gatch to Bryan, October 16, 1932, C286, InU-Ar. Gatch estimated that the medical school and hospitals needed a minimum of $315,025 to remain in operation (Gatch to Bryan, April 2, 1932, C286, InU-Ar).

89. Gatch to Bryan, April 2, 1932, C286, InU-Ar. Gatch to Bryan, May 5, 1932; Gatch to Bryan, May 18, 1932; Gatch to Bryan, August 18, 1932, C286, InU-Ar. Gatch to Bryan, April 21, 1937. Following an emergency measure approved by the IU BOT in September 1932, the salaries of those earning $5,000 or more at the university were decreased by another 2.5 percent. These measures reduced the budget by $30,000, leaving another $33,000 to be cut from other budget areas.

90. Gatch, Report to the IU Board of Trustees, June 7, 1934; Gatch to Bryan, October 16, 1932; E. B. H. Martin, Annual Report to the RMA, January 28, 1936, C286, InU-Ar. Gatch to Wells, August 27, 1938, Box 2, Herman B Wells papers, Collection C75, Indiana University Archives, Bloomington.

91. Gatch, Report to the IU Board of Trustees, June 7, 1934, C286, InU-Ar.

92. The inclusion of the hospitals in the medical school budget was a consistent problem because both excesses in expenses and revenues could widely shift the budgets. Gatch, Report to the IU Board of Trustees, June 7, 1934; Gatch to Bryan, October 1932.

93. "$75,000 Given for Oxygen Treatment Room at Riley Hospital by Sorority," *Indianapolis Star*, June 23, 1931; "Sorority Will Aid in Equipping Riley Hospital with Light Therapy Division," *Indianapolis Star,* February 16, 1935; Annual Meeting Minutes, RMA, January 14, 1932, RMA; J. W. Carr, Secretary's Report, January 28, 1936, RMA. Minutes, Joint Executive Committee, December 10, 1934; March 18, 1935; May 13, 1935; June 11, 1935, RMA. "Therapeutic Pool at Riley Hospital Assured US Aids," *Indianapolis Star*, August 2, 1934; "Tribute Paid to Riley's Memory," *Indianapolis News*, October 7, 1935; Van Allen et al., *Keeping the Dream*, 19; Ludmerer, *Time to Heal*, 53. The total cost of the pool was $69,040. The federal government provided $59,651 (Report of the State of the Medical Center [June 1936], C286, InU-Ar).

94. Thurman Brooks Rice, "History of the Medical Campus, Chapter VI," 142.

95. "New $600,000 IU Clinical Building"; "State Medical Center Augmented by Modern Building"; "IU Departments Ready to Occupy New Clinical

Building on West Side"; "Dedication of Clinical Building"; Gatch to Wells, September 14, 1938, Box 37—79, C213, InU-Ar.

96. "IU Medical Center Wins Recognition at Dedication of $600,000 Clinical Unit," May 15, 1938; "Dedication of Clinical Building," *Indiana University Alumni Quarterly* 25 (Summer 1938): 358–60; Gatch to Franklin Crockett, September 23, 1938; Myers, *Medical Education*, 190.

97. "New $600,000 IU Clinical Building to House Latest Type of Equipment for Never-Ending Campaign on Disease," *Indianapolis Times*, February 19, 1938; "State Medical Center Augmented by Modern Building Co-ordinating Administrative and Clinical Division," *Indianapolis News*, February 19, 1938; "IU Departments Ready to Occupy New Clinical Building on West Side," *Indianapolis Star*, February 21, 1938.

98. Gatch to Bryan, April 21, 1937; Gatch to Wells, September 14, 1938; Gatch to Albert Rabb, September 29, 1938, UA 073, InUI-Ar. Matthew Winters, J. O. Ritchey, Culbertson, Report of the Self-Survey Committee of the Medical Center [January 9, 1939], Box 377–79, C213, InU-Ar.

99. Gatch to Wells, September 14, 1938; Report of the Self-Survey Committee of the Medical Center [January 9, 1939].

100. Gatch to Wells, October 28, 1938, UA 073, InUI-Ar; Wells to Crockett, September 28, 1939, Box 377–79, C213, InU-Ar; "Medical School Merger Studied"; Clark, *Indiana University*, 3: 144.

101. "Medical Center Costs Discussed," *Indiana Alumni Magazine* 1 (January 1939): 6–7.

102. [Gatch], Memoranda on the Financial Return of the Indiana University School of Medicine in Case House Bill 74 Is Passed; Minutes, Executive Committee of the IU Medical Center, March 14, 1939, UA 073, InUI-Ar.

103. A Bill for An Act to Provide Medical Care and Surgical Care and Hospitalization for Indigent Persons [January 13, 1939], Box 377–79, C213, InU-Ar; [Gatch], Memoranda on Proposed Plan for Meeting Cost of Eighty-five Charity Beds in the New Building [1939], UA 073, InUI-Ar; [Gatch], Memoranda on the Financial Return of the Indiana University School of Medicine in Case House Bill 74 Is Passed, UA 073, InUI-Ar; Frederick E. Jackson to George R. Hays, January 11, 1939 [read before Wayne Union County Medical Society January 12, 1939, and referred to the legislative committee], UA 073, InUI-Ar; Martin to Gatch, May 3, 1940, Box 377–79, C213, InU-Ar; "Hospital Expense," *Franklin Star*, February 28, 1940.

104. [Gatch], Report on the Medical Center for the Year 1939, [January 15, 1940], Box 377–79, C213, InU-Ar; Martin to Bryan, February 26, 1936, C286, InU-Ar; Report of the State of the Medical Center [June 1936].

105. Gatch to Wells, September 14, 1938; [Gatch], Report on the Medical Center for the Year 1939; Rice, "History of the Medical Campus, Chapter X," 236–38; Martin, "The Medical Center of the University of Indiana," [reprint] *Hospital Management* (November 1938), Box 377–79, C213, InU-Ar; IU BOT Minutes, May 18, 1959.

106. Day interview.

107. IU BOT Minutes, June 1, 1920; Myers, Indiana University School of Medicine, Bloomington, 1940 [October 5, 1940]; "Dr. B. D. Myers," 6. With the

exception of the American Board of Ophthalmology and the American Board of Otolaryngology, most specialty boards were created during the 1930s. Ludmerer, *Time to Heal*, 88; Battersby, *Dr. Gatch as I Knew Him*, 1.

108. Wells to the IU Board of Trustees, April 20, 1940, Box 377–79; Wells to Gatch, May 8, 1940, Box 377–79, C213, InU-Ar. IU BOT Minutes, June 1, 1940; "President Wells Outlines IU Progress Since 1938," *Indiana Alumni Magazine* 3 (January 1941): 4.

109. Medical School Problem [July 2, 1940], Box 377–79, C213, InU-Ar; "Medical Research Here at Home" [November 11, 1939], Reference File, InU-Ar.

110. Memorial Resolution on the Death of John Ditmar Van Nuys, February 1965, Box 11, Indiana University Faculty Council records, Collection C181, Indiana University Archives, Bloomington. See next chapter for more on Van Nuys. For background on the Epileptic Village, see Loofbourrow, "The Indiana Village for Epileptics."

111. [Gatch], Report on the Medical Center for the Year 1939. Although some sources state that Van Nuys became director of hospital admissions in 1941, the minutes of the IU Board of Trustees show that this appointment began in June 1940. IU BOT Minutes, June 1, 1940; "University Shocked by Death of Dean Van Nuys," 13.

112. Gatch to Wells, November 3, 1941; Wells to Gatch, September 28, 1942, Box 377–79, C213, InU-Ar.

113. 1931 Report on Administration of IUSM.

114. 1931 Report on Administration of IUSM; Gatch to Bryan, December 16, 1931, C286, InU-Ar; Gatch, Harold M. Trusler, "The Research Division," *QB* 1 (January 1939): 19; Ludmerer, *Time to Heal*, 30.

115. Gatch and Harold M. Trusler, "The Research Division," *QB* 1 (January 1939): 19–20; Ludmerer, *Time to Heal*, 30–31. The sources of funding for IUSM faculty were as follows: $3,000 for Huesmann Fund; $5,000 for Eli Lilly Corp.; $10,000 for Landon Fund.

116. "IU Medical Center Develops Revolutionary Method of Treating Burned Persons," *Indianapolis Star*, December 14, 1939; Elizondo et al., "Physiology at Indiana University-Bloomington," 321.

117. Report on the Medical Center for the Year 1939; Summary of Research at the IU School of Medicine, 1938–40.

118. Besch et al., "Outline of the Historical Development of the Department of Pharmacology and Toxicology, 1906–1993," Center and Departmental Histories, UA 073 InUI-Ar; Harger, "'Debunking' the Drunkometer," 497–506. For background, see Lerner, *One for the Road*. On Mazzini, see Bodenhamer, Barrows, and Vanderstel, *The Encyclopedia of Indianapolis*, 983.

119. "The Research Division," 20; [Gatch], Report on the Medical Center for the Year 1939; Summary of Research at the IU School of Medicine, 1938–40, Box 377–79, C213, InU-Ar; "Indiana University Foundation," 502; Minutes, Executive Committee of the IU Medical Center, July 30, 1937, UA 073, InUI-Ar; Myers to Wells, May 3, 1940, Box 377–79, C213, InU-Ar.

120. [Gatch], Report on the Medical Center for the Year 1939; [Summary of Research at the IU School of Medicine], [1938–1940], Box 377–79, C213, InU-Ar; "Indiana University Foundation," 502.

7. The Medical Center at War and After, 1941–1946

1. For an overview, see Cooter, "Medicine and the Goodness of War," 147–59.
2. Thomas A. Hendricks to Gatch, January 13, 1943, UA 073, Indiana University School of Medicine Records, 1848–2005, University Library Special Collections and Archives, University Library, Indiana University Purdue University Indianapolis (hereafter cited as UA 073 InUI-Ar). Wells to C. Anderson Ketchum, January 18, 1943, Box 2; [Gatch], Report to the President and the IU Board of Trustees, June 3, 1944, Box 34, Herman B Wells Papers, Collection C75, Indiana University Archives, Bloomington (hereafter cited as C75, InU-Ar). "Outstanding Service of the 32d General Hospital," 9; Ludmerer, *Time to Heal*, 125.
3. Wells to Gatch, August 10, 1938, Box 377–79, Indiana University President's Office records, Collection C213, Indiana University Archives, Bloomington (hereafter cited as C213, InU-Ar). Minutes, Executive Committee of the IU Medical Center, July 25, 1940; January 22, 1942. Sanders, "The Relation of the University in the National Defense Plan," 6.
4. Wells to Ketcham, October 24, 1940; Wells to J. W. Carr, December 23, 1940, Box 377–79, C213, InU-Ar.
5. Gatch to Bryan, December 28, 1941, William Lowe Bryan papers, Collection C69, Indiana University Archives, Bloomington; Gatch to Wells, June 12, 1942, UA 073, InUI-Ar; Rice, "History of the Medical Campus, Chapter XV: The Medical Campus in Wartime," 68.
6. Gatch to Wells, June 12, 1942, UA 073, InUI-Ar; Minutes, Executive Committee of the IU Medical Center, January 20, 1942, UA 073, InUI-Ar; Rice, "History of the Medical Campus, Chapter XV: The Medical Campus in Wartime," 68; "Medical Center Plans for Raid," *Indianapolis Star*, December 11, 1941.
7. Gatch to Wells, December 28, 1941; Minutes, Executive Committee of the IU Medical Center, January 20, 1942.
8. Executive Committee of the IU Medical Center, January 20, 1942.
9. AAMC, "Proceedings of the Special Meeting Held February 14, 1942," accessed June 13, 2016, https://www.aamc.org/download/173476/data/aamc_proceedings_of_the_special_meeting_1942.pdf. For background, see Ludmerer, *Time to Heal*, 125–31.
10. Bowen interview; "The Indiana University War Service Plan," *Indiana University Newsletter* 30 (January 1942).
11. "Medical Students and Hospital Interns May Join the Enlisted Reserve Corps and Be Discharged by Local Board from Service in the National Army," 1917/1918, UA 073, InU-Ar.
12. Harold M. Manifold, interview by Chad Berry, November 16, 1994, Indiana Medicine, 1993, Indiana University Center for the Study of History and Memory (hereafter CSHM), Bloomington.
13. Bowen interview.
14. Minutes, Executive Committee, January 20, 1942.
15. See World War 2 Medical Research Centre, "WW2 Military Hospitals," accessed June 14, 2016, https://www.med-dept.com/articles/ww2-military-hospitals-zone-of-interior.

16. "47 IU Officers Join Army Today," *Indianapolis Star*, May 13, 1942; "47 Doctors, 72 Nurses Inducted into Army," Gatch to Wells, June 12, 1942; "Medical Center Load Is Normal," *Indianapolis Star*, July 20, 1942. See also the following materials, all in C213, InU-Ar: [Gatch], Report to the President and Trustees of Indiana University on the Work of the Indiana University Medical Center, The Medical Department at Bloomington, and the Student Health Center, September 1, 1942, to August 31, 1943, Box 377–79; [Gatch], Report on the First Five Years of President Herman B Wells Administration, August 29, 1944, Box 377–79 [Transcript Hearing of State Senate Commission to Investigate Indiana Medical Center, February 26, 1945], [enclosure]: Gatch to Wells, March 1, 1945, Box 377–79; [Gatch], "Report on School of Medicine and the Medical Center for Year 1944–1945," September 17, 1945, Box 377–79.

17. "Indiana General Hospital No. 32," *Quarterly Bulletin Indiana University Medical Center* (hereafter cited as QB) 8 (1946): 4–7.

18. Paul R. Hawley to [Wells], July 1, 1945, Reference files, Indiana University Archives, Bloomington (hereafter cited as Reference files, InU-Ar). For more, see "US Army 32d General Hospital, Indiana University Affiliate Is First Major Medical Installation to Move into Germany," Press Release, Headquarters Communications Zone, European Theater Operations, US Army, Reference files, InU-Ar; "47 IU Officers Join Army Today," *Indianapolis Star*, May 13, 1942; "47 Doctors, 72 Nurses Inducted into Army," *Indianapolis Star*, May 14, 1942; "Outstanding Service of 32d General Hospital," 9; Clark, *Indiana University* 3: 395. For a list of the military hospital's personnel see "Outstanding Service of 32d General Hospital," 13–14; "Indiana General Hospital No. 32," 17.

19. Gatch to Wells, June 12, 1942.

20. "47 IU Officers Join Army Today," *Indianapolis Star*, May 13, 1942; "47 Doctors, 72 Nurses Inducted into Army"; Gatch to Wells, June 12, 1942; "Medical Center Load Is Normal," *Indianapolis Star*, July 20, 1942; [Gatch], Report to the President and Trustees of Indiana University on the Work of the Indiana University Medical Center, the Medical Department at Bloomington, and the Student Health Center, September 1, 1942–August 31, 1943, C75, InU-Ar.

21. [Gatch], Report to the President and Trustees of Indiana University on the Work of the Indiana University Medical Center; Minutes, RMA Annual Meeting, April 25, 1945, RMA; Philip Kalisch and Kalisch, *American Nursing*, 472–73; Clark, *Indiana University* 3: 394.

22. [Gatch], Report to the President and Trustees of Indiana University on the Work of the Indiana University Medical Center, September 1, 1942–August 31, 1943.

23. Gatch to Wells, June 12, 1942; "Medical Center Load Is Normal"; Gatch to George B. Darling, October 24, 1942, UA 073, InUI-Ar; Ludmerer, *Time to Heal*, 128.

24. Ludmerer, *Time to Heal*, 127.

25. Charles Fisch, interview by Chad Berry, September 2, 1992, Indiana Medicine 1993, CSHM.

26. Medical Advisory Council, Box 2, Gatch to Victor Johnson, July 19, 1943, UA 073, InUI-Ar; [Gatch], Report to the President and Trustees of Indiana University on the Work of the Indiana University Medical Center, September

1, 1942–August 31, 1943; Minutes, Medical Advisory Council, March 6, 1943; Maurice Early, "The Day in Indiana," *Indianapolis Star*, March 21, 1943; Wells to C. Omer Free, January 25, 1945, Box 377–79, C213, InU-Ar.

27. Clark, *Indiana University* 3: 130–33.

28. Gatch to Wells, January 13, 1943, with enclosure "Procurement and Assignment Service for Physicians, Dentists and Veterinaries," December 29, 1942; Willard C. Rappleye Memorandum to Medical School Deans, December 30, 1942, Box 377–79, C213, InU-Ar. For a national comparison, see Ludmerer, *Time to Heal*, 126–31.

29. Lukemeyer interview; Morris Green, interview by Chad Berry, February 1, 1993, CSHM. Maurice Early, March 21, 1943; Gatch to Thomas A. Cookson, October 17, 1944, Box 377–79, C213, InU-Ar.

30. Rice, "History of the Medical Campus, Chapter XV: The Medical Campus in Wartime," 68.

31. Gatch to Wells, January 28, 1942; Wells to Gatch January 30, 1942, Box 377–79, C213, InU-Ar.

32. Walter B. Tinsley, interview by Angela Potter, May 19, 2015, UA 073, InUI-Ar.

33. Gatch to Wells, June 12, 1944; [Gatch], Report to the President and Trustees of Indiana University, June 3, 1944; Lukemeyer interview; Green interview; Glenn W. Irwin Jr., interview by Elizabeth van Allen, November 30, 2000, UA 073, InUI-Ar; Rappleye, "Effects to Date of the Wartime Program of Medical Education," 48; Ludmerer, *Time to Heal*, 128.

34. Rock, "A History of the Indiana University Training School for Nurses," 88–89.

35. Ibid., 69–81.

36. C. G. Culbertson to Gatch, March 25, 1943; Dean Gatch Correspondence, Cr-D, 1942–1943 folder, Box 52, ISOM Records, InIP-Ar. Rock, "A History of the Indiana University Training School for Nurses," 87–88.

37. Rock, "A History of the Indiana University Training School for Nurses," 82–85.

38. Ibid., 88–89.

39. Ibid., 87–90.

40. Minutes, Executive Committee of the IU Medical Center, 20 January 1942; "Medical Center Research Shifts to War Projects," *Indianapolis News*, April 18, 1942; Minutes, Research Committee, April 2, 1942, Research 1942, UA 073, InUI-Ar; Publications from the IUMC since the Organization of the Research Division in 1931; [Gatch], Report to the President and Trustees of Indiana University on the work of the Indiana University Medical Center, the Medical Department at Bloomington, and the Student Health Department, September 1, 1942–September 1, 1944, Box 377–79, C213, InU-Ar; Ludmerer, *Time to Heal*, 131–33.

41. [Gatch] Report to the President and Trustees of Indiana University, September 1, 1942–September 1, 1944; Bowman, "The Dean's Intuition," November 1985, Box 1, Dept. of Biochemistry Records, UA-63, University Library Special Collections and Archives, University Library, Indiana University Purdue University Indianapolis; "Dr. Donald Bowman Discovered Bowman-Birk

Protease Inhibitor," *Indianapolis Star*, October 9, 2002; Battersby, *Dr. Gatch as I Knew Him*, 8.

42. Andrus, "Forward"; Schneider, "The Origin of the Medical Research Grant," 279–311.

43. [Gatch] Report to the President and Trustees of Indiana University, September 1, 1942–September 1, 1944; Wells to J. W. Carr, January 10, 1946, Box 1, C75, InU-Ar. Harmon to Gatch, January 14, 1942, Box 377–79, IU Research Contracts/Total of Research Contracts since the War Started, December 19, 1944, Box 377–79, C213, InU-Ar. Maurice Early, "The Day in Indiana," *Indianapolis Star*, April 26, 1942; Schneider, "The Origin of the Medical Research Grant," 301–9.

44. Leathers, "The Association of American Medical Colleges and Some Postwar Medical Problems," 3.

45. Bush, *Science, the Endless Frontier*. The quote is from the November 1944 letter sent by Roosevelt to Bush asking him to investigate lessons for the postwar period from the work of the OSRD, but Bush drafted the letter for the president.

46. Joint Resolution, January 30, 1945, Box 377–79; [Gatch], "Report on School of Medicine and the Medical Center for Year 1944–1945," Medical Schools in the United States, Graduates from July 1, 1945 to June 30, 1945, Box 377–79, Indiana University, No. of "Medical" Degrees, [1933–1934 to 1943–1944], Box 377–79, C213, InU-Ar.

47. Transcript Hearing of State Senate Commission to Investigate Indiana Medical Center [February 26, 1945]; Free, Samuel E. Johnson et al., "Report of Commission to Investigate Indiana Medical Center," February 28, 1945, Box 377–79, C213, InU-Ar; IU BOT Minutes, February 10, 1945.

48. *QB* 2 (1940): 159. For national comparison, see Ludmerer, *Let Me Heal*, 113–17. "Medical Class Rosters, 1911–1956," UA 073, InI-U-Ar.

49. *IU School of Medicine Bulletin*, 1931, 1940.

50. Resolution, IU Board of Trustees, September 1, 1944, "Post War Plans for the Indiana University School of Medicine."

51. "Post War Plans for the Indiana University School of Medicine"; IU BOT Minutes, June 23, 1945.

52. "Post War Plans for the Indiana University School of Medicine."

53. Ibid.

54. Ibid.

55. Indiana University Institutional Research and Reporting, "Historical Student Enrollment at Indiana University," accessed April 29, 2018, https://uirr.iu.edu/facts-figures/enrollment/historical/index.html.

56. IU BOT Minutes, September 11, 1943; [Wells], IU BOT Minutes, November 2–3, 1945; Notes re. phone conversation with Gatch [November 6, 1945]; Hastings interview. Part of the confusion came from a phased in change in retirement age of deans from seventy to sixty-five, passed by the IU BOT [Minutes] on September 11, 1943, which stated, "Those reaching the age of 69 by July 1, 1944 will be retired from administrative duties on that date, those reaching 68 by July 1, 1945 will be retired from administrative duties then, and so on until July 1, 1948 when those reaching 65 will be so retired."

57. [Wells], Notes re: phone conversation with Gatch [November 6, 1945]; Hastings interview.

58. [Wells], Notes re: phone conversation with Gatch [November 6, 1945]; Hastings interview.

59. In his history of IU, Clark stated that "Dean Gatch's precipitate resignation, June 26, 1946, caught the Trustees by surprise." However, Minutes of the Board of Trustees clearly reveal that a special committee asked for Gatch's resignation on this date (IU BOT Minutes, June 27, 1946; Clark, *Indiana University* 3: 402.

60. Wells to Wildermuth, June 6, 1947, Box 49, C75, InU-Ar.

61. Rice to Wells, September 5, 1946; Wells President Papers, InU-Ar.

62. Dr. John Ditmar Van Nuys was born in New Castle, Indiana, on October 10, 1907. He was the son of Dr. W. C. Van Nuys and Mrs. Margaret Sevoid Van Nuys. He completed high school at New Castle High and received his AB in 1929 from Wabash College. He graduated from the IUSM with his MD in 1936 and continued his residency at the Medical Center until 1939. He served as director of admissions and was the chief resident physician medical director of the university hospitals until June 30, 1946. Van Nuys became the executive secretary of this committee on July 1, 1946, serving until June 11, 1947, when he was appointed dean of the Indiana University School of Medicine, in which position he remained until his death, February 15, 1965. "Memorial Resolution on the death of John Ditmar Van Nuys," February 1965, Indiana University Faculty Council records, 1947–1970, InU-Ar; Clark, *Indiana University* 3: 411–12.

63. Rice to Wells, September 5, 1946; Notes on interview with Kenneth G. Kohlstaedt [September 1946]; Notes on interview with Frank Forry [September 1946]; H. E. Klepinger, October 4, 1946; Notes on interview with [Maynard] Hine [September 1946]; Notes on interview with Dr. Sherman Jones-Hammond; Notes on interview with Dr. Herman M. Baker re: medical deanship; Notes on interview with Roy Smith, September 13, 1946; Wells to the IU Board of Trustees, September 28, 1946, Box 377–79, C213, InU-Ar. IU BOT Minutes, September 9, 1946.

64. IU BOT Minutes, April 14, 1947; Wells to Board of Trustees, June 12, 1947.

65. Jack Porter to Hastings, May 23, 1947, Box 377–79, C213, InU-Ar; Taylor to Wells, August 13, 1946.

66. Van Nuys was not formally added to the faculty until his appointment as associate professor of medicine in December 6, 1947. He became professor of medicine in December 1955. "Memorial Resolution on the Death of John Ditmar Van Nuys," Box 11, Indiana University Faculty Council records, Collection C181, Indiana University Archives, Bloomington; Harger to Wells, June 3, 1947, Box 377–79, C213, InU-Ar.

67. Wildermuth to Wells, June 5, 1947; IU BOT Minutes, June 13, 1947.

8. Crossing the New Frontier, 1946–1963

1. Burnham, "American Medicine's Golden Age," 1474–79; Brandt and Gardner, "The Golden Age of Medicine?" 21–37.

2. For national comparisons, see Ludmerer, *Time to Heal*, 139–79.

3. "School of Medicine Admits Record Class of 202," *The Quarterly Bulletin of the Indiana University Medical Center* (hereafter cited as *QB*) 24 (Summer 1962): 27–28; "Medical School Enlarges Faculty," *QB* 24 (Summer 1962): 34–35; IU BOT September 20, 1963, October 25, 1963.

4. Lull, "Fifty Thousand Doctors," 91–108; Weisz, *Divide and Conquer*, 135–46; Starr, *The Social Transformation of American Medicine*; Ludmerer, *Time to Heal*, 98–100.

5. Fuchs, "Major Trends in the U. S. Health Economy since 1950," 973–77.

6. Glickman et al., "United We Stand," 903–4; Braunwald, "Cardiology—Division or Department?" 1887–1890; Anderson, "Subspecialization in Internal Medicine," 74–81.

7. For a comparison, see Solberg, *Reforming Medical Education*.

8. "Medical Center Expansion Bill Near Final Vote," *Indianapolis News*, March 8, 1947; "Biennial Budget," 7; Rice, "History of the Medical Campus, Chapter X," 238–39; Ralph F. Gates to Wells, April 24, 1947, Box 377–79, Indiana University President's Office records, Collection C213, Indiana University Archives, Bloomington (hereafter cited as C213, InU-Ar).

9. Van Nuys to Wells, January 29, 1947, Box 377–79, C213, InU-Ar. Wells to John J. Mahoney, March 21, 1947; Van Nuys to Wells, July 22, 1947; IU BOT Minutes, September 12, 1947.

10. "IU Medical School Faces Student Flood," *Indianapolis Star*, February 9, 1947; IU BOT Minutes, May 16, 1947.

11. Admissions Figures, Notes for Remarks to Budget Committee [October 18, 1945], Box 377–79, C213, InU-Ar; Clark, *Indiana University* 3:148–49; "Historical Student Enrollment at Indiana University," accessed May 3, 2018, https://uirr.iu.edu/facts-figures/enrollment/historical/index.html.

12. J. B. H. Martin, "Annual Report of the Administrator of the Indiana University Medical Center to the Board of Governors of the James Whitcomb Riley Memorial Association," April 24, 1946; April 30, 1947, Records of the James Whitcomb Riley Memorial Association, Indianapolis (hereafter cited as RMA). Legislative Budget, 1945–1947, Box 377–79, C213, InU-Ar.

13. Schneider, "The Men Who Followed Flexner," 7–60.

14. *Encyclopedia of Indianapolis*, 1197. On Ritchie's role as mentor of Dean Glen Irwin, see Gray, IUPUI, 137–38.

15. Ludmerer, *Time to Heal*, 43–44, 157.

16. "Thurman Brooks Rice," 400; Hull, "History of the Department of Pathology."

17. See chapter 4.

18. Rice to Wells, August 20, 1947; Wells to Rice August 27, 1947, Box 377–79, C213, InU-Ar. "School of Public Health," *Indianapolis Star*, January 27, 1947. For an open letter to the public by Rice see, "The Proposed School of Public Health at the Medical Center," *Monthly Bulletin Indiana State Board of Health*, December 1947. Clark states that a later attempt to revive the proposal for the school might have fallen victim to the budget compromise of 1949. Clark, *Indiana University* 3: 153, 405.

19. On the trustees' decision, see BOT minutes, September 23, 1946. The HPER School was established at the September meeting in 1945. The HPER

degree was supported by Rice, and the last year of coursework was to be taken at the medical school in Indianapolis, but unpublished correspondence with Stephen Jay, July 17, 2017, suggests that Rice's proposal elicited contentious debate.

20. Gebbie et al., *Who Will Keep the Public Healthy?* 41–51. For a contemporary view of the earlier period, see Bigelow, *Health Education*.

21. During the period from 1951 to 1956, both programs were offered, but the diploma was discontinued in 1957, with the last diploma graduates in 1960. "Emily Holmquist," Box 14, UA 025, Indiana University School of Nursing Records, 1914–2002, University Library Special Collections and Archives, University Library, Indiana University Purdue University Indianapolis; Flowers, *A Legacy of Leadership*, ch. 3.

22. Annual Report of the Indiana University School of Medicine 1956–1957 (IUSM AR), Box 377–79, C213, InU-Ar. IU BOT Minutes, July 27, 1956; October 12, 1957; September 25, 1959. Andrew L. Andrews, "Undergraduate Health Science Curricula at the Indiana University Medical Center, Proposed Development," November 7, 1957, Indiana University President's Office records, Collection C304, Indiana University Archives, Bloomington (hereafter cited as C304, InU-Ar; Wells, "A Proposal on the Organization and Administration of the Undergraduate Health Science Curricula of the Medical Center Campus," January 20, 1958, C304, InU-Ar; Carol Nathan, "History, Occupational Therapy Program, Indiana University, 1924–1981," Box 207, Records of the Office of the Executive Vice Chancellor/Dean of the Faculties, UA-44, InUI-Ar; Ruth L. Ladue, "History of Physical Therapy Department, Division of Allied Health, Indiana University School of Medicine, 1924–1982," Box 12, Department of Physical Therapy Records, UA-30, InUI-Ar. In addition to Occupational and Physical Therapy, the allied health programs included Medical Record Library Science, Medical Technology, Dental Hygiene, Health Education, Sanitary Science, and X-ray Technology.

23. Randall L. Thompson to Van Nuys, March 7, 1947, Box 377–79, C213, InU-Ar; Van Nuys to Wells, March 14, 1947, Box 377–79, C213, InU-Ar; Wells to Randall L. Thompson, June 17, 1947, Box 377–79, C213, InU-Ar. IU BOT Minutes, September 9, 1925; February 28, 1938; June 30, 1947; July 21, 1947. "New Departments," *Indiana Alumni Magazine* 10 (September 1947): 15; Ludmerer, *Time to Heal*, 148–49. Clinical, surgical, and anatomical pathology were combined into one department in 1951 (A Brief History of the Pathology Department). [Conference Wells and Van Nuys], School of Medicine, [May 12, 1947]; Van Nuys to Hastings, February 2, 1948, Box 377–79, C213, InU-Ar; Van Nuys, Indiana University School of Medicine, 1948–49.

24. Van Nuys to Wells, October 13, 1947, Box 377–79, C213, InU-Ar. IU BOT Minutes, November 5, 1947; December 16, 1947.

25. On the national trend, see Ludmerer, *Time to Heal*, 72–77; Merton et al. *The Student-Physician*.

26. "Ranking of Medical Schools on Basis of Total Enrollment," *QB* 14 (October 1952): 91.

27. At the end of 1948, the IU administration claimed that Indiana University spent 40 percent less per medical student than other state universities in the region. The expansion of classroom and laboratory space was hampered by a lack

of building funds. In the three years after the war, Indiana University received about $1 million for permanent building construction, whereas eight other Midwestern state universities had been voted an average of over $10 million. "A Nine-Million-Dollar Budget," *Indiana University Bulletin* (Alumni Edition), December 1948, Box 377–79, C213, InU-Ar; "Lack of Space Makes Other Difficulties," *Indiana University Bulletin* (Alumni Edition), December 1948; "Protecting a Precious Stake," *Indianapolis News*, January 29, 1949; "Two Million Cut from Budget," *Indiana University Bulletin* (Alumni Edition), April 1949, Box 377–79, C213, InU-Ar; Clark, *Indiana University* 3: 151–52.

28. IU BOT Minutes, May 16, 1947; June 13, 1947. Statement on Medical and Dental Schools, Admissions for September 1947, Box 377–79, C213, InU-Ar; "Medical School Will Admit 141," *Indianapolis Star*, August 8, 1947; "IU Medical School Faces Student Flood"; Ludmerer, *Time to Heal*, 163, 209–10.

29. George Rawls, interview by Kendra Clauser, March 29, 2012, Collection # SC 3091 DVD 0654, IHS; William Paynter, interview by Chad Berry and Patrick Ettinger, January 13, 1993, interview 93–002, transcript, 8, Indiana Medicine, 1993, Indiana University Center for the Study of History and Memory, Bloomington (hereafter CSHM).

30. "School of Medicine Accepts 150 Applicants for Fall Enrollment," *QB* 17 (October 1955): 80; Indiana University School of Medicine Records, 1848–2005, University Library Special Collections and Archives, University Library, Indiana University Purdue University Indianapolis, Box 31.

31. Annual Report of the Indiana University Medical Center to the James Whitcomb Riley Memorial Association, April 29, 1953; IUSM AR 1956–57, Box 377–79, C213, InU-Ar; "Are We Losing Our Best Doctors," *Indianapolis Times*, December 25, 1960; Ludmerer, *Time to Heal*, 207–8.

32. Black Graduates of Indiana University School of Medicine, 1908–1989, unprocessed papers, UA 073, Indiana University School of Medicine Records, 1848–2005, University Library Special Collections and Archives, University Library, Indiana University Purdue University Indianapolis (hereafter cited as UA 073 InUI-Ar); Rawls interview; "4 IU Girls Don't Mind 38 to 1 Odds," *Indianapolis News*, April 20, 1956; "School of Medicine Admits Record Class of 202"; "Women in Medicine," *Indianapolis Times*, September 22, 1963; Ludmerer, *Time to Heal*, 206–7, 249–50; Cogan, *Negroes for Medicine*; Pulos, "A Study of Some Measured Characteristics," 80.

33. Meyers, "Doing the 'Not Possible,'" 351.

34. Stern, "Against the Odds," 325, 327.

35. Robert F. Reed, interview by Patrick Ettinger, February 15, 1995, interview 93–050, transcript, 17, Indiana Medicine, 1993, CSHM; Morantz-Sanchez, *Sympathy and Science*.

36. Robert Holden, interview by Elizabeth J. Van Allen, November 28, 2000, UA 073, InUI-Ar.

37. Meyers, 351; Paynter interview.

38. Reed interview.

39. Charles A. Bonsett, interview by Steven Stowe, May 27, 1992, interview 92–002, transcript, 14, Indiana Medicine, 1993, CSHM. On Kime and Harmon, see *The Indiana University Catalogue . . . Register . . . Announcements*, 1922, 288–36.

40. Reed interview.

41. Paynter interview.

42. Bonsett interview.

43. Van Nuys to Wells, March 21, 1949, Box 377–79, C213, InU-Ar.

44. Ibid.

45. Ibid.

46. Ludmerer, *Let Me Heal*, 139, inter alia; Rothstein, *American Medical Schools*, 310–12.

47. IU BOT Minutes, December 16, 1947; IUSM AR 1948–1949; Minutes, Executive Committee of the IU Medical Center, November 5, 1945, UA 073, InUI-Ar; Ludmerer, *Time to Heal*, 180–86.

48. Stoelting, *History of the Department of Anesthesiology*; *Oral History of Vergil K. Stoelting, M.D.* (Park Ridge, IL: The Library-Museum, 1985).

49. King and Schmetzer, *Dr. Edenharter's Dream*; John I. Nurnberger and Hugh C. Hendrie, "History of the Department of Psychiatry," 1990, IUSM Center and Departmental Histories, UA 073 InUI-Ar.

50. Van Nuys, Indiana University School of Medicine, 1948–1949; "Alumni Organization Formed by Physicians," *QB* 10 (July 1948): 61–62.

51. Conference Wells and Van Nuys, School of Medicine [May 12, 1947]. IU BOT Minutes, December 16, 1947; November 18, 1949. Ward W. Moore, interview by Elizabeth Van Allen, November 8, 2000, UA 073, InUI-Ar; Report of the Indiana University Medical Center to the James Whitcomb Riley Memorial Association, April 22, 1959, RMA; Alan Gregg to Wells, December 15, 1950, Box 377–79, C213, InU-Ar; Ludmerer, *Time to Heal*, 149. Dennis E. Jackson earned his PhD under William J. Moenkhaus in 1908. Elizondo, and Moore, "Physiology at Indiana University-Bloomington," 323.

52. Report of Indiana University Medical School Expansion Study Committee, October 6, 1952, Box 377–79, C213, InU-Ar; Gregg to Wells, December 15, 1950.

53. For example, just on Shumacker, see "Harris B. Shumacker, Jr., MD, Appointed Chairman of the Department of Surgery," *QB* 10 (July 1948): 55; "New Surgery Chairman," *Indiana Alumni Magazine* 11 (September 1948): 9–10; "Heart Surgery Gives New Life to City Woman," *Indianapolis Times*, December 21, 1952; "IU Surgeon Mends Child's Defective Heart," *Indianapolis News*, January 2, 1953; "Six Delicate Grafts to Ruptured Arteries Performed at IU Center," *Indianapolis Star*, October 7, 1954; "Hoosier Medic Makes Tots' Hearts 'New,'" *Indianapolis News*, November 19, 1954; "IU Med Center Works on Spare Parts for People," *Indianapolis Times*, January 26, 1958; Shumacker to J. W. Carr, January 19, 1953, Box 377–79, C213, InU-Ar; Shumacker to J. W. Carr, December 17, 1958, Box 377–79, C213, InU-Ar; "Harris B. Shumacker, Jr., M.D., National Spotlight on IU Surgeon," *Indianapolis Times*, July 14, 1963; "Pioneer Hoosier Surgeon Recalls Open-Heart Triumph," *Indianapolis Star*, November 22, 2002.

54. Ludmerer, *Time to Heal*, 131–35; Strickland, *Politics, Science, and Dread Disease*; Zachary, *Endless Frontier*, 13–16; A. N. Richards, "The Impact of the War on Medicine," *Science* 103, no. 2680 (May 10, 1946): 578, doi:10.1126/science.103.2680.575.

55. "Med Center Research Program Hits $2 Million," *Indianapolis Times*, June 5, 1960. Admittedly starting from a small base, this was a twentyfold increase over external funds received in 1950.

56. "Alumni Hear Dean's Review, Forecast of Medical School Plans, Activities," *QB* 23 (Summer 1961): 35; "Indiana University School of Medicine, General Research Program"; "University Shocked by Death of Dean Van Nuys"; Ludmerer, *Time to Heal*, 144.

57. W. D. Gatch and H. M. Trusler, "The Research Division," *QB* 1 (January 1939): 19–21.

58. Shryock, *American Medical Research*, Bush, *Science, the Endless Frontier*, 13–16; Ludmerer, *Time to Heal*, 132–35; Dupree, *Science in the Federal Government*; Philip Scarpino, Oral History with Glenn Irwin, former dean of IUSM, UA 041, InUI-Ar. The importance of the prewar federal investments in science is evident in the use of the Northern Regional Laboratory of the US Department of Agriculture in Peoria, Illinois, created under the Agricultural Adjustment Act of 1938, as the primary research site for industrialization of penicillin production.

59. Van Nuys to J. W. Carr, April 19, 1950, Box 377–79, C213, InU-Ar; Research Unit, April 25, 1951, Annual Meeting Minutes, RMA; "Cancer Expert Joins IU Medical Faculty," *Indianapolis News*, January 1, 1950; "Dr. Edwin A. Lawrence Is Professor of Surgery and Cancer Coordinator," *QB* 12 (January 1950): 19; "Cancer Campaign" *Indiana Alumni Magazine* 12 (February 1950): 8; "Cancer Grant," *Indiana Alumni Magazine* 12 (March 1950): 13; IU BOT Minutes, October 21, 1949; Ludmerer, *Time to Heal*, 146; Van Allen et al. *Keeping the Dream*, 33.

60. [Conference Wells and Van Nuys], School of Medicine, [May 12, 1947]; Randall L. Thompson to Van Nuys, March 7, 1947, Box 377–79, C213, InU-Ar.

61. Report of the Secretary, James Whitcomb Riley Memorial Association, April 28, 1948; "Riley Memorial Gives IU $50,000 for Clinical Research," *Indianapolis News*, November 20, 1947; "Grant Aids Endocrinal Research," *Indianapolis Star*, November 20, 1947; "Research Grants Enable IU Medical Center to Expand," *Indianapolis News*, December 31, 1947; "IU School Probes Many Mysteries of Science," *Indianapolis News*, February 24, 1948; "Gifts Start Medical Center on Wide Research Program," *Indianapolis Star*, December 12, 1948; "Lions' $25,000 Gift Doubles Cancer Facilities of IU," *Indianapolis News*, June 13, 1949; Van Nuys, Indiana University School of Medicine, 1948–1949.

62. Report of the Secretary, April 28, 1948, RMA; "Riley Memorial Gives IU$50,000 for Clinical Research"; "Grant Aids Endocrinal Research." This was part of a broader national trend; see Creager, "Mobilizing Biomedicine."

63. "Research Grants Enable IU Medical Center to Expand"; "IU School Probes Many Mysteries of Science."

64. Radiology/Cancer Control Material, 1946–1990s, UA 073, InUI-Ar.

65. "Cancer Expert Joins IU Medical Faculty," *Indianapolis News*, January 1, 1950; "Dr Edwin A. Lawrence Is Professor of Surgery and Cancer Coordinator," *QB* 12 (January 1950): 19; "Cancer Campaign," *Indiana Alumni Magazine* 12 (February 1950): 8; "Cancer Grant," *Indiana Alumni Magazine* 12 (March 1950): 13; Minutes, IU Board of Trustees, October 21, 1949.

66. IU BOT Minutes, October 21, 1949; Deitrick, *Medical Schools in the United States at Mid-Century,* 159–60.

67. Van Nuys to J. W. Carr, January 12, 1948, Box 377–79, C213, InU-Ar; Report of the Secretary, April 28, 1948, RMA.

68. IU BOT Minutes, February 6, 1948; Report to the Board on Proposals for the Creation of the James Whitcomb Riley Centennial Fund for Medical Research in the Diseases of Children and Adults in the James Whitcomb Riley Hospital for Children, September 12, 1948, RMA; Questions and Answers Relative to the Historical Background and the Operation of a Proposed Center of Research in Association with the James Whitcomb Riley Hospital for Children, [1948], Box 377–79, C213, InU-Ar; Van Allen et al. *Keeping the Dream,* 22–23.

69. "Cancer Wing Grows," *Indiana Alumni Magazine* 15 (November 1952): 12.

70. "Larue Depew Carter," *Encyclopedia of Indianapolis,* 387.

71. *Rockefeller Foundation Annual Report for 1952,* 79–80.

72. Van Nuys to Gregg, October 12, 1950, Box 377–79, C213, InU-Ar; "Rockefeller Grant," *Indiana Alumni Magazine* 15 (October 1952): 16; Doris H. Merritt, "The Progress of Research," *QB* 25 (Fall 1963): 70; Van Nuys to Wells, May 8, 1952, Box 377–79, C213, InU-Ar; Clark, *Indiana University* 3:101, 255; Gathorne-Hardy, *Alfred C. Kinsey,* 226. IU BOT Minutes, June 14, 1952; September 19, 1952. "The History of the Department of Psychiatry at the Indiana University School of Medicine," IUSM Center and Departmental Histories, UA 073 InUI-Ar.

73. King and Schmetzer, *Dr. Edenharter's Dream.*

74. Van Nuys to Briscoe, September 10, 1954, Box 377–79, C213, InU-Ar; IU BOT Minutes, July 30, 1955; "State Takes $1,500,000 Mental Research Stride," *Indianapolis Star,* December 14, 1956; "Psychiatric Research Unit Dedicated to Basic Studies of Mental Illnesses," *QB* 19 (January 1957): 13; Clark, *Indiana University* 3: 427; "3 Psychiatrists Quit in IU Medical Row," *Indianapolis News,* August 14, 1954; IU BOT Minutes, October 27, 1955; "Appointment of Dr. John Nurnberger Fills Psychiatric Chairmanship," *QB* 17 (October 1955): 77, 84; "The History of the Department of Psychiatry," Center and Departmental Histories, UA 073 InUI-Ar; John I. Nurnberger Sr., "The Psychiatric Research Institute—A Statement of Aims and Purposes," *QB* 19 (April 1957): 21–23, 25; "First Annual Report, The Institute of Psychiatric Research of the Department of Psychiatry, IU Medical Center, and Division of Mental Health of the State of Indiana," July 1, 1957–June 30, 1958, Box 377–79, C213, InU-Ar; Coons and Bowman, *Psychiatry in Indiana.*

75. "New Medical Science Building Construction Starts in Indianapolis," *Indiana Alumni Magazine* 17 (January 1955): 12; "Promise Fulfilled," *Indiana Alumni Magazine* 24 (March 1962): 26; "School of Medicine Admits Record Class of 202," *Indiana Alumni Magazine* 25 (November 1962): 19; Irwin, "Years as Dean of Medicine"; Clark, *Indiana University* 3: 426.

76. Wells to William M. M. Kirby, February 27, 1957, Box 377–79, C213, InU-Ar; Kirby to Van Nuys, October 5, 1956, Dean's Office Files, IUSM; Kenneth G. Kohlstaedt to Wells, March 11, 1957, Box 377–79, C213, InU-Ar; Shumacker to Wells, March 1, 1957, Box 377–79, C213, InU-Ar; Kirby to Behnke, June 7, 1957, Dean's Office Files, IUSM; Kirby to Irwin, June 7, 1957, Dean's

Office Files, IUSM; "Department of Medicine Headed by W. M. M. Kirby," *Indiana Alumni Magazine* 19 (April 1957): 11.

77. Lukemeyer interview; Elizabeth Van Allen, notes on conversation with Walter J. Daly, August 1, 2001; Ludmerer, *Time to Heal*, 143, 150.

78. McIntosh, "Memorial: John Bamber Hickam, M.D.," ix–ixii. See also Jay, "Legacies of Hoosier Aviation," 25–33.

79. Charles Clark Jr., quoted in Ford et al., *Regenstrief*, 66; Fisch interview; Walter J. Daly, interview by Elizabeth J. Van Allen, May 2, 2001, UA 073; "Dr. John B. Hickam Dies Suddenly," *QB* 31 (Fall 1969): 12–13.

80. Knoebel, "Profiles in Cardiology: Charles Fisch," 782–83.

81. Van Nuys to [Wells], January 14, 1958, Box 377–79, C213, InU-Ar; Van Nuys, "Annual Report of the Dean to the James Whitcomb Riley Memorial Association," April 24, 1963, RMA; James A. Stuart, Merrill S. Davis, Daniel I. Glossbrenner to RMA Board of Governors, April 17, 1959, Box 377–79, C213, InU-Ar; John A. Campbell, "Progress Report of Riley Memorial Association Grant-in-Aid for Cineradiography," January 29, 1960, Box 377–79, C213, InU-Ar; Lukemeyer interview; Daly interview, May 2, 2001; Fisch interview; Paul R. Lurie, "Medical Center Grows and Grows," *Indianapolis Times*, August 30, 1961; "IU Medical Center Gets $4,600 Grant," *Indianapolis Star*, March 21, 1958; "Kidney Machine," 8; "Artificial Kidney Unit Expands Clinical and Research Facilities," *QB* 18 (April 1956): 47; Ford et al., *Regenstrief*, 65–66; Ludmerer, *Time to Heal*, 143; Clark, *Indiana University* 3: 426.

82. Fisch interview; Daly interview, May 2, 2001; "Dr. John B. Hickam Dies Suddenly," *QB* 31 (Fall 1969):12.

83. "Editorial," *QB* 21 (Winter 1958): 2; "Med Center Research Program Hits $2 Million," *Indianapolis Times*, June 5, 1960; Ludmerer, *Time to Heal*, 145–46.

84. Bowman, "Summary of the First Five Years of the Department of Biochemistry, 1958–1963," 1963, Center and Departmental Histories, UA 073 InUI-Ar; [David M. Gibson], "Up Here in Biochemistry," Department of Biochemistry and Molecular Biology, IUSM, [1993], Center and Departmental Histories, UA 073 InUI-Ar; "The Atom," *Indianapolis Star Magazine*, November 8, 1959.

85. Ochs and Knoebel, "History of the Department of Physiology and Biophysics," Center and Departmental Histories, UA 073 InUI-Ar; Glenn W. Irwin Jr. et al., "A Brief History of the Indiana University School of Medicine," 8, unprocessed papers, UA 073, InUI-Ar; "Cancer Research" [1962], Box 377–79, C213, InU-Ar; Moore interview.

86. Lautzenheiser to J. A. Franklin, June 8, 1950, Box 377–79, C213, InU-Ar.

87. IUSM AR 1960–1961; "Indiana University School of Medicine Cardiovascular Research," [1962], Box 377–79, C213, InU-Ar; "IU Work Finds Help for Heart," *Indianapolis Times*, October 29, 1960; Stuart Bondurant, "National Space Program and Heart Research," *QB* 24 (Fall 1963): 42; "4.5 Million in Medical Research," *Indianapolis News*, March 14, 1962.

88. "Indiana University School of Medicine Proposal for Heart Research Center," October 17, 1960, Box 377–79, C213, InU-Ar; IUSM AR 1960–1961; "Indiana University School of Medicine Cardiovascular Research"; IUSM AR 1961–1962, Box 377–79, C213, InU-Ar; Bondurant, "National Space Program

and Heart Research"; "$4.3 Million Given IU for Heart Study," *Indianapolis News*, June 20, 1961; "Here's What Heart Grant to IU Will Do," *Indianapolis Times*, September 29, 1961; "4.5 Million in Medical Research."

89. IUSM AR 1960–1961; IUSM AR 1961–1962; "Indiana University School of Medicine, Mental Health, Neurological Diseases, and Vision," [1962]; "New Grant Backs IU Disturbed Child Study," *Indianapolis Times*, July 1961; "School to Begin Center for Schizophrenia Study"; "IU Research Aids Mentally Ill Child," *Indianapolis News*, May 15, 1963; "Indiana University School of Medicine, Mental Health, Neurological Diseases, and Vision"; "4.5 Million in Medical Research"; "IU Scientists Exploring Brain's Effect on Behavior."

90. "Cancer Research," [1962]; "IU Tries to Learn How to Starve Cancer," *Indianapolis News*, March 15, 1962; James A. Stuart, Merrill S. Davis, Daniel I. Glossbrenner to RMA Board of Governors, April 17, 1959, Box 377–79, C213, InU-Ar; Report of the Indiana University Medical Center to the James Whitcomb Riley Memorial Association, April 25, 1962, RMA.

91. For more on this trend which continues to this day, see Schneider, "The Origin of the Medical Research Grant," 279–81.

92. "Med Center Research Program Hits $2 Million"; Van Nuys, "Report to the Alumni—The Indiana University School of Medicine," *QB* 22 (Spring 1960): 23; Petersdorf, "Medical Schools and Research," 101–3; Ludmerer, *Time to Heal*, 143–44, 196; Kerr, *The Uses of the University*, 27–28, 41–45.

93. Rice to Wells, April 26, 1950, Box 377–79, C213, InU-Ar; Van Nuys to Wells, September 28, 1950, Box 377–79, C213, InU-Ar; Briscoe to Wells, October 4, 1950, Box 377–79, C213, InU-Ar; Ludmerer, *Time to Heal*, 158.

94. J. A. Franklin to Wells, January 3, 1950; Post War Plans for the Indiana University School of Medicine. IU BOT Minutes, November 18, 1949; January 19, 1950; March 17, 1950; June 10, 1950; October 20, 1950. Cookson to Wildermuth, January 26, 1951, Box 377–79, C213, InU-Ar; Wells to Wildermuth, January 27, 1951, Box 377–79, C213, InU-Ar; "Indiana University News and Notes," 499; Wells, "Dedication of Student Union and Food Services Building," September 30, 1953, Box 10, C137, InU-Ar; "Med Union Dedicated," 4–5; Stevens, *In Sickness and in Wealth*, 216–19; Ludmerer, *Time to Heal*, 163.

95. IU BOT Minutes, February 1, 1947; J. A. Franklin to Wells, January 3, 1950, Box 377–79, C213, InU-Ar; Rice, "History of the Medical Campus, Chapter X," 238–39; Van Nuys to Wells, October 13, 1947, Box 377–79, C213, InU-Ar; [Conference Wells and Van Nuys], School of Medicine [May 12, 1947]; Van Nuys to F. T. Reed, April 19, 1947, Box 377–79, C213, InU-Ar. Van Nuys to Wells, March 21, 1949; Wells to Van Nuys, March 27, 1949, Box 377–79, C213, InU-Ar.

96. Van Nuys to Wells, October 13, 1947, Box 377–79, C213, InU-Ar; [Conference Wells and Van Nuys], School of Medicine [May 12, 1947]; Van Nuys to F. T. Reed, April 19, 1947, Box 377–79, C213, InU-Ar; "New Quarters," 12; "Hospital Expanded," 22; Van Nuys, Indiana University School of Medicine, 1948–1949, Box 377–79, C213, InU-Ar.

97. "City to Get 1,000-Bed VA Hospital," *Indianapolis Star*, January 27, 1946; Minutes, Executive Committee of the IU Medical Center, March 14, 1946; "Mayor Offers Hospital Site"; "2d VA Hospital for Indianapolis Is Approved," *Indianapolis News*, April 23, 1946.

98. "VA Hospital Plans Changed"; "Medical Care Second to None," 102, 116–17; "V. A. Plans Dedication Today of New Hospital," *Indianapolis Star*, February 3, 1952.

99. IU BOT Minutes, June 15, 1951.

100. Hale, *Caring for the Community*, 182; Van Allen et al., *Keeping the Dream*, 112.

101. For comparisons to the national environment, see Ludmerer, *Time to Heal*, 260–88.

102. IU BOT Minutes, June 15, 1951

103. Abstract of the Survey by James M. Hamilton and Associates, Minneapolis Minnesota, "A Hospital Plan for the Indianapolis Area, Indiana," July 12, 1951, Box 377–79, C213, InU-Ar; J. W. Carr to Wells, November 20, 1951, Box 377–79, C213, InU-Ar. For national trends in hospital construction, see Risse, *Mending Bodies, Saving Souls*, 514–77; Ludmerer, *Time to Heal*, 163.

104. Abstract of the Survey by James M. Hamilton and Associates, Minneapolis Minnesota, "A Hospital Plan for the Indianapolis Area, Indiana," July 12, 1951, Box 377–79, C213, InU-Ar; Carr to Wells, November 20, 1951, Box 377–79, C213, InU-Ar; "Programming for New University Hospital, Stage I," March 1958, folder 5, AG93-85, InUI-Ar; J. A. Franklin to Marc Waggener, March 3, 1952, Box 377–79, C213, InU-Ar. IU BOT Minutes, July 12, 1951; April 18, 1952. Stevens, *In Sickness and in Wealth*, 220, 223.

105. Schneider, "Hoosier Health Philanthropy."

106. Van Nuys to J. A. Franklin, July 18, 1950, Box 377–79, C213, InU-Ar; "Patient Shortage Threatens Cut in IU Output of Doctors," *Indianapolis Times*, December 23, 1951.

107. IU BOT Minutes, May 20, 1952; Van Nuys to J. A. Franklin, July 18, 1950.

108. Herschell, "They Just Must Get Well," 16–18, 55–56.

109. Annual Report of the Administrator of the Indiana University Medical Center to the James Whitcomb Riley Memorial Association, April 26, 1944, RMA; The Role of the Convalescent Hospital [October 1, 1951], Box 377–79, C213, InU-Ar; IU BOT Minutes, July 13, 1951; Interview with John R. Scott, December 7, 1993, RMA; Van Nuys to Franklin, July 18, 1950; Van Allen et al., *Keeping the Dream,* 23–24.

110. IU BOT Minutes, May 20, 1952; June 13, 1952. Van Nuys to J. W. Carr, January 8, 1951, Box 377–79, C213, InU-Ar. For specific statistics regarding the downward trend in patient occupancy at Riley Hospital see Van Nuys to J. A. Franklin, June 3, 1952, Box 377–79, C213, InU-Ar.

111. "Rotary Convalescent Home (a brief history)," March 1984, Box 38, UA 073, InUI-Ar. E. J. Shea to J. W. Carr, January 11, 1952; Van Nuys to J. A. Franklin, June 5, 1952; J. W. Carr to William T. Gruber, August 12, 1957, Box 377–79, C213, InU-Ar.

112. Report of the Indiana University Medical Center to the James Whitcomb Riley Memorial Association, April 25, 1956, RMA; Minutes, RMA Board of Governors, April 24, 1957, RMA; "The Life of Riley," *The Kiwanis Magazine* (February 1959): 26; Lorin J. Badsky to Indiana Kiwanis Club Presidents, September 25, 1957, Box 377–79, C213, InU-Ar; Van Allen et al., *Keeping the Dream,* 24–25.

113. Oral History of Morris Green, Indiana Medicine Oral History Project, Collection# M697, IHS.

114. Report . . . to the James Whitcomb Riley Memorial Association, April 25,1956; Badsky to Indiana Kiwanis Club Presidents; Morris Green to J. W. Carr, March 4, 1959, Box 377–79, C213, InU-Ar. Minutes of the Forty-Second Annual Meeting of the James Whitcomb Riley Memorial Association, April 24, 1963, RMA; "Riley Leadership," *Riley Memorial Association News* (June 1960).

115. Minutes, RMA Board of Governors, October 26, 1960; January 11, 1961; April 26, 1961; RMA. IU BOT Minutes, November 26, 1960; March 17–18, 1961. Van Allen et al., *Keeping the Dream*, 25.

116. Shumacker, "Advanced Ideas Incorporated in New Riley Hospital Operating Room Plans," Riley Surgery Construction, 1961–1965, UA 073, InUI-Ar; Minutes, RMA Board of Governors, October 26, 1960; RMA Annual Meeting Minutes, April 28, 1965, RMA; Heimburger to Charles G. Drake, April 27, 1965, folder 10, Box 3, A89–35, InUI-Ar; Van Allen et al., *Keeping the Dream*, 25–26.

117. Arthur D. Lautzenheiser to J. A. Franklin, June 8 June, 1950, Box 377–79, C213, InU-Ar.

118. IU BOT Minutes, April 20, 1951; April 17, 1953; April 30, 1955; July 27, 1956; September 20, 1963. Buildings and Grounds, Indianapolis, Annual Report, 1956–1957, Box 377–79, C213, InU-Ar.

119. Resolution adopted by the House of Delegates of the Indiana State Medical Association, October 31, 1946, Box 377–79, C213, InU-Ar; "Urge to Move to MC," 22; IU BOT Minutes, February 1, 1947; J. A. Badertscher et al., to Wells, July 15, 1947, Box 377–79, C213, InU-Ar.

120. Ludmerer, *Time to Heal*, 149; Van Nuys to Wells, October 13, 1947, Box 377–79, C213, InU-Ar; IU BOT Minutes, October 17, 1947; Conference [Wells and Van Nuys], School of Medicine [May 12, 1947]; Van Nuys to Hastings, February 2, 1948, Box 377–79, C213, InU-Ar; Van Nuys, Indiana University School of Medicine, 1948–1949.

121. Minutes of the Indiana University Medical School Expansion Study Committee, May 21, 1952, Box 377–79, C213, InUI-Ar.

122. To Wells [handwritten memorandum], [July 8, 1950], Box 377–79, C213, InU-Ar; Wells to Wildermuth, January 27, 1951; Minutes of the Indiana University Medical School Expansion Study Committee, May 21, 1952, Box 377–79, C213, InU-Ar; Report of Indiana University Medical School Expansion Study Committee; "Patient Shortages Threatens Cut in IU Output of Doctors," December 23, 1951; Roehr, *Trustees and Officers of Indiana University, 1950 to 1982*, 116.

123. Minutes of Meeting of the Medical School Expansion Committee, Box 377–79, C213, InU-Ar; Report of Indiana University Medical School Expansion Study Committee; Post War Plans for the Indiana University School of Medicine; Report of Indiana University Medical School Expansion Study Committee; "Committee Studies Expansion," 17; Van Allen et al., *Keeping the Dream*, 91–94.

124. Gregg to Wells, December 15, 1950; Minutes of the Indiana University Medical School Expansion Study Committee, May 21, 1952; Ludmerer, *Time*

to Heal, 129, 144–45; Report of Indiana University Medical School Expansion Study Committee; Minutes of the Indiana University Medical School Expansion Study Committee, May 21, 1952; "Committee Studies Expansion."

125. Report of Indiana University Medical School Expansion Study Committee; Van Nuys to Wells, January 18, 1951, Box 377–79, C213, InU-Ar; Van Nuys to Claude Rich, April 20, 1951, Box 377–79, C213, InU-Ar; Minutes of the Indiana University Medical School Expansion Study Committee, May 21, 1952; Ludmerer, *Time to Heal*, 207–8.

126. Kassebaum, "Origin of the LCME," 85–87; Eaglen, *Academic Quality and Public Accountability in Medical Education.*

127. Edward L. Turner and William N. Hubbard, "Report of Survey, Indiana University School of Medicine October 21–23, 1954," Box 233, UA 073, InUI-Ar.

128. Ibid.

129. One of the most important of these traditions was the Med-Law Boress, which had taken place during homecoming weekend each year since 1920. The event "included raids by the 'Laws' on Owen Hall (after 1937 on Myers Hall), and by the 'Meds' on Maxwell Hall (after 1956 on the School of Law Building)." Later, hundreds of students gathered in front of the Indiana Memorial Union Building in Bloomington to witness law and medical students exchanging "taunts, jibes, and jeers, delivered with passionate oratory, songs, [and] chants." Medical students "generally wore white lab coats and waved large bones," whereas Law students "wore black coats and derbies and carried canes and umbrellas." On Saturday morning, before the regular homecoming football game, students from both schools participated in athletic contests. The winner "became the owner of the 'Thundermug Trophy.'" The *Indiana Daily Student* once claimed that because of its many colorful attributes, the Med-Law Borress created "The World's Most Pornographic Weekend." Alvin J. Haley, "Reminiscences of Medical School" [2001]; files of *Indiana University Arbutus, 1921* (Bloomington: Indiana University, 1921); "An Era Ends," *Indiana Alumni Magazine* 20 (November 1957): 7.

130. Ludmerer, *Time to Heal*, 207–8.

131. "Teaching-Juniors, 1954–1960"; "Teaching-Seniors, 1954–1957," UA 073, InUI-Ar. USM AR 1956–1957.

132. IUSM AR 1956–1957; IUSM AR 1958–1959, Box 377–79, C213, InU-Ar. Daly interview, May 2, 2001; Ludmerer, *Time to Heal*, 197–99; Rothstein, 310–12.

133. "Medical Science Building to Be Dedicated April 22," *IDS* (April 16, 1959); "Medical Science Building Being Readied for Fall Opening," *QB* 20 (Summer 1958): 39–45; Wells, "Dedication Convocation of Medical Science Building," April 22, 1959, Box 17, C137, InU-Ar; "Dedication of the Medical Science Building," *QB* 21 (Spring 1959): 19–23; "Medical Science Building Renaming, 1988," UA 083, InUI-Ar.

134. Van Nuys, "Indiana's Progress in Medical Education Reviewed in Dean's Report to Alumni," 61. Wishard died in January 1941, and Bryan died in November 1955. "Dr. Wishard, 'Grand Old Man' of Indiana Medicine, Is Dead," *Indianapolis Times*, January 23, 1941; Van Allen et al., *Keeping the Dream*, 88.

135. Report of the Indiana University Medical Center to the James Whitcomb Riley Memorial Association, April 25, 1956, RMA; Van Nuys, "Indiana's Progress in Medical Education Reviewed in Dean's Report to Alumni," *QB* 20 (Fall 1958): 62.

136. Abstract of the Survey by James M. Hamilton and Associates; "Programming for New University Hospital, Stage I"; IUSM AR 1956–1957; IU BOT Minutes, December 13, 1958.

137. Gray, *IUPUI,* 42–44.

138. John V. Wilson, "IU Back Again with Request for Hospital," *Indianapolis Times,* June 13, 1960; "Mickey McCarty Says," *Indianapolis News,* November 28, 1960; Minutes, IU Board of Trustees, March 17–18, 1961; "Indiana University School of Medicine, Annual Report, 1960–1961."

139. "Programming for New University Hospital, Stage I"; IUSM AR 1959–1960; "Research Work Is Expanded"; "IU Back Again with Request for Hospital," *Indianapolis Times,* June 18, 1960; Gray, *IUPUI,* 58.

140. "To Clinical Heads, Heads of Departments and/or Services," February 3, 1962, folder 10, Box 3, A89–35, InUI-Ar (emphasis in the original); IU BOT Minutes, September 21, 1962.

141. Elvis J. Stahr Jr. to Eldon F. Lundquist, March 7, 1963, C304, InU-Ar; Wells, *Being Lucky,* 417; "'I Belong Here. Besides, I'm Not a Politician'— Wells," *Indianapolis Times,* November 19, 1961; IU BOT Minutes, May 31– June 3, 1963; Press Release, News Bureau, July 27, [1962], C304, InU-Ar; Wells, *Being Lucky,* 155–63; Roehr, 127–31.

142. Wesley Bowers to Stahr, December 28, 1962, "Indiana Higher Education is at the Crossroads" [1962–1963], C304, InU-Ar; IUSM AR 1961–1962; Stahr, "State of the University," December 18, 1963, Stahr Speeches, InU-Ar.

143. "First Hold the Line, Then Take a Look," *Indianapolis Star,* January 11, 1963.

144. Bowers to Stahr, December 28, 1962; Stahr to Lundquist, March 7, 1963; Stahr to Robert P. O'Bannon, March 3, 1963; Stahr to W. Wayne Townsend, March 7, 1963, C304, InU-Ar. J. A. Franklin to Alvin C. Cast, March 18, 1963, C304, InU-Ar. IU BOT Minutes, March 22, 1963; January 17, 1964. Stahr, "State of the University," December 28, 1963; "Statement by Elvis J. Stahr, Jr., President of Indiana University," Press Release, April 22, 1963, News Bureau, IU Bloomington, folder 155, Box 155, Matthew E. Welsh Papers, InU-Ar; "First Hold the Line, Then Take a Look," *Indianapolis Star,* January 11, 1963. J. A. Franklin to A. C. Offut, January 15, 1964; J. A. Franklin to Wells, October 14, 1964, C304, InU-Ar. "Construction Started on New Teaching Hospital at Center," *Indiana Alumni Magazine* 27 (June–July 1965): 28; "4 Hoosiers Get Honorary Degrees at New I. U. Hospital Dedication," *Indianapolis Star,* April 30, 1970, 46.

145. "Liaison Committee on Medical Education, Report of the Survey of the Indiana University School of Medicine, December 12, 1963," Box 234, UA 073, InUI-Ar; IUSM AR 1963–1964; "University Shocked by Death of Dean Van Nuys."

146. "Bigger 'n Better 'n Ever: Medical School Enrolls 214 First-Year Students; Largest Freshman Class in School's History," *QB* 25 (Fall 1963): 39.

147. "University Shocked by Death of Dean Van Nuys"; "Advanced Medical Education in Demand," *Indiana Alumni Magazine* 24 (January 1962): 14; Thomas A. Hanna, September 24, 1963, C304, InU-Ar; Report of the IU Medical Center to the James Whitcomb Riley Memorial Association, April 29, 1964, RMA.

9. The Indiana Plan: Statewide Medical Education, 1964–1974

1. Edward L. Turner, William N. Hubbard, Report of Survey, Indiana University School of Medicine (Bloomington-Indianapolis), Oct. 21–23, 1954, Box 377–79, Indiana University President's Office records, Collection C213, Indiana University Archives, Bloomington (hereafter cited as C213, InU-Ar); Van Nuys to Stahr, November 12, 1963, Collection No. C304, Box 180, Indiana University President's Office Records, 1962–68, InU-Ar (hereafter cited as C304, InU-Ar).

2. See chapter 10 for more information about growth.

3. LCME Report, 1963; Mahoney to Van Nuys, January 16, 1964, InU-Ar; Sorensen, "Black Americans and the Medical Profession," 337–42; "Bigger 'n Better 'n Ever: Medical School Enrolls 214 First-Year Students"; Largest Freshman Class in School's History," *Quarterly Bulletin of the Indiana University Health Center* (hereafter cited as *QB*) 25 (Fall 1963): 39. Although 214 students initially were admitted, 216 freshmen enrolled in fall 1963 (Press Release, March 30, 1965, Box 131, C304, InU-Ar).

4. "Advanced Medical Education in Demand, 14; Thomas A. Hanna, September 24, 1963, Box 77–79, C304, InU-Ar; VanNuys, Indiana University Annual Report, 1959–60; Report of the IU Medical Center to the James Whitcomb Riley Memorial Association, April 29, 1964, Records of the James Whitcomb Riley Memorial Association, Indianapolis (hereafter cited as RMA).

5. LCME Report, 1963.

6. LCME Report, 1963; National Institutes of Health. Division of Research Grants, *A Guide to Public Health Service Grants and Awards*, Washington, DC: Public Health Service Publication no. 1067, 1963; National Institutes of Health, Division of Research Grants, *Research Grants and Fellowships Awarded by the Public Health Service, Fiscal Year 1955 Funds*, Washington, DC: Public Health Service Publication no. 469, 1956.

7. LCME Report, 1963.

8. Ibid.

9. IU BOT Minutes, January 17, 1964; "University Shocked by Death of Dean VanNuys"; Ludmerer, *Time to Heal*, 158–59; Edward L. Turner and William N. Hubbard, Report of Survey, Indiana University School of Medicine (Bloomington-Indianapolis), October 21–23, 1954, p. 7; Box 377–79, C213, InU-Ar; LCME Report 1963.

10. LCME Report 1963; Nurnberger, IUSM AR 1963–64; "University Shocked by Death of Dean Van Nuys."

11. "University Shocked by Death of Dean Van Nuys"; Memorial Resolution on the death of John Ditmar Van Nuys, February 1965, Indiana University Faculty Council records, 1947–1970, Box 11, Indiana University Faculty Council records, Collection C181, Indiana University Archives, Bloomington, InU-Ar.

12. IU BOT Minutes, February 21, 1964; LCME Report, 1979; Van Nuys to Stahr, October 5, 1962, C304, InU-Ar. As dean for research and sponsored programs at IUPUI, she helped launch education programs including the Consortium for Urban Education. National Library of Medicine, "Living Legends of Medicine." See also http://www.nlm.nih.gov/locallegends/Biographies /Merritt_Doris.html.

13. IU BOT Minutes, September 25–26, 1964.

14. Although there are no surviving minutes from the search committee, oral histories describe the search process. Walter J. Daly, interview by Kevin Grau, November 1, 2005, IUSM Oral History Collection, InUI-Ar; Lukemeyer interview.

15. IU BOT Minutes, September 25–26, 1964; IU BOT Minutes, January 14–15, 1965; Nurnberger to Stahr, September 8, 1964, C304, InU-Ar; Irwin, Oral History, October 12, 2005; Lukemeyer, interview.

16. Report of Indiana University Medical School Expansion Study Committee; Van Nuys to Wells, January 18, 1951, Van Nuys to Claude Riche, April 20, 1951, Box 377–79, C213, InU-Ar; Minutes of the Indiana University Medical School Expansion Study Committee, May 21, 1952.

17. Surgeon General's Consultant Group, *Physicians for a Growing America*; "Eisenhower Plans Talks to Nation on Urgent Issues," *New York Times*, October 23, 1957. For background, see Eli Ginzberg, "The Politics of U. S. Physician Supply," *Health Policy* 55 (1990): 237–39.

18. See, for example, Christopher C. Fordham, "The *Bane Report* Revisited," *JAMA* 244, no. 4 (July 25, 1980): 354–57.

19. Ginzberg, "The Politics of U. S. Physician Supply," 242–44. The most comprehensive and dramatic revision was the *Report of the Graduate Medical Education National Advisory Committee to the Secretary, Department of Health and Human Services* (September 30, 1980), which predicted "70,000 more physicians than required in 1990" and called for a 17 percent decrease in medical school enrollments. https://files.eric.ed.gov/fulltext/ED210990.pdf (accessed May 12, 2018).

20. The seven states were Florida, Indiana, Michigan, New Jersey, Ohio, Texas, and Washington. Minutes, IU Trustees, November 12, 1959; Van Nuys to Wells, October 28, 1959, Herman B Wells Papers, Collection C75, Indiana University Archives, Bloomington.

21. Van Nuys to Stahr, September 9, 1962; IU BOT Minutes, December 14, 1962, and September 20, 1963; Medical Center Executive Committee Minutes, October 12, 1962, Box 27, C304, InU-Ar. A 2017 report by the AAMC found that "overall, 54.5% of the individuals who completed residency training from 2007 through 2016 are practicing in the state of residency training." For Indiana, the figure was 56.6 percent. AAMC, *Report on Residents*, 2017 edition, accessed May 12, 2018, https://www.aamc.org/data/484710/report-on-residents. html.

22. IU BOT Minutes December, 14 1962; Indianapolis Hospital Redevelopment Association report, November 1962.

23. "Welsh sees second medical school needed," *Indianapolis Star*, August 21, 1963.

24. Daniel Martin, "The Medical Center in a Community," 1056–60. Stahr to Franklin, October 12, 1963; Wells to Franklin, November 2, 1963; Stahr to Matthew E. Walsh, November 18, 1963; John R. Emens to Stahr, November 27, 1963, C304, InU-Ar.

25. Rothstein, 225. For a list of all accredited medical schools by state and their founding date, see LCME, "Accredited U. S. Programs," accessed June 17, 2016, https://www.printfriendly.com/p/g/dy4Dw6#.

26. LCME, "Accredited U. S. Programs."

27. IU News Bureau, Press Release, November 15, 1963.

28. H. Lawrence Wilsey to Stahr, January 10, 1964, C304, InU-Ar.

29. Coggeshall, *Planning for Medical Progress through Education*; Howell, "Lowell Coggeshall," 711–18. Coggeshall to George Beadle, October 1964, Beadle, George Wells. Papers [Box 20, Folder 1], Special Collections Research Center, University of Chicago Library.

30. Johnson, "The Study of Applicants," 1017–30.

31. The median attrition rate was 13.7 percent per class in the "freshman" year, compared to a national average under 10 percent. About two-thirds of attrition occurred during the first year, with continued decrease for each class through fourth year.

32. Shumacker to Shultz, June 8, 1964; Ganz to Nurnberger, November 16, 1964; Stahr to Wilsey, November 5, 1964, C304, InU-Ar.

33. "Development of Medical Education in Indiana," Booz, Allen and Hamilton, December 8, 1964, Box 27, C 304, InU-Ar.

34. Ibid.

35. Alvin Eurich, "A Commentary on Medical Education in Indiana," South Bend: AED, February 1965; "You, Your Family Doctor, and the Doctor Shortage" (Muncie: Ball State University, 1965); Statement from John R. Emens, January 20, 1965, Memo, Joint Sub-Committee Hearing on SB 366, January 18, 1965, C304, InU-Ar.

36. Kenneth Penrod, Draft Discussion Paper, Committee on Medical Education, June 2, 1965, C304, InU-Ar. For national reaction to the plan, see Penrod, "The Indiana Program for Comprehensive Medical Education," 868–70; Penrod and Irwin, "A Proposed Statewide Medical School for Indiana," 1030–36; K. E. Penrod, "The Indiana University Medical Center, a Decade Ahead," 4 passim.

37. Penrod, Draft Discussion Paper; Jordan to Wilsey, June 7, 1965, Irwin to Stahr, June 10, 1965, C304, InU-Ar.

38. Irwin to Stahr, March 17, 1965; "Future Medical Education in Indiana— The Indiana Plan," April 12, 1966, Box 111, C304, InU-Ar.

39. "Future Medical Education in Indiana."

40. Irwin to Committee [Beneville], July 22, 1966, "Future Medical Education in Indiana," Box 111, C 304, InU-Ar; "Divided on Medical School," *The Republic* (Columbus, Indiana) December 29, 1966.

41. Stahr, Remarks to Indianapolis Chamber of Commerce, December 12, 1966; Stahr, Remarks to Medical Alumni Association, May 12, 1965; Remarks to Lake County Medical Society, September 21, 1966; Presentation to Indiana Pre-Legislative Conference, December 1, 1966, C304, InU-Ar.

42. Irwin to Stahr, January 22, 1967, SB 359, Medical Education Board Statement of Policy, November 1, 1967, Box 145, C304, InU-Ar.

43. Irwin to Stahr, June 28, 1968, C304, InU-Ar.

44. "Medical Education in Indiana: A Presentation for the State Policy Commission on Post-High School Education," 3–5; August 1, 1968, Box 1, A7930, InU-Ar.

45. State Policy Commission on Post High School Education, *An Indiana Pattern for Higher Education, Indianapolis,* (Indianapolis, 1968).

46. Ibid., 59–64.

47. There was no allocation of funds for the operation of the commission, so SerVaas began using his own funds to pay for its activities. Executive Order 23–69; Armstrong to Clark, August 22, 1969; Clark to Sutton, August 27, 1969, InU-Ar.

48. Hine, Notes from Commission meeting, September 24, 1969, C304; Glenn Irwin, Notes on Indiana Statewide Medical Education InU-Ar; Lukemeyer interview.

49. LCME Report, 1971.

50. "Statewide Medical Education Programs in Indiana," July 1971, in Maynard Hine Papers, Box 4, Office of the Chancellor Records, 1914–2006, University Library Special Collections and Archives, IUPUI University Library, Indiana University Purdue University Indianapolis, Indianapolis (hereafter cited as UA 041, InUI-Ar).

51. "Statewide Medical Education in Indiana"; Progress Report on the Indiana Statewide Medical Education System, Summer 1971, "Centers for Medical Education Program," July 22, 1971, Box 22, UA 041.

52. Fordham, "The *Bane Report* Revisited," 357.

53. Mallon et al., *Regional Medical Campuses*, 63. See also Ramsey et al., "From Concept to Culture," 76–775.

54. Mallon, 3–4. As of 2006, a number of states had regional campuses but they were typically for clinical teaching of third and fourth year medical students.

55. Robert Cook-Deegan and Michael McGeary, "The Jewel in the Federal Crown?" 176, 189.

56. This and other information about the medical research philanthropy are from Lupton, "Local Foundations."

57. Leonard Betley, interview by Suzann Lupton, October 29, 2014, in Lupton, "Local Foundations."

58. Ford et al., *Regenstrief*.

59. For the changing relationships between IUSM and Krannert, see "Krannert Charter, 1962–1987," "Krannert Institute, ca. 1967–2000," "Krannert Pavilion, 1964–1993." For NIH center fundings, see LCME Report, 1963; "Krannert Institute Marks 50 Years of Leading Cardiovascular Research: Stories: Weekly Features: InScope: Indiana University," accessed August 7, 2017, http://inscopearchive.iu.edu/features/stories/2013–11–14-krannert-institute-inscope.shtml; Bodenhamer, Barrows, and Vanderstel, *The Encyclopedia of Indianapolis,* 879.

60. "History of the Department of Medicine," IUSM Center and Departmental Histories, UA 073 InUI-Ar.

61. Betley interview, in Lupton, "Local Foundations."

62. Harvey Feigenbaum, interview by Suzann Lupton, October 24, 2014, in Lupton, "Local Foundations"; Henry Feigenbaum, interview by Kendra Clauser, May 10, 2012, SC 3095, Indiana Historical Society.

63. Lupton, "Local Foundations."

64. Ford et al., *Regenstrief*, 54.

65. Memo to Sam Regenstrief, April 24, 1967, Regenstrief Foundation documents, folder 1.

66. "Memorial Resolution," Professor Emeritus Raymond Gorbold Murray (May 12, 1916–October 7, 1998), Indiana University Bloomington Faculty Council, September 19, 2000, Box 11, C 181, InUI-Ar.

67. See Annual Reports for listings of publication, and grant projects, which begin to appear regularly during this period. For context, see Walter J. Daly, interview by Philip Scarpino, May 10, 2017, IUSM Oral History Collection, InUI-Ar; Holden interview.

68. Holden interview; Daly interview, 2017; Badertscher, "A New Wishard Is on the Way," 345–82; Robert B. Jones, interview by Kevin Grau, April 22, 2008, IUSM Oral History Collection, InUI-Ar. For a look at Wishard during this period, see "Wishard Scrapbook," Indiana Medical History Museum, accessed August 7, 2017, http://indiamond6.ulib.iupui.edu/cdm/ref/collection /IMHM/id/299.

69. McDonald and Tierney, "The Medical Gopher," 823–29; Ford et al., *Regenstrief*.

70. Minutes of the Showalter Trust Selection Committee, July 10, 1973, Showalter files, folder 2.

71. Ibid.

72. Walther authored an autobiography whose title reflected his lack of modesty: *A Life Like None Other: Recollections of a Maverick Hoosier Physician*.

73. Web pages for individual department histories can be found at History of the Indiana University School of Medicine Materials, accessed June 6, 2018, https://archives.iupui.edu/handle/2450/11448.

74. For a recent application of Hickam's dictum, see Borden and Linklater, "Hickam's Dictum," 164. For more on Hickam, see, Hickam, "Periodic Recertification," 1657–58; Ross, "John Bamber Hickam," 571–73; Hickam and Close, "Symposium on Medical Education," 907–9; Trobe, "Noble J. David, MD, Reminisces," 240–46.

75. IUSM AR, 1969–73, passim, Daly interview, 2017; "History of the Department of Medicine"; Ross, "John Bamber Hickam," 571–73.

76. The divisions were formed over time, so it was a gradual process rather than a comprehensive decision to reorganize. Hickam appointed directors for each division usually as they were hired, and the organization continued under his successor, Walter Daly. These included (in 1958) Joseph C. Ross in Pulmonary Disease, Philip A. Christiansen in Gastroenterology, and William P. Deiss, Jr. in Endocrinology, followed (in 1961) by Charles Fisch in Cardiology and (in

1967) by Arthur C. White in Infectious Diseases and Stuart A. Kleit in Nephrology. See "History of the Department of Medicine."

77. Ibid.

78. Ross, "John Bamber Hickam," 571; Augustus Watanabe, interview by Kevin Grau, April 15, 2008, IUSM Oral History Collection, InUI-Ar; Daly interview, 2017; Daly interview, 2005.

79. Watanabe, Oral History.

80. Daly interview, 2017; Baker, Mamlin, and Daly, "Simulation Modeling," 836.

81. Elizondo, and Moore, "Physiology at Indiana University-Bloomington," 319–24.

82. History of the Indiana University School of Medicine Materials, Departmental and Center Histories, accessed June 6, 2018, https://archives.iupui.edu /handle/2450/11448.

83. "A Brief History of the Department of Pediatrics, Indiana University School of Medicine," Departmental and Center Histories; Office of the Chancellor, and James Whitcomb Riley Memorial Association, *Report of the Chancellor's Office to the James Whitcomb Riley Memorial Association* (Indianapolis: IUPUI, 1971).

84. Robert Garrett, "Urology at Indiana University," 1993, IUSM Center and Departmental Histories, UA 073, InUI-Ar.

85. Jesseph also was an avid historian and maintained his ties with the military. His contributions are celebrated in the Jesseph Memorial Lectures. Canal and Lillemoe, "The Department of Surgery," 11–12; Grillo, "To Impart This Art: The Development of Graduate Surgical Education in the United States," 1–14; "Memorial Resolution on Behalf of John E. Jesseph, M.D.," (1982), IUSM Collection, UA 073, InUI-Ar.

86. After working more than fifteen years in the department, John Campbell took over as chair in 1971. The Radiation Therapy Building was built in 1974 and dedicated in 1977. Hale and Wilson, *Through the Years*; IUSM Center and Departmental Histories, UA 073 InUI-Ar.

87. Hale and Wilson, *Through the Years*, 92–110.

88. In 1976, Norins succeeded Hackney as chairman, and the number of faculty continued to grow.

89. Hickam and Close, "Symposium on Medical Education."

90. McKusick and Harper, "History of Medical Genetics," 1–39; Rimoin and Hirschhorn, "A History of Medical Genetics in Pediatrics," 150–59; Peggy Knople, "History of Medical Genetics at Indiana University School of Medicine" (2014), IUSM Center and Departmental Histories UA 073, InUI-Ar.

91. "History of the Department of Medicine."

92. Nurnberger and Hendrie, "History of the Department of Psychiatry"; Angela Potter, Oral History with Alan Schmetzer, former Chairman of Department of Psychiatry, June 15, 2015, UA 073 Oral History, InUI-Ar; DeMyer, Hingtgen, and Jackson, "Infantile Autism Reviewed," 388–451.

93. Potter, "Learning Human Anatomy." Examples of the large literature on the broader context are Bickel, "Gender Equity in Undergraduate Medical

Education," 261–70, and "A Half Century of Progress of Black Students," 28–31.

94. Ralph D. Gray, *IUPUI*; Lantzer, "The Other Side of Campus," 153–78; Wynkoop, *Dissent in the Heartland*.

95. Watanabe interview. See also Mellisa K. Klein, "The Legacy of the 'Yellow Berets': The Vietnam War, the Doctor Draft, and the NIH Associate Training Program" (manuscript, 1998, NIH History Office, National Institutes of Health, Bethesda, MD), https://history.nih.gov/research/downloads/Yellow Berets.pdf.

96. "Medical Students Win National Recognition," *QB* 22, no. 2 (Spring 1960): 29–30.

97. SAMA, Box 23, 1961–64, UA 041, InUI-Ar.

98. "Medical Students Turn on to Start New Health Center," *QB* 30, no. 3–4 (Summer and Fall 1968): 21.

99. *Journal of the Indiana SMA* [Student Medical Association] (September 1969): 1168–69.

100. "Medical Students Turn on to Start New Health Center," *QB* 30, no. 3–4 (Summer and Fall 1968): 21.

101. "SAMA News," *Auxesis* (June 1969).

102. George Lukenmeyer to Chancellor Hine, May 18, 1970, Box 3, UA 041, InUI-Ar.

103. "Report of the Survey of IUSM by Liaison Committee on Medical Education presented to AMA and the Association of American Medical Colleges," May 17–20, 1971, 19, Box 15, UA 041, InUI-Ar.

104. "Summary of Meeting between the Black Health Students and Dr. MK Hine," May 12, 1970, Box 3, UA 041, InUI-Ar.

105. Gray, *IUPUI*, 46–47.

106. Ibid.

107. LCME Report, 1963.

108. Indiana University—Indianapolis Campus Master Plan, July 1966, unprocessed papers, UA 073, InUI-Ar.

109. Elvis Stahr, "Development of the Indianapolis Campus," remarks at the Indianapolis Chamber of Commerce, (December 12, 1966), C304, InU-Ar; Gray, *IUPUI*, 84–85.

110. Gray, *IUPUI*, 85.

111. Richard Lugar, "A Great University for Greater Indianapolis," (December 14, 1968), IUPUI University Library University Library Special Collections and Archives, eArchives, accessed May 17, 2018, https://archives.iupui.edu/handle /2450/7555.

112. Gray, *IUPUI*, 83.

113. Gray, *IUPUI*, 83; "Background Information Indiana University-Purdue University at Indianapolis," Box 3, Annual Report for 1968–1969, Indiana University–Purdue University at Indianapolis, Box 15, UA 041, InUI-Ar.

114. Hine to Sutton, Box 22, C268. For enrollment statistics, see IUPUI Office of the Registrar, "Enrollment Statistics—1968 to Present," accessed February 22, 2017, http://registrar.iupui.edu/genealogy/enroll.html.

10. The Medical Center, 1975–1995:
Administration and Medical Education

1. Community Health Services was founded as a section in Department of Medicine in 1968 as part of Hickam's initiatives. In 1971, it became its own department under Raymond Murray, head of the Krannert Institute, as part of a slate of organizational changes, including the creation of the Family Practice Program and the Faculty Practice Plans. When Daly took over as head of Regenstreif, he returned the organization to the Regenstrief Institute, Wishard and Outpatient Clinics. He felt that many of the planned initiatives were duplicating efforts, and he focused on the Indianapolis clinics.

2. Because the hospital was renamed in 1975, henceforward it will be referred to as Wishard. In 2013, the hospital moved into new facilities and was renamed for Sidney and Lois Eskenazi, who donated $40 million. "A heart for the Poor," *Indianapolis Star*, June 22, 2011; "Eskenazi Health Is Here Thanks to the Community," *Indianapolis Star*, December 6, 2013. For national context on these changes, see Ludmerer, *Learning to Heal*, 366–48; Rothstein, *American Medical Schools*, part V.

3. Gray, *IUPUI*, 135–37.

4. As an indication of Irwin's conciliatory skills, he appointed Moore as the executive vice chancellor at IUPUI. See "Historical Note," Finding Aid, Office of the Dean of Faculties/Executive Vice Chancellor, 1966–2007, UA 044, University Library Special Collections and Archives, IUPUI University Library, Indiana University Purdue University Indianapolis, Indianapolis (hereafter cited as InUI-Ar); Steven C. Beering, oral history interview, November 15, 2006, Purdue University Oral History Program Collection, Virginia Kelly Karnes Archives and Special Collections Research Center; Lora Posey, "John William Ryan—Indiana University Archives," accessed March 15, 2017, https://blogs.libraries .indiana.edu/iubarchives/tag/john-william-ryan; Gray, *IUPUI*, 138.

5. Lukemeyer spent his entire career at IU, earning a BS degree in 1944 and an MD degree in 1947. He began as an instructor of Internal Medicine in 1954 and established the artificial kidney laboratory. As an administrator, he played a key role in the development of the Statewide Medical Education System as associate dean of the School of Medicine in 1966 and was the executive associate dean and medical director of the University Hospitals from 1972 to 1990. Lukemeyer served on the Medical School Admissions Committee beginning in 1960, and he served as chair from 1982 to 2000. He played an active role nationally, including the American Medical Association Council on Medical Education (1986–95), the LCME (1994–97), the National Board of Medical Examiners (1991–96), chairman of the Accreditation Council on Graduate Medical Education (ACGME), and the American Medical Association Council on Medical Education. See "George T. Lukemeyer," Box 121, UA 041, InUI-Ar. Lukemeyer, interview; Daly interview, 2005; Stephen C. Beering, interview by Elizabeth J. Van Allen, December 7, 2000, UA 073, InUI-Ar.

6. The IUSM Search Committee Files were not preserved in the Chancellor's Office Records (UA 041 InUI-Ar) for this search, and oral histories are noticeably silent on this transition of deans. For studies on the changing role of the

dean in schools of medicine, and academic medical centers, see Schieffler, "The Evolution of the Medical School Deanship."

7. Beering does not talk in detail about his time at IUSM in most of his oral histories. Beering interview, Purdue University; Holden interview.

8. "Beering, Steven C., President of Purdue University, 1983–2006," UA 073, InUI-Ar.

9. Wm. Hugh Headlee, "Representation of the IUSM Faculty in Faculty Organizations and Affairs," May 3, 1973, UA 073, InUI-Ar.

10. Ibid.

11. Gray, *IUPUI*, 135–43. Glenn W. Irwin, interview by David Zubke, November 12, 19; December 2, 1996, UA 041, InUI-Ar. Headlee was the head of the IUPUI Faculty Council in 1973.

12. For a national perspective, see Ludmerer, *Time to Heal*, 214, 395.

13. LCME Self-Study, 1979; Gray, *IUPUI*, 251–60; Ludmerer, *Time to Heal*, 337–48.

14. LCME Self-Study, 1979.

15. LCME Self-Study, 1979; IUSM Annual Reports, passim.

16. Appointments at this time included Roger Hunt as director of Indiana University Hospitals, Sally Knox as associate director of the University Hospitals for Nursing Services, and Fred Ficklin as assistant dean for Student Affairs and assistant professor of health administration; IUSM Annual Reports, passim.

17. School of Health and Rehabilitation Science Records 1955–1995, University Library Special Collections and Archives, University Library, Indiana University Purdue University Indianapolis (UA 029, InUI-Ar). In 2002, the school was restructured to focus on graduate degrees in health and rehabilitation science disciplines, whereas the undergraduate allied health sciences degrees migrated to other home academic units on the IUPUI campus. In 2003, the name was changed to the School of Health and Rehabilitation Sciences. LCME Self-Study, 1979, 1987, 1994.

18. From 1943 to 1946, Bowen served in the Medical Corps of the navy, rising from the rank of first lieutenant to captain. This experience connected him with many of the top leaders at IUSM, who had also gone through the army program in medical school. He was on the staff of various hospitals in Indiana and served as coroner for Marshall County, Indiana. Bowen, *Doc: Memories from a Life in Public Service*; Bowen interview.

19. "Bowen, Otis, 1985," "IUPUI Self-Study, 1982–1992," "Bowen Research Center, 1990–1991," Box 204; "Bowen Research Center," UA 073 InUI-Ar; Wailoo, *Pain: A Political History*; Oberlander, *The Political Life of Medicare*, 54–60; Blumenthal and Morone, *The Heart of Power*, 300–314; Bowen, *Doc*; Bowen interview.

20. The name of the Bowen Research Center was changed to Bowen Center for Health Workforce Research & Policy and became housed in the Fairbanks School of Public Health. Bowen Research Center, 1990–1991," UA 073 InUI-Ar; Evans interview.

21. Clarian Health changed to IU Health in 2010. Daniel Evans Jr., interview by Kevin Grau, February 6, 2008, IUSM Oral History Collection, UA 073, InUI-Ar; "End of an Era at IU Health: CEO Daniel Evans to Retire,"

Indianapolis Star, September 1, 2015; Bowen, *Doc*, 140. For the importance of local and national politics in health care reform, see Oberlander, "Learning from Failure in Health Care Reform," 1677–79.

22. "Purdue's New President to Take Office July 1," *Lafayette Journal and Courier*, February 4, 1983 "14 Months of Travel and Talk Involved in Purdue Hunt," *Journal and Courier*, February 5, 1983; "Beering Era Starts Today at Purdue," *Lafayette Journal and Courier*, July 1, 1983; IU BOT Minutes, February 4, 1983; Beering interview, Purdue University; Beering interview, UA 073, InUI-Ar.

23. Daly, "Presidential Address," 10.

24. Walter J. Daly, interview by Jean Freedman, June 27, 1994, Indiana University Oral History Archive, 1991–98, Oral History Research Center, Indiana University, Bloomington; Daly interview, 2005; Daly interview, 2017.

25. Daly interview, 2017; Daly interview, 2005; Snodgrass, *A Life in Academic Medicine*.

26. Ora Pescovitz, interview by Kevin Grau, April 17, 2008, IUSM, UA 073, InUI-Ar; Daly interview, 2017; LCME Self-study, 1987; Indiana University School of Medicine, "Annual Reports—IU School of Medicine, 1993" UA 073, InUI-Ar.

27. For examples of studies, showing the complexities of the Dean's Office, see "Indiana University Medical Education Study, 1982–1983," "IU Medical Center Strategic Planning Committee, 1983–1984," "IU Hospitals Inpatient Task Force, Medical Staff Survey, 1984," "IU Hospitals Competitor Analysis Report, 4/13/1984," "IU Hospitals Referral Physician Study, 3/1984," "IUMC Medical Staff Survey, 4/9/1984," UA 073, InUI-Ar.

28. Bepko, a former special agent with the Federal Bureau of Investigation, joined the law school's faculty in 1973. He became an associate dean in 1979 and dean in 1982. Like Irwin, Bepko was an IU vice president with supervisory authority over both campus and system-wide schools. In 1991, Bepko became chair of the University Operations Cabinet, which reviewed and revised IU's nonacademic policies with the goal of controlling costs and increasing efficiencies. For more on Bepko see, Gray, IUPUI, 248–54. For examples of biomedical initiatives, see "Biomedical Research, 1988–2000," Box 326–7, UA 041, InUI-Ar.

29. Thomas Ehrlich, "One University," 1988; "Thomas Ehrlich, 1987–1994," UA 073, InUI-Ar.

30. LCME Self-Study, 1993.

31. Daly interview, 2017.

32. "Deans of School of Medicine—Office of Gift Development, "Campaign Book for IU School of Medicine," Box 180; "Dean's Gift Office," Box 209; "History of Medicine," Box 327–23, UA 041. "John Shaw Billings," UA 073, InUI-Ar.

33. "Master Plan/Facilities Plan, Space Plan, 1991–1995," Box 122, UA 041, InUI-Ar. "University Hospital Dedication, 1970," "Class of 1961 30th Anniversary Class Gift Campaign, 1991," "Dedication Ceremony, Addition to the James Whitcomb Riley Hospital for Children, 1986," "Medical Research Building and Library Dedication, 1988–1989," Box 229; "Medical Science Center Dedication,

1998," Box 255; "Medical Sciences Naming Ceremony—John D. VanNuys, 5/1988," UA 073, InUI-Ar. Holden interview.

34. LCME Self-Study, 1979.

35. An example was a Grievance Committee that examined the complaints made by a female faculty member who claimed that her work environment was hostile, that she was the victim of gender discrimination, and that she had been unfairly removed from her original position. The committee (made up of five women and three men) acknowledged that it would have been helpful if there had been a mentor to guide the junior faculty member through these department difficulties, and that she may have received some mixed messages that compounded her problems. Nonetheless, the committee found no documentary evidence of sexual discrimination or harassment, and it concluded that ultimately, the division leadership was well within their rights to reassign her to a different position. Chancellor's records UA 041 128–12. This was just one of a number of cases that reached the status of a disciplinary hearing. See, for example, letters from a group of women who consulted a lawyer about harassment. "Sexual Harassment," Box 128–7, UA 041, InUI-Ar.

36. Daly interview, 1994.

37. LCME Self-Study, 1993.

38. Mallon, *Mini-Med*. On national notoriety, see "Medical School Expands off Campus," *American Medical News*, October 1, 1973.

39. "History of Statewide Medical Education," LCME Self-Study, 1993; Daly interview, 2017.

40. See chapter 7 for more information.

41. LCME Self-Study, 1963; Lukemeyer and Irwin, "Statewide Medical Education in Indiana," 264–70.

42. As mentioned in earlier chapters, there is a long tradition of preceptorship in medical education, going back to the apprentice model of the nineteenth century. Although twentieth-century reforms called for more full-time faculty, the increased emphasis on clinical instruction was solved by use of "volunteers" often in the clinical setting. Local physicians volunteered their time for a variety reasons ranging from altruistic to the prestige of affiliation with a medical school. See Ryan et al., "Benefits and Barriers among Volunteer Teaching Faculty." As the statistics show, the Indiana statewide program was also heavily dependent on volunteers for preclinical instruction at the regional centers.

43. For overall histories of the system and the individual centers, see "Statewide Medical Education, 1972," "Statewide Medical Education Evansville Center, 1972–1981," "Statewide Medical Education Ft. Wayne Center, 1973–1976," "Statewide Medical Education Muncie Center, 1971–1975," "Statewide Medical Education Southwest Center, 1972–1981," "Statewide Medical Education Lafayette Center, 1972–1975," "Statewide Medical Education Terre Haute Center, 1972–1980," "Statewide Medical Education South Bend Center, 1974–1980," UA 073 InUI-Ar. In that same collection, see also "The Serendipitous Creation of the Indiana Statewide System of Medical Education," "Statewide Medical Education, Annual Reports, 1972–2003," Reports—Study Council-IU Statewide Medical Education System," "Study Council-IU Statewide Medical Education

System—Final Report, 1991," and "Statewide Medical Education in Indiana, 1964–2005."

44. LCME Self-Study, 1971, 1978, 1987, 1983.

45. LCME Self-Study 1987.

46. To avoid confusion with IUPUI and the long rivalries including over the medical school, the center located in West Lafayette was called "Lafayette." Most of the medical facilities affiliated with the center were in Lafayette, although Purdue now hosts third- and fourth-year students and has close connections to other life science initiatives on campus through Discovery Park. "History of Regional Medical Campus System—IU School of Medicine—Lafayette," 2014, Departmental Histories, UA 073, InUI-Ar.

47. "I. U. Med·School Expands," Your University, UA 073, InUI-Ar; "History—IU School of Medicine—South Bend," "History of Regional Medical Campus System—IU School of Medicine—Lafayette," UA 073, InUI-Ar.

48. "Indiana University School of Medicine Evansville 1972–2012," Departmental Histories, UA 073, InUI-Ar.

49. Commission on Higher Education, "Summary of the Report of the Council to Study the Future of IU System of Statewide Medical Education" (Indianapolis: Indiana General Assembly, October 30, 1991), UA 073, InUI-Ar.

50. O'Hara, "The Very Model of Modern Urban Decay," 135–54; Catlin, *Racial Politics and Urban Planning: Gary, Indiana.*

51. "History of the Reginal Medical Campus System"; LCME Self-Study, 1993; Brokaw et al., "The Influence of Regional Basic Science Campuses," 29.

52. Sivam and Vaughn, "Integration of Pharmacology into a Problem-Based Learning Curriculum," 289–96; Robin Biesen, "A New Breed of Student. IUN Medical Program Takes Hands-On," *The Times* (Munster, IN), 2012; "IU School of Medicine—Northwest Celebrates 40 Years of Physician Education—Indiana University Northwest," Departmental Histories, UA 073, InUI-Ar. For the national context, Ludmerer, Time to Heal, 304–6.

53. Myers Hall was originally completed as the Medical Building in 1936, and then it was named for Dean Burton D. Myers in 1958. The renovated building was finished in 2002. "Myers Hall to Be Rededicated Friday: IU News Room: Indiana University," "Indiana Molecular Biology Institute," departmental histories, UA 073, InUI-Ar; LCME Self-Study 1993.

54. "Indianapolis," *Caduceus (Indiana University School of Medicine)* (Indianapolis: Indiana University, School of Medicine, 1991).

55. As late as 1993, most of the other centers relied heavily on volunteer faculty affiliated with local hospitals for the second year of instruction. LCME Self-Study, 1993. It took years to regularize the faculty appointments from the central medical school administration, including hiring and tenure decisions, although as late as 1993, all instruction at Lafayette was by Purdue faculty.

56. LCME Self-Study, 1987; Daly interview, 1994; Commission on Higher Education, "Summary of the Report of the Council to Study the Future of IU System of Statewide Medical Education"; "Future Directions for Indiana's System of Medical Education: Myers Hall to Be Rededicated Friday: IU News Room: Indiana University," Indiana Molecular Biology Institute, departmental histories, UA 073, InUI-Ar; "A Policy Paper" (Indianapolis: Indiana General Assembly, October 9, 1992), UA 073, InUI-Ar.

57. The Gary and Bloomington centers were on Indiana University campuses, which simplified space allocation, but because budgets were kept separate, the medical centers were largely run independently. As late as the 1993 self-study for accreditation, the space at centers at Bloomington and South Bend was described as "inadequate." In addition to classroom space, each campus needed laboratory and research space, often in short supply in some of the smaller campus, requiring the eventual construction of new facilities. LCME Self-Study, 1993, part XIII, 6.

58. Ibid. For examples of communications with regional centers, see "Statewide Medical Education in Indiana, Quarterly Newsletter, Speeches, Correspondence, 1972–1982," UA 073, InUI-Ar.

59. LCME Self-Study, 1987, 1993; Daly interview, 2017; Brokaw et al., "The Influence of Regional Basic Science Campuses"; Commission on Higher Education, "Summary of the Report of the Council to Study the Future of IU System of Statewide Medical Education."

60. LCME Report, 1971, 1979, 1987, 1994.

61. "The Early Development of Indiana Statewide Medical Education, 1967–1991," UA 073, InUI-Ar; "Statewide Medical Education in Indiana, 1964–2005," UA 073, InUI-Ar.

62. LCME Self-Study, 1987; Brokaw et al., "The Influence of Regional Basic Science Campuses"; Commission on Higher Education, "Report of the Council to Study the Future of IU System of Statewide Medical Education" (Indianapolis: Indiana General Assembly, October 30, 1991), Box 203, UA 071, InUI-Ar.

63. Joseph Grady, "Evansville," "South Bend," "Muncie," "Fort Wayne," *Caduceus*, 1994, 13–17. For a national periodical article on the new program with additional student opinions, see "Medical School Expands off Campus," *American Medical News*, October 1, 1973, 13–15.

64. Students at the Fort Wayne center expressed a sentiment that was likely shared by others about their placement regional centers: "Although Fort Wayne may not have been the first campus choice for many of us, we persevered, perhaps even prospered, under the guidance of our caring faculty and with the support of our fellow classmates." One student who took his freshman year at Muncie wrote, "There is so much caring here. If you skip a class, you're missed. If you're worried, someone notices. If you make a mistake, it's right out in the open." Grady, "Fort Wayne," "Evansville," "Gary," *Caduceus*, 1991, 18; "I. U. Med School Expands," *Your University*, September–October 1971, Box 76, UA 041, InUI-Ar.

65. Reflecting the growing autonomy, the regional centers were elevated to the status of "schools" with the renaming of the Evansville Center, for example, to the "Indiana University School of Medicine- Evansville" (IUSM-E) in 2005. In 2013, IUSM and ISUM-E announced that they would expand to a four-year medical school with multiple residency opportunities. Third-year students began the summer of 2013 and continued as fourth-year students in 2014, as well as expanding incoming enrollments. "Press Release IU Trustees Approve Design of IU School of Medicine-Evansville Multi-Institutional Academic Health Science and Research Center," 2012, Departmental Histories, UA 073, InUI-Ar; "Indiana University School of Medicine Evansville 1972–2012"; John Martin,

"Ground Broken for 'Transformative' Downtown IU Med School," *Evansville Courier Press*, October 23, 2015.

66. Brokaw et al., "The Influence of Regional Basic Science Campuses"; Wade et al., "Influence of Hometown," 248–54.

67. Institute of Medicine (US) Division of Health Sciences Policy, ed., *Medical Education and Societal Needs: A Planning Report for the Health Professions* (Washington, DC: National Academies Press, 1983), unprocessed papers, UA 073, InUI-Ar; Ludmerer, *Time to Heal*, 210–19; Mallon, ed., *Mini-Med*; Cheifetz et al., "Regional Medical Campuses," 1140–43.

68. Crowley "Graduate Medical Education," 1585–93; Britt, "Graduate Medical Education," 136–39. For the example of the GMENAC, see *Report of the Graduate Medical Education National Advisory Committee to the Secretary, Department of Health and Human Services* (September 30, 1980), accessed May 12, 2018, https://files.eric.ed.gov/fulltext/ED210990.pdf.

69. Cooper, "Medical Schools and Their Applicants," 71–84; Ludmerer, *Time to Heal*, 295–301.

70. Application numbers from IUSM annual reports. IUSM analysis shows there were a variety of ways to look at the data, including student characteristics (race, gender, ethnicity, age), grades, state of residence. Application acceptance rates were also of critical concern. George Lukemeyer, "A Look into the Future: The Decline in the Applicant Pool," paper delivered at Central Association of Advisors for the Health Professions meeting, Mayo Clinic, 1979, Lukemeyer papers (in process), UA 073, InUI-Ar; Cooper, "Medical Schools and Their Applicants."

71. IUSM AR passim; LCME Self-Study, 1979, 1995.

72. Lukemeyer, "A Look into the Future."

73. Ibid.; Institute of Medicine Division of Health Sciences Policy, *Medical Education and Societal Needs*; IUSM Annual Report, 1987–88; Singer, "The Effect of the Vietnam War on Numbers of Medical School Applicants," 567–73; Lohr, Vanselow, and Detmer, *U. S. Physician Supply and Requirements*.

74. Thomas Ehrlich, interview by Philip Scarpino, February 9, 2007, Randall L. Tobias Center for Leadership Excellence, IUPUI, Indianapolis, IN; Daly interview, 2017; Daly interview, 1994.

75. Daly interview, 2017; Commission on Higher Education, "Report of the Council to Study the Future of IU System of Statewide Medical Education."

76. Ibid.; "Consolidation of Regional Medical Centers," third draft, May 10, 1991, in Lukemeyer papers.

77. Handel et al., "The Development and Maturation," 230–35; "Summary of the Report of the Council to Study the Future of the Indiana University System of Statewide Medical Education," UA 073, InUI-Ar.

78. IUSM AR 1974–1995; IU Council Minutes. For national comparisons, see Lohr, Vanselow, and Detmer, *U. S. Physician Supply and Requirements*.

79. LCME Self-Study, 1977.

80. LCME Self-Study, 1977, 1987, 1995; Indiana University School of Medicine, "Annual Reports—IU School of Medicine." The transition from a DNS program to the current PhD program was approved in 1995, with the first students enrolling in 1996.

81. Nationally IUSM ranked forty-seventh out of 127 schools as reported in the Association of American Medical Colleges report 1995, as quoted in LCME Self-Study, 1993.

82. LCME Self-Study, 1979.

83. Indiana University School of Medicine, "Annual Reports—IU School of Medicine."

84. Crowley, "Graduate Medical Education"; Donini-Lenhoff and Hedrick, "Growth of Specialization in Graduate Medical Education," 1284–89; Rich et al., "Medicare Financing of Graduate Medical Education," 283–92; Ludmerer, *Time to Heal*.

85. *Center* (magazine of IU Medical Center) (spring/summer 1990): 28; LCME Self-Study, 1979, 1987, 1994; Daly interview, 2017; Indiana University School of Medicine, The Indiana Initiative; "Summary of the Report of the Council to Study the Future of the Indiana University System of Statewide Medical Education," UA 073, InUI-Ar.

86. In addition to Ginzberg, 242–44, for analysis of the national trends, see Ludmerer, *Time to Heal*, 209–15; Rothstein, *American Medical Schools*, 283–86.

87. For contemporary and self-assessments, see George Lukemeyer, "A Look into the Future"; "IU System celebrates 25 years of innovative medical education," *Statewide Medicine* (IUSM Newsletter) 2, no.1 (winter 1996); Health Services Management, "Indiana Physician Profile" (Indianapolis, 1975), Unprocessed Files, IUSM History, UA 073, InUI-Ar. For national context, see Rothstein, *American Medical Schools*, 291–93; Ludmerer, *Time to Heal*, ch. 13. Not until 2002 was there enough interest to create a professional group, the Organization of Regional Medical Campus Deans (OMCD). See Donini-Lenhoff and Hedrick, "Growth of Specialization in Graduate Medical Education," 1284–89.

88. Affirmative Action Committee Reports, 1974–93, UA 073, InUI-Ar; LCME Self-Study, 1979; IUSM AR 1974–81.

89. Lukemeyer, "A Look into the Future." Lukemeyer's study is the first time of note that MCATs are cited by the school, in an effort to demonstrate the quality of students in the expanded IUSM at a time of declining applicants. Before that, the concern focused on the quantity of medical students enrolled in response to pressure from the state legislature. The exams began in 1926 as the SAT for Medical Students and then were revamped in 1946. For background, see McGaghie, "Assessing Readiness for Medical Education," 1085–90.

90. Potter, "Learning Human Anatomy." For examples describing the broader national setting, see Morantz-Sanchez, *Sympathy and Science*; Ludmerer, *Time to Heal*; Wendy Kline, *Bodies of Knowledge*; More, *Restoring the Balance*; More et al., *Women Physicians*.

91. "IUPUI Office for Women: Online Archive: Women Creating Excellence at IUPUI," accessed March 10, 2017, https://ofw.iupui.edu/Leadership/Online-Archive-Women-Creating-Excellence-at-IUPUI; Pescovitz interview; More et al., *Women Physicians*; "Women in Medicine: Are We 'There' Yet?" *Medscape*, accessed March 3, 2017, http://www.medscape.com/viewarticle/732197.

92. *Medical Class of 1973*; *Caduceus*, 1981, 95.

93. "Ann Slanders: Sexism in Medicine," in *Retrospectoscope* (Indianapolis: Indiana University, School of Medicine, 1979), 44.

94. Ibid.

95. Ibid.

96. The new associate dean was charged with dealing with a variety of student issues including counseling, financial aid, retention, developing other resources to help recruiting, and diversity programs.

97. "Griffin, Linda B., 1987–2000," "Affirmative Action Office & Committees, 1974," UA 073, InUI-Ar.

98. "Affirmative Action Committee Reports, 1974–1993," Box 247, UA 073, InUI-Ar; IUSM Annual Reports, 1974–1995; AAMC, "Assessment of Minority and Nonminority U. S. Medical School Graduates"; Langsley, *Trends in Specialization.*

99. "American Association of University Professors (AAUP) files of Elizabeth Solow" UA 073, InUI-Ar; Faculty Women's Club of IU School of Medicine, Misc., 1973–1979, UA 073, InUI-Ar; Research & Sponsored Programs—Correspondence, Doris Merritt, UA 073, InUI-Ar; Frances Rhome, "Affirmative Action Register/Indiana Alumni," UA 073, InUI-Ar; Faculty Women's Club of IU School of Medicine, Misc., 1973–1979, UA 073, InUI-Ar; Doris H. Merritt, Interview by Philip Scarpino, July 17, 2007, IUPUI Oral History Project, InUI-Ar.

100. "Suzanne Knoebel," *Indianapolis Star*, July 13, 2014. On Allen, see, "School of Medicine Distinguished Alumni Award (1993)," accessed July 2, 2018, https://honorsandawards.iu.edu/search-awards/honoree.shtml?honoree ID=2046.

101. AAMC, "U. S. Medical Students First-Year Enrollment by Race and Ethnicity, 1968–69 to 2002–03," accessed September 22, 2017, http://www.aamc diversityfactsandfigures2016.org/report-section/section-5/applicants-enrollment. In contrast, the percentage of women accepted to US medical schools rose steadily from 9.7 percent in 1968–69 to 31.5 percent in 1982–83.

102. Indiana Commission on Higher Education, "Progress Report on State Policy Recommendations on Medical Education," May 4, 1994, UA 073, In-U-Ar in process of accession.

103. Robert DeFrantz, "Two Recent Photos Are Worth Thousands of Words," *Indianapolis Recorder*, February 12, 1977, 9

104. James E. Carter, MD, Associate Dean, to Walter J. Daly, MD, Dean, School of Medicine, June 4, 1984, Indiana University School of Medicine Records, 1848–2005, University Library Special Collections and Archives, University Library, Indiana University Purdue University Indianapolis, Box 161, Folder: Student Affairs Office, 1979–1989; "Affirmative Action Office & Committees, 1974," UA 073, InIU-A; Indiana University School of Medicine, "Annual Reports—IU School of Medicine." During the same period, the proportion of women entrants at IUSM almost exactly matched the national trend, more than tripling from 9.0 percent to 31.7 percent between 1968 and 1982. The figures for the 1990s are from Indiana Commission on Higher Education, "Additional Progress Report on State Policy Recommendations on Medical Education," October 4, 1994, UA 073, InIU-A, in process of accession.

105. "Basic Sciences," *Caduceus*, 1985.

106. *Indiana University School of Medicine Student Manual, 1977/78*; *Indiana University School of Medicine Student Manual, 1986/87*, UA 073, InUI-Ar.

107. Mark Mattern, *Caduceus*, 1994, 3–4.

108. "The Wards: Junior & Senior Year," *Caduceus*, 1985.

109. "The Making of a Doctor: Junior Year: Rotations Provide Clinical Insight," *Caduceus*, 1991.

110. "I. U. M. C. 81–85," *Caduceus*, 1985, 10.

111. "And the O.R.," *Caduceus*, 1985.

112. "The Making of a Doctor: Senior year: Electives Allow Seniors Freedom" (Indianapolis: Indiana University, School of Medicine, 1991), 9.

113. "Senior Year: Looking for the Perfect Match," *Caduceus*, 1991; "Senior Year: Getting Serious," *Caduceus*, 1991.

114. "Senior Year: The Big Day . . . And More," *Caduceus*, 1991.

115. "The Making of a Doctor: Family Life: Providing Escape from Med School," *Caduceus*, 1991.

11. Tower of Babel or Paper Tiger: Research, Hospitals, and Clinical Practice at the Medical Center, 1975–1995

1. "Rotary to Build Hospital Unit," *Greencastle Herald*, July 29, 1930, 4. Although Columbia claims to be the country's first medical center, as mentioned in chapter 3, when Dean Emerson dedicated the Medical Sciences Building in 1919, he called it part of a "great medical center in Indianapolis." See, "Indiana University School of Medicine, in Its New Home, Joins in the Great Work of the R. W. Long Hospital," *Indianapolis Star*, November 2, 1919.

2. Merritt, "Present-Day Medical Education," 1194–97; Rothstein, *American Medical Schools*, 177; Ludmerer, *Time to Heal*, 114.

3. IU BOT, April 6, 1936.

4. Daly, "Presidential Address," 10–14.

5. Ibid. See also Daly, "Essay on Medical Education," in process, Indiana University School of Medicine Records, 1848–2005, University Library Special Collections and Archives, University Library, Indiana University Purdue University Indianapolis (hereafter cited as UA 073, InUI-Ar); Daly interview, 2017. For background, see Mallon, "Benefits and Challenges of Research Centers."

6. Daly interview 2017.

7. LCME Self-Study, 1971, 1994, UA 073, InUI-Ar. For national comparisons, see Ludmerer, *Time to Heal*, 280–87.

8. Ludmerer, *Time to Heal*, 283–84.

9. See chapter 6 for more information on these centers.

10. LCME, 1971.

11. For each LCME accreditation, the research program of the school was evaluated, which gives general and specific information on research activity. Each IUSM Annual Report provides more detailed information on research, including principal investigators, publications, and granting agencies. Annual reports became available to the public and used for development under Daly (e.g., IUSM AR 1980–85). Although departments submitted annual reports to the dean annually from the 1950s, in the 1980s many departments began to make their annual reports more formal and available to the public. See for example "Dept. of Psychiatry Annual Reports, 1991–1997," UA 073, InUI-Ar.

12. Feigenbaum "Evolution of Echocardiography," 1321–27. See also Weyman, "Harvey Feigenbaum: A Retrospective," 3–6; Feigenbaum and Hyde, "Ultrasound Diagnosis of Pericardial Effusion," 711–14.

13. Daly interview, 2017; Feigenbaum, "The Origin of Echocardiography," 87–88; Harvey Feigenbaum, interview by Kendra Clauser, May 10, 2012, SC 3095, Indiana Historical Society.

14. "An Interview with Lawrence Einhorn, MD," 167.

15. Lupton, "Local Foundations." On the growth of NIH, see Schneider, "The Origin of the Medical Research Grant," 279–81.

16. Regenstrief Institute Board Minutes, September 5, 1978; Lupton, "Local Foundations." In 2000, the board decided that the institute should stand more on its own as an independent legal organization. The Regenstreif Foundation therefore once again became a private grant-making foundation with a funding strategy focused on "sustained, long-term funding of a small number of programs, with an emphasis on informatics, epidemiology, economics, and innovations in health care delivery." "The Regenstreif Foundation Strategic Direction," report, 1979, 1, Regenstrief Archives, Indianapolis, Indiana; "Regenstrief Institute, 1967–1973," "Memorandum of Understanding, 1969–1972," Box 19; Regenstrief Health Center, 1973–1999," Box 230, UA 041, InUI-Ar; Ford et al., *Regenstrief*; Daly interview, 2017; Holden interview.

17. Regenstreif Foundation Board Minutes, June 14, 1978, Regenstreif Archives, Indianapolis, Indiana.

18. See, for example, Scientific Advisory Committee, Letter to the Regenstreif Foundation Board, June 6, 1980, Regenstrief Archives.

19. Lupton, "Local Foundations."

20. Lupton, "Local Foundations"; "Showalter Professor of Biochemistry, 1973," Box 22, UA 041, InUI-Ar; "Showalter Committee, 1975–1981," "Showalter Trust, 1973–1974, 1980–1989," UA 073, InUI-Ar. For an example of early research projects, see "Showalter Trust-Ultrasonic Exam of Female Breast, 1974–1975" and "Showalter Trust- Ultrasonic Diagnosis & Treatment of Brain Tumors, 1975," UA 073, InUI-Ar.

21. LCME Self-Study, 1994; Daly interview, 2017; Watanabe interview.

22. "Li, Ting-Kai, 1988–2002," Box 118, UA 041, InUI-Ar; Diamond et al., "Recognizing Dr. Ting-Kai Li," 2029; "Ting-Kai Li, M. D. Named New Director of NIH's Alcohol Research Institute | National Institute on Alcohol Abuse and Alcoholism (NIAAA)," accessed June 14, 2017, https://www.niaaa.nih.gov/news-events/news-releases/ting-kai-li-md-named-new-director-nih-alcohol-research-institute; Daly interview, 2017; Watanabe interview.

23. In 1987, the LCME visitors found that "even though research programs have generally increased, there remains a serious unevenness in research productivity among various departments. Some departments have minimal research programs." The report called for more effort to promote research across the school. During the interim, Daly and Li's initiative bore fruit. Internal grant funding supported eight faculty members, although the total number of principal investigators with grants was 374. LCME Report, 1987, 1994; Daly interview, 2017.

24. LCME Self-Study, 1994.

25. Richard T. Miyamoto and Raleigh E. Lingeman, "The History of the Department of Otolaryngology Head and Neck Surgery," 2016, Departmental Histories, UA 073, InUI-Ar; Houston et al., "The Ear Is Connected to the Brain," 446–63; Eisenberg and Johnson, "Audiologic Contributions to Pediatric Cochlear Implants," 10–13; Osberger et al., "Effect of Age at Onset of Deafness," 883–88.

26. Ballen, Gluckman, and Broxmeyer, "Umbilical Cord Blood Transplantation," 491–98; Elizabeth Hunt, "Lifeline," IU Research and Creative Activity Magazine (Fall 2003).

27. "IU Simon Cancer Center, Nation's Cancer Centers Jointly Endorse Updated HPV Vaccine Recommendations," January 11, 2017, accessed January 16, 2020, http://news.medicine.iu.edu/releases/2017/01/hpv-statement.shtml.

28. "Institute of Psychiatric Research, 1988–1995," "Larue Carter Child Service, 1996," "Larue D. Carter Memorial Hospital—Blueprint for Future Excellence, ca. 1993," "Larue Carter Memorial Hospital Correspondence, 1991–1995," "Hendrie, Hugh—Correspondence & Papers, 1983–1984," UA 073, InUI-Ar; John I. Nurnberger and Hugh C. Hendrie, "History of the Department of Psychiatry," 1990, IUSM Departmental Histories, UA 073, InUI-Ar. An indication of the leading role of IUSM in psychological research was Hendrie's 2017 Alzheimer's Association International's Lifetime Achievement Award. Among his achievements, he served as a principal investigator for the largest and longest National Institute on Aging (NIA)–funded study at the time on aging.

29. There were a number of changes in the divisions' chiefs. Lawrence Lumeng followed Christiansen in the Gastroenterology Division in 1984. In 1988, T. Dwight McKinney succeeded Kleit in Nephrology, Robert B. Jones replaced White in Infectious Diseases, and William J. Martin II became director of the Pulmonary Division. Charles Fisch retired as director of Cardiology in 1990 and was followed by David R. Hathway. "History of IUSM Department of Medicine," 1993 Departmental Histories, UA 073, InUI-Ar.

30. Grosfeld completed his general surgical training in 1966 in New York City, served in the US Army Medical Corps from 1966 to 1968, and then completed pediatric surgical training at the Columbus Children's Hospital, Ohio. Grosfeld returned to New York for two years, at which time he was recruited by Jesseph to come to Indiana and become professor and director of Pediatric Surgery. At IUSM he developed a neonatal surgery program, a postgraduate residency training program in pediatric surgery, and pediatric anesthesiology and pathology programs. "History of the Department of Surgery," 2013, Departmental Histories, UA 073, InUI-Ar.

31. Department of Medical and Molecular Genetics, "Historical Overview," Departmental Histories, UA 073, InUI-Ar.

32. "Riley Hospital Adding Disease Research Center," *Seymour Tribune*, November 10, 1986, Clipping File, "Wells Center for Pediatric Research, 1988–2000," Box 200, UA 041.

33. George Weiss, *Divide and Conquer*.

34. On translational research, "Bench to bedside" as emphasized by NIH director Elias A. Zerhouni, see Butler, "Translational Research," 840–42; IUSM, LCME Self-Study, 1994; Daly interview, 2017; "University Lab's Building

Block? It's Space," *Indianapolis Star*, May 17, 1995. This was part of a series of reports aimed at calling attention to the IUSM before the announcement of the merger.

35. "And Learning," *Caduceus*, 1985; "The Wiz," *Caduceus*, 1982.

36. "The White Castle," *Caduceus*, 1982.

37. "And Learning."

38. "The Riley," *Caduceus*, 1982.

39. Handel et al., "The Development and Maturation," 230.

40. Ibid.

41. Stuart Kleit received his DDS from the University of Pennsylvania in 1957 and his MD from the University of Florida in 1961. After residency, fellowship, and military service, he was recruited in 1967 by Hickam to the IU School of Medicine to become the founder and first division chief of Nephrology in the Department of Medicine, a position he held until his retirement in 1998. In 1985, he became associate dean for Clinical Affairs, overseeing all graduate medical education and clinical programs. "School of Medicine Glenn W. Irwin Jr. Distinguished Faculty Award (1998)," accessed July 4, 2018, https://honorsandawards.iu.edu/search-awards/honoree.shtml?honoreeID=5343. See also Daly interview, 2017; Holden, interview; Handel et al., "The Development and Maturation," 230–35.

42. Badertscher, "A New Wishard Is on the Way," 345–82; Hale, *Caring for the Community*; Holden interview; Daly interview; Stephen C. Beering, interview by Elizabeth J. Van Allen, December 7, 2000, UA 073, InUI-Ar; "IU Trustees Spurn Partial Deal to Man Wishard for County," *Indianapolis Star*, May 7, 1983; "IU Gets Right to Control Wishard," *Indianapolis Star*, June 16, 1983.

43. Indiana Perinatal Quality Improvement Collaborative, "Addressing Infant Mortality in Indiana" (Indianapolis, March 26, 2014); "City Offered Plan to Lower Black Infant Death Rate," *Indianapolis Star*, February 25, 1989; "Marion County Short in Infant-Mortality Goal," *Indianapolis Star*, February 10, 1999.

44. Holden interview; Beering interview, 2000; "History of the Department of Medicine," 1993, IUSM Departmental Histories, UA 073, InUI-Ar; Daly interview, 2017; Daly interview, 2005.

45. Holden interview.

46. Ibid.

47. Hale, *Caring for the Community*. See chapter 3 for more information.

48. LCME, Self-Study, 1979, 1987, 1994; Holden interview.

49. Gray, *IUPUI*, 140; Holden interview; Philip Snodgrass, *A Life in Academic Medicine* (iUniverse, 2007); "Indianapolis Medical Center—The City Health Care Built," *Indianapolis Star*, November 14, 1976; Damon, "To Care for Him Who Shall Have Borne the Battle."

50. "A Brief History of the Department of Pediatrics, Indiana University School of Medicine"; *IUMC Center Magazine* (fall 1990): 17.

51. *IUMC Center Magazine* (spring 1992): 4.

52. IUSM, Department of Medicine, Annual Reports, 1970–83; Department of Medicine History (1993).

53. IU School of Medicine, Faculty Records Management System report, March 9, 2017.

54. Personal communication, former Dean Robert Holden, May 23, 2017. On national trends, see Cluff, "Economic Incentives of Faculty Practice," 2931–34; Ludmerer, *Learning to Heal*, 176.

55. Daly interview, 2017.

56. Department of Medicine History (1993), History of the Indiana University School of Medicine Materials, InUI-Ar, accessed June 6, 2018, https://archives .iupui.edu/handle/2450/11448. The 2015 IRS filing for University Medical Diagnostics was $61,682,966.

57. IUSM, Department of Medicine, annual reports and Department of Medicine History.

58. Departmental Histories Amended Articles of Incorporation and Code of Bylaws, August 18, 1977. See Hull, "History of the Department of Pathology."

59. "History of Dermatology," History of the Indiana University School of Medicine Materials, InUI-Ar.

60. John I. Nurnberger Sr. and Hugh C. Hendrie, "History of the Department of Psychiatry." See also Coons and Bowman, *Psychiatry in Indiana*.

61. Alan Schmetzer, interview by Angela Potter, June 15, 2015, UA 073, InUI-Ar.

62. Coons and Bowman, *Psychiatry in Indiana*, 289; Spurlock, *Black Psychiatrists and American Psychiatry*, 14; Potter, "Learning Human Anatomy."

63. Daly interview, 2017.

64. Ibid.

65. "Pediatrics, Department of: A Brief History," History of the Indiana University School of Medicine Materials, InUI-Ar.

66. Ibid.

67. All subspecialty outpatient programs at Riley Hospital were consolidated in the new Riley Outpatient Center (ROC) in 2000. At the time of the opening, the center was considered the largest, most modern pediatric outpatient building in the country. A new pediatric hospitalist program grew to fifteen faculty.

68. Examples of sources, among many, are White's autobiography, *Ryan White: My Own Story*; a recent work by a reporter who covered the story, Price, *The Quiet Hero*; and Brown, "Mothers Against AIDS," 81–114.

69. Interview with Pam Perry, May 2017.

70. Ibid.

71. *Indianapolis Star*, February 17–18, 1974.

72. Perry interview. For more on Julie Nixon Eisenhower, see "Eisenhower, Julie Nixon—Stay at Krannert Pavilion, 1974," UA 073, InUI-Ar.

73. See Walter J. Daly, "Indiana University Medical Center, 1903–1993."

74. Daly interview, 2017.

75. Handel et al., "The Development and Maturation," 230–35.

76. Ibid.; Indiana University School of Medicine, "IU-Methodist-Riley Consolidation Reports (Media Information)," May 1996, UA 071, InUI-Ar; "Hospitals Work Together to Adapt to New Markets," *Indianapolis Star*, October 27, 1993, http://www.newspapers.com/image/107372774/?terms=hospital %2Bmerger%2Bnetwork. The IUSM hospitals were noticeably missing from the discussions with hospitals in Indianapolis.

77. Indiana University School of Medicine, "IU-Methodist-Riley Consolidation Reports (Media Information)"; "Hospitals Work Together to Adapt to New Markets."

78. Handel et al., "The Development and Maturation," 230–35; Indiana University School of Medicine, "IU-Methodist-Riley Consolidation Reports (Media Information)"; "Hospitals Work Together to Adapt to New Markets"; Indiana University School of Medicine, "IU-Methodist-Riley Consolidation Reports (Media Information)"; "Hospitals Work Together to Adapt to New Markets."

79. Handel et al., "The Development and Maturation," 231.

80. Planners argued that other models such as a merger or an operating agreement would not be acceptable because of the strong identity of both operations, the perceived quality of the partners, and the need for cohesiveness and institutional integration. From the administrative perspective, essential to the agreement was creation of a new board of directors that would represent key community constituents of both partners. Handel et al., "The Development and Maturation," 230–35; Evans interview.

There is a long list of publications on mergers. See, for example, Van Etten, "Camelot or Common Sense?" 143–48; Bauer, "The Folly of Teaching-Hospital Mergers," 1762–63; Kastor, *Mergers of Teaching Hospitals*; Mallon, "The Alchemists," 1090–104.

81. Handel et al., "The Development and Maturation," 230–35.

82. "The Benefits of Merging Methodist with IU," *Indianapolis Star*, April 7, 1995.

83. IU BOT, May 2, 1996. "IU, Methodist Finalize Merger of Hospitals," *Indianapolis Star*, May 3, 1996.

84. IU press release May 2, 1996, materials related to Clarian agreement, UA 073, InUI-Ar, in process.

85. Loveday had been at Methodist as CEO since 1988, coming from hospital management in California. He was a national leader in hospital interest and reform groups, as well as in community organizations in Indiana.

86. Handel, director of IUMC since 1985, came from hospital operations at Vanderbilt.

87. Daly interview, 2017.

88. Personal communication from Robert Holden, May 23, 2017; Holden interview.

12. Into the Second Century

1. LCME Self-Study, 1994.
2. Ibid.
3. LCME Self-Study, 2017.
4. LCME Self-Study, 1994.
5. LCME Self-Study, 2008.
6. AAMC, "Trends in Income," accessed June 8, 2018, https://www.aamc.org/download/381720/data/fy2013_trends.pdf, and https://www.aamc.org/data/finance/480320/fig8–9.html.
7. The American Hospital Association defines health-care systems as a "more concrete relationship, usually bounded by common ownership, leasing,

sponsoring, or a contract." Accessed July 9, 2018, https://pdfs.semanticscholar.org/3b0e
/4dbedbd93342cb1f581a4e6d117e6c5a1a23.pdf.

8. Ibid.

9. Holden received his BS in pharmacy from Purdue University in 1958 and his MD from Indiana University in 1963. He began as an assistant professor of radiology at IUSM following completion of a diagnostic radiology residency at Vanderbilt University in 1973. He moved through the academic ranks, attaining associate professor in 1977, professor in 1982, and chair of Radiology in 1991. Oral history of Robert Holden by Elizabeth Van Allen, November 28, 2000, UA 073, InUI-Ar.

10. Handel et al., "The Development and Maturation," 232. Most of what follows is a summary of their article.

11. Handel et al., 233–34.

12. Department of Veterans Affairs, "Combined Assessment Program Review of the Richard L. Roudebush VA Medical Center Indianapolis, Indiana," Report No. 04–01852–115, March 28, 2005.

13. Accessed July 22, 2017, http://www.eskenazihealth.edu/about/history.

14. "Simon Family Tower Opens for Hoosier Children and Beyond," January 27, 2011, accessed, July 26, 2017, http://iuhealth.org/news-hub/detail/simon-family-tower-opens-for-hoosier-children-and-beyond/#.WXjkmHeZPeQ.

15. Oral History of D. Craig Brater by Kevin Grau, February 19, 2008, UA 073, InUI-Ar.

16. Stark Neurosciences Research Institute History, accessed July 27, 2017, http://snri.medicine.iu.edu/about/history. Stark and his wife donated $15 million, Clarian Health Partners contributed $10 million, and the Riley Children's Foundation donated $2 million. "New Institute Promises Stellar Medical Research, Innovation," IUSM Press Release, November 2, 2000.

17. "Newly Created Clarian Sees Benefits in Hospital Merger," Indianapolis Star, January 19, 1997.

18. "Mid America Adolescent STD Cooperative Research Center," IUSM press release, September 30, 1998, accessed October 4, 2017, https://indiana.pure.elsevier.com/en/projects/pyschophysical-partner-specific-coitus-specific-risk-protective-f.

19. The center is currently called the Center of Excellence in Molecular Hematology (CEMH) "CEMH Indianapolis—Center of Excellence in Molecular Hematopoiesis," accessed December 11, 2015, http://www.cemh.pediatrics.iu.edu/index.html.

20. Simon J. Atkinson et al., "Indiana O'Brien Center for Advanced Microscopic Analysis," accessed July 9, 2018, https://scholarworks.iupui.edu/handle/1805/5262.

21. Since then, additional economic development centers and business incubators have been established in Indianapolis and around the state. "Life Sciences Get a Boost at IU," Indianapolis Star, July 2, 2002; "The Evolution of BioCrossroads 2002-2012," BioIntellex, accessed December 7, 2015, http://www.biointellex.com/the-evolution-of-biocrossroads-2002-2012.

22. Ora Pescovitz was appointed executive associate dean of Research in 2000, following in the tradition of Suzanne Noble and Doris Merritt. After her

unsuccessful candidacy for medical school dean, she left IUSM in 2009 to head the University of Michigan Medical School. For more on Pescovitz, who became president of Oakland University in 2017, see https://ofw.iupui.edu/Leadership /Online-Archive-Women-Creating-Excellence-at-IUPUI/Women-Creating -Excellence/OraPescovitz, accessed July 2, 2018.

23. In fact, new centers were created as a result of the grant, such as the IU Center for Bioethics, whereas existing ones such as the Center for Medical Genomics were able to expand significantly. See http://www.forwardlegacytrust .com/lilly-endowment-awards-105-mm-grant-to-indiana-universitys-genomics -initiative; Lilly Endowment Annual Report, 2007, 6–7, http://www .lillyendowment.org/annualreports/2007/2007_Report.pdf. See also "Indiana Genomics Initiative, 2001–2003," Box 262, UA 044, InUI-Ar; "Life Sciences Initiative Research: Indiana Genomics Initiative (INGEN), Progress Reports," "Genomics Initiative, Indiana (INGEN), 2000–2008," UA 073, InUI-Ar.

24. Nathan and Benz, "Comprehensive Cancer Centres," 240–45.

25. Ibid., 242.

26. "Indiana University Cancer Center Receives National Cancer Institute Designation," press release, September 30, 1999, accessed July 27, 2017, https:// www.eurekalert.org/pub_releases/1999-09/IU-IUCC-300999.php. See also NCI Fact Books, 1992–2002, accessed July 27, 2017, https://www.cancer.gov/about -nci/budget/fact-book/archive; "Cancer Center, 1995–2002," "Cancer Center Program, 1987–1996," "Clinical Cancer Center, 7/1995," "Cancer Center, Historical, 1978–80," UA 073, InUI-Ar.

27. The gift included $20 million for a building to house an expanded eye clinic and $10 million for a research endowment. See IU press release, "IU School of Medicine's Glick Eye Center to Be Dedicated Today," August 19, 2011, accessed July 20, 2018, http://newsinfo.iu.edu/news/page/normal/19317 .html?emailID=19317.

28. "Indiana University, Clarian Health Dedicate IU Simon Cancer Center's New Patient Building on Aug. 21," press release, August 18, 2008, accessed July 27, 2017, http://cancer.iu.edu/news-publications/article.shtml?id=1933.

29. For a history of this work, see Quigley, *Walking Together, Walking Far.*

30. Two major archival collections include "Indiana University's University of Karachi Jinnah Postgraduate Medical Center Project records, 1955–1967," Collection 511, In-U-Ar, and the papers of Headlee in UA 073, InUI-Ar.

31. AMPATH's collaborative research involves investigators from more than fifteen institutions in Africa, Europe, and North America, including active research partnerships with Brown University, Duke University, University of Massachusetts, University of Notre Dame, Purdue University, University of Toronto, and the University of California San Francisco. As of this writing, PEPFAR alone has contributed over $140 million, and in 2015, AMPATH received approximately $10 million in other grants.

32. "Department of Biostatistics: History," accessed October 4, 2017, https:// biostat.iupui.edu/about-us/history.

33. Interview with D. Craig Brater, July 21, 2017; "AAMC Calls for 30 Percent Increase in Medical School Enrollment," June 19, 2006, accessed July 21, 2017, https://www.aamc.org/newsroom/newsreleases/2006/82904/060619.html.

See also "AAMC Statement on the Physician Workforce," June 2006, accessed July 21, 2017, https://www.aamc.org/download/55458/data.

34. IUSM press release, "IU Should Graduate More Physicians to Meet Indiana's Needs, Study Group Concludes," December 19, 2006, accessed July 21, 2017, http://www2.indstate.edu/thcme/Web_Center_Line/IUSM-THExpansion/Press%20release.htm. An example of an earlier report was the January 2005 US Council on Graduate Medical Education (COGME) Report, "U. S. Likely to Face a Shortage in 2020." For a broader historical perspective, see Dalen, "The Moratorium on US Medical School Enrollment," 1–2.

35. Scott Olsen, "IU Seeking Funding to Help Alleviate Doctor Shortage: Medical school Wants Extra $5 Million from Legislature to Tackle Projected Shortfall of 1,300 Physicians by 2025," *Indianapolis Business Journal*, October 20, 2008.

36. Brater interview, 2017; "IUSM-Muncie expansion to four year program slated for June," INScope, February 20, 2014, accessed July 21, 2017, http://inscopearchive.iu.edu/headlines/2014–02–20-headline-iusm-muncie-inscope.shtml.

37. "Marian University to Launch State's Second Medical School," *Indianapolis Business Journal*, January 15, 2010.

38. AAMC, *State Physician Workforce Data Book*, accessed June 22, 2017, https://www.aamc.org/data/workforce/reports/442830/statedataandreports.html.

39. AAMC, *State Physician Workforce Data Book*, accessed June 22, 2017, https://www.aamc.org/data/workforce/reports/442830/statedataandreports.html.

40. Interview, July 24, 2017, with Joyce McKinnon, School of Health and Rehabilitation Science, who headed a study committee to determine guidelines for reorganization in 2000.

41. Ibid.

42. For more, see, "Undergraduate & Graduate Program in Public Health (Environmental Health), 1978–1982," Box 9, "MHA (IUPUI) Masters in Health Administration, 1979–1993," Box 5, C 108, Indiana University School of Public and Environmental Affairs records, 1969–2007, 1971–89, InU-Ar.

43. Bepko to Daly, March 3, 1993; Bepko Memorandum to Ad Hoc Committee on a School of Public Health," February 3, 1994; personal communication from Stephen Jay, July 18, 2017.

44. Personal communication from Stephen Jay, July 18, 2017; "School of Public Health at IUPUI Named for Fairbanks in Honor of Foundation's $20 Million Gift," September 27, 2012, accessed July 28, 2017, http://newscenter.iupui.edu/index.php?id=5794; "Halverson Named Founding Dean of Richard M. Fairbanks School of Public Health at IUPUI : Headlines: InScope: Indiana University," February 21, 2013, accessed December 11, 2015, http://inscopearchive.iu.edu/headlines/2013-02-21-headline-halverson-dean-fairbanks-inscope.shtml.

45. "Program Designed to Attract More Doctors to Indiana's Rural Areas," March 18, 1997, IUSM Press Release.

46. Other examples include the opening of the Riley Hospital Outpatient Center in 2000 and the Clarian Cardiovascular Center in 2001.

47. "Indiana University Methodist Family Practice Center Opens Its Doors to Patients," IUSM Press Release, September 22, 1998; "First Indiana University Faculty Named to Otis R. Bowen Professorship," IUSM Press Release, August 31, 1998. Dr. Allen also became director of the Bowen Research Center at IU; the center is a collaborative program between the IU Schools of Medicine and Public and Environment Affairs.

48. "IU School of Medicine Department of Family Medicine Receives Bronze Achievement Award," IUSM Press Release, June 2, 1998.

49. AAMC, "Diversity in Medical Education, Facts and Figures, 2008," 109, accessed July 10, 2018, https://www.aamc.org/download/386172/data/diversity inmedicaleducation-factsandfigures2008.pdf.

50. For example, each year, three Indiana University School of Medicine students are the recipients of a George and Lula Rawls Award of Excellence to minority students for academic achievement. George Rawls, MD, is a retired Indianapolis surgeon, assistant dean, and associate clinical professor of surgery at the IU School of Medicine. "Indiana University Medical School Honors Three Minority Students with Awards of Excellence," IUSM Press Release, November 23, 1998.

51. AAMC, "Applicant, Matriculant, & Graduation, by Medical School Tables, Table 33. Medical School Matriculants by State, Medical School, Sex, Race, and Ethnicity, 2015," accessed July 10, 2018, https://www.aamcdiversity factsandfigures2016.org/report-section/medical-schools/#tablepress-33.

52. For current statistics, see "FACTS: Applicants, Matriculants, Enrollment, Graduates, MD/PhD, and Residency Applicants Data—Data and Analysis—AAMC."

53. "Affirmative Action Office & Committees, 1974," Box 51, UA 073, InUI-Ar; IUSM Annual Reports, 1974–95; Daly interview, 2017.

54. Nationally, debt levels of medical graduates from public medical schools increased 59.2 percent between 1985 and 1995. Greysen et al., "A History of Medical Student Debt," 840–45; Kassebaum et al., "On Rising Medical Student Debt," 1124–34; Rohlfing et al., "Medical Student Debt," 10.3402/meo. v19.25603.

55. Brokaw et al., "Impact of a Competency-Based Curriculum," 213.

56. Ludmerer, *Let Me Heal*, 280–84; "Joined Hospitals in Bumpy Phase of Honeymoon," *Indianapolis Star*, March 15, 1998; H. J. Ralston et al., "Capturing the Promise of Science in Medical Schools," 1314–23; Bauer, "The Folly of Teaching-Hospital Mergers," 1762–63.

57. Burnham, "American Medicine's Golden Age," 1474–79.

58. The Accreditation Council for Graduate Medical Education (ACGME) has established six general competencies for residents, which have considerable overlap with the IUSM competencies. Swing, "The ACGME Outcome Project," 648–54.

59. Alpert Medical School at Brown University continues to use the "nine abilities" competency-based curriculum that was officially launched in 1996. Smith and Fuller, "MD2000: A Competency-Based Curriculum," 292–98.

60. Bell et al., "Medical Students' Reactions to a Competency-Based Curriculum," 21–27; Gunderman, "Competency-Based Training," 324.

61. Brokaw et al., "Impact of a Competency-Based Curriculum," 207–14.

13. The Case of IU Medical School

1. Association of American Medical Colleges, "U. S. Medical School Applications and Matriculants by School, State of Legal Residence, and Sex, 2017–2018," accessed June 20, 2018, https://www.aamc.org/download/321442/data/factstable1.pdf.

2. Banaszak-Holl and Greer, "Turnover of Deans of Medicine," 1–7. There are numerous other assessments of deans' roles in US medical schools, ranging from the particular, such as Graham, "UNC's Deans of Medicine," 562–68, to more general analyses in the journal *Academic Medicine*. Examples of the latter are Levin et al., "Organizational, Financial, and Environmental Factors," 640–64, and Petersdorf, "Deans and Deaning," 953–58.

BIBLIOGRAPHY

Abbreviations

AAMC	Association of American Medical Colleges
CSHM	IU Oral History Research Center (Indiana University Center for the Study of History and Memory, Bloomington
InUI-Ar	University Library Special Collections and Archives, University Library, Indiana University Purdue University Indianapolis
In-U-Ar	University Archives, Wells Library, Indiana University, Bloomington
LCME	Liaison Committee for Medical Education
IU AR	*Indiana University Annual Report*
IU BOT	Indiana University Board of Trustees Minutes
PU-Ar	Purdue University Archives and Special Collections
QB	*Quarterly Bulletin of the Indiana University Medical Center* (succeeded by *Medical Quarterly of the Indiana University School of Medicine*)
RMA	Riley Memorial Association Papers, Riley Memorial Hospital, Indianapolis, Indiana

Archives

University Archives, Wells Library, Indiana
University, Bloomington (In-U-Ar)

Burton Dorr Myers papers, Collection C82 (Burton Dorr Myers papers, 1906–1956)

Collection C126 (old E126, Box 1) [*Note*: old E126 Box 2–4 are in UA 073, InUI-Ar.]

Herman B Wells papers, Collection C75 (Herman B Wells papers, 1819–2001)

Indiana University Board of Trustees minutes, Collection C218 (Indiana University Board of Trustees minutes, 1838–1859, 1883–2017)

Indiana University Faculty Council records, Collection C181

Indiana University President Emeritus John W. Ryan papers, Collection C456, (Indiana University President Emeritus John W. Ryan papers, 1944–2011)

Indiana University President's Office correspondence, Collection C270, (Indiana University President's Office correspondence, 1902–1913)

Indiana University President's Office correspondence, Collection C286 (Indiana University President's Office correspondence, 1913–1937)

Indiana University President's Office records, Collection C213, (Indiana University President's Office records, 1937–1962)

Indiana University President's Office records, Collection C304, (Indiana University President's Office records, 1962–1968)

Indiana University President's Office records, Collection C501, (Indiana University President's Office records, 1976–1995)

President Herman B Wells speeches, Collection C137 (President Herman B Wells speeches, 1937–1962)

President William Lowe Bryan speeches, Collection C71 (President William Lowe Bryan speeches, 1903–1937)

Presidents' Reports to the Indiana University Board of Trustees, Collection C654

Reference files (collection of miscellaneous items being processed)

Speeches of President Elvis J. Stahr (Speeches of President Elvis J. Stahr, 1962–1968)

William Lowe Bryan papers, Collection C69, Indiana University Archives, Bloomington (William Lowe Bryan papers, 1830–1960)

University Library Special Collections and Archives, University Library, Indiana University Purdue University Indianapolis (InUI-Ar)

American Association of University Professors (AAUP) Records, 1961–1977. UA 070.

Departmental and Center Histories, "History of Indiana University School of Medicine Materials," available in eArchives of University Library Special Collections and Archives, https://archives.iupui.edu/handle/2450/11449, unless otherwise indicated.

Departmental and Center Histories, History of the Department of Medicine, eArchives.

Besch, Jr., H. R., Shreepad Wagle, and Robert B. Forney. "Outline of the Historical Development of the Department of Pharmacology and Toxicology, 1906–1993." UA 073, InUI-Ar.

Bowman, Donald E. "Summary of the First Five Years of the Department of Biochemistry, 1958–1963." 1963. UA 073, InUI-Ar.

Garrett, Robert. "Urology at Indiana University." 1993. IUSM Departmental and Center Histories, eArchives.

Gibson, David M., "Up Here in Biochemistry." Department of Biochemistry and Molecular Biology, IUSM, 1993. UA 073, InUI-Ar.

Grayson, Merrill. *Development of the Department of Ophthalmology, Indiana University School of Medicine, 1908–2006.* Indianapolis: Indiana University School of Medicine, 2007. eArchives.

Hale, Hester Anne, and Susan Overs Wilson. *Through the Years: A Living History of the Indiana University, School of Medicine, Department of Radiology, 1906–2004.* Bloomington, IN: AuthorHouse, 2004. eArchives.

Holden, Robert W., Eugene C. Klatte, et al. "History of the Indiana University School of Medicine's Department of Radiology, 1915–1993." UA 073, InUI-Ar.

Hull, Kathleen Warfel. "History of the Department of Pathology and Laboratory Medicine." *Department of Pathology Newsletter*, 2004–2013. eArchives.

Knople, Peggy. "History of Medical Genetics at Indiana University School of Medicine," 2014. UA 073, InUI-Ar

Ladue, Ruth L. "History of Physical Therapy Department, Division of Allied Health, Indiana University School of Medicine, 1924–1982." Box 12, Department of Physical Therapy Records, UA-30, InUI-Ar.

Miyamoto, Richard, and Raleigh Lingeman. "History of the Department of Otolaryngology." 2016. eArchives.

Nurnberger, John I., and Hugh C. Hendrie. "History of the Department of Psychiatry." 1990. eArchives.

Ochs, Sidney, and Leon K. Knoebel. "History of the Department of Physiology and Biophysics." Department of Physiology and Biophysics, IUSM, 1993. UA 073, InUI-Ar.

Stoelting, Vergil K. *History of the Department of Anesthesiology at Indiana University School of Medicine: The First 30 Years.* Indianapolis: Indiana University, 1977. UA 073, InUI-Ar.

Thompson, Joseph F. *"This Important Trust": A History of the Department of Obstetrics and Gynecology, Indiana University School of Medicine and Medical Center, 1909–1992.* Indianapolis: University Obstetricians and Gynecologists, 1993. UA 073, InUI-Ar.

Hine, Maynard. Papers (being processed).

Indiana University Office of the Chancellor Records, 1914–2006. UA 041.

Indiana University Office of the Dean of Faculties/Executive Vice Chancellor, 1966–2007. UA 044.

Indiana University School of Dentistry Records, 1934–2003. UA 035.

Indiana University School of Health and Rehabilitation Sciences Records, 1955–95. UA 029.

Indiana University School of Medicine Records, 1848–2005. UA 073.

Indiana University School of Nursing Records, 1914–2002. UA 025.

IUPUI Faculty Council Records, 1968–2001. UA 042.

Lukemeyer, George. Papers (being processed).

Oral Histories and Interviews

Abbreviations

CSHM-MP   Medical Profession in Indiana, 1975, 1976, 1978, Indiana
         University Center for the Study of History and Memory,
         Bloomington

CSHM-IM   Indiana Medicine, 1993, Indiana University Center for the Study
         of History and Memory, Bloomington

CSHM-IU   History: Indiana University, 1968–1981, Indiana University
         Center for the Study of History and Memory, Bloomington

CSHM-OH   Indiana University Oral History Archive, 1991–1998, Indiana
         University Center for the Study of History and Memory,
         Bloomington

IUSM-OH   History of IUSM oral histories, History of Indiana University
         School of Medicine Materials eArchives of University Library
         Special Collections and Archives, IUPUI, Indianapolis

OHP   IUPUI Oral History Project, University Library Special
         Collections and Archives, University Library, IUPUI,
         Indianapolis

Tobias   Tobias Leadership Center, IUPUI, Indianapolis

IHS   Indiana Historical Society

Purdue   Purdue University

Interview Subjects

Ade, Mary Keller: CSHM-IM
Albertson, Frank P.: CSHM-IM
Beering, Steven C.: IUSM-OH (2000); Purdue (2006)
Bonsett, Charles A.: CSHM-IM
Bowen, Otis: Tobias
Brater, D. Craig: IUSM-OH
Chattin, Herbert O.: CSHM-IM
Compton, George L.: CSHM-IM
Culbertson, Clyde G.: CSHM-IM
Dalton, Naomi: CSHM-IM
Day, William D.: CSHM-IM
Daly, Walter J.: IUSM-OH (2001, 2005, 2017); CSHM-OH (1994)
Ehrlich, Thomas: Tobias
Evans Jr., Daniel: IUSM-OH
Feigenbaum, Harvey: IHS
Fisch, Charles: CSHM-IM
Fitzgerald, Brice E.: CSHM-IM
Green, Morris: IHS; IUSM-OH (2000); CSHM-IM (1993)
Hastings, John S.: CSHM-IU
Holden, Robert: IUSM-OH
Irwin, Glen: CSHM-OH
Jones, Robert B.: IUSM-OH

Kilgore, Byron: CSHM-IM
Link, Goethe: CSHM-MP
Lukemeyer, George T.: IUSM-OH
Macy, George W.: CSHM-IM
Manifold, Harold M.: CSHM-IM
McNutt, Ruth J.: CSHM-IU
Merritt, Doris H.: OHP
Miller, L. B.: CSHM-IM
Moore, Ward W.: IUSM-OH
Newhouse, Margaret M.: CSHM-IM
Paris, Durward W.: CSHM-IM
Paynter, William: CSHM-IM
Pescovitz, Ora: IUSM-OH
Ramsey, Frank: CSHM-IM
Rawls, George: IHS
Reed, Robert F.: CSHM-IM
Richter, Arthur B.: CSHM-IM
Schmetzer, Alan: IUSM-OH
Schuman, Edith: CSHM-IM
Sholty, William M.: CSHM-IM
Tinsley, Walter B.: IUSM-OH
Watanabe, Augustus: IUSM-OH
Vollrath, Victor J.: CSHM-IM
Van Buskirk, Edmund L.: CSHM-IM

Additional Miscellaneous Interviews

D. Craig Brater, interviewed by William Schneider, July 21, 2017
Joyce McKinnon, interviewed by William Schneider, July 24, 2017
Pam Perry, interviewed by William Schneider and Angela Potter, May 2017

Selected Newspapers and Periodicals

Bloomington Telephone, 1907
Central States Medical Monitor, 1907
Indiana Daily Student (IDS), 1906–1907
Indiana Magazine of History, 1862–1994
Indiana Medical History Quarterly, 1982
Indiana Medical Journal, 1862–1907
Indiana University Alumni Quarterly, 1914–1951
Indianapolis Journal 1862–1865
Indianapolis News, 1894–1915
Indianapolis Sentinel, 1894–1903
Indianapolis Star, 1905–1944
Journal of the Indiana State Medical Association, 1911–1933
Lafayette Courier and Journal 1906–1997
Monthly Bulletin, Indiana State Board of Health, 1947–1952

Medical and Surgical Monitor, 1902–1904
Medical Student, 1902–1907
News Gazette (Indiana University), 1915
Transactions of the Indiana State Medical Society 1868

Selected References

AAMC. *Assessment of Minority and Nonminority U. S. Medical School Graduates' Premedical and Medical School Specialty Selection, and Success in Obtaining Choice of Residency Training: Final Report.* Edited by Charles D. Killian and Wendy L. Colquitt. Washington, DC: AAMC, 1991.

AAMC. "FACTS: Applicants, Matriculants, Enrollment, Graduates, MD/PhD, and Residency Applicants Data—Data and Analysis—AAMC." Accessed December 16, 2015. https://www.aamc.org/data/facts.

AAMC. "Medicare's Graduate Medical Education Policy: Its Inception and Congress' Clear and Persistent Commitment." Accessed November 2015. https://www.aamc.org/download/449774/data/medicaresgraduatemedical educationpolicyitsinceptionandcongresss.pdf.

AAMC. "Minutes of the Fifteenth Annual Meeting, April 10, 1905." Chicago: AMA, 1905.

Aaron, Henry J. "The Plight of Academic Medical Centers." *Brookings*, November 30, 2001. https://www.brookings.edu/research/the-plight-of-academic -medical-centers.

Ackerknecht, Erwin H. "Diseases in the Midwest." In *Essays in the History of Medicine in Honor of David J. Davis, M.D., M.P.H.*, 168–81. Chicago: University of Illinois Press, 1965.

Anderson, Lee. *Internal Medicine and the Structures of Modern Medical Science: The University of Iowa, 1870–1990.* Ames: Iowa State University Press, 1991.

Anderson, Odin Waldemar. *The Uneasy Equilibrium: Private and Public Financing of Health Services in the United States, 1875–1965.* New York: College & University Press, 1968.

Anderson, Ronald J. "Subspecialization in Internal Medicine: A Historical Review, an Analysis, and Proposals for Change." *American Journal of Medicine* 99, no. 1 (July 1995): 74–81.

Andrus, E. C. "Forward." In *Advances in Military Medicine*, edited by E. C. Andrus et al., 1: xlii–xliii. Boston: Little, Brown, 1948.

Apple, Rima. *Perfect Motherhood: Science and Childrearing in America.* New Brunswick, NJ: Rutgers University Press, 2006.

Badertscher, Kathi. "A New Wishard Is on the Way." *Indiana Magazine of History* 108, no. 4 (December 1, 2012): 345–82.

Baker, D. H., J. J. Mamlin, and W. J. Daly. "Simulation Modeling—A Tool for Medical Planning." *Journal of Laboratory and Clinical Medicine* 78, no. 5 (November 1971): 836.

Banaszak-Holl, Jane, and David S. Greer. "Turnover of Deans of Medicine during the Last Five Decades." *Academic Medicine* 69 (January 1994): 1–7.

Bannister, Samuel, ed. *Indiana University, 1820–1904*. Bloomington: Indiana University, 1904.

Barnhill, John F. "An Epoch of Medical Education." *Indiana Medical History Quarterly* 1 (July 1974): 52–63.

Battersby, J. Stanley. *Dr. Gatch as I Knew Him*. Indianapolis: Indiana University–Purdue University at Indianapolis, 1989.

Bauer, E. A. "The Folly of Teaching—Hospital Mergers." *New England Journal of Medicine* 336, no. 24 (June 12, 1997): 1762–63.

Beecher, Henry K., and Mark D. Altschule. *Medicine at Harvard: The First Three Hundred Years*. Hanover, NH: University Press of New England, 1977.

Bell, Mary A., et al. "Medical Students' Reactions to a Competency-Based Curriculum." *Medical Science Educator* 18, no. 1 (2008): 21–27.

Bennett, Jeff, and Richard D. Feldman. "'The Most Useful Citizen of Indiana': John N. Hurty and the Public Health Movement." *Traces of Indiana & Midwestern History* 12, no. 3 (July 2000): 34–43.

Bernheim, Bertram Moses. *The Story of the Johns Hopkins; Four Great Doctors and the Medical School They Created*. New York: Whittlesey House, 1948.

Bickel, Janet. "Gender Equity in Undergraduate Medical Education: A Status Report." *Journal of Women's Health and Gender-Based Medicine* 10, no. 3 (May 2001): 261–70.

Biesen, Robin. "A New Breed of Student. IUN Medical Program Takes Hands-On." *The Times* (Munster, IN), May 31, 1993. Accessed June 1, 2020. https://www.nwitimes.com/uncategorized/a-new-breed-of-student-iun -medical-program-takes-hands-on/article_6c04a56e-27dc-54c8-9b56 -55906cc301f0.html.

Bigelow, Maurice A. *Health Education in Relation to Venereal Disease Control Education*. New York: American Social Hygiene Association, 1941.

Blake, Israel George. *Paul V. McNutt: Portrait of a Hoosier Statesman*. New York: Central, 1966.

Blumenthal, David, and James Morone. *The Heart of Power: Health and Politics in the Oval Office*. Berkeley: University of California Press, 2010.

Bobbs, John S. "Address at the Opening of the Indiana Medical College." Indianapolis: Douglass & Conner, Printers, 1870.

———. "Introductory Lecture." Indianapolis: Douglass & Elder, 1849.

———. "President's Address, the Origin, Objects, and Progress of the Indiana State Medical Society." *Transactions of the Indiana State Medical Society* 18 (May 19–20, 1868): 11–12.

Bodenhamer, David J., Robert Graham Barrows, and David Gordon Vanderstel. *The Encyclopedia of Indianapolis*. Indianapolis: Indiana University Press, 1994.

Bonner, Thomas Neville. *Becoming a Physician: Medical Education in Great Britain, France, Germany, and the United States, 1750–1945*. New York: Oxford University Press, 1996.

———. *To the Ends of the Earth: Women's Search for Education in Medicine*. Cambridge, MA: Harvard University Press, 1995.

Bonsett, Charles A. "Medical Museum Notes." *Indiana Medicine* 77, no. 1 (June 1984): 425.

Borden, Nathan, and Derek Linklater. "Hickam's Dictum." *Western Journal of Emergency Medicine* 14, no. 2 (March 2013): 164.

Bowen, Otis R., and William Du Bois. *Doc: Memories from a Life in Public Service*. Bloomington: Indiana University Press, 2000.

Brandt, Alan M., and Martha N. Gardner, "Antagonism and Accommodation: Interpreting the Relationship between Public Health and Medicine in the United States during the 20th Century." *American Journal of Public Health* 90 (2000): 707–15.

———. "The Golden Age of Medicine?" In *Medicine in the Twentieth Century*, edited by Roger Cooter and John Pickstone, 21–37. Netherlands: Harwood Academic, 2000.

Braunwald, Eugene. "Cardiology—Division or Department?" *New England Journal of Medicine* 329, no. 25 (December 16, 1993): 1887–1890.

Brayton, A. W. "History of the Indiana Medical College." *Medical Student* 1 (November 1902): 5–6.

Brayton, J. H. "Development of Medical Education in Indiana." MA thesis, Indiana University 1929.

A Brief History of the Indiana University School of Medicine. Indianapolis: Indiana University School of Medicine, 1994.

Britt, L. D. "Graduate Medical Education and the Residency Review Committee: History and Challenges." *American Surgeon* 73, no. 2 (2007): 136–39.

Brokaw, James J., et al. "The Influence of Regional Basic Science Campuses on Medical Students' Choice of Specialty and Practice Location: A Historical Cohort Study." *BMC Medical Education* 9 (June 6, 2009): 29.

Brokaw, James J., et al. "Impact of a Competency-Based Curriculum on Medical Student Advancement: A Ten-Year Analysis." *Teaching and Learning in Medicine* 23, no. 3 (July 2011): 207–14.

Brown, E. Richard. *Rockefeller Medicine Men: Medicine and Capitalism in America*. Berkeley: University of California Press, 1979.

Brown, H. E. "Training the Next Generation of Doctors and Nurses." *Peace Corps*. Accessed July 21, 2017. https://www.peacecorps.gov/stories/training-next-generation-doctors-and-nurses/.

Brown, Nancy E. "Mothers against AIDS in Kokomo, Indiana." *Indiana Magazine of History* 114 (June 2018): 81–114.

Burnham, John C. "American Medicine's Golden Age: What Happened to It?" *Science* 215 (March 19, 1982): 1474–79.

Burrow, Gerard N. *A History of Yale's School of Medicine: Passing Torches to Others*. New Haven, CT: Yale University Press, 2008.

Bush, Monique, et al. "Indiana University School of Social Work: 90 Years of Professional Education." *Advances in Social Work* 2 (2001): 83–100.

Bush, Vannevar. *Science, the Endless Frontier: A Report to the President on a Program for Postwar Scientific Research*. Washington, DC: National Science Foundation, 1960.

Bush, Vannevar, Richard Bush, and John Bush. *Modern Arms and Free Men: A Discussion of the Role of Science in Preserving Democracy*. New York: Simon and Schuster, 1949.

Butler, Decian. "Translational Research: Crossing the Valley of Death." *Nature* 453 (June 11, 2008): 840–42.

Canal, David F., and Keith Lillemoe. "The Department of Surgery, Indiana University School of Medicine, Indianapolis." *Archives of Surgery* 141, no. 1 (January 2006): 11–12. doi:10.1001/archsurg.141.1.11.

Capshew, James H. *Herman B Wells: The Promise of the American University.* Bloomington: Indiana University Press, 2012.

Carlson, Elof Axel. "The Hoosier Connection: Compulsory Sterilization as Moral Hygiene." In *A Century of Eugenics in America: From the Indiana Experiment to the Human Genome Era*, edited by Paul A. Lombardo, 11–25. Bloomington: Indiana University Press, 2010.

"The Carnegie Foundation Report on Medical Education." *JAMA* 54, no. 24 (1910): 1949.

Carr, Jack D. "History of the Indiana Dental College, 1879–1925." MA thesis, Butler University, 1957.

Catlin, Robert A. *Racial Politics and Urban Planning: Gary, Indiana, 1980–1989.* Lexington: University Press of Kentucky, 1993.

Catlin-Leguto, Cinnamon. *The Art of Healing: The Wishard Art Collection.* Indianapolis: Indiana Historical Society, 2004.

Carpenter, Coy Cornelius. *The Story of Medicine at Wake Forest University.* Chapel Hill: University of North Carolina Press, 1970.

Cheifetz, Craig E., et al. "Regional Medical Campuses: A New Classification System." *Academic Medicine* 89, no. 8 (August 2014): 1140–43.

Chesney, Alan M. *The Johns Hopkins Hospital and the Johns Hopkins University School of Medicine: A Chronicle.* Baltimore, MD: Johns Hopkins University Press, 1943.

Clark, Thomas D. *Indiana University: Midwestern Pioneer.* 4 vols. Bloomington: Indiana University Press, 1970–77.

Cleland, Ethel. "The Mural Decorations of the City Hospital." *Modern Hospital* 12, no. 6 (1919): 395–99.

Cluff, Leighton E. "Economic Incentives of Faculty Practice. Are They Distorting the Medical School's Mission?" *JAMA* 250, no. 21 (1983): 2931–34.

Cogan, Lee. *Negroes for Medicine. Report of the Macy Conference on Negroes for Medicine, Ft. Lauderdale, FL 1967.* Baltimore, MD: Johns Hopkins University Press, 1969.

Coggeshall, Lowell. *Planning for Medical Progress through Education.* Evanston, IL: Association of American Medical Colleges, 1965.

Cohen, Arthur M. *The Shaping of American Higher Education: Emergence and Growth of the Contemporary System.* San Francisco: Josey-Bass, 1998.

Cohen, Jordan J., and Elisa K. Siegel. "Academic Medical Centers and Medical Research: The Challenges Ahead." *JAMA* 294, no. 11 (September 21, 2005): 1367–72. doi:10.1001/jama.294.11.1367.

Cohen, Richard L. *House Officer: Becoming a Medical Specialist.* New York: Plenum Medical, 1988.

"Coleman Hospital, 1927–1967." *Medical Quarterly of the Indiana University School of Medicine* (formerly *Quarterly Bulletin of the IU Medical Center*) 29 (Fall 1967): 13–18.

Combs, Charles N., "History of the Indiana State Medical Association." In *100 Years of Indiana Medicine*, edited by Dorothy Ritter Russo, 7–29. Indianapolis: Indiana State Medical Association, 1949.

Constantine, Norman A. "Converging Evidence Leaves Policy Behind: Sex Education in the United States." *Journal of Adolescent Health* 42, no. 4 (April 2008): 324–26.

Cook-Deegan, Robert, and Michael McGeary. "The Jewel in the Federal Crown? History, Politics and the National Institutes of Health." In *History and Health Policy in the United States*, edited by Rosemary A. Stevens et al., 176–201. Piscataway, NJ: Rutgers University Press, 2006.

Coons, Philip M., and Elizabeth S. Bowman. *Psychiatry in Indiana: The First 175 Years.* New York: iUniverse, 2010.

Cooper, Richard A. "Medical Schools and Their Applicants: An Analysis." *Health Affairs* 22, no. 4 (July 1, 2003): 71–84. doi:10.1377/hlthaff.22.4.71.

Cooter, Roger. "Medicine and the Goodness of War." *Canadian Bulletin of Medical History*, 7 (Fall 1990): 147–59.

Cottman, George Streibey. *Centennnial History of Indiana.* Indianapolis: Max R. Hyman, 1916.

Creager, Angela. "Mobilizing Biomedicine: Virus Research between Lay Health Organizations and the U. S. Federal Government, 1935–1955." In *Biomedicine in the Twentieth Century: Practices, Policies, and Politics*, edited by Caroline Hannaway, 171–202. Washington, DC: IOS, 2008.

Crowley, A. E. "Graduate Medical Education in the United States, 1984–1985." *JAMA* 254, no. 12 (September 27, 1985): 1585–93.

Curran, Robert S. *Introductory Lecture Delivered at the Opening of the Second Session of the Indiana Central Medical College.* Indianapolis: Douglass & Elder, 1850.

Dalen, James E. "The Moratorium on U. S. Medical School Enrollment from 1980 to 2005: What Were We Thinking?" *American Journal of Medicine* 121, no. 2 (2008): 1–2.

Dalton, Martin L. *The History of the Mercer University School of Medicine, 1965–2007.* Macon, GA: Mercer University Press, 2009.

Daly, Walter J. "Indiana University Medical Center, 1903–1993." Address to the Newcomen Society, held in Indianapolis March 17, 1993. Newcomen Publication Number 1399.

———. "The Origins of President Bryan's Medical School." *Indiana Magazine of History* 97 (2002): 266–84.

———. "Presidential Address: A Personal Testament—Reflections on the Tower of Babel." *Journal of Laboratory and Clinical* Medicine 99, no. 1 (January 1982): 10–14.

Damon, Bradley K. "'To Care for Him Who Shall Have Borne the Battle': A History of the Indianapolis Veterans Administration Hospitals, 1928–1988." MA thesis, Indiana University, 1990.

Davenport, Horace W. *Not Just Any Medical School: The Science, Practice, and Teaching of Medicine at the University of Michigan, 1850–1941.* Ann Arbor: University of Michigan Press, 1999.

Deitrick, John E., and Robert C. Berson. *Medical Schools in the United States at Mid-Century.* New York: McGraw-Hill, 1953.

DeMyer, M. K., J. N. Hingtgen, and R. K. Jackson. "Infantile Autism Reviewed: A Decade of Research." *Schizophrenia Bulletin* 7, no. 3 (1981): 388–451.

Devers, Kelly J., Linda R. Brewster, and Lawrence P. Casalino. "Changes in Hospital Competitive Strategy: A New Medical Arms Race?" pt. 2. *Health Services Research* 38, no. 1 (February 2003): 447–69. doi:10.1111/1475-6773.00124.

Diamond, Ivan, Harriet De Wit, and Jan B. Hoek. "Recognizing Dr. Ting-Kai Li for a Job Well Done." *Alcoholism: Clinical and Experimental Research* 32, no. 12 (December 1, 2008): 2029.

Dishman, Madge. "Coleman Hall: A Monument to Indiana Medicine." *Indiana Medicine* 77 (1984): 621–23.

Donini-Lenhoff, F. G., and H. L. Hedrick. "Growth of Specialization in Graduate Medical Education." *JAMA* 284, no. 10 (September 13, 2000): 1284–89.

Dowling, Harry F. *City Hospitals: The Undercare of the Underpriveleged.* Cambridge, MA: Harvard University Press, 1982.

Dunn, Jacob Piatt. *Greater Indianapolis: The History, the Industries, the Institutions, and the People of a City of Homes.* Chicago: Lewis, 1910.

Dupree, A. Hunter. *Science in the Federal Government: A History of Policies and Activities.* Baltimore, MD: Johns Hopkins University Press, 1986.

Eaglen, Robert H. *Academic Quality and Public Accountability in Medical Education: The 75-Year History of the LCME.* Washington, DC: Liaison Committee on Medical Education, 2017.

Earp, Samuel E. "Joseph Eastman, M.D., L.L.D." *The Medical and Surgical Monitor* 5 (June 15, 1902): 207.

———. "Death of Robert W. Long—His Life History." *Indianapolis Medical Journal* 16 (July 15, 1915): 314–18.

Edmondson, Edna H. "The Indiana Child Welfare Association." *Bulletin of the Extension Division, Indiana University* 5, no. 5 (1920). https://scholarworks.iu.edu/journals/index.php/imh/article/view/6188.

Eisenberg, Laurie S., and Karen C. Johnson. "Audiologic Contributions to Pediatric Cochlear Implants." *ASHA Leader* 13, no. 4 (March 1, 2008): 10–13. doi:10.1044/leader.FTR1.13042008.10.

Elizondo, R. S., N. Jacobs, and W. W. Moore. "Physiology at Indiana University-Bloomington. A History." *Physiologist* 27, no. 5 (October 1984): 319–24.

Emerson, Charles P. "Indiana University School of Medicine." *Journal of the Indiana State Medical Association* 8 (January 1915): 40.

———. "Medical Social Services of the Future." *Transactions of the American Hospital Association,* 21 (1919): 333–42.

Erickson, Norma. "African-American Hospitals and Health Care in Early Twentieth Century Indianapolis, Indiana, 1894–1917." MA thesis, IUPUI, 2016.

Essays in the History of Medicine in Honor of David J. Davis, M.D., M.P.H., 168–81. Chicago: University of Illinois Press, 1965.

Etheridge, Jr., J. E. "Graduate Medical Education: Then and Now." *Virginia Medical Quarterly* 121, no. 3 (1994 Summer 1994): 166–67.

Fee, Elizabeth. "History." In *Who Will Keep the Public Healthy? Educating Public Health Professionals for the 21st Century,* edited by K. Gebbie,

L. Rosenstock, and L. M. Hernandez, 41–60. Washington, DC: National Academies Press, 2003.

Feigenbaum, Harvey. "Evolution of Echocardiography." *Circulation* 93, no. 7 (1996): 1321–27.

———. "The Origin of Echocardiography?" *Texas Heart Institute Journal* 35, no. 1 (2008): 87–88.

Feigenbaum, Harvey, J. A. Waldhausen, and L. P. Hyde. "Ultrasound Diagnosis of Pericardial Effusion." *JAMA* 191 (March 1, 1965): 711–14.

Fenton, R. A. "A Brief History of Otolaryngology in the United States from 1847 to 1947." *JAMA Otolaryngology—Head & Neck Surgery* 46, no. 2 (August 1, 1947): 153–62.

Fishbein, Morris. *Doctors at War.* New York: Books for Library Press, 1972.

Flexner, Abraham. *Medical Education in the United States and Canada: A Report to the Carnegie Foundation for the Advancement of Teaching.* New York: Carnegie Foundation for the Advancement of Teaching, 1910.

Flowers, Leslie. *A Legacy of Leadership: Indiana University School of Nursing, 1914–2014.* Indianapolis: Indiana University Press, 2014.

Ford, Wendy, Joanne Fox, and Julie Sturgeon. *Regenstrief: Legacy of the Dishwasher King.* Indianapolis: Regenstrief Foundation, 1999.

Fordham, Christopher C. "The *Bane Report* Revisited." *JAMA* 244, no. 4 (July 25, 1980): 354–57.

Fosdick, Raymond B. *Adventure in Giving: The Story of the General Education Board, a Foundation Established by John D. Rockefeller.* New York: Harper & Row, 1962.

Foucault, Michel. *The Birth of the Clinic: An Archaeology of Medical Perception.* New York: Pantheon Books, 1973.

Fuchs, Victor R. "Major Trends in the U. S. Health Economy since 1950." *New England Journal of Medicine* 366, no. 11 (March 15, 2012): 973–77. Accessed May 1, 2018. https://www.nejm.org/doi/suppl/10.1056/NEJMp1200478/suppl_file/nejmp1200478_appendix.pdf.

Gathorne-Hardy, Jonathan. *Alfred C. Kinsey: Sex the Measure of All Things* (London: Chatto & Windus, 1998).

Gebbie, Kristine, Linda Rosenstock, Lyla M. Hernandez, eds. *Who Will Keep the Public Healthy? Educating Public Health Professionals for the 21st Century.* Washington, DC: National Academies, 2003.

Geiger, Roger L. *To Advance Knowledge: The Growth of American Research Universities, 1900–1940.* New York: Oxford University Press, 1986.

Germano, Nancy M. "A View of the Valley the 1913 Flood in West Indianapolis." MA thesis, Indiana University, 2009.

Ginzberg, Eli. "The Politics of U. S. Physician Supply." *Health Policy* 55 (1990): 233–46.

Glickman, R. M., J. C. Bennett, and J. P. Nolan. "United We Stand." *Annals of Internal Medicine* 118 (1993): 903–4.

Gordon, Linda. *Pitied but Not Entitled: Single Mothers and the History of Welfare, 1890–1935.* Cambridge, MA: Harvard University Press, 1995.

Gordon, Robert Boyd, and Patrick M. Malone. *The Texture of Industry: An Archaeological View of the Industrialization of North America.* New York: Oxford University Press, 1997.

Graham, John B. "UNC's Deans of Medicine. Reminiscences of a Septuagenarian." *North Carolina Medical Journal* 56 (November 1995): 562–68.

Grauer, Neil A. *Leading the Way: A History of Johns Hopkins Medicine.* Baltimore, MD: Johns Hopkins University Press, 2012.

Gray, Ralph D. *IUPUI—The Making of an Urban University.* Bloomington: Indiana University Press, 2003.

Greysen, S. Ryan, Candice Chen, and Fitzhugh Mullan. "A History of Medical Student Debt: Observations and Implications for the Future of Medical Education." *Academic Medicine* 86, no. 7 (July 2011): 840–45.

Grillo, H. C. "To Impart This Art: The Development of Graduate Surgical Education in the United States." *Surgery* 125, no. 1 (January 1999): 1–14.

Gugin, Linda C., and James E. St. Clair. *The Governors of Indiana.* Indianapolis: Indiana Historical Society, 2006.

Gunderman, Richard B. "Competency-Based Training: Conformity and the Pursuit of Educational Excellence." *Radiology* 252, no. 2 (August 1, 2009): 324–26.

Haber, Samuel. *The Quest for Authority and Honor in the American Professions, 1750–1900.* Chicago: University of Chicago Press, 1991.

"A Half Century of Progress of Black Students in Medical Schools." *Journal of Blacks in Higher Education* 30 (Winter 2000–2001): 28–31.

Hale, Hester Anne. *Caring for the Community: The History of Wishard Hospital.* Indianapolis: Wishard Memorial Foundation, 1999.

Haller, John S. *The History of American Homeopathy: From Rational Medicine to Holistic Health Care.* New Brunswick, NJ: Rutgers University Press, 2009.

———. *A Profile in Alternative Medicine: The Eclectic Medical College of Cincinnati, 1845–1942.* Kent, OH: Kent State University Press, 1999.

Halpern, Sydney Ann. *American Pediatrics: The Social Dynamics of Professionalism, 1880–1980.* Berkeley: University of California Press, 1988.

Handel, David J., Stuart A. Kleit, and Daniel A. Handel. "The Development and Maturation of a Statewide Academic Health Care System: Clarian Health Partners/Indiana University Health." *Academic Medicine* 89, no. 2 (February 2014): 230–35.

Harger, R. N. "'Debunking' the Drunkometer." *American Journal of Police Science* 40 (1949): 497–506.

Harling, Samuel Bannister, ed. *Indiana University, 1820–1904, Historical Sketch, Development of the Course of Instruction, Bibliography.* Bloomington: Indiana University, 1904.

Harrington, Thomas Francis. *Harvard Medical School: A History, Narrative and Documentary. 1782–1905.* Vol. 1. New York: Lewis, 1905.

Harvey, A. McGehee. *Adventures in Medical Research: A Century of Discovery at Johns Hopkins.* Baltimore, MD: Johns Hopkins University Press, 1976.

Henry, Edna G. "Dedication of the Robert W. Long Hospital." *Indiana University Alumni Quarterly* 1 (October 1914): 407.

Herschell, William. "They Just Must Get Well." *The Rotarian* 40, no. 1 (January 1932): 16–18, 55–56.

Hickam, John B. "Periodic Recertification." *JAMA* 213, no. 10 (September 7, 1970): 1657–58.

Hickam, John B., and W. D. Close. "Symposium on Medical Education—No. 3. V. The Proposed Indiana Family Practice Program." *JAMA* 176, no. 11 (1961): 907–9. doi:10.1001/jama.1961.03040240013005.

Hitz, Benjamin D. *A History of Base Hospital 32.* Indianapolis: Edward Kahle American Legion Post, 1922.

Houston, Derek M., et al. "The Ear Is Connected to the Brain: Some New Directions in the Study of Children with Cochlear Implants at Indiana University." *Journal of the American Academy of Audiology* 23, no. 6 (June 2012): 446–63. doi:10.3766/jaaa.23.6.7.

Howell, Joel D. "Lowell Coggeshall and American Medical Education: 1901–1987." *Academic Medicine* 67, no. 11 (November 1992): 711–18.

———, ed. *Medical Lives and Scientific Medicine at Michigan, 1891–1969.* Ann Arbor: University of Michigan Press, 1994.

"Indiana as a Factor in Medical Education: A Medical Department for the State University." *Indiana Medical Journal* (August 1903): 65–71.

Indiana Centennial Celebration Committee. *Suggestive Plans for a Historical and Educational Celebration in Indiana in 1916.* Indianapolis, 1912.

Indiana Committee on Mental Defectives. *Mental Defectives in Indiana. Third Report.* Indianapolis: W. B. Burford, 1922.

Indiana Perinatal Quality Improvement Collaborative. "Addressing Infant Mortality in Indiana." Indianapolis, March 26, 2014.

Indiana University Catalog. Bloomington: Indiana University, 1915.

Inghram, Mrs. W. H. "Formal Opening of the New Home of the Central College of Physicians and Surgeons." *The Medical and Surgical Monitor* 5 (November 15, 1902): 395–97.

Inlow, William DePrez. "The Indiana Physician in World War I." In *One Hundred Years of Indiana Medicine,* edited by Dorothy R. Russo, 92–105. Indianapolis: Indiana State Medical Association, 1949.

Institute of Medicine Division of Health Sciences Policy. *Medical Education and Societal Needs: A Planning Report for the Health Professions.* New York: National Academies, 1983.

"An Interview with Lawrence Einhorn, MD: Testicular Cancer—Don't Settle for the Status Quo." *Journal of Oncology Practice* 1, no. 4 (November 1, 2005): 167.

"Is Medicine Attractive to Scholarly Men?" *JAMA* 41, no. 1 (August 1903): 317.

Jacobson, Timothy C. *Making Medical Doctors: Science and Medicine at Vanderbilt since Flexner.* Tuscaloosa: University of Alabama Press, 1987.

Jay, Steven J., "Legacies of Hoosier Aviation and Medical Science Visionaries." *Traces of Indiana and Midwesten History* 30 (Spring 2018): 25–33.

Johnson, Davis G. "The Study of Applicants, 1964–1965." *Journal of Medical Education* 40, no. 11 (1965): 1017–30.

Jones, Amanda. "The Greatest Outrage: Military Park, Long Hospital, and Progressive Era Notions of Urban Space." MA thesis, Indiana University, 2009.

Kalisch, Philip Arthur, and Beatrice J Kalisch. *American Nursing: A History.* Philadelphia: Lippincott Williams & Wilkins, 2004.

Kassebaum, Donald G. "Origin of the LCME, the AAMC–AMA Partnership for Accreditation." *Academic Medicine* 67, no. 2 (February 1992): 85–87.

Kassebaum, Donald G., P. L. Szenas, and M. K. Schuchert. "On Rising Medical Student Debt: In for a Penny, in for a Pound." *Academic Medicine* 71, no. 10 (October 1996): 1124–34.

Kastor, John Alfred. *Mergers of Teaching Hospitals in Boston, New York, and Northern California.* Ann Arbor: University of Michigan Press, 2009.

Katz, Michael B. *In the Shadow of the Poorhouse: A Social History of Welfare in* America. New York: Basic Books, 1996.

Kaufman, Martin. *American Medical Education, the Formative Years, 1765–1910.* Westport, CT: Greenwood, 1976.

Kemper, G. W. H. *A Medical History of Indiana.* Chicago: American Medical Association, 1911.

Kerr, Clark. *The Uses of the University.* Cambridge, MA: Harvard University Press, 2001.

King, Lucy Jane, and Alan D. Schmetzer. *Dr. Edenharter's Dream: How Science Improved the Humane Care of the Mentally Ill in Indiana 1896–2012.* Carmel, IN: Hawthorne, 2012.

Kirk, Ruth V. "The State Board of Medical registration and Examination." In *100 Years of Indiana Medicine,* edited by Dorothy Ritter Russo, 51–53. Indianapolis: Indiana State Medical Association, 1949.

Kleiman, Martin B. "The Media and Illness in a Public Figure: Enough Is Never Enough." *Pediatric Infectious Disease Journal* 11, no. 7 (July 1992): 513–15.

Klein, Mellisa K. "The Legacy of the 'Yellow Berets': The Vietnam War, the Doctor Draft, and the NIH Associate Training Program." Bethesda, MD: National Institutes for Health, 1989. https://history.nih.gov/research/downloads/YellowBerets.pdf.

Kline, Wendy. *Bodies of Knowledge: Sexuality, Reproduction, and Women's Health in the Second Wave.* Chicago: University of Chicago Press, 2010.

Knoebel, Suzanne B. "Profiles in Cardiology: Charles Fisch." *Clinical Cardiology* 14 (1991): 782–83.

Koch, Amanda Jean. "Not a 'Sentimental Charity': A History of the Indianapolis Flower Mission, 1876–1993." MA thesis, Indiana University, 2010.

Kohler, Robert E. *Partners in Science: Foundations and Natural Scientists, 1900–1945.* Chicago: University of Chicago Press, 1991.

Kotlowski, Dean J. *Paul V. McNutt and the Age of FDR.* Bloomington: Indiana University Press, 2015.

Kovac, Anthony, Nancy Hulston, Grace Holmes, and Frederick Holmes. "'A Brave and Gallant Company': A Kansas City Hospital in France during the First World War." *Kansas History* 32, no. 3 (September 2009): 168–85.

Kunzel, Regina G. Fallen *Women, Problem Girls: Unmarried Mothers and the Professionalization of Social Work, 1890–1945.* New Haven, CT: Yale University Press, 1995.

Langsley, Donald G., James H. Darragh. *Trends in Specialization: Tomorrow's Medicine.* Evanston, IL: American Board of Medical Specialties, 1985.

Lantzer, Jason S. "The Indiana Way of Eugenics: Sterilization Laws, 1907—74." In *A Century of Eugenics in America: From the Indiana Experiment to the Human Genome Era,* edtied by Paul A. Lombardo, 26–42. Bloomington: Indiana University Press, 2010.

———. "The Other Side of Campus: Indiana University's Student Right and the Rise of National Conservatism." *Indiana Magazine of History* 101, no. 2 (June 1, 2005): 153–78. https://scholarworks.iu.edu/journals/index.php/imh/article/view/12120.

Lears, Jackson. *Fables of Abundance: A Cultural History of Advertising in America*. New York: Basic Books, 1994.

Leathers, W. S. "The Association of American Medical Colleges and Some Postwar Medical Problems." *Academic Medicine* 19 (January 1944): 1–7.

Lerner, Barron H. *One for the Road: Drunk Driving Since 1900*. Baltimore, MD: Johns Hopkins University Press, 2011.

Levin, Rebecca, et al. "Organizational, Financial, and Environmental Factors Influencing Deans' Tenure." *Academic Medicine* 73 (June 1998): 640–44.

Lister, J. "The History of Postgraduate Medicine Education." *Postgraduate Medical Journal* 70, no. 828 (October 1994): 728–31.

Lohr, Kathleen N., Neal A. Vanselow, and Don E. Detmer. *U. S. Physician Supply and Requirements: Match or Mismatch?* Bethesda, MD: National Academies, 1996.

Lombardo, Paul A., ed. *A Century of Eugenics in America: From the Indiana Experiment to the Human Genome Era*. Bloomington: Indiana University Press, 2011.

Loofbourrow, Rebecca L. "The Indiana Village for Epileptics, 1907–1952: The Van Nuys Years." MA thesis, Indiana University, 2008.

Lovett, Laura L. *Conceiving the Future: Pronatalism, Reproduction, and the Family in the United States, 1890–1938*. Chapel Hill: University of North Carolina Press, 2009.

Lucas, Christopher J. *American Higher Education: A History*. 2nd ed. New York: Palgrave Macmillan, 2006.

Ludmerer, Kenneth M. *Learning to Heal: The Development of American Medical Education*. Baltimore, MD: Johns Hopkins University Press, 1996.

———. *Let Me Heal: The Opportunity to Preserve Excellence in American Medicine*. New York: Oxford University Press, 2014.

———. *Time to Heal: American Medical Education from the Turn of the Century*. New York: Oxford University Press, 2005.

Lukemeyer, George T., and Glenn W. Irwin. "Statewide Medical Education in Indiana." *Indiana Medicine* 89, no. 3 (May–June 1996): 264–70.

Lull, George F. "Fifty Thousand Doctors and Half a Million Personnel." In *Doctors at War*, edited by Morris Fishbein, 91–108. New York: Books for Library, 1972.

Lupton, Suzann Weber. "Local Foundations and Medical Research Support in Indianapolis after 1945." PhD diss., Indiana University, 2019.

Lynch, Charles, Frank W. Weed, and Loy McAfee, eds. *The Medical Department of the United States Army in the World War*. Vol. 1. Washington, DC: Government Printing Office, 1923.

MacDougall, John D. "Joseph Eastman, M.D., L.L.D.: Citizen, Soldier, Surgeon and Medical Educator." *Indiana Medical History Quarterly* 1 (October 1974): 28.

Madison, James H. *Hoosiers: A New History of Indiana*. Bloomington: Indiana University Press, 2014.

———. *Indiana through Tradition and Change: A History of the Hoosier State and Its People, 1920–1945*. Indianapolis: Indiana Historical Society, 1982.

———. *The Indiana Way: A State History*. Bloomington: Indiana University Press, 1990.

Mallon, William T. "The Alchemists: A Case Study of a Failed Merger in Academic Medicine." *Academic Medicine* 78, no. 11 (November 2003): 1090–1104.

———. "The Benefits and Challenges of Research Centers and Institutes in Academic Medicine: Findings from Six Universities and Their Medical Schools." *Academic Medicine* 81, no. 6 (June 2006): 502–12.

———, ed. *Mini-Med: The Role of Regional Campuses in U. S. Medical Education*. Washington, DC: Association of American Medical Colleges, 2003.

Mallon, William T., M. Liu, R. F. Jones, and M. E. Whitcomb, *Regional Medical Campuses: Bridging Communities, Enhancing Mission, Expanding Medical Education*. Washington, DC: Association of American Medical Colleges, 2006.

Markel, Howard. "The University of Michigan Medical School, 1850–2000." *JAMA* 283, no. 7 (February 16, 2000): 915.

Manhart, George B. "The Indiana Central Medical College, 1849–1852." *Indiana Medical History Quarterly* 8: 105–22.

Marriner-Tomey, Ann, ed. *Nursing at Indiana University: 75 Years at the Heart of Health Care*. Indianapolis: Indiana University School of Nursing, 1989.

Martin, Daniel. "The Medical Center in a Community." *JAMA* 190 (December 21, 1964): 1056–60.

Martin, John Bartlow. *Indiana: An Interpretation*. Bloomington: Indiana University Press, 1947.

McDonald, Clement J., and William M. Tierney. "The Medical Gopher—A Microcomputer System to Help Find, Organize and Decide about Patient Data." *Western Journal of Medicine* 145, no. 6 (December 1986): 823–29.

McDonell, Katherine Mandusic. "Care of the Sick Poor of Indianapolis to 1915." Unpublished manuscript, Indiana Historical Society.

———. "The Indianapolis City Hospital, 1833–1866." *Indiana Medical History Quarterly* 9, no. 2 (June 1983): 3–23.

McGaghie, William C. "Assessing Readiness for Medical Education: Evolution of the Medical College Admission Test." *JAMA* 288, no. 9 (September 4, 2002): 1085–90.

McIntosh, Henry D. "Memorial: John Bamber Hickam, M.D." *Transactions of the American Clinical Climatological Association 1971* 82: ix–lxii.

McKusick, Victor A., and Peter S. Harper. "History of Medical Genetics." In *Emery and Rimoin's Principles and Practice of Medical Genetics*, 6th ed., edited by David L. Rimoin et al., 1–39. Philadelphia: Churchill Livingstone Elsevier, 2013.

Meckel, Richard A. *Save the Babies: American Public Health Reform and the Prevention of Infant Mortality, 1850–1929*. Ann Arbor: University of Michigan Press, 1990.

"Medical Activity in the State Universities." *JAMA* 40, no. 25 (June 20, 1903): 1726.

"The Medical College of Indiana of the University of Indianapolis." *Indiana Medical Journal* (1899–1900): 89–91.

Merritt, H. Houston. "Present-Day Medical Education and the Medical-Center Concept." *New England Journal of Medicine* 271 (December 3, 1964): 1194–97.

Merton, Robert K., George G. Reader, and Patricia Kendall, eds. *The Student-Physician: Introductory Studies in the Sociology of Medical Education.* Cambridge, MA: Harvard University Press, 1957.

Meyers, Elsie F. "Doing the 'Not Possible': The Memoirs of Elsie F. Meyers, M.D.," *Indiana Magazine of History* 104, no. 4 (December 2008): 329–66.

Moore, Leonard Joseph. *Citizen Klansmen: The Ku Klux Klan in Indiana, 1921–1928.* Chapel Hill: University of North Carolina Press, 1991.

Morantz-Sanchez, Regina. *Sympathy and Science: Women Physicians in American Medicine.* New York: Oxford University Press, 1985.

More, Ellen S. *Restoring the Balance: Women Physicians and the Profession of Medicine, 1850–1995.* Cambridge, MA: Harvard University Press, 2009.

More, Ellen S., Elizabeth Fee, and Manon Parry. *Women Physicians and the Cultures of Medicine.* Baltimore, MD: Johns Hopkins University Press, 2009.

Myers, Burton D. *History of Medical Education in Indiana.* Bloomington: Indiana University Press, 1956.

Nathan, David, and Edward J. Benz. "Comprehensive Cancer Centres and the War on Cancer." *Nature Reviews: Cancer* 1 (December 2001): 240–45.

Nora, L. M. "Sexual Harassment in Medical Education: A Review of the Literature with Comments from the Law." Supplement, *Academic Medicine* 71, no. 1 (January 1996): S113–18.

O'Hara, S. Paul. "'The Very Model of Modern Urban Decay': Outsiders' Narratives of Industry and Urban Decline in Gary, Indiana." *Journal of Urban History* 37, no. 2 (2011): 135–54.

Oberlander, Jonathan. "Learning from Failure in Health Care Reform." *New England Journal of Medicine* 357, no. 17 (October 25, 2007): 1677–79.

———. *The Political Life of Medicare.* Chicago: University of Chicago Press, 2003.

"Opening of the Indiana Medical College, University of Indianapolis." *Indiana Medical Journal* 15 (1896–1897): 158–61.

Osberger, Mary Joe, et al. "Effect of Age at Onset of Deafness on Children's Speech Perception Abilities with a Cochlear Implant." *Annals of Otology, Rhinology & Laryngology* 100, no. 11 (November 1, 1991): 883–88. doi:10.1177/000348949110001104.

Osgood, Robert L. "The Menace of the Feebleminded: George Bliss, Amos Butler and the Indiana Committee on Mental Defectives." *Indiana Magazine of History* 97, no. 4 (December 2001): 253–77.

———. "Education in the Name of 'Improvement': The Influence of Eugenic Thought and Practice in Indiana's Public Schools, 1900–1930." *Indiana Magazine of History* 106, no. 3 (September 1, 2010): 272–99.

Penrod, Kenneth E. "The Indiana Program for Comprehensive Medical Education." *JAMA* 210, no. 5 (November 3, 1969): 868–70. doi:10.1001/jama.1969.03160310056011.

———. "The Indiana University Medical Center, a Decade Ahead." *Alumni Bulletin—School of Dentistry*, Indiana University (1968): 4 passim.

Penrod, K. E., and G. W. Irwin. "A Proposed Statewide Medical School for Indiana." *Journal of Medical Education* 41, no. 11 (November 1966): 1030–36.

Pernick, Martin S. "Eugenics and Public Health in American History." *American Journal of Public Health* 87 no. 11 (1997): 1767–72.

Petersdorf, Robert G. "Deans and Deaning in a Changing World." *Academic Medicine* 72 (November 1997): 953–58.

———. "Medical Schools and Research: Is the Tail Wagging the Dog?" *Daedalus* 115 (Spring 1986): 101–3.

Phillips, Clifton Jackson. *Indiana in Transition: The Emergence of an Industrial Commonwealth, 1880–1920*. Indianapolis: Indiana Historical Bureau & Indiana Historical Society, 1968.

Pickard, Madge E., and R. Carlyle Buley. *The Midwest Pioneer, His Ills, Cures, & Doctors*. New York: Henry Schuman, 1946.

Piepho, Lois Ann. "The History of the Social Service Department of the Indiana University Medical Center, 1911–1932." MA thesis, Indiana University, 1950.

Pinel, Philippe. *The Clinical Training of Doctors. An Essay of 1793*. Baltimore, MD: Johns Hopkins University Press, 1981.

Posey, Author Lora. "John William Ryan—Remembering IU's 14th President." Accessed March 15, 2017. https://blogs.libraries.indiana.edu/iubarchives /tag/john-william-ryan.

Potter, Angela B. "From Social Hygiene to Social Health: Indiana and the United States Adolescent Sex Education Movement, 1907–1975." MA thesis, Indiana University, 2015.

———. "Learning Human Anatomy: Women and the Changing Student Body at the Indiana University School of Medicine, 1907–2007." In *Women at Indiana University: Views of the Past and the Future*, edited by Andrea Walton. Bloomington: Indiana University Press, forthcoming.

Potter, Theodore. "A Brief History of the Medical College of Indiana." *The Medical Student* 3 (April 1905): 11.

———. "Microscopic Laboratories of the College." *The Medical Student* 1 (November 1902): 7–8.

Preston, Samuel H., and Michael R. Haines. *Fatal Years: Child Mortality in Late Nineteenth-Century America*. Princeton, NJ: Princeton University Press, 2014.

Price, Nelson. *The Quiet Hero: A Life of Ryan White*. Indianapolis: Indiana Historical Society, 2015.

Pulos, William Leroy. "A Study of Some Measured Characteristics of an Entering Class of the Indiana University Medical School." PhD diss., Indiana University, 1957.

Quigley, Fran. *Walking Together, Walking Far: How a U. S. and African Medical School Partnership Is Winning the Fight against HIV/AIDS*. Bloomington: Indiana University Press, 2009.

Ralston, H. J., et al. "Capturing the Promise of Science in Medical Schools." *Academic Medicine* 71, no. 12 (December 1996): 1314–23.

Ramsey, Paul G., et al. "From Concept to Culture: The WWAMI Program at the University of Washington School of Medicine." *Academic Medicine* 76, no. 8 (August 2001): 765–75.

Rappleye, Willard C. "Effects to Date of the Wartime Program of Medical Education." *Academic Medicine* 19, no. 1 (January 1944): 46–48.

Rawls, George H. *History of the Black Physician in Indianapolis 1870 to 1980.* Indianapolis: N.p., 1984.

Reiser, Stanley Joel. *Technological Medicine: The Changing World of Doctors and Patients.* Cambridge, UK: Cambridge University Press, 2014.

"Relation of the Indiana Medical College to the State University." *Indiana Medical Journal* 24 (February 1906): 347–50.

Rice, Thurman B. *History of the Medical Campus, Indianapolis, Indiana.* Indianapolis: 1949. Published in earlier installments in *Monthly Bulletin, Indiana State Board of Health,* from January 1947 through December 1948.

———. "History of the Medical Campus, II: Dr. Burton Dorr Myers." *Monthly Bulletin. Indiana State Board of Health* 50 (February 1947): 35–40.

———. "History of the Medical Campus, IV: The Origin and Development of the City Hospital." *Monthly Bulletin. Indiana State Board of Health* 50 (April 1947): 91–93.

———. "History of the Medical Campus, Chapter V: The Medicine School Building of the Medical Campus," *Monthly Bulletin. Indiana State Board of Health* 50 (May 1947): 117–20.

———. "History of the Medical Campus, Chapter VI: Indiana University Chooses a Medical Campus." *Monthly Bulletin. Indiana State Board of Health* 50 (June 1947): 139–42.

———. "History of the Medical Campus, Chapter VIII: The School of Nursing." *Monthly Bulletin. Indiana State Board of Health* 50 (August 1947): 185–88; 193–94.

———. "History of the Medical School Campus, Chapter IX: The Dental College." *Monthly Bulletin. Indiana State Board of Health* 50 (September 1947): 211–16.

———. "History of the Medical Campus, Chapter X: The State Board of Health on the Medical Campus." *Monthly Bulletin. Indiana State Board of Health* 51 (October 1947): 235–39.

———. "History of the Medical Campus, Chapter XV: The Medical Campus in Wartime." *Monthly Bulletin. Indiana State Board of Health* 51 (March 1948): 68.

———. *The Hoosier Health Officer: A Biography of Dr. John N. Hurty and the History of the Indiana State Board of Health to 1925.* Indianapolis: Indiana State Board of Health, 1946.

———. *One Hundred Years of Medicine: Indianapolis, 1820–1920.* Indianapolis: Indiana State Board of Health, 1944.

———. "One Hundred Years of Medicine in Indianapolis." *Monthly Bulletin. Indiana State Board of Health* 54 (November 1951): 255–62.

———. *Racial Hygiene: A Practical Discussion of Eugenics and Race Culture.* New York: Macmillan, 1929.

Rich, Eugene C., et al. "Medicare Financing of Graduate Medical Education." *Journal of General Internal Medicine* 17, no. 4 (April 2002): 283–92.

Richards, A. N. "The Impact of the War on Medicine." *Science* 103, no. 2680 (May 10, 1946): 575–78. doi:10.1126/science.103.2680.575.

Rimoin, David L., and Kurt Hirschhorn. "A History of Medical Genetics in Pediatrics." *Pediatric Research* 56, no. 1 (July 2004): 150–59.

Risse, Guenter B. *Mending Bodies, Saving Souls a History of Hospitals.* New York: Oxford University Press, 1999.

Ritchie, J. O. "Obituary: Dr. Ada Estelle Schweitzer." *Annals of Internal Medicine* 36, no. 1 (January 1952): 221.

Rock, Dorcas Irene. "A History of the Indiana University Training School for Nurses." MA thesis, Butler University, 1956.

Roehr, Eleanor L. *Trustees and Officers of Indiana University, 1950 to 1982.* Bloomington: Indiana University Press, 1983.

Rogers, Helen Cintelda. *Seventy Years of Social Work at Indiana University.* Indianapolis: Indiana University School of Social Work, 1982.

Rogers, Helen Worthington. *A Digest of Laws Establishing Reformatories for Women in the United States.* New York City: Bureau of Social Hygiene, 1923.

Rogers, Naomi. *An Alternative Path: The Making and Remaking of Hahnemann Medical College and Hospital.* New Brunswick, NJ: Rutgers University Press, 1998.

Rohlfing, James, et al. "Medical Student Debt and Major Life Choices Other than Specialty." *Medical Education Online* 19 (November 2014). doi:10.3402/meo.v19.25603.

Rosenberg, Charles E. *The Care of Strangers: The Rise of America's Hospital System.* Baltimore, MD: Johns Hopkins University Press, 1995.

Rosenstock, Linda, Karen Helsing, and Barbara K. Rimer. "Public Health Education in the United States: Then and Now." *Public Health Reviews* 33, no. 1 (2011): 39–65.

Ross, Joseph C. "John Bamber Hickam: Physician, Educator, Investigator." *Archives of Internal Medicine* 127, no. 4 (April 1, 1971): 571–73.

Rothman, David J. *Beginnings Count: The Technological Imperative in American Health Care.* New York: Oxford University Press, 1997.

Rothstein, William G. *American Medical Schools and the Practice of Medicine: A History.* New York: Oxford University Press, 1987.

Rudolph, Frederick, and John R. Thelin. *The American College and University: A History.* Reissue edition. Athens: University of Georgia Press, 1990.

Russo, Dorothy Ritter. "Pioneer Medicine in Indiana." In *One Hundred Years of Indiana Medicine*, edited by Dorothy Ritter Russo, 4–5. Indianapolis: Indiana State Medical Association, 1949.

Ryan, Michael S., Allison A. Vanderbilt, Thasia W. Lewis and Molly A. Madden, "Benefits and Barriers among Volunteer Teaching Faculty: Comparison between Those Who Precept and Those Who Do Not in the Core Pediatrics Clerkship." *Medical Education Online* 18, no. 1 (May 2013). doi: 10.3402/meo.v18io.20733.

Safianow, Allen. "Ryan White and Kokomo, Indiana." *Traces of Indiana & Midwestern History* 25, no. 1 (2013): 14–26.

Sanders, Chauncey. "The Relation of the University in the National Defense Plan." *Indiana Alumni Magazine* 3 (April 1941): 6.

Sappol, Michael. *"A Traffic of Dead Bodies": Anatomy and Embodied Social Identity in 19th-Century America.* Princeton, NJ: Princeton University Press, 2002.

Scherrer, Simon P. "A True Statement of Facts Relating to the Coalition of the Central College of Physicians and Surgeons with Indiana University, 1905." *Indiana Medical History Quarterly* 1 (February 1975): 63.

Schieffler, Danny A., Philip M. Farrell, Marc J. Kahn, and Richard A. Culbertson. "The Evolution of the Medical School Deanship: From Patriarch to CEO to System Dean." *The Permanente Journal* 21 (2017). doi:10.7812/TPP/16–069.

Schneider, William H. "Hoosier Health Philanthropy: Understanding the Past." In *Hoosier Philanthropy: Understanding the Past, Present and Future*, edited by Gregory Witkowski. Bloomington: Indiana University Press, forthcoming.

———. "The Men Who Followed Flexner: Richard Pearce, Alan Gregg, and the Rockefeller Foundation Medical Divisions, 1919–1951." In *Rockefeller Philanthropy and Modern Biomedicine: International Initiatives from World War I to the Cold War*, edited by William H. Schneider, 7–60. Bloomington: Indiana University Press, 2002.

———. "The Origin of the Medical Research Grant in the United States: The Rockefeller Foundation and the NIH Extramural Funding Program." *Journal of the History of Medicine and Allied Sciences* 70 (2015): 279–311.

Shryock, Harold. *Modern Medical Guide.* Rev. ed. Manila: Philippines Publishing House, 1986.

Shryock, Richard Harrison. *American Medical Research, Past and Present.* New York: Commonwealth Fund, 1947.

Singer, A. "The Effect of the Vietnam War on Numbers of Medical School Applicants." *Academic Medicine* 64, no. 10 (October 1989): 567–73.

Sivam, S. P., P. G. Iatridis, and S. Vaughn. "Integration of Pharmacology into a Problem-Based Learning Curriculum for Medical Students." *Medical Education* 29, no. 4 (July 1995): 289–96.

Smiley, Dean F. "History of the Association of American Medical Colleges 1876–1956." *Academic Medicine* 32, no. 7 (July 1957): 512–25.

Smith, Andrew F. "'The Diploma Peddler': Dr. John Cook Bennett and the Christian College, New Albany, Indiana." *Indiana Magazine of History*, 90, no. 1 (1994): 26–47.

Smith, Jason Scott. *Building New Deal Liberalism: The Political Economy of Public Works, 1933–1956.* Cambridge, UK: Cambridge University Press, 2006.

Smith, S. R., and B. Fuller. "MD2000: A Competency-Based Curriculum for the Brown University School of Medicine." *Medicine and Health, Rhode Island* 79, no. 8 (August 1996): 292–98.

Snell, Ronald. "State Finance in the Great Depression." National Conference of State Legislatures, 2009. Accessed June 29, 2018. http://www.ncsl.org/print/fiscal/statefinancegreatdepression.pdf.

Snodgrass, Philip. *A Life in Academic Medicine.* New York: iUniverse, 2007.

Snyder, Thomas D., ed. *120 Years of American Education: A Statistical Portrait.* Washington, DC: National Center for Educational Statistics, 1993. Accessed June 29, 2018. https://nces.ed.gov/pubs93/93442.pdf.

Solberg, Winton U. *Reforming Medical Education: The University of Illinois College of Medicine, 1880–1920.* Champaign: University of Illinois Press, 2009.

Sorensen, Andrew A. "Black Americans and the Medical Profession, 1930–1970." *Journal of Negro Education* 41, no. 4 (Autumn, 1972), 337–42.

Sowder, Charles R. "Address, The Central College of Physicians and Surgeons and Medical Education in Indiana." *The Medical and Surgical Monitor* 7 (June 16, 1904): 242–43.

Spurlock, Jeanne, ed. *Black Psychiatrists and American Psychiatry.* Washington, DC: American Psychiatric Association, 1999.

Starr, Paul. *The Social Transformation of American Medicine: The Rise of a Sovereign Profession and the Making of a Vast Industry.* New York: Basic Books, 1984.

Steinecke, Ann, and Charles Terrell. "Progress for Whose Future? The Impact of the Flexner Report on Medical Education for Racial and Ethnic Minority Physicians in the United States." *Academic Medicine* 85, no. 2 (February 2010): 236–45.

Stern, Alexandra Minna. "Making Better Babies: Public Health and Race Betterment in Indiana, 1920–1935." *American Journal of Public Health* 92, no. 5 (May 2002): 742–52.

———. "'We Cannot Make a Silk Purse Out of a Sow's Ear,' Eugenics in the Hoosier Heartland." *Indiana Magazine of History* 103, no. 1 (March 2007): 3–38.

———. "Against the Odds: Becoming a Female Physician in Midcentury Indiana," *Indiana Magazine of History* 104, no. 4 (December 2008): 323–38.

Stevens, Rosemary. *American Medicine and the Public Interest.* New Haven, CT: Yale University Press, 1971.

———. "Graduate Medical Education: A Continuing History." *Journal of Medical Education* 53, no. 1 (January 1978): 1–18.

———. *In Sickness and in Wealth: American Hospitals in the Twentieth Century.* Baltimore, MD: Johns Hopkins University Press, 1999.

Stevens, Thaddeus M. "Synopsis of Early Laws of Indiana Enacted to Regulate the Practice of Medicine in the State, with Comments; Also, a Synopsis of a Bill Proposed to Be Drafted, Having the Same Objects in View." *Indiana Medical Journal* 3 (1884–1885): 21–22.

Stoelting, Vergil K. *History of the Department of Anesthesiology at Indiana University School of Medicine: The First 30 Years.* Indianapolis: Indiana University, 1977.

Stone, Winthrop E. "The New School of Medicine." *The Medical Student* 4 (October 1905).

———. "The Evolution of Medical Education in Indiana." *Indiana Medical Journal* 25 (June 1907): 471.

Strickland, Stephen P. *Politics, Science, and Dread Disease: A Short History of United States Medical Research Policy.* Cambridge, MA: Harvard University Press, 1972.

Stump, Albert, "Regulation of the Practice of Medicine in Indiana since 1897." In *100 Years of Indiana Medicine*, edited by Dorothy Ritter Russo, 53–59. Indianapolis: Indiana State Medical Association, 1949.

Stypa, Caitlyn. "Purdue Girl: The Female Experience at a Land-Grant University, 1887–1913." MA thesis, Indiana University, 2013.

Sulgrove, Berry Robinson. *History of Indianapolis and Marion County.* Philadelphia: L. H. Everts, 1884.

Surgeon General's Consultant Group on Medical Education. *Physicians for a Growing America.* Washington, DC: US Department of Health, Education, and Welfare, Public Health Service, 1959.

Swing, Susan R. "The ACGME Outcome Project: Retrospective and Prospective." *Medical Teacher* 29, no. 7 (January 2007): 648–54.

Tani, Karen M. "An Administrative Right to Be Free from Sexual Violence? Title IX Enforcement in Historical and Institutional Perspective." *Duke Law Journal* 66, no. 8 (2017): 1847–903.

"Thurman Brooks Rice." *JAMA* 151, no. 5 (January 31, 1953): 400.

Topping, Robert W. *A Century and Beyond: The History of Purdue University.* West Lafayette, IN: Purdue University Press, 1988.

Trobe, Jonathan D. "Noble J. David, MD, Reminisces." *Journal of Neuro-Ophthalmology* 22, no. 3 (September 2002): 240–46.

Van Allen, Elizabeth J. *James Whitcomb Riley: A Life.* Bloomington: Indiana University Press, 1999.

Van Allen, Elizabeth J., and Omer H. Foust, eds. *Keeping the Dream, 1921–1996: Commemorating 75 Years of Caring for Indiana's Children.* Indianapolis: James Whitcomb Riley Memorial Association, 1996.

Van Etten, P. "Camelot or Common Sense? The Logic behind the UCSF/Stanford Merger." *Health Affairs* 18, no. 2 (April 1999): 143–48.

Veysey, Laurence R. *The Emergence of the American University.* Chicago: University of Chicago Press, 1970.

Vogel, Morris J. *The Invention of the Modern Hospital: Boston, 1870–1930.* Chicago: University of Chicago Press, 1980.

Wade, Michael E., et al. "Influence of Hometown on Family Physicians' Choice to Practice in Rural Settings." *Family Medicine* 39, no. 4 (April 2007): 248–54.

Wailoo, Keith. *Pain: A Political History.* Baltimore, MD: Johns Hopkins University Press, 2015.

Walther, Joseph E. *A Life Like None Other: Recollections of a Maverick Hoosier Physician.* Indianapolis: Jostens, 2003.

Warner, John Harley. *Against the Spirit of System: The French Impulse in Nineteenth-Century American Medicine.* Baltimore, MD: Johns Hopkins University Press, 2003.

———. "The Fall and Rise of Professional Mystery: Epistemology, Authority, and the Emergence of Laboratory Medicine in Nineteenth-Century America." In *The Laboratory Revolution in Medicine*, edited by Andrew Cunningham and Perry Williams, 310–41. Cambridge, UK: Cambridge University Press, 1992.

———. "The Maturation of American Medical Science." In *Sickness and Health in America: Readings in the History of Medicine and Public Health*, 2nd ed., edited by Judith Walzer Leavitt and Ronald L. Numbers, 113–25. Madison: University of Wisconsin Press, 1985.

———. *The Therapeutic Perspective: Medical Practice, Knowledge, and Identity in America, 1820–1885*. Cambridge, MA: Harvard University Press, 1986.

Warner, John Harley, and Lawrence J. Rizzolo. 2006. "Anatomical Instruction and Training for Professionalism from the Nineteenth to the Twenty-First Centuries." *Clinical Anatomy* 19 (2006): 403–14.

Weiskotten, Herman G., Alphonse M. Schwitalla, William D. Cutter, and Hamilton H. Anderson. *Medical Education in the United States, 1934–1939*. Chicago: American Medical Association, 1940.

Weisz, George. *Divide and Conquer: A Comparative History of Medical Specialization*. New York: Oxford University Press, 2005.

Wells, Herman B *Being Lucky: Reminiscences and Reflections*. Bloomington: Indiana University Press, 2012.

Weyman, A. E. "Harvey Feigenbaum: A Retrospective." *Journal of the American Society of Echocardiogry* 21, no. 1 (2008): 3–6.

Wheatley, Steven Charles. *The Politics of Philanthropy: Abraham Flexner and Medical Education. History of American Thought and Culture*. Madison: University of Wisconsin Press, 1988.

White, Ryan, and Ann Marie Cunningham. *Ryan White: My Own Story*. New York: Dial, 1991.

Witte, Florence M., Terry D. Stratton, and Lois Margaret Nora. "Stories from the Field: Students' Descriptions of Gender Discrimination and Sexual Harassment during Medical School." *Academic Medicine* 81, no. 7 (July 2006): 648–54.

"Women in Medicine: Are We 'There' Yet?" *Medscape*. Accessed March 3, 2017. http://www.medscape.com/viewarticle/732197.

Woodburn, James Albert, D. D. Banta, and Burton Dorr Myers. *History of Indiana University, 1820–1902*. Bloomington: Indiana University Press, 1940.

Wooten, Heather Green. *Old Red: Pioneering Medical Education in Texas*. Denton: Texas State Historical Association, 2012.

Wynkoop, Mary Ann. *Dissent in the Heartland: The Sixties at Indiana University*. Bloomington: Indiana University Press, 2002.

Wynne, Frank B. "Dr. Theodore Potter." *Journal of the Indiana State Medical Association* 8 (1915): 192–93.

Xu, Xiaoqun. *Chinese Professionals and the Republican State: The Rise of Professional Associations in Shanghai, 1912–1937*. Cambridge, UK: Cambridge University Press, 2000.

Zachary, G. Pascal. *Endless Frontier: Vannevar Bush, Engineer of the American Century.* Cambridge, MA: MIT Press, 1999.

Zapffe, Fred C. "Study of Student Accomplishment in Seventy-nine Medical Schools in the United States." *Journal of the Association of American Medical Colleges* 8 (1933): 331–46.

Zerfas, L. G. "Medical Education in Indiana As Influenced by Early Indiana Graduates in Medicine from Transylvania University." *Indiana Magazine of History* 30, no. 2 (1934): 139–48.

Zerhouni, Elias A. "Translational and Clinical Science—Time for a New Vision." *New England Journal of Medicine* 353, no. 15 (October 13, 2005): 1621–23. doi:10.1056/NEJMsb053723.

INDEX

WILLIAM H. SCHNEIDER, PhD, is Professor Emeritus of History and Medical Humanities at Indiana University–Purdue University Indianapolis. He is author of *The History of Blood Transfusion in Sub-Saharan Africa* and editor of *Rockefeller Philanthropy and Modern Biomedicine*. His research has been supported by multiple grants from the National Endowment for the Humanities, National Institutes of Health, and Fulbright fellowships, plus research grants from the National Science Foundation and the Henry Luce Foundation.

ELIZABETH J. VAN ALLEN is managing editor of the *Encyclopedia of Indianapolis* at the Indianapolis Public Library. She is contributing author to *Hoosier Philanthropy: Understanding the Past, Planning the Future* (Indiana University Press, forthcoming) and author of *James Whitcomb Riley: A Life* (Indiana University Press, 1999).

KEVIN T. GRAU is a former doctoral candidate in the Department of the History and Philosophy of Science and Medicine at Indiana University.

ANGELA B. POTTER is a doctoral candidate in history at Purdue University focusing on the history of mental illness and public health. She is also a graduate student in Medical Humanities at IUPUI with a focus on history of medicine and medical education.